To Health… *Naturally!*

John Goetz

DISCLAIMER

"To Health… *Naturally!*" does not directly or indirectly dispense medical advice or prescribe the use of vitamins, minerals, herbs or any other nutrients or drugs. This book is for informational purposes only, and expresses the point of view of a new theory of human health without any intent to advise, diagnose or prescribe to the reader on matters of health. The author and publisher shall have no liability or responsibility to any person or entity with respect to any loss, damage or injury, or alleged loss, damage or injury caused directly or indirectly by the information in the book. The information presented herein is not a substitute for medical counseling. Always consult your physician on matters of health.

Library of Congress CN: 2004096325
ISBN 0-9675434-5-2
Shadow Publishing
Clearwater, Florida

Cover art by Joseph Duhamel, Avalon Design Unlimited Inc.
www.joedu.com

Printed in the United States of America

How to Order this Book:
visit www.tohealthnaturally.com

Dedication

To Dorothy, who gave up her dream of writing the
great American novel to raise the kids. Thanks, Mom.

Acknowledgements

The author expresses sincere thanks to the following people for their help in bringing this book to life:

- Bill Goetz, my brother, for his advice, encouragement, support and invaluable editing of the manuscript.
- Barbara Harrington, Henry Kreider, Yvonne Ludwick, Marie Goetz and Will Goetz for their advice and editing help.
- Joe Duhamel for his excellent artwork and formatting of the book.
- Many friends for their support, especially Harry and Rose Brown, Jackie Royal, Don Voytish, Cy and Joanne Lessig, Carol Michaud and Ruth McGrath.
- Dr. J. Stein, who saved my life twenty-five years ago.
- The thousands of dedicated medical researchers and scientists referenced in this book and their research, which has changed nutrition from art to science.

CONTENTS

List of Tables

List of Figures

INTRODUCTION

Kirk Douglas observed that life is "a B-picture script." Like most people, my life story would not be a compelling Hollywood movie, but it is a true story of "health lost," a 10-year odyssey to "health regained" and a second chance at life. The health misadventures began with undiagnosed and misdiagnosed hyperthyroidism. Unfortunately, this led to severe liver and pancreas damage and eventually to life-threatening acute hypoadrenal crises. My second chance came when I discovered an important new principle underlying human health and disease. That new principle is called Equilibrium Theory, and its simple, common sense method to build health and eliminate disease can help others with severe health problems get a second chance at life.

Two unusual circumstances came together and enabled me to discover Equilibrium Theory. First, I was trained in science. I have a degree from Case Western Reserve University in Cleveland Ohio, and following that many years of scientific research. In my quest for recovery, I used my expertise in examining published papers in the scientific literature to research the medical literature relating to my condition and human health in general. The study of nutrition turned out to be most important, as this science investigates the basic building blocks of health. This book presents the results of what I found at the medical library – "just the facts" distilled from over 2000 references reporting what medical experts have proven on the safety and efficacy of nutrition.

The second unusual circumstance that led to Equilibrium Theory presented itself after my health stabilized at a very low functioning level. Using nutrition, I slowly and steadily improved the dysfunctions in the thyroid, liver, pancreas and adrenal gland – initially from *do something* and suffer now, to *do something* and suffer tomorrow, and finally to *do something* without any aftereffects. During this 10-year journey back to health, the two approaches to nutrition – one from science, the other from experience – came into agreement and merged to form a more fundamental and general approach, that is, Equilibrium Theory.

Equilibrium Theory is a revolutionary new solution to human health and chronic diseases. See if you don't find value in its common sense simplicity.

John Goetz
St. Petersburg, Florida
November 2004

1. HEALTH and HARMONY

Significant advances in science often come through theories, for example Pasteur's germ theory, Darwin's theory of evolution and Einstein's theory of relativity. In these and many other theories, an underlying general principle explains complicated observations and phenomena. By finding the general principle, a theory organizes and simplifies knowledge in a particular field. It transforms thinking – the old familiar world gives way to new understanding.

This book presents a breakthrough theory of human health, "Equilibrium Theory," which condenses the large body of medical knowledge on human physiology into an easy-to-understand, easy-to-use general principle. The theory conforms to medical science, and goes beyond that science to decipher baffling physiological evidence. Two major findings come from the theory. First, Equilibrium Theory identifies human nutritional requirements exactly. The resulting nutritional program provides simple and flexible complete nutrition that adjusts easily for lifestyle and current needs. Second, Equilibrium Theory solves the longstanding mystery of chronic diseases, revealing the mechanisms behind and solutions to osteoarthritis, rheumatoid arthritis, multiple sclerosis (MS), lupus, fibromyalgia, chronic fatigue syndrome and many more!

Except for genetic and environmental factors, physiology and nutrition control health. Physiology is internal functions and activities, especially how glands and organs work. Nutrition provides the raw materials, vitamins and so forth, for glands and organs to manufacture and secrete hormones and other end products necessary for life. Targeted nutrition for each function in the body builds vigorous health and long life, and eliminates diseases and their root causes.

The sciences of physiology and nutrition currently exist in isolation. Equilibrium Theory marries these two fundamental health providers with precise correlations, thereby enabling you to truly live Hippocrates' words, "Let food be your medicine." To achieve this coupling, the theory further defines and characterizes the medical term, "HOMEOSTASIS: stability and equilibrium in a physiological system through feedback." Homeostasis is the internal dialogue of harmony going on in all living things. The great philosophers throughout history teach harmony too – in your life, in your mind and in your relations with others. Equilibrium Theory extends that work in progress to the delicate, complicated physical self. And physical harmony, working with and not against your own internal homeostasis, promotes mind-body-spirit wellness.

The physical world confounds and thwarts the human mind at every turn, but it often hides a solution in plain sight. Not so many centuries ago, our ancestors looked up at the sun and full moon in wonder and saw only round, sacred objects. A new perspective would change the world forever. During the Renaissance, a corps of discoverers saw spheres and the shadow of a sphere on the moon, and realized that that said something profound about the earth and its place in the solar system. Somewhere health hides a similar secret and simple key… perhaps as follows.

The delicate, complicated physical body lives a hard reality indeed. Eat, drink and breathe or there's no thinking, acting, living output. Food is the primary input, and food consists of four distinct compositional types: carbohydrates, proteins, fats and fibers. Why four, and does that say something profound about the human body, how it developed and how it handles the challenges of life?

The general principle of Equilibrium Theory is the following new understanding of the inner workings of homeostasis. Within the human body and its network of glands and organs, four interconnected functions – ENERGY, HEALING, STRESS and IMMUNE – work in healthy equilibrium, or internal balance. The body's response to all internal needs and external forces lies within and must adhere to this four-part harmony. Moreover, these tasks are the template for all nutrition. Thus with the perfect symmetry of nature, each food type nourishes one of the four functions: carbohydrates for energy, proteins for healing, fats for stress (cells burn fat instead of glucose, a true definition of stress!), and fibers for immune. The same direct relationship and necessary equilibrium apply to all other raw material nutrients.

Western medicine has gone astray. Drugs rule instead of nutrition. Health care has become the #3 killer in America,[1] behind only cardiovascular disease and cancer. Up to one hundred and eighty thousand patients die from medical malpractice in US hospitals each year.[2] Adverse drugs events (ADE) such as adverse and allergic reactions, drug interactions and medication errors kill approximately one hundred thousand hospitalized Americans every year.[3] "Safe and effective" is the Food and Drug Administration (FDA) standard, but these words doublespeak a dark language. Society will continue to suffer terrible consequences for some time to come. Individuals can walk away from perverted science, and chart a new course. Instead of today's money-driven *patent medicine,* nature's chemistry holds the true solution to nature's human body.

"To Health… *Naturally!*" is a handbook of nature's chemistry, presenting concise reviews of the scientific medical literature for all vitamins, fatty acids, minerals (trace metals), and many herbs. With over 2000 references, here is the first comprehensive, up-to-date summary of nutritional knowledge since the 1960s and Adelle Davis. And one giant leap in the truth about nutrition, as medical experts report proven, peer-reviewed findings on fruits and vegetables, whole-grain cereals, Vitamin E, Vitamin C, bioflavonoids and many more of nature's finest raw materials. Unique and valuable insights emerge from seldom-seen scientific papers. For example, Vitamin A is necessary for resistance to and recovery from infection.[4] Tumor cells are always low in manganese, specifically the protective enzyme manganese superoxide dismutase.[5] The herb Bilberry, rich in special anthocyanin flavonoids, improves microvascular health including the capillary aneurysms and hemorrhages of diabetic retinopathy.[6] An extensive index at the end of the book brings the entire nutritional medical literature alive, so you can learn directly from the medical experts.

The search for truth remains the grand adventure of life. The human mind has two ways of thinking and coming to the truth about anything in existence, and the ancient Greeks were the first to describe and put names to both methods: (1) empiricism is practical experience – what your senses, observations and experiences tell you about this complicated world. Your mind interprets these facts; therefore empiricism is subjective. And (2) rationalism is the search for truth independent of experience. Rationalism is objective, i.e. evidence determines true or false. It is reason over opinion and belief. These two different ways of thinking can be at loggerheads, or they can be combined to solve difficult problems. This combined effort is the essence and purpose of a theory – integrate proven, objective science with subjective insight and discovery to explain the currently unexplainable and understand the world more completely. Rationalism supplies the pieces to a jigsaw puzzle; empiricism can put the puzzle together to form a beautiful picture!

The medical literature and its many scientific papers are pieces of the health jigsaw puzzle. Equilibrium Theory puts this puzzle together beautifully to reveal a true solution to human health and chronic diseases. The theory transforms thinking about life's inscrutable chemistry, and becomes a straightforward (or if necessary – a detailed) "how to" guide. Nature is at once complex and simple, complex in trying to understand human chemistry, but simple in finding the nutrition to run that chemistry successfully. Unfortunately, nature does not adhere to the human desire for a pill to fix everything. Patience is necessary. Nutrition does not give instant results; rather it's a slow building process of one nutritional factor upon another until there is synergy, a nutrition and resulting health effect much greater than the sum of the parts. Good raw material input equals good end product output – here is the inviolable rule of all chemical systems including life's most advanced creation.

The storm and stress of life often leave no safe harbor. Still, you can survive inevitable gales and doldrums and thrive on great adventures if you possess the inner world of health too. This is a book of discovery about that strange inner world and your most precious asset – GOOD HEALTH – how to keep it, and how to get it back if you have lost it. Life doesn't have to become a shipwreck. Western medicine is fixated on disease. The better course is a healthy lifestyle including an "on target" nutritional program for your crucial energy, healing, stress and immune systems. Perfect nutrition is life giving, restorative and forgiving. Start with the fundamentals; learn and apply the major points of physiology and nutrition. These are the touchstones to health… naturally. Then if necessary, get into the details of solving complex dysfunctions and diseases. Confirm Equilibrium Theory's usefulness in your life step by step. The truth of anything lies in its consequences.

***

2. ADRENAL GLAND PRESCRIBES HEALTH

Health begins with physiology, your body's internal functions and activities. Everything you do in life, from tentative first steps to self-confident quests for the impossible dream, depends on physiology. How do these functions and activities accomplish each and every goal? The answer is chemistry, nature's chemistry. The process begins in your brain when YOU decide to "Do this" or "Do that." Complex chemical reactions then take over to accomplish these tasks. Messengers called hormones rush around the bloodstream chemically expressing "do this," "do that." Key hormones are manufactured and secreted by five special glands – pituitary, adrenal, thyroid, pancreas and liver – each of which handles part of the task and all of them together achieve the goal. They literally perform magic... the magic that is YOU!

Figure 2-A shows the location of these five glands in your body. By definition, a gland secretes substances, such as hormones, for use elsewhere in the body or for elimination from the body. An organ is distinct, large in size and specialized for some particular function. Liver is both gland and organ. The pituitary, adrenal, thyroid, pancreas and liver do not perform alone, but they are the protagonists of the human drama. Other glands act in supporting roles: hypothalamus, pineal gland, sex glands (ovaries or testes), parathyroid gland and the lymphatic system including thymus and spleen. All of these glands secrete hormones or other substances into blood or lymph, therefore they are "internally secreting" or from Greek "endocrine," *endo-* meaning "internal" and *-krinein* "to separate." And this interconnected network of glands and organs is called the endocrine system.

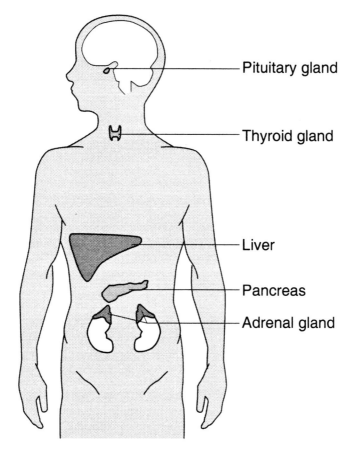

FIGURE 2-A. THE ENDOCRINE SYSTEM.
Location of major glands: pituitary, adrenal, thyroid, pancreas and liver.

Complications, complications… Endocrine communication is not limited to hormones; neurotransmitters handle some tasks. The nervous system directly links the brain to a number of glands and body parts much like long telegraph wires. Along these *wires*, neurotransmitters, chemical substances just as hormones are, carry nerve impulse messages across the synapse (small gap) between the many connecting neurons (nerve cells). Neurotransmitters generate almost instantaneous gland response, while hormones are slower acting, but more long lasting in their effect. As science learns more about endocrine expression, the distinction between hormone and neurotransmitter is increasingly a blurred one. The brain and central nervous system begin the action and to a significant degree direct the hormonal system.

And what is endocrinology? It's Greek to almost everybody! However, the suffix *-logy* simply means "the study of." So, endocrinology is the study of pituitary, adrenal, thyroid, pancreas and liver anatomy (structure) and physiology (functions and activities) including hormones and neurotransmitters. There may be over one hundred endocrine hormones and neurotransmitters, many still unknown. Each year, thousands of new scientific papers enlarge the field and human knowledge. As with all sciences, endocrinology is a work in progress.

Endocrine glands are highly specialized units. Pituitary is crew chief, overseeing all others and uniting them into a single, cohesive force. The adrenal gland directs energy, healing, stress and immune functions. Thyroid adjusts metabolic rate, or how fast cells burn fuel. Pancreas has both endocrine and digestive duties; its endocrine function maintains normal blood sugar levels. Liver is involved in thousands of chemical reactions, making new molecules for use throughout the body and breaking down many more old, worn-out ones. It stores hundreds of compounds, and serves as the filtering plant for blood, removing impurities and detoxifying harmful substances. Liver oversees numerous body processes, including contributing crucially to fat digestion.

While the pituitary gland regulates this complicated endocrine system, the physiology of the adrenal gland dictates the action – how the body responds to ALL internal needs and external forces. This is why the adrenal gland prescribes health! And why it will be studied first and foremost in this book.

ADRENAL PHYSIOLOGY... how it works

Adrenal tissues consist of a pair of small slender glands, approximately two inches long, one inch wide and one-quarter inch thick, located on the upper end of each kidney (renal), hence "ad-renal." For purposes of reading ease, these two adrenals will be referred to simply as the adrenal gland.

The adrenal gland is divided in two distinct and identifiable physical parts, the medulla and the cortex. "Medulla" is a medical term indicating the center of a gland, organ or body structure, and "cortex" the surrounding outer regions. Structurally, 90% of the adult adrenal gland is cortex.

Functions

Functions are tasks that the creator, evolution or the life force have programmed into the human body to meet all challenges of our environment. The adrenal gland runs the most important task program, with four primary functions – Energy for today's activities, Healing of the body, whether normal breakdown and repair or from injury, Stress, i.e. handling stress, and Immune response and system – and many lesser or subfunctions within these primary ones. In the pages and chapters ahead, the term "primary function" signifies one of the four principals here, and not a subfunction. When indicating a primary function, Energy, Healing, Stress and Immune are capitalized to distinguish them for our general use of these words.

Reading Your Adrenal Health. Figure 2-B is a construct, a simple model to explain and predict how the complex adrenal gland works. The figure does not depict physical structure; rather it is a schematic of the primary functions, dependent body systems and normal functional flow or communication within the endocrine system, pituitary → adrenal medulla → adrenal cortex → pituitary feedback. Figure 2-B is the most important discovery in this book; understand it and you understand everything that follows. For this reason, adrenal mechanisms are described in considerable detail. At times, these explanations may seem complicated, but *hang in there* because applying this knowledge pays life dividends.

Figure 2-B reveals a four-part harmony in the adrenal tasks of Energy, Healing, Stress and Immune. This is the central concept of Equilibrium Theory and the key to internal balance in your life. Your adrenal gland works four jobs, often at the same time: energy czar, healing supervisor, stress manager and minister of defense. You can help it perform flawlessly by providing the specific raw materials (nutrition) used for each job. These nutrients, the wellspring for life and health, are introduced later in this chapter following the mechanics and dynamics of adrenal physiology.

Adrenal Medulla is divided into two functional (not physical) parts, Energy and Healing. These parts have to be in balance or equilibrium with each other as represented by "⇌" in Figure 2-B. Neither primary function dominates over the other. Basically, Energy and Healing share medulla resources in a give-and-take relationship, going back and forth depending on current body needs. Energy comes principally from the medulla hormone adrenaline. The medical profession now calls

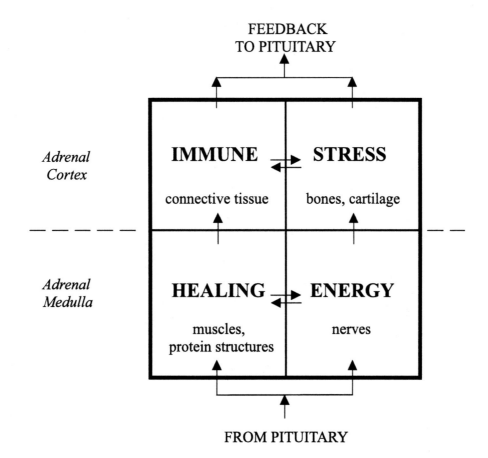

FEEDBACK
TO PITUITARY

Adrenal
Cortex

IMMUNE → STRESS

connective tissue   bones, cartilage

Adrenal
Medulla

HEALING → ENERGY

muscles,   nerves
protein structures

FROM PITUITARY

FIGURE 2-B. ADRENAL GLAND PHYSIOLOGY.

Two identifiable physical parts: medulla and cortex. Four primary functions: ENERGY, HEALING, STRESS and IMMUNE with "dependent body systems" listed under each. Arrows indicate normal functional flow; equilibrium arrows ($\rightleftharpoons$) denote balance between functions within the medulla and cortex.

adrenaline, "epinephrine." However, everyone knows the meaning of "get the adrenaline flowing," so this book sticks with the old familiar term. The nervous system is interconnected with and dependent upon Energy/adrenaline, thus the term "dependent body system." If something goes wrong with Energy functioning, something will go wrong with your nerves! The other half of medulla equilibrium is Healing (primary adrenal function) and muscles and protein structures in the body (its dependent body system). All muscle diseases lie in this Healing province.

Common medical knowledge… Adrenal medulla receives pituitary instructions (signified by →) through the central nervous system and neurotransmitters. Reacting, it manufactures and secretes two major hormones, epinephrine (adrenaline) and nor-epinephrine. Adrenaline directs *fight or flight* response, increasing heart rate, cardiac output, blood pressure and carbohydrate metabolism. Norepinephrine, both hormone and neurotransmitter, has like but limited hormonal action, constricting blood vessels and dilating bronchial tubes. Meanwhile, Healing activities largely take place outside of the adrenal gland. Remember, Figure 2-B does not clarify chemistry or where that chemistry takes place; it models functions and how they interact.

Adrenal Cortex is similarly divided into two functional parts, Stress and Immune, which have to be in equilibrium. Neither primary function has an absolute right to cortex resources. Stress and Immune are coupled in a dance for life, as are medulla Energy and Healing. Stress, or better said, "your ability to handle stress," comes from the cortex hormone cortisol. The often-prescribed steroid cortisone is an imperfect copy of cortisol, and an imperfect attempt to restore proper function here. The dependent body system of Stress is bones and cartilage. Stress diseases manifest in bone and cartilage, typically arthritis. Immune system is the other primary function in the back and forth cortex equilibrium *tango*. Connective tissue is its dependent body system.

Common medical knowledge… Adrenal cortex manufactures and secretes two steroidal hormones: cortisol (known as a glucocortiocoid) for fighting stress and for inflammatory and immune system suppression, and aldosterone (mineralocorticoid) to control sodium/potassium and water balance in the body. The cortex also releases some male hormones. In both sexes, the cortex is directly involved in sexual func-tioning and connected to the ovaries or testes. Immune system activities occur most-ly outside of the adrenal gland and within bone marrow, thymus, spleen and the lym-phatic system, there producing B-lymphocytes, T-lymphocytes and other white blood cells. More on these defense specialists ahead in subfunctions.

Dependent Body Systems

Dependent body systems are systems seemingly in no way connected to the adre-nal gland, yet they require proper adrenal functioning and health to maintain their own well being. How can this be? How can these distant, large systems – nerves, muscles and protein structures, bones and cartilage, and connective tissue (from Figure 2-B) – be brought down to dysfunction and disease by the tiny adrenal gland?

The best explanation is an example, the common worldwide scenario of a lifetime of too much stress wearing out the Primary Stress Function and causing permanent imbalance between Immune $\rightleftharpoons$ Stress. Immune system dominates, leading to autoimmune diseases, i.e. the body attacks itself. Responding all the time but with no foreign invaders to fight, Immune instead attacks injured tissue. In this case, the autoimmune complaint is arthritis, an attack on bone cartilage, which in Figure 2-B is the dependent system of a worn-out, exhausted Stress function. In essence, <u>Figure 2-B predicts where the attack will occur and what the underlying cause is; therefore the figure becomes a powerful tool in understanding and solving this and many other chronic diseases</u>!

Rheumatoid arthritis involves Stress exhaustion and resulting Immune $\leftarrow$ Stress imbalance (instead of normal, healthy Immune $\rightleftharpoons$ Stress). Osteoarthritis adds a dominating Healing exhaustion. Constant inflammation from the attack and mounting cartilage damage produce painful symptoms. Nonsteroidal anti-inflammatory drugs (NSAIDs) can temporarily relieve the pain and inflammation, but with harmful side effects including gastrointestinal ulcers and bleeding. Treating symptoms is endless folly and in the end counterproductive. Cure comes only by correcting the adrenal exhaustion and imbalance, the underlying cause. Restore cortex equilibrium and the attack on cartilage will instantly stop. Then, you can begin healing.

Stress-arthritis is the archetype for chronic diseases. In the same way, other primary functions and subfunctions give rise to distant dependent-body-system diseases. Energy function disorders can lead to serious nerve diseases such as multiple sclerosis (MS) and amyotropic lateral sclerosis (Lou Gehrig's disease). Healing problems can manifest in muscles with fibromyalgia and other muscle diseases. For Immune, lupus (systemic lupus erythematosus) is an autoimmune assault on connective tissue. Like arthritis, lupus is autoimmune in character, but the initiating cause is too much Immune with hyperactivity in one or more lymphocyte types, not an exhausted or hypoactive Stress function. At the other extreme, an exhausted hypoactive Immune function wreaks primary – NOT dependent body system – havoc with susceptibility to infections, colds and flu, candidiasis (yeast infection), shingles (herpes zoster), Legionnaire's bacteria, cancers, etc.

Where any dependent body system attack comes depends on where the adrenal gland first goes *haywire*. Sometimes, though, "where" is more complicated than the dependent systems of Figure 2-B. Interactions occur, and other dependent systems exist and are tied to adrenal functions in more complex ways. For example, skin depends upon total medulla health, Energy and Healing together. Heart and red blood cells rely mostly on Stress mechanisms, while white blood cells obviously require well-maintained Immune mechanisms.

Where exactly chronic disease strikes also depends on specific underlying adrenal causes, including subfunction variations and multiple dysfunctions of first cause (the setup for disease) and second cause (precipitating event, often trauma). All these contribute to unique final outcomes and explain the myriad of disease possibilities. The modus operandi of attack on a dependent system is almost always hyperactive Immune (autoimmune) or hypoactive Healing (degenerative) in character, or both.

To cite a complex disease process, osteoarthritis actually develops from two separate dysfunctions. First-cause Stress exhaustion induces arthritis, an autoimmune attack on cartilage. Subsequently, a dominating second-cause Healing exhaustion modifies the disease to a degenerative attack on the protein structures (Healing's dependent system) of cartilage. And, in fact, this is the exact pathology of osteoarthritis reported in the scientific medical literature! Dependent body systems, their diseases and initiating adrenal causes are discussed in great depth in coming chapters, especially Chapter 12 "Correcting Dis-ease" where the Gordian knot of chronic disease is solved.

Normal Functioning

The arrows (→, ⇒) in Figure 2-B indicate the course or flow of functioning or tasking. The adrenal gland receives instructions via neurotransmitters and hormones from the pituitary, the master control gland of the body. General instructions come first to the adrenal medulla as indicated in Figure 2-B. The medulla in turn can stimulate the cortex, which then sends feedback to the pituitary to further regulate adrenal response to exactly meet body needs.

This 'feedback loop' is one of thousands in the human body; many involve pituitary oversight. Feedback produces stability and equilibrium in a physiological system, and is technically known as homeostasis or homeostatic mechanism. Loss of homeostasis leads directly to poor health and disease.

The usual work of the adrenal gland, such as handling the daily stress (cortex) of life must first involve energy and adrenaline (medulla). In like manner, the immune system must be brought to action by healing, and in fact healing and immune activities together share the inflammation mechanism. Thus, a natural division exists in adrenal functioning, not between medulla and cortex, but between the two functional sides of medulla and cortex. Energy and Stress functions go together to form one "action plan" (from one set of general instructions), and likewise for Healing and Immune.

Adrenal equilibriums, Healing $\rightleftharpoons$ Energy and Immune $\rightleftharpoons$ Stress in Figure 2-B, operate at cross-purposes to and yet blend with the two actions plans of Energy $\rightarrow$ Stress and Healing $\rightarrow$ Immune. Good adrenal health requires both equilibriums, which move back or forth as needed, and the action plans. Complicated? A little. Adrenal functioning is woven like tapestry, producing a beautiful design in form and function.

The pituitary gland at any time can override general instructions (the two action plans) and adrenal equilibriums, and write specific instructions to achieve any task, for example, *"Immune Function: URGENT, fight the flu!"* Or, pituitary ACTH (adrenocorticotropic hormone) orders the Stress hormone cortisol into action. Direct feedback to the pituitary on specific instructions guarantees a correct, measured response. Again, pituitary regulates and controls, but the physiology of the adrenal gland dictates the action. In effect, it is easier to think of the adrenal gland, say, adjusting Healing $\rightleftharpoons$ Energy to fix a skinned knee.

An adrenal equilibrium can be temporarily out of balance. Recovering from surgery, Healing function dominates over Energy function and you feel like staying in bed – no energy! Fighting that flu, Immune function dominates over Stress function, and the stress of your job is just too much that day. If you decide to go to work anyway, your adrenal gland will try to adjust to these two opposites, probably with poor results for both. Not surprisingly, the adrenal gland and body have great difficulty achieving opposite functions in the extreme.

Worse than opposites, however, is one constant effort. For example, workaholism

– constant job stress, bringing it home, taking it to bed – can leave you susceptible to minor immune lapses and in time to serious disease. The cornerstone of good health is TEMPORARILY out of balance. When temporarily becomes CONSTANTLY, your health gets out of sync and falls apart. Adrenal equilibriums plead for equilibrium in your life. Balance, equanimity, harmony – the spiritual teachings of the great philosophers may be rooted in our physical nature, the internal physiology and homeostasis of the four primary adrenal functions!

Most of life's tasks are easily handled by the adrenal gland, even opposite functions. Only in the extreme are internal mechanisms revealed. To illustrate, consider Immune again and various degrees of difficulty. If healthy, your immune response to the everyday environment is not a problem. It involves killing bacteria viruses, fungi and other pathogens that attempt to invade your body all the time, and with no apparent effect on Stress ability, the opposite function. However, as the difficulty increases – cold, flu, pneumonia – Primary Stress Function loses importance as the endocrine system marshals all its forces to fight the invader. Immune ⇌ Stress equilibrium swings more and more resources to the immune system and attempting any stressful activity at this time proves counterproductive to disastrous. Your approach to health should always be… Don't get in the way of your body's natural response.

How well your adrenal gland handles opposite functions is a good measure of how healthy you are. When young, the two adrenal equilibriums rest on a broad plain. When old and frail, these equilibriums sit on a knife-edge – you're up, you're down! Good nutrition, employing the raw materials that power adrenal functions, can maintain and rebuild youthful response.

Circadian Cycle

The human body has its own biological clock, a rhythmic cycle of approximately 24 hours, or circadian. The two adrenal action plans, Energy → Stress and Healing → Immune, are part of this circadian rhythm or wave. In the morning, your adrenal gland stirs before you wake and begins to prepare for the day ahead with energy hormones. When night comes, the bias shifts toward healing and immune, their tasks and sleep, *going gently into that good night*. This natural ebb and flow between action plans – a dance to the music of time – is regulated by the pineal gland in the brain, which then influences the pituitary gland and, in turn, adrenal equilibriums (details in

Chapter 8). People who work night shifts are fighting their own internal clock, as are those suffering jet lag, a shift in time zones.

Energy and its Subfunctions

When your body needs energy for work or play, the adrenal medulla responds with just the right amount of adrenaline. Adrenaline is the first hormone you use in the morning. It gets your head off the pillow, and gives children their boundless energy. If your adrenaline response is insufficient or worse, hardly there, then the cause is nutritional. You have a deficiency or imbalance, a chronic failure to meet medulla needs. The deprivation may be mild or severe. Either way, damage has been done to the medulla. Fortunately, the adrenal gland is amazingly resilient and much or all of this function can be restored. The nutritional raw materials required for energy, pep, vigor, motivation and drive are introduced in the next section of the chapter.

Energy, or lack of it, is more complicated than just adrenaline response. Several other subfunctions lie within this primary designation and affect energy output. Surprisingly, the nervous system is one of them. The nervous system is the only dependent body system that is also an actor, not just a receiver of action. Nerves and energy/adrenaline are intertwined as follows:

> Epinephrine [adrenaline] is synthesized and stored in the adrenal medulla and released into the bloodstream to influence tissues throughout the body. Epinephrine is also a neurotransmitter in certain regions of the central nervous system. The adrenal medulla and sympathetic nervous system make up an anatomical and physiological unit, which is often referred to as the sympathoadrenal system.[1]

This excerpt from "*Williams Textbook of Endocrinology*," an authoritative text/reference, requires definition of the term, 'sympathetic nervous system.' The sympathetic nervous system originates in the thoracic and lumbar spinal cord and regulates involuntary actions – breathing rate, heart rate, cardiac output and blood pressure – the fight or flight response associated with get the adrenaline flowing!

How nerves affect energy output can be seen with caffeine consumption. In small amounts, caffeine is actually a nerve nutrient/raw material. With frequent large doses however, it becomes a nerve stimulant, which triggers adrenaline flow. Millions of people around the world employ cups of Java in the morning to wake up their energy. It works, but not without mild addiction and side effects that grow worse over time. Chapter 7 describes this caffeine fix syndrome in detail, including how to overcome it.

Two other subfunctions lie within Primary Energy Function, also with mutual interactive effects. These are sex, or more correctly the start of sex, involving nervous energy; and mood including feelings, emotions, depression and anxiety. Phobias are extreme anxiety. Feeling down, the blues, mild and severe depression, and manic-depression all involve energy, nerve health, related body chemistry, mental processes and external factors. Depression is a complex interaction of these elements, often requiring professional help. In its simplest characterization, however, depression is not enough energy and mania is too much energy.

To review, the four subfunctions within Primary Energy Function are:

– energy: adrenaline response (includes epinephrine and norepinephrine),
– nervous system (dependent body system too),
– start of sex (nervous energy),
– mood: feelings, emotions, depression, mania and anxiety.

Healing and its Subfunctions

Healing originates in the adrenal medulla too, the second partner in the medulla equilibrium dynamic. Cut your finger, recover from surgery or just repair the body after a day's work, Healing does the job – an intricate, not well-understood process of repair and replacement of injured and worn-out cells and tissue. Cells breakdown; cells are repaired or replaced continuously, every moment of every day. How well you heal determines how young you feel, or stated another way, how much of you is still you and not scar tissue. Scar tissue is dead, gone forever, the result of cell oxidation, which occurs not only with skin, but inside too. Improving healing and preventing cell oxidation slow aging. Therefore, healing and antioxidation are two subfunctions within the primary Healing designation. Further explanation of these processes is given in the "Breakdown and Repair" section at the end of this chapter, and in Chapter 3 "Protein Metabolism."

Two other Healing subfunctions, inflammation and vasoconstriction, are shared with Immune. Inflammation is the body's response to injury (healing required) or infection (immune system required) and involves the following activities in a localized area: swelling from the opening of the blood vessels (vasodilation), fever or temperature rise, and redness, which signifies corrective action. Vasoconstriction is the narrowing of blood vessels, the opposite of what happens at the beginning of inflammation, and these two must be in balance so the body can adjust blood flow to tissues as needed:

$$vasoconstriction \rightleftharpoons vasodilation.$$

Loss of this equilibrium increases susceptibility to infections, aggravates inflammation diseases, those ending in the suffix "-itis" such as arthritis and bursitis, contributes to varicose veins, and may be a factor in migraine headaches[2, 3] and other afflictions where blood vessels open uncontrollably. In the chapters ahead, inflammation and vasoconstriction are always presented under Healing, but apply equally to Immune.

In review, the four subfunction tasks within Primary Healing Function are:

– healing: repair and replace cells and tissue,
– antioxidation: protect cells and tissue,
– inflammation including vasodilation (Immune too),
– vasoconstriction (Immune too).

Stress and its Subfunctions

"Life is just one damn thing after another." No matter the source of stress – mental or physical – problem, worry, effort or struggle – the adrenal cortex responds with just the right amount of the natural steroidal hormone cortisol. Of course, stress can go on and on, eventually wearing down and overwhelming the cortisol response. Fortunately, nature installed a backup system. This backup exists within Primary Stress Function and is called fatigue function here. Actually, temporary exhaustion is its definable symptom, but this creates confusion with permanent exhaustion of functions and accompanying chronic diseases in dependent body systems, as investigated in Chapter 12.

Fatigue function has its own cortex hormone, aldosterone. When you begin to feel fatigue and temporary exhaustion from prolonged stress, aldosterone kicks in with relief. Fatigue function comprises: (1) the body's salt balance of sodium (Na) $\rightleftharpoons$ potassium (K); (2) water balance, a dependent system of the salt balance that prevents dehydration or the opposite, edema (accumulation of fluid in tissues); and (3) a link to the thyroid gland via the pituitary gland for even more backup. Thyroid hormones can boost metabolism to meet any level of stress. The adrenal-pituitary-thyroid connection is explored in the "Stamina" section later in the chapter. Chapter 9 explains thyroid functions and dysfunctions.

As fatigue approaches, aldosterone holds sodium and water in tissues, preventing dehydration. The liver keeps additional sodium and potassium in reserve. With severe fatigue, adrenal cortex *calls up* the liver to send over more sodium. If the liver is damaged or the amount of sodium needed is beyond its ability, then heat exhaustion develops: pale and damp skin, rapid pulse, dizziness, nausea, and finally collapse. Sodium and fluids are lost mainly through sweat. Accordingly, ingesting sodium salt (regular table salt, NaCl) early into these warning signs and symptoms will support aldosterone and the liver and help prevent fatigue and heat exhaustion. Taking salt tablets is common practice in hot, stressful environments such as steel mills.

Feeling too hot or too cold is related to aldosterone, thyroid function, or both. If you are briefly too hot or too cold, this is due to severe stress. Permanently too hot or too cold signifies aldosterone or thyroid dysfunction. Edema usually indicates permanent aldosterone exhaustion, although serious disorders such as congestive heart failure, kidney disease and cirrhosis may be causative.[4] If drinking a lot of water brings on nausea or headache, then water balance and controlling aldosterone are impaired. Chapter 12 "Correcting Dis-ease" gives aldosterone/fatigue cures.

Another function within primary Stress is the conclusion of sex, which generates cortisol and aldosterone action. Sex has four distinct phases: excitement, plateau, orgasm and resolution.[5] Excitement and plateau involve nervous energy and the adrenal medulla. Plateau and orgasm are stressful; orgasm and resolution reflect temporary exhaustion/fatigue. Sexual response is a natural flow of events and hormones, not unlike many activities that begin with energy (medulla) and progress to (→) stress and fatigue (cortex).

Cortex sexual function is connected to the ovaries or testes. These glands produce sex hormones for growth and development, procreation, secondary sex characteristics and behavior. Ovaries secrete several estrogens, progesterone for the menstrual cycle, and relaxin for the reproductive/birth canal. Testes produce testosterone and less-potent androsterone. The health of female and male structures is cortex related, and so included in later chapters under the Stress designation.

Two final functions within the Stress galaxy are small but necessary parts of glucose (sugar) metabolism. Generally, glucose metabolism is thought of as a pancreas function with insulin controlling blood glucose levels (see Chapter 10), but some function also lies in the liver, adrenal medulla with an adrenaline response, and adrenal cortex. Cortex glucose metabolism involves: (1) gluconeogenesis, and (2) glucose tolerance factor. Gluconeogenesis is counterregulation to insulin, raising blood glucose levels and preventing hypoglycemia. The word "gluconeogenesis" means new glucose from sources other than current digestion. The adrenal cortex contributes new glucose after the liver and adrenal medulla and suffers the consequences of gluconeogenesis failure, as hypoglycemia is massive stress.

Glucose tolerance factor (GTF) partners with insulin in regulating glucose fueling of cells. The adrenal cortex processes the trace metal chromium into metabolically active GTF and other metabolites, with excess then stored in the liver for ready use. Later chapters examine these complex glucose mechanisms fully.

To review, five functions lie within Primary Stress Function:

– stress: cortisol response,
– fatigue: aldosterone response,
– conclusion of sex (involving stress and fatigue and connected to ovaries/testes),
– gluconeogenesis: glucose counterregulation,
– glucose tolerance factor (GTF), initial metabolism of chromium.

Immune and its Subfunctions

The immune system is a complicated defense system with many ways to kill bacteria, viruses, fungi, other foreign invaders, and infected and malignant cells. Basically, Immune attacks anything alive or from life that isn't you, your normal healthy cells. Immune response involves the thymus at the base of the neck (producing T-lymphocytes, also called T-cells), lymphatic system (producing B-lymphocytes or B-cells), spleen and bone marrow; however, control and responsibility lie in the adrenal cortex function.

Lymphocytes are white blood cells derived from stem cells (undifferentiated cells) manufactured in the bone marrow. Each lymphocyte type matures into its special role at a different location (T = thymus). T-lymphocytes kill invaders directly; they are strong against cancers, viruses, fungi, parasites and other foreign cells. HIV develops into full-blown AIDS from a lack of T-cells. The T-system, known as "cell-mediated immunity" or "cellular immunity," coordinates immune response and can stimulate B-lymphocyte production.

B-lymphocytes kill indirectly by first producing antibodies (antibody proteins/ immunoglobulins) upon encountering a foreign invader, and these antibodies then search and destroy. Any invader eliciting an antibody response is generically known as an antigen. When activated, B-lymphocytes are particularly effective against bacteria and allergies. B-system responses are called "humoral immunity," humoral meaning "of or from a body fluid."

This is only the beginning of self vs. nonself. Lymph, a clear yellowish fluid, occupies the space between structures in the body with its own lymphatic vessels along side of arteries, veins and blood vessels. Besides T- and B-lymphocytes, lymph contains NK (natural killer) lymphocytes, which are strong against cancer and viruses. NK cells are the first line of defense against cancer.[6, 7] Lymph nodes filter the lymph, trapping foreign substances. The spleen filters blood, stores extra blood cells and eliminates aging ones. Many lymphocytes mature in the spleen. Thymus and spleen are usually considered part of this lymphatic system.

Lymphocytes operate both in lymph and blood. In blood, they are one type of white blood cell. There are four other types: neutrophils, strong against bacteria;[8] eosinophils and basophils, which release histamines and other inflammatory compounds (part of the inflammation mechanism) and breakdown antibody-antigen complexes; and monocytes, the clean-up crew. When damaged, mast cells, a type of basophil, release too much histamine causing allergic reaction.[9] Here the inflammation mechanism is taken over and misused by allergies and autoimmune diseases. Phagocyte is a general term denoting a white blood cell that engulfs and devours microorganisms and cell fragments. Neutrophils, eosinophils and macrophages (long-living, large white blood cells derived from monocytes) are crucial phagocytes. In total, white blood cells number one or two for every one thousand red blood cells.

Cortex Immune is organized differently than the other three primary adrenal functions, with multiple ways to accomplish the same function or task of killing bacteria, viruses, fungi, allergens or cancers. Of course, one could consider T-, B- and NK-lymphocytes, neutrophils, eosinophils, basophils, monocytes, macrophages and phagocytes as immune tasks, but this requires expensive scientific measurement to determine which lymphocyte is malfunctioning and extensive knowledge of how to manipulate that lymphocyte and the immune system as a whole with efficacy. Such understanding is in its infancy, for now only a worthy scientific goal.

Nature has an easier solution, recommending bacteria, viruses and the other *bad guys* as tasks, since many vitamins and foods have proven efficacy against them. For example, Vitamin A kills bacteria, Vitamin C kills viruses, and fruits and vegetables are effective against numerous cancers. The scientific evidence on these defense nutrients is provided in upcoming chapters. For now, focusing on end results rather than on complicated lymphocyte mechanisms is the way to proceed. Therefore in this book, Primary Immune Function and tasks are defined as:

– bacteria,
– viruses,
– fungi,
– allergens,
– cancers.

With two shared functions:

– inflammation including vasodilation (Healing too),
– vasoconstriction (Healing too).

NUTRITION

Equilibrium Theory is a major advance in our understanding of human physiology. The four primary adrenal functions of Energy, Healing, Stress and Immune play a central role in health and disease. The body's response to all internal needs and external forces lies within and must adhere to their four-part harmony. This internal balance is nature's imposed moderation on life and its appetites and activities.

Once you understand how the adrenal gland works, how your actions and goals affect its well being, and what nutrition it requires for proper functioning, you can start building health and preventing or eliminating dysfunctions and related diseases. Energy, Healing, Stress and Immune tasks are the key to health and the template for all nutrition. One common sense concept is fundamental – good raw material input equals good end product output. Nutrition supplies the raw materials, and physiology turns out the end products of life's amazing chemistry.

Table 2-1 outlines the complete nutritional program of Equilibrium Theory, the raw materials your crucial Energy, Healing, Stress and Immune functions and systems need to make all hormones and other end products and to perform properly under all circumstances. Simple and flexible in its application, this program adjusts easily for lifestyle and current needs. Of course, nutrition does not give instant "pill" results. Patience is necessary for the slow building process of one nutritional factor upon another until there is synergy, a nutrition and resulting health effect much greater than the sum of the parts. Take time to do it right.

As a topic, nutrition is so large that each of five raw materials of Table 2-1 is presented in its own separate chapter, a comprehensive how-to guide. In these chapters, Equilibrium Theory integrates nutrition and physiology with precise correlations, thereby enabling you to live Hippocrates' wisdom, "Let food be your medicine."

A brief introduction to macronutrients, B vitamins, fatty acids, trace metals and herbs is given below. This essential nutrition sustains not only adrenal gland, but also the entire endocrine system and human body.

Macronutrients

Food carbohydrates, proteins, fats and fibers are much more than just calories. Each of these four distinct compositional food types matches up with one of the four primary adrenal functions, and greatly contributes to its performance and well-being. Specifically, carbohydrates produce energy, proteins supply healing substrates, fats are burned by cells to meet the demands of stress, and fibers including phyto-compounds (*phyto-* prefix meaning "plant") empower immune defense. The better the quality and variety of each macronutrient, the better the corresponding adrenal function and system will serve you.

TABLE 2-1. THE COMPLETE NUTRITIONAL PROGRAM.
Energy, Healing, Stress and Immune Raw Materials

Raw Material	Description	Presented in
Macronutrients	Carbohydrates, proteins, fats and fibers power the four primary adrenal functions and their metabolisms.	Chapter 3
B Vitamins	Water-soluble building blocks for adrenal and endocrine end products. Needed daily.	Chapter 4
Fatty Acids	Fat-soluble building blocks for adrenal and endocrine end products. Vegetable oils, fish oils, Vitamins A, D, E and beta-carotene. Needed daily.	Chapter 5
Trace Metals	Minerals — necessary for all chemical reactions to proceed normally and efficiently. Needed occasionally.	Chapter 6
Herbs	Herbs contain potent vitamin factors that adjust functioning and get things running right. Needed occasionally.	Chapter 7

B Vitamins

Only the adrenal gland, pancreas and liver use B vitamins, but their role and importance cannot be overemphasized. The human body is made up of both water-soluble and fat-soluble tissues. B's supply the water-soluble building blocks for adrenal gland, pancreas and liver hormones, neurotransmitters, enzymes, coenzymes and cofactors. To illustrate, pantothenic acid (B5) has the chemical composition $C_9H_{17}NO_5$, and the adrenal medulla hormone adrenaline of Primary Energy Function is $C_9H_{13}NO_3$. The difference between the two is $2H_2O$ or two water molecules.

$$\text{pantothenic acid} \rightarrow \text{adrenaline} + \text{water}$$
$$C_9H_{17}NO_5 \rightarrow C_9H_{13}NO_3 + 2H_2O$$

Most of adrenal and endocrine chemistry is this easy. Supply the raw materials and your glands and organs will do their jobs.

Because B vitamins are water-soluble, many B factors can be and quite literally are washed away by blood. Consequently, they need to be replenished daily.

Fatty Acids

Fatty acids supply the fat-soluble building blocks for adrenal and endocrine hormones, neurotransmitters, enzymes, coenzymes and cofactors, as well as for gland maintenance. Fatty acids also become essential components of cell membranes. These end products are made in sufficient amounts only from: (1) vegetable oils including olive oil, safflower oil, sunflower oil, soy oil and evening primrose oil, collectively known as Omega 6 oils; (2) fish oils, collectively known as Omega 3 oils, and eating fish and seafood; and (3) special vitamins isolated from these oils, the well-known fat-soluble vitamins: Vitamins A, D, E and beta-carotene. No other oils or fats, in particular animal fats, dairy fats and man-made fats such as partially hydrogenated, are needed by or in fact beneficial to endocrine machinery, although such fats can be burned as fuel by cells or stored as weight gain for future use.

Unlike water-soluble B vitamins, fatty acids are not flushed from the body so easily. However, daily supply is often best, especially if you have experienced fatty acid deprivation in the past.

Trace Metals

Trace metals facilitate all chemical reactions in the body. They act in three ways:

– Becoming metalloenzymes in the functioning of the adrenal gland or other gland or organ. An example is copper, which becomes part of adrenal medulla Energy/nerve function. Nature chose copper here, the best electrical conductor to go with nerves, the electrical conductor in the body! Copper wiring in the home is a good analogy.

– As catalysts throughout the body. A catalyst is necessary for a chemical reaction to proceed, but is not part of that reaction. For instance, molybdenum is the catalyst for all protein processes including protein digestion.

So, protein indigestion or protein diseases in muscles and protein structures of glands and organs may need molybdenum to restore normal function.

– As special messengers, forming complex molecules with special duties. Glucose Tolerance Factor (GTF) is the chromium complex that partners with insulin to regulate glucose metabolism.

Trace metals are needed in very small amounts, hence the modifier *trace*, and much less often than B vitamins and fatty acids. Occasional use (defined in Chapter 6) is best. The important point is not to run out of them, and not to overdose – keep your nutritional reservoirs filled. This concept of nutrient reservoir is a good way to view nutrition and to meet adrenal, endocrine and body needs.

Herbs

Herbs are vitamins too. Or more precisely, they contain vitamin/nutritional factors. Herbs provide critical nutrition, sometimes very potent nutrition, to a specific adrenal or endocrine part. Their targeted nutrients and assortment of therapeutic actions, ranging from stimulation to suppression to "get things running right," can correct adrenal and endocrine imbalances and exhaustions and restore health.

With all the good herbs can do, there's one problem. Too much of an herbal factor produces negative overdose consequences. The notorious example is caffeine in coffee. Caffeine can be considered herbal because, in fact, the nervous system needs it in small amounts. Too much, however, generates nerve and energy problems, allergic sensitivity and dependency – that caffeine fix syndrome. Therefore, use herbs occasionally, although there are some exceptions such as taking St. John's Wort every day to alleviate mild depression and *the blues*.

Drugs, Hormones and Gland Extracts

Energy, Healing, Stress and Immune tasks run on the five raw materials of Table 2-1 and NOTHING ELSE! They do not run on facsimiles of adrenal hormones such as cortisone and prednisone. These unnatural steroid drugs are the often-prescribed MD treatments for adrenal dysfunction. However, they act only on the adrenal cortex and lead to serious side effects, not long-term solutions. When a physician prescribes steroids, they are officially called glucocorticoids. Whatever they are called, the medical literature describes their debilitating side effects as follows:

> Glucocorticoid administration causes Cushing's syndrome (hyperactive adre-
> nal cortex functioning) and hypothalamic-pituitary-adrenal axis suppression,
> which in turn leads to cataracts, aggravation of glaucoma, hypertension [high
> blood pressure], pancreatitis, panniculitis [inflammatory reaction in subcuta-
> neous fat; skin nodules develop], and death of femoral and humeral bone
> heads. Osteoporosis is the most common complication. Other possible side
> effects include weakness, loss of muscle mass, worsening diabetes, poor
> wound healing, excessive weight gain, increased susceptibility to infection,
> activation of latent tuberculosis or histoplasmosis [fungus disease caused by
> phagocyte dysfunction; symptoms are cough, fever, anemia and malaise], lack
> of linear growth in children and psychiatric disturbances. Herpetic keratitis
> [cornea inflammation caused by herpes virus type I] may also accelerate,
> bringing on blindness.[10]

Look again at Figure 2-B with the four primary adrenal functions and their dependent body systems. The above side effects, as documented by the medical profession, reflect three hypoactive functions – Energy, Healing and Immune – and one hyperactive Stress function, manifesting Cushing's syndrome. Moreover, glucocorticoid therapy causes pituitary shutdown (hypothalamic-pituitary-adrenal axis suppression) and, with continued use, atrophy.

Nature's perfect pituitary-adrenal physiology is knocked out of commission, and for what? Side effects eventually become the dominant clinical feature. All pharmaceutical drugs act in a similar harsh manner, delivering powerful action/proven efficacy for one specific complaint within the tens of thousands of interconnected activities in the body, all of which need to work in perfect harmony. Drugs are miserable comforters. In reality, they treat symptoms, not underlying causes. "Cause and effect" is basic tenet of science, yet consistently ignored and violated by Western medicine. The better solution is to gently nourish functions and activities back to health with nature's raw materials targeted to each gland and task.

The adrenal gland and endocrine system do not run on the latest health-food fad hormones either, such a DHEA (dehydroepiandrosterone), CoQ10 (Coenzyme Q10) and melatonin, the pineal gland hormone. Favorably, these hormones are exact copies of the real thing and very limited use can get things running right. The best illustration here is melatonin, which can reset your circadian clock and bring on sleep. Take a small dose, 2 mg of melatonin an hour or two before bedtime, then not again for several weeks. Melatonin is discussed in Chapter 8. Another use exception is treatment of disease, for example CoQ10 eases the neurological deficits of Parkinson's disease.[11] For healthy individuals, however, abuse of these natural hormones quickly interferes with normal internal production and homeostasis. Where disease has not ravaged function, on-target macronutrients, B vitamins, fatty acids, trace metals and herbs can rebuild deficient output.

The adrenal gland and endocrine system do not run on gland extracts such as desiccated bovine adrenal gland. All gland extracts soon prove counterproductive. In general, drugs, hormones and ground-up glands are end products, and not in any way raw materials. End products upset endocrine balance and mechanisms – and force functioning.

Good raw material input equals good end product output. This basic fact of all chemical systems is the secret to vigorous health and long life. Supply the right raw materials and your adrenal gland and endocrine system will do its job naturally, perfectly. Good nutrition empowers glands and organs, whereas drugs, hormones and gland extracts stimulate without nourishing, knock delicate physiology and homeostasis out of commission, and create harsh to debilitating side effects. Nature designed the raw materials, nature designed the endocrine system – it's a perfect fit. Nature's chemistry is millions of years old, modern man-made chemistry less than 200 years old. You decide.

STAMINA

Real life and dictionary definitions of energy, stress and fatigue are reflected in the adrenal hormones adrenaline, cortisol and aldosterone, respectively, and in their adrenal functions. The human body starts all of life's physical and mental tasks in the same way, in the adrenal medulla with energy from adrenaline. If the task becomes stressful, adrenal cortex cortisol kicks in, doubling metabolism (as explained in Chapter 3). When stress gets to be too much and fatigue sets in, then aldosterone takes over, adjusting salt (sodium $\rightleftharpoons$ potassium) and water balances so the body can cope. Beyond that, through a link to the thyroid gland via the pituitary gland, fatigue can trigger thyroid hormones to raise your metabolism to the level of any task. At this point, you also get your "second wind." In reality, what you get is nature's back-up system of stored food energy (weight-gain carbohydrates and fats) to help overcome the rigors of planet earth. This girthy reserve is released and turned back into energy and stress action. Figure 2-C diagrams this back-system and loop, which reflects the real life and dictionary definition of STAMINA!

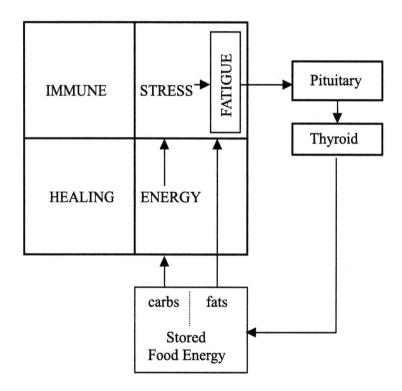

FIGURE 2-C. STAMINA.

NATURE'S BACK-UP SYSTEM: energy → stress → fatigue → pituitary → thyroid → stored food energy (carbohydrate and fat reserves) → energy and stress again, or SECOND WIND.

Weight Loss

Stamina is the only healthy way to lose weight. Your body withdraws stored car-bohydrate and fat substrates from *that spare tire*, *those love handles*, and converts them back into chemical energy, just as if they came directly from the digestive system. Stamina can go on and on. Once around this back-up loop is second wind, twice around the loop, third wind, and so on. Cardiovascular exercise is the best and safest way to melt extra pounds. Stick with second wind exercising, as this is sufficient to raise thyroid metabolism and make weight gain harder and weight loss easier. Physical workouts, recreational running and good sex are examples of stamina in action. Third wind and beyond lie in the region of marathons.

Slow, steady dieting can be successful too, especially in conjunction with raised thyroid basal metabolism. Eat mainly proteins lean in fat and fiber-rich fruits and vegetables, encouraging your body to withdraw those stored carbohydrates and fats. Severe or rapid weight-loss diets put protein and fiber needs at risk and can lead to muscle and connective tissue losses – a very bad result. And a result your body tries to correct by *screaming* for these food types, but this craving, if satisfied with carbohydrate and fat goodies, produces yo-yo dieting and failure, not to mention poor health and premature aging.

There are no easy answers to weight loss. Using the Figure 2-C stamina loop requires healthy energy, stress and fatigue functions. If you have no energy, if your ability to handle stress is worn out, if fatigue function is itself permanently exhausted, then forcing them to give what they don't have will only injure these tissues. First and foremost, the health of your adrenal gland and its energy-stress action plan must be restored with good nutrition as outlined in Table 2-1 and explained throughout Chapters 3-7. Adrenal dis-ease also may have to be corrected according to Chapter 12. Then, you can begin cardiovascular exercising. Exercising without weight concerns or goals is worthwhile and rewarding too. USE IT OR LOSE IT! Putting adrenal Energy and Stress functions through physical paces is an important counterpoint to the modern rat race. Why not vigor, vim, better trim?

Weight loss using drugs is the forced employment of the Figure 2-C stamina loop. Forced functioning is always harmful. The often-prescribed MD treatments of the recent past such as Fen-phen (fenfluramine and phentermine) have proven in hindsight to have life-threatening side effects, specifically pulmonary hypertension and heart valve disease.[12-14] Avoiding such forced functioning is foresight. The Chinese herb Ma Huang (ephedra) works in this same forced way. Of ephedra case reports submitted to the Food and Drug Administration (FDA), severe hypertension is the most frequent adverse effect followed by tachycardia (rapid heartbeat), heart attack, stroke and seizure with permanent impairment and possibly death.[15] Avoid ephedra except under medical supervision.

BREAKDOWN and REPAIR

All machines – your TV, refrigerator, car and your body – share the common frailty and fate of breakdown and repair (or replacement). In the human body, break-down of cells comes: (1) when they're old and worn out (the initial step in healing), or (2) prematurely aged as a result of stress. Actually, being old and worn-out is due to a lifetime of little stresses, therefore repair/replacement is the same for both mech-anisms. Stress just increases the load on healing. In essence, Primary Stress and Healing Functions are paired together in a marriage for life.

Handle stress better and there's less breakdown; heal better and there's more repair and replacement – and breakdown doesn't get out of control and lead to cell oxidation, a major contributor to aging. Consider the legendary, hearty breakfasts of past generations: lots of protein for healing, lots of fat to handle stress, something like a double order of bacon and eggs got our grandparents through farm chores or hard labor without fatigue, which is palpable cell breakdown. Vegetarianism is fine theory, but past generations got through the day by eating meat and other animal products because they provide protein and fat together. Today, we can achieve the same goal in a smarter way, avoiding all the cholesterol and saturated fats of the worst meats and animal products, instead using lean meats, vegetarian and fish choices, and new and some very old sources of protein for healing and fatty acids for stress (fat burning). Fatty acids, as we shall see in Chapter 5, are also powerful healers.

<u>Aldosterone fatigue = palpable cell breakdown</u>. However, these two stress events don't have to lead to aging. Fatigue can again be that "tired but good feeling" we remember from our youth. Cell breakdown can take two courses – with or without oxidation of the cell. Oxygen is the Jekyll and Hyde of our internal life. Every cell in the body needs oxygen, inside the cell, to perform its duties including burning glucose and fats. This could be best described as controlled use of a dangerous sub-stance. Oxygen is dangerous outside the body and in the larger world because it is the one necessary ingredient for fire, uncontrolled oxidation.

The same uncontrolled oxidation can happen inside the body too. Instead of cells using oxygen, oxygen uses cells, literally burning or oxidizing them, partially (causing injury) or completely (creating scar tissue). Scar tissue is dead, never to return, and you've gotten a little older in that moment. When you become mostly scar tissue... well, *hello* nursing home. Aging involves a number of known and unknown mechanisms; cell oxidation is the most pernicious.

Primary Healing Function normally prevents cell oxidation, especially when young and at its best. Somehow stress, LOTS OF STRESS, can overwhelm this preventative mechanism, and things get out of control. That somehow happens approximately as follows: oxygen and other unstable compounds becomes ionized in the blood or inside cells. Ions are electrically charged particles with free electrons. These oxygen ions and other ions, collectively known as free radicals, are highly reactive and can easily injure or kill cells by chemical reaction: healthy cell + free radical → scar tissue.

The cell components most susceptible to free radical damage are proteins, DNA and lipids (fats and fat-related compounds), principally through oxidation of fatty acid cell membranes.[16,17] Free radicals are a causative factor in over one hundred diseases including arthritis, atherosclerosis (depositing of plaque on artery walls, which leads to cardiovascular disease), ischemic (insufficient blood supply) injury, gastrointestinal disorders, carcinogenesis, Alzheimer's and Parkinson's diseases, and aging.[18]

Antioxidants

In recent years, science has discovered that many natural vitamin and herb substances are powerful free radical destroyers. These substances, called antioxidants, sweep the body clean of free radicals and relieve the symptoms of stress. Apparently, when you feel stressed, in large part you are feeling the buildup of free radicals, a monkey wrench in the breakdown and repair system. Some antioxidants protect cells at the point of attack, cell membranes and within cell structures; others search and destroy free radicals in the blood. Antioxidants separate the previously inseparable fatigue (palpable cell breakdown) and cell oxidation (injury or scar tissue) into two distinct phenomena. Now, you can return to those thrilling days of yesteryear, your youth, when fatigue was a pleasant experience. Antioxidants are a major health breakthrough and should be a part of everyone's health plan, every day.

You can demonstrate the power of antioxidants in your own life and activities. Antioxidants change bad stress (oxidative stress) into good stress. Sore muscles are nothing more than new scar tissue in the muscle. Strenuous activity, whether work or play, causes muscle breakdown and some scarring. Select an activity – physical labor, yard work or sports – where sore muscles are an unfortunate and recurring consequence. Then, add antioxidants to your diet, and see if you can separate these two phenomena of cell breakdown (fatigue) and cell oxidation. Take both water-soluble and fat-soluble antioxidants for best results, since each protects different cell parts. Chapter 5 fat-soluble antioxidant Vitamin E safeguards cell membranes, while Chapter 7 water-soluble antioxidant Vitamin C defends internal cell machinery such as mitochondria, the cell *organ* responsible for respiration and energy production. In addition, many trace metals become protective enzyme antioxidants. And food antioxidants from Table 3-3 also slow the sands of time.

Athletes know the nature of strenuous exercise and being "in shape." Getting in shape involves lots of sore muscles, particularly the initial workouts after a time away from the field. Once in shape, however, soreness eases significantly. Apparently, the human body and adrenal functions can adjust and regain proper, youthful breakdown and repair functioning through exercise! This is another powerful, persuasive reason for cardiovascular workout. Here too though, antioxidants give extra benefit. Everything is relative; game day on the field or in life is more stressful than practice.

***

3. MACRONUTRIENTS

Food… glorious food

Food is taste and pleasure, sustenance and culture – part of life's rich pageant. Inside of you, food becomes chemical energy to power your muscles, thoughts, hopes and dreams, your entire body including the remarkable adrenal gland, whose design, as we learned in Chapter 2, dictates how the body responses to all internal needs and external forces. Food supplies the basic construction materials that the four primary adrenal functions – Energy, Healing, Stress and Immune – use to carry out their tasks.

Food consists of four distinct compositional types: carbohydrates, proteins, fats and fibers. These are the macronutrients of food. Carbohydrates include sugars, a type of carbohydrate. Fats encompass vegetable, fish, animal and even man-made fats such as partially hydrogenated and trans fat, since all of these can become chemical energy. Vegetable and fish oils and their vitamins, collectively known as fatty acids, play two roles, one here as fat and chemical energy, and a second separate role as a special adrenal and endocrine nutrient (see Chapter 5).

Food macronutrients become Energy, Healing, Stress and Immune construction materials through digestion (below). They then fulfill their destiny with metabolism, specialized endocrine processing to final use (later in the chapter). Digestion takes place during the transit of food from mouth to stomach to small and large intestines, with the liver and pancreas adding bile and digestive enzymes, respectively. Technically, the digestive system or alimentary canal and the bile and enzymes secreted into it are considered external to the body, part of the exocrine system (externally secreting) and the specialized field of gastroenterology. However, this is a somewhat arbitrary distinction. Here exocrine and endocrine processes are closely linked, and rise and fall together.

The digestive system handles each food type differently, as follows.

Carbohydrate Digestion

Carbohydrates begin their journey by reacting with water and ptyalin, an enzyme in saliva, which starts the process of breaking down complex carbohydrates and sugars into simpler molecules. The stomach mixes and mashes these ingredients from three-quarters to four hours, depending on amount and type of carbohydrate and food in general, after which the pancreas secretes amylase digestive enzymes into the duodenum, the first part of the small intestine, to continue and complete carbohydrate breakdown to simple sugars. The final product is glucose ($C_6H_{12}O_6$), the simplest sugar, which is absorbed across the intestine wall and into the bloodstream for cell metabolism.

Lactose (milk sugar, $C_{12}H_{22}O_{11}$) and sucrose (common table sugar, also $C_{12}H_{22}O_{11}$, i.e. an isomer or different arrangement of atoms), along with maltose (malt sugar, $C_{12}H_{22}O_{11} \cdot H_2O$), must be broken down to glucose by special intestinal enzymes in the following reaction: $C_{12}H_{22}O_{11} + H_2O \rightarrow 2C_6H_{12}O_6$. Lactose intolerance results from a deficiency in the intestinal enzyme lactase. Between 70% and 90% of Asian, African, Mediterranean and American Indian adults lack this secretion. Fortunately, lactase supplements are now available, enabling digestion of milk and dairy products by these adults. Fructose (fruit sugar) and galactose (another milk sugar derivative) are isomers of glucose. They are absorbed directly into the blood and later converted to glucose by the liver.

Protein Digestion

In the stomach, hydrochloric acid of 1.5-2.5 pH (strongly acidic) together with two stomach protein-digesting enzymes, pepsin and protease, split long chains of protein molecules called polypeptides into smaller lengths. After pancreatic juices neutralize stomach acids in the duodenum, pancreatic digestive enzymes, notably trypsin and chymotrypsin, along with intestinal protease enzymes reduce peptides to their simplest molecules, amino acids, which are absorbed and put to use throughout the body.

Approximately 80 amino acids exist in nature. Of the eighty, the human body can make all needed molecules for protein metabolism from the following eight "essential amino acids."

– threonine	$C_4H_9NO_3$
– valine	$C_5H_{11}NO_2$
– methionine	$C_5H_{11}NO_2S$
– leucine	$C_6H_{13}NO_2$
– isoleucine	$C_6H_{13}NO_2$ (isomer)
– lysine	$C_6H_{14}N_2O_2$
– phenylanine	$C_9H_{11}NO_2$
– tryptophan	$C_{11}H_{12}N_2O_2$

These eight essential amino acids are derived from classical studies of nitrogen balance. Using more modern methods, histidine and during disease and certain stages of development arginine, citrulline, cysteine, ornithine, taurine and tyrosine also become essential.[1] Foods that contain all the essential amino acids are called complete protein. Foods lacking in one or more of the essential amino acids are incomplete protein.

Animal proteins such as meat, dairy products and eggs, and fish and seafood provide complete protein. Plant proteins from grains (wheat, rice, oats and other cereals), nuts and seeds, and legumes (beans, soybean, peas, peanut and alfalfa) are incomplete. Vegetarians must mix and match plant proteins to create complete nutrition.

Fat Digestion

Chewing food helps to separate fats from the other macronutrients. The stomach secretes the fat-digesting enzyme lipase to begin the chemical breakdown of fats. Bile from the liver and stored in the gallbladder is released to emulsify these fats, reducing them to small globules and making them water-soluble (actually a suspension of one liquid in another). Pancreatic lipase then completes the final breakdown of emulsified fats into esters and glycerol, which are absorbed for metabolism.

Ester or fatty acid. Ester is the general scientific term for a digested fat; fatty acid is the same thing but more specific. In common usage, fatty acid describes an ester of vegetable and fish oils and their naturally occurring vitamins: Vitamins A, D, E and beta-carotene, and will be reserved exclusively for that purpose in this book.

Two bad actors come along with the digestion of animal and dairy fats: cholesterol and triglycerides. Cholesterol can deposit on artery walls causing arteriosclerosis and heart disease.[2] High cholesterol is also implicated in gallstones.[3] Chapter 11 on the liver and bile gives important answers on how to control cholesterol naturally. Triglycerides are the worst kind of saturated fat. Definitions for all actors in the fat domain are presented in Chapter 5 "Fatty Acids."

Fiber Digestion

Fiber digestion is largely non-digestion. Most fibers such as cellulose and hemicellulose remain chemically inert during transit from mouth to stomach to intestines. Cows need three stomachs (four, depending on how you count) and cud chewing to digest fiber. Human beings, instead of digesting fiber, benefit from its ability to bind to large amounts of water, thereby increasing food transit through the intestines and helping to prevent constipation, diverticulosis and other gastrointestinal disorders.[4, 5] A high fiber diet also reduces cholesterol levels[6, 7] and colorectal cancers,[8, 9] and improves the glucose profile of diabetics.[7]

Medical experts agree that fiber digestion does not exist at all. This author has a slightly different point of view, and the difference may just be a matter of definition. Phytochemistry (plant biochemistry) involves thousands of naturally occurring plant compounds beyond cellulose and basic fibers. These "phyto-compounds" protect cells from oxidation and aid in defense. Many do not fit into carbohydrate, protein or fat classification. The best known are bioflavonoids, also called Vitamin P, and commonly found in rose hips and citric pulp. Phyto-compound technical names include flavonoids, carotenoids, plant lignans, phytosterols, saponins, coumarins, curcumins, phthalides, sulfides and terpenoids. Most, however, remain anonymous. For all practical purposes, digestion and absorption of phyto-compounds is fiber digestion.

Adrenal Functioning and Metabolism

Macronutrients are much more than just calories. Digested carbohydrates, proteins, fats and fibers play specific roles in adrenal functioning and metabolism. With the perfect symmetry of nature, each of the four food types "powers" one of the four primary adrenal functions, as shown in Table 3-1.

TABLE 3-1. FOOD TYPES "POWER" ADRENAL FUNCTIONS.

Food Type		Adrenal Function
CARBOHYDRATES	→	ENERGY
PROTEINS	→	HEALING
FATS	→	STRESS
FIBERS	→	IMMUNE

The verb "powers" has three precise meanings here:

Definition (1)—Each food type activates the corresponding Table 3-1 adrenal function to make all its adrenal hormones and other end products by utilizing the other four adrenal raw materials: B vitamins, fatty acids, trace metals and herbs (Table 2-1) in the following chemical reaction:

$$\text{RAW MATERIALS} \quad \xrightarrow{\frac{\text{FOOD}}{\text{TYPE}}} \quad \text{ADRENAL HORMONES}$$
$$\text{recently supplied *}$$

* B vitamin, fatty acid, trace metal and herb usage according to Table 2-1 guidelines, daily or occasionally, but most importantly, "Keep nutrient reservoirs filled."

Each food type acts as a catalyst, helping a particular function (for example Energy) to process raw materials (such as B vitamin pantothenic acid) into end product hormones (adrenaline). Of course, adrenal functions manufacture and secrete not only hormones, but also neurotransmitters, enzymes, coenzymes, cofactors and other effectors. All of these are brought to action in a concerted effort to accomplish the assigned task.

Definition (2)—Same as Definition (1) above, but <u>without</u> B vitamin, fatty acid, trace metal and herb raw materials recently supplied:

HEALTHY FUNCTION $\xrightarrow[\text{TYPE}]{\text{FOOD}}$ ADRENAL HORMONES

When you're young and healthy, your adrenal gland can do amazing things on poor nutrition. Not so, as you get older. Only so much adrenal abuse is tolerated before mild to severe adrenal exhaustion develops, after which no amount of that food type will generate the corresponding adrenal hormones and response. A good example is simple sugars for quick energy – candy, sweets, soft drinks and the ubiquitous high-fructose corn syrup. These empty calories sooner or later wear out adrenaline response, not to mention pancreatic insulin. Then you're in *big trouble*, and superior nutrition is required to rebuild the exhausted adrenal function back to vigorous health (details in Chapter 12).

Definition (3)—After adrenal hormones are produced according to Definition (1) or (2), each digested food type combines with those activated adrenal hormones to generate metabolism, or function (task) accomplished:

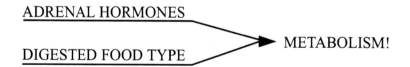

ADRENAL HORMONES

DIGESTED FOOD TYPE → METABOLISM!

To illustrate, adrenaline + carbohydrates = energy, while no adrenaline + carbohydrates = no energy, and no carbohydrates = no energy. Cortisol (adrenal cortex hormone) + fats = stress ability, and so on. Of course, these characterizations are oversimplified in their process description, but essentially correct.

The four primary adrenal metabolisms are examined below. These metabolisms can be further subdivided into catabolism and anabolism. Catabolic processes involve breaking down compounds, cells and tissue. Anabolic processes involve construction, building up compounds, cells and tissue.

Carbohydrate Metabolism

Glucose, the final product of carbohydrate digestion, combines with adrenal medulla Energy hormones, principally adrenaline, to produce metabolism, or in this case energy. Glucose is the preferred fuel of every cell in your body and oxidizes or "burns" according to this formula:

$$glucose + oxygen \rightarrow water + carbon\ dioxide,$$
$$C_6H_{12}O_6 + 6O_2 \rightarrow 6H_2O + 6CO_2$$

releasing 4 calories of energy per gram of original carbohydrate to power cells. Oxygen comes from the lungs, and carbon dioxide is expelled by the lungs.

If needed, cells can also burn...

2nd choice: fats (esters) releasing 9 calories per gram of original fat. As revealed in Table 3-1, fats power Stress and fat burning is the means. Stress demands high-energy fuel, and fats give over twice the metabolism of carbohydrates. Adrenaline instructs cells to burn glucose; cortisol tells them to burn esters.

3rd choice: proteins (amino acids) releasing 4 calories per gram of original protein.

Complex carbohydrates require up to four hours to digest in the stomach, and so deliver a slow, steady stream of glucose to the blood and all body cells. Simple sugars, on the other hand, dump too much glucose into the bloodstream, too quickly. Glucose metabolism, or how fast cells burn this fuel, is regulated by the pancreas hormone insulin (Chapter 10) and by Glucose Tolerance Factor (GTF, Chapter 6). Simple sugars and their resulting spikes in blood glucose wear out pancreatic insulin over time, bringing on hypoglycemia and eventually diabetes.[10, 11] Obesity and cardiovascular disease can also develop as consequences.[10] Simple sugars are TWICE BAD, wrecking both the pancreas and adrenal medulla Primary Energy Function, as explained in Definitions (2) and (3) above. When no adrenaline = no energy, the sugar/energy high of simple sugars disappears, and your health is worse for having employed this tempting energy shortcut.

Overall, carbohydrate metabolism is mostly catabolic, glucose breaking down and releasing energy. However, anabolic processes do occur. Excess glucose and calories are stored as weight gain, and a few carbohydrate substrates become part of nerves, muscles, organs and other tissues.

Protein Metabolism

Digested proteins (amino acids) activate Primary Healing Function and almost all of them go into repair and replacement of injured and worn out cells and tissue. After water, protein is the most plentiful substance in the human body. Muscles and tendons, organs and glands, brain, blood, skin, hair, nails and many hormones, enzymes and antibodies contain mostly protein, with fatty acid cell membrane components and some carbohydrate and fiber structural elements. The making of new tissue occurs on site, controlled by cell DNA (deoxyribonucleic acid), which unzips its double helix permitting exact copies. RNA (ribonucleic acid) then collects amino acids and other nutrients from the bloodstream and supervises construction of needed life molecules.

The healing described above is all anabolic, with newly digested amino acids going into building block repair and replacement. Of course, any replacement necessarily involves first catabolic breaking down of worn out cells and tissue. Thus, healing is actually a two-step metabolism. Beyond normal maintenance lies tissue reconstruction following injury, a much bigger Healing project with visible inflammation as an essential part of the effort.

Amino acids can also be used as fuel for cells (3rd choice above), catabolically releasing 4 calories per gram of original protein. However, this is very rare, limited to emergency situations such as trauma.

Table 3-2 gives a partial list of individual essential amino acid metabolisms and resulting activities and effects. Descriptions in this table involve considerable scientific complexity and are presented only to highlight the size and scope of the human puzzle. Combined amino acid metabolisms are even more complicated.

TABLE 3-2. INDIVIDUAL ESSENTIAL AMINO ACID ROLES.

ESSENTIAL AMINO ACIDS and their various metabolisms	Resulting Activities and Effects, including errors and diseases
THREONINE serine-threonine kinase [an enzyme transfers a phosphate group from ATP to another molecule]. Serine: non-essential amino acid; ATP: adenosine triphosphate, primary energy source within all living cells.	repairs DNA double-strand breaks.[12] TGF-beta (Transforming Growth Factor beta) signaling, which mediates cell growth and differentiation, embryonic development and immune response,[13] including inflammatory response.[14]
VALINE RNA editing of DNA	isoleucine/valine substitution error,[15] in glutathione S-transferases gene mutation causes testicular, bladder and lung cancer,[16] and in amyloid precursor protein (APP) gene mutation causes familial Alzheimer's disease.[17, 18] methionine/valine gene mutation causes most common hereditary amyloidosis [protein deposited in organs and tissues],[19] also with valine/glycine gene mutation causes dementia.[20] methionine/valine gene mutation causes prion diseases ('Mad Cow') including Creutzfeldt-Jakob and fatal familial insomnia.[21]
branched-chain amino acids (BCAA: valine, leucine and isoleucine).	become muscle protein.[22] synthesis of Coenzyme A [derived from ATP], involved in many metabolic pathways.[23] synthesis of brain glutamate, a fast, excitatory central nervous system (CNS) neurotransmitter.[24] provide energy and other amino acids independent of liver function; regulate protein synthesis, which is helpful in liver disease, sepsis [pathogens in the blood], trauma and burns.[25] liver regeneration.[26] recovery from hepatic encephalopathy [liver failure generates CNS/brain dysfunction; confusion to unresponsive coma].[27]
hemoglobin	high valine content.[28]

ESSENTIAL AMINO ACIDS and their various metabolisms	Resulting Activities and Effects, including errors and diseases
METHIONINE methionine ⇌ homocysteine equilibrium; each is precursor and detoxifier of the other.[29] Homocysteine: sulfhydryl non-essential amino acid.	hyperhomocysteinemia [-emia: of the blood] causes cardiovascular disease, thrombosis [blood clot],[30] neurodegenerative diseases,[31] and in pregnancy: miscarriage, pre-eclampsia, placenta abruptio, thrombosis and neural tube defects.[32]
as the only sulfur-containing essential amino acid.	enhances gene transcription.[33] protects heart from oxygen free radicals.[23] methionine + ATP → SAMe (next); this reaction is impaired by liver disease.[34] Vitamin B12 and folic acid deficiencies impair SAMe.[35]
SAMe (S-adenosylmethionine)	transmethylation in DNA, proteins and phospholipids; gives cell membranes their fluidity; faulty methionine metabolism here causes cancer, heart disease, obesity, aging and Parkinson's disease.[36] transsulfuration to cysteine, precursor of glutathione, a major cellular antioxidant[37] and immune modulator;[38] dysfunction here causes mitochondria [cell *organ* responsible for respiration and energy production] death, as in alcohol cirrhosis[39] and drug-induced hepatotoxicity.[40] ameliorates cholestasis [arrest of normal bile flow].[40] reduces liver fibrosis.[41]
Initiator tRNA(Met) = Methionine-isoaccepting tRNA (t = transfer).	increases DNA encoding of new cells; liver cell proliferation/regeneration.[42]
methionine + lysine → carnitine. Often considered an amino acid by itself, carnitine transports esters across the mitochondrial membrane for use as cell fuel; see "Fat Metabolism" ahead.	cell energy production.[43] high concentrations in human skeletal and cardiac muscles.[44]
methionine + glycine + arginine → creatinine.	becomes skeletal muscle.[45]

neuropeptide methionine enkephalin.	immunomodulatory signaling.[46]

LEUCINE

leucine zipper (bZIP) transcription factors.	regulates gene expression, DNA binding and transcriptional activation; cell differentiation into blood, liver, pancreas, skin, etc.[47] neuroendocrine functions.[48]
leucine-rich NES (nuclear export signal) proteins.	transports proteins out of the cell nucleus.[49]
branched-chain amino acids (BCAA: valine, leucine and isoleucine).	See valine above, plus... in brain glutamate synthesis, leucine particularly important.[24] in liver disease, increased leucine flux indicates protein breakdown, muscle wasting.[50]
leucine-rich repeat (LRR structure) glycoprotein superfamily, operates outside of the cell.	cell proliferation, differentiation, recognition, adhesion, and migration; regulates development, tissue repair, and metastasis [transfer from one organ/part to another].[51] transmembrane signaling, innate immune response.[52] blood platelet membrane activity; dysfunction causes Bernard-Soulier syndrome, hereditary bleeding disorder [no adhesion].[53] gonadotropin [pituitary sex hormone] receptors.[54]
hemoglobin	high leucine content.[28]

ISOLEUCINE

peptide histidine-isoleucine (PHI)	in the parasympathetic nervous system, vasodilator of cerebral circulation.[55] in pineal gland nerve fibers, innervates the gland.[56] neuromediator secreted by nerve fibers in the skin, modulates immune system through receptors; dysfunction causes inflammatory psoriasis and dermatitis.[57]
peptide tyrosine-isoleucine-glycine-serine-arginine (YIGSR).	inhibits tumor angiogenesis [new capillary blood vessels].[58]

ESSENTIAL AMINO ACIDS and their various metabolisms	Resulting Activities and Effects, including errors and diseases
LYSINE	
acetylation of lysine residues within the amino-terminal tails of core histones [five basic proteins around which DNA winds].	regulates gene transcription.[59]
lysine or arginine	dilates cerebral arterioles.[60]
lysine/arginine ratio	affects serum cholesterol levels.[61]
antimicrobial peptides are lysine- or arginine-rich.	quickly available to battle microbes.[62]
lysyl oxidase	this enzyme oxidizes lysine in collagen and elastin substrates generating the cross-linking matrix of tissue repair.[63] Steroids alter this collagen metabolism, leading to hepatic and pulmonary fibrosis.[64]
PHENYLANINE	
RNA editing of DNA	phenylalanine/lycine gene mutation of amyloid precursor protein (APP) gene causes familial Alzheimer's disease.[17]
phenylalanine derivatives	reduces sickling of red blood cells, useful in sickle cell disease.[65]
tetrahydrobiopterin cofactor (BH4), stimulated by phenylalanine.	various enzyme activities.[66]
phenylalanine hydroxylase (PAH). PAH enzyme and BH4 are part of phenylalanine-hydroxylating system.	dysfunction causes neurological deterioration.[67]
phenylketonuria (PKU) [-uria: present in the urine].	mental retardation;[68] newborn screening for this metabolic error is necessary, successful treatment with low phenylanine formulae.[69]
TRYPTOPHAN	
serotonin precursor. Serotonin: 5-hydroxytryptamine; CNS neurotransmitter especially important in the brain, also vasoconstrictor.	seratonin is a factor in sleep regulation, depression, anxiety, aggression, appetite, temperature, sexual behavior and pain sensation.[70]

	anorexia nervosa is consistent with increased serotonin activity; binging consistent with reduced serotonin.[71] African trypanosomiasis or sleeping sickness is related to reduced tryptophan, then serotonin.[72] low tryptophan = low serotonin and causes delirium and psychosis.[73] low serotonin, factor in action myoclonus [abrupt muscle twitching/spasms].[74]
tryptophan supplementation	for mild cases of depression including bipolar disorder, also mental disorders induced by levodopa [L-dopa drug: dopamine/Parkinson's treatment].[75]
excess tryptophan	most important essential amino acid for growth of viruses, bacteria and certain parasites; locally depleted tryptophan within inflammation is part of natural immune defense.[76]
tryptophan and tyrosine O-quinone cofactors.	improve B- and T-lymphocyte response, and neurologic, growth and reproductive function, etc.[77]

NOTE: Histidine, arginine, citrulline, cysteine, ornithine, taurine and tyrosine can also become essential amino acids.

The complexity of Table 3-2 amino acids demands respect. These eight essential amino acids need to be in perfect balance to achieve proper healing and the other vital metabolisms listed in the table. Complicated equilibriums and interactions exist here that only nature fully understands. If just one amino acid is missing, processes grind to a halt. Similarly, upsetting amino acid balance with too much of just one produces adverse consequences. Therefore, long term let Mother Nature supply your complete protein needs from nutritious high-protein meals. Multi-amino acid supplements can build muscle mass quickly, but they do so only with major disturbance to nature's perfection. In addition to amino acids, two other raw materials form impossibly complex equilibriums and interactions: B vitamins (next chapter) and trace metals (Chapter 6). These also require natural management long term, not all-knowing human intervention. It's not nice to fool Mother Nature!

Short term, individual amino acid supplements can provide health saving, even life-saving, answers for some unmanageable disorders. Examples indicated in Table 3-2 are:

Methionine. The liver is the only organ in the body that can regenerate itself, however, accumulating environmental toxins, jaundice, hepatitis and cirrhosis disable this mechanism. Methionine supplementation puts a failed regeneration mechanism back to work! SAMe and branch-chain amino acids (next) also aid in rebuilding liver function. "How to" is explained in Chapter 11.

Branched-chain amino acids (BCAA) valine, leucine and isoleucine can prevent protein breakdown/muscle wasting associated with liver disease.

Lysine + Vitamin C for herpes simplex (cold sores, canker sores and genital herpes) and herpes zoster (shingles). Lysine-rich antimicrobial peptides fight the herpes infection[78-80] and supercharge Vitamin C's general virus fighting and herpes-specific action,[81, 82] bringing virulent herpes outbreaks under control.

Phenylanine for sickle cell disease.

Tryptophan for sleep, mild depression and anxiety. Regrettably, the FDA continues to ban tryptophan in the United States despite strong evidence now that contaminated tryptophan from Japanese manufacturer Showa Denko caused the 1989 eosinophilia-myalgia syndrome (EMS) epidemic.[83]

Fat Metabolism

Fat metabolism involves catabolism and anabolism separately in two essential, but completely different tasks. Catabolically, fat burning (using any ester) occurs during stress, when the body needs high-energy fuel (9 calories per gram) to satisfy increased cell metabolism. Pundits have offered many definitions of "stress" over the years. The true definition, the one your body uses, is a simple one: when cells have to switch from burning glucose to burning fat, that's STRESS! Diabetes, for instance, is a stressful disease because impaired glucose metabolism forces cells to burn fat most of the time. The Atkins low-carbohydrate, high-fat diet is also very stressful. Internal balance between your energy and stress systems is fundamental to good health and long life.

Fat (ester) burning by cells produces by-product ketones, which become toxic at high blood concentrations.[84, 85] The kidneys attempt to flush these ketones, however, this can cause dehydration and, in the extreme, kidney failure and coma. Therefore, you must step in and help out. Excessive stress, particularly from diabetes, requires drinking extra fluids to keep ketones at safe levels. Another example, football players and other athletes know to drink plenty of fluids during the game.

A further concern, too much fat in the diet or too little fat burning can lead to unused calories and their storage as weight gain. Fat in food, because it contains 9 calories per gram, requires careful management especially with sedentary ways. Cardiovascular exercise can burn off these digested and stored fats, and is good stress if no adrenal function is exhausted and all nutritional needs are met. Review "Stamina" in Chapter 2.

The carnitine question: carnitine, a natural amino acid combination of methionine and lysine (Table 3-2), plays a crucial role in fat metabolism, transporting esters across the mitochondrial membrane. Mitochondria are the cell *organ* responsible for respiration (oxygen use with the oxidation/burning of glucose and esters) and chemical energy production. In a sense, carnitine is a catalyst for fat burning, necessary to but not part of the reaction. Normally present in abundance from internal manufacture and animal food sources, carnitine can become depleted with untreated diabetes, cirrhosis, kidney dialysis, intravenous feeding, malnutrition and various genetic, endocrine, neuromuscular and reproductive disorders.[86] Health food stores carry carnitine supplements, which should be considered whenever your stress ability is impaired. However, supplement only short term to rebuild reserves since carnitine upsets the body's complex amino acid balance in the same way that individual amino acids do. The herb Hydrangea of Chapter 7 also catalyzes fat metabolism.

Anabolically, fats (esters, but here ONLY fatty acids) become essential components of cell membranes, blood, tissue and organ structures, muscles and tendons, and the nervous system. The myelin sheath surrounding and insulating nerves is a soft white fatty acid tissue, destruction of which leads to the neuromuscular impairment multiple sclerosis (MS).[87, 88] Fatty acids are also necessary for the internal manufacture of Vitamin D, various hormones and enzymes, and prostaglandins, which control inflammation, pain and body temperature. These are but a few of the many anabolic fat metabolisms. With the exception of weight gain, anabolic use is only satisfied by fatty acids and not by esters in general. Chapter 5 reports the complete fatty acid story.

Lastly, fat digestion produces esters – and glycerol. Glycerol is an important substrate for gluconeogenesis.[89] For an explanation of gluconeogenesis, see Chapter 2 "Stress and its Subfunctions."

Fiber Metabolism

Fiber metabolism is immune defense! Phyto-compounds of all types are proven bacteria, virus, fungus and cancer fighters, as well as disease combatants. Table 3-3 gives a partial list of their amazing abilities with supporting medical evidence from human studies. Review papers also include animal studies.

TABLE 3-3. PHYTO-COMPOUND SOURCES AND EFFECTS.

Major phyto-compounds are polyphenolics (general term), flavonoids, carotenoids, plant lignans, phytosterols, saponins, coumarins, curcumins, phthalides, sulfides and terpenoids. Over 4000 flavonoids exist.

Phyto-Compound and/or Source	Proven Efficacy with respect to...
fruits and vegetables	cancers of lung, stomach, esophagus, pharynx, oral cavity, endometrium, pancreas and colon (review of 206 human epidemiologic studies, 22 animal studies).[90]
fruits and vegetables	antioxidation.[91]
many vegetables	antioxidation (review).[92]
cruciferous vegetables, broccoli and cabbage.	bladder cancer risk.[93]
broccoli	antioxidant,[94] coronary heart disease deaths.[95]
broccoli sprouts	chemical carcinogens.[96]

Flavonoids are polyphenolic compounds present in high concentration in many fruits and vegetables particularly citrus, grapes, apples, soybeans and tea leaves. Subclasses: flavonols and flavones.

flavonoids, citrus	anti-inflammatory,[97] antitumorigenic,[98, 99] anticancer (review).[100]
hesperidin, citrus flavonoid	anti-inflammatory and analgesic.[101]
flavonoids, citrus especially tangeretin and nobiletin.	antimutagenic,[102] squamous [scaly, platelike] cell carcinoma.[103]
tangeretin	cancer cell growth.[104]
naringin, white grapefruit	lung cancer risk.[105]
flavonoids, grape juice	LDL [low-density lipoprotein] antioxidation;[106] platelet aggregation, decreased risk of coronary thrombosis [blood clot formation] and myocardial infarction [heart attack].[107]

red wine	antioxidant,[108] LDL/HDL antioxidation,[109] LDL antioxidant, reduced atherosclerotic [depositing plaque on artery walls] complications,[110] antioxidant cardioprotection (review),[111] platelet aggregation.[112]
resveratrol, red wine	cardiovascular diseases (review),[113] antitumorigenic.[114]
red wine, resveratrol and quercetin	oral squamous carcinoma cells.[115]
any alcohol (approx. two drinks), red wine provides extra benefits.	cardioprotective effects (review).[116]
flavonols and flavones in wine, tea, fruits and vegetables.	free radical scavengers, metal chelators, anti-thrombotic agents, non-fatal myocardial infarction.[117]
tea flavonoids	LDL antioxidation,[118] severe aortic atherosclerosis.[119]
catechins in teas	antioxidants;[120] lipid peroxidation, blood platelet aggregation.[121]
green tea (Camellia sinensis) and black tea.	UV-B light-induced oxidative DNA damage and skin carcinogenesis.[122]
green tea, catechins	apoptosis [programmed cell death] of human stomach cancer cells,[123] cancer preventive (review),[124, 125]
green tea	oral leukoplakia [pre-cancerous growth, thick white patches],[126] leukemic cells,[127] prostate cancer,[128] skin cancer (review).[129]
flavonoids	chronic venous insufficiency [inadequate blood flow, most often manifesting in the legs with swelling, pain and muscle cramps; can lead to venous thrombosis].[130]
flavonoids, diosmin and hesperidin	chronic venous insufficiency (review),[131] hemorrhoidal disease.[132]
flavonoids including myricetin	lymphocyte antioxidant.[133]
flavonoids, mosses	antibacterial.[134]
fumaric acid, found in the lichen Iceland moss and the herb Shepherd's Purse.	cancer chemoprevention (review).[135]

Phyto-Compound and/or Source	Proven Efficacy with respect to...

Quercetin is a flavonoid ($C_{15}H_{10}O_7$). Many vegetables contain quercetin and related polyphenolic compounds.

quercetin	antioxidant (review),[136] anti-inflammatory,[137] chronic prostatitis,[138] colorectal carcinogenesis,[139, 140] anticancer and anti-metastasis.[141]
quercetin, green beans	antioxidant.[142]
quercetin, onions and apples	lung cancer risk.[105]

Soybean is a major source of the isoflavonoids daidzein and genistein – and phytoestrogen.

soybean, genistein and isoflavones	urinary tract cancer.[143]
genistein	lung cancer cells,[144] anticarcinogenic.[145]
soy, genistein and phytoestrogen	breast and prostate cancer (review).[146]
genistein, daidzein, biochanin A and coumestrol.	MCF-7 and T-47D breast cancer, genistein both inhibits and stimulates some breast cancer cell lines.[147]
soybean/avocado unsaponifiables	osteoarthritis.[148]

Phytoestrogens are of three principal types: flavonoids, isoflavonoids and lignans (also described ahead).

phytoestrogen	prostate cancer, [149] inhibits cancer formation and growth (review).[150]
estrogenic kaempferol, a flavonoid	antioxidant.[151]
bee propolis: kaempferol, quercetin and galangin.	herpes simplex virus type1.[152]
bee propolis	antibacterial, antifungal, antiviral.[153]

Rutin is a flavonoid. Best source: buckwheat.

rutin	antioxidant.[154]
oxerutins	chronic venous insufficiency.[155, 156]

Luteolin (flavone) and silymarin (flavonoid).

luteolin	lymphocyte antioxidant,[133] anticancer, anti-metastasis.[141]
luteolin and apigenin, a flavone	thyroid cancer.[157]
luteolin-rich artichoke extract	LDL oxidation,[158] hepatobiliary dysfunction and digestive complaints (review).[159]

silymarin, an artichoke flavonoid   skin cancer (review).[129]
silymarin, milk thistle. More in   liver antioxidant.[160]
  Chapter 11.

Carotenoids are red, orange and yellow food pigments. Major sources of lutein, a carotenoid, are spinach, broccoli, lettuce, tomatoes, oranges and orange juice, carrots, celery, and greens. Lycopene is the principle carotenoid in tomato. See Chapter 5 regarding beta-carotene and Vitamin A carotenoids.

carotenoids   antioxidant (review).[161]
carotene-containing fruits and   lung cancer.[162]
  vegetables.

lutein and zeaxanthin, the two   oxidative eye damage.[163]
  main pigments in 'macula lutea'
  membranes of the human eye.
lutein   colon cancer.[164]

tomato, carrot and spinach   DNA antioxidation.[165]
tomato   antioxidant, [166] lymphocyte antioxidant,[167]
                                             T-lymphocyte function,[168] anticarcinogenic
                                             (review),[169] prostate cancer,[170] cancers espe-
                                             cially prostate, lung and stomach (review of
                                             35 studies).[171]

Plant lignans are found in many cereals, grains, fruits and vegetables, and give rise to the human lignans, enterodiol and enterolactone. Richest source is linseed (flaxseed) and other oilseeds.

lignans   antioxidant,[172] colon tumor cells.[173]
twelve lignan derivatives   breast carcinoma cell growth.[174]
lignans, flaxseed   anticancer (review).[175]

arctigenin, a lignan   regulates immune response.[176]
dibenzylbutane, a lignan   priming human neutrophils.[177]

Phytosterols are unsaturated solid alcohols of the steroid group. Plant oils are excellent sources; nuts and seeds contain moderate levels, fruits and vegetables generally low concentrations.

phytosterols   antiviral, [178] cholesterol-lowering (review),[179]
                                             lowering total and LDL cholesterol
                                             (review),[180] cholesterol-lowering, reduced
                                             risk of coronary heart disease.[181, 182]
beta-sitosterol and its glycoside   improved T-lymphocyte and natural killer (NK)
                                             cell activity, dampening effect on overactive
                                             antibody responses (review);[183] adjuvant in
                                             treatment of pulmonary tuberculosis.[184]

Phyto-Compound and/or Source	Proven Efficacy with respect to...
azuprostat, a beta-sitosterol	benign prostatic hyperplasia [nonmalignant enlargement].[185]

Saponins are glycoside surfactants found principally in medicinal plants, for example American Ginseng, Sarsaparilla and Yucca of Chapter 7.

saponins and sapogenins	venous insufficiency.[186]
horse-chestnut seed extract	venous edema.[187]
sapogenins from Agave desert plants.	anti-inflammatory.[188]
saponins from South American tree Quillaja saponaria.	adjuvant for immune response to hepatitis B antigen.[189]
triterpenoid saponins	cytotoxic against tumor cells.[190]

Coumarins are pleasant smelling compounds (released on wilting) found in many plants. Over 300 coumarins have been identified.

simple coumarins	lipid peroxidation (review).[191]
coumarin derivatives	ischemic retinopathy, anticoagulant of marginal efficacy.[192]
coumarin (1,2-benzopyrone)	lymphoedema [swelling caused by obstruction in lymphatic drainage and at lymph nodes] (review).[191]
osthole	hypotension, inhibits platelet aggregation and smooth muscle contraction (review).[191]

Curcumin is abundant in the spice turmeric.

curcumin	antioxidation,[193] cancer chemoprevention (review).[135]
turmeric root extract	biliary dyskinesia [dysfunction in muscle controlling bile release].[194]

Sulfides. More on the power of sulfur nutrition later in this chapter. Green Cabbage and Raw Garlic are discussed in Chapter 7.

sulfhydryl compounds of Vitamin U/green cabbage.	bind free radicals and improve protein synthesis, heal gastric and duodenal ulcers,[195] and gastritis with bleeding;[196] protect against ulcerative colitis.[197]
S-alkyl cysteine sulfoxides of garlic and onions.	antibiotic, hypocholesterolemic [lowering blood cholesterol], fibrinolytic [breaking down blood clots], antidiabetic (review).[198]
garlic organosulfides	anticarcinogenic.[199]

Your mother was right when she said, "Eat your vegetables." To that can be added, "fruits and other phyto-compound fiber foods." A wide variety of these foods is essential for an effective immune system and disease prevention. The more different, unusual, *weird*, fiber and phyto-compound foods you eat, the more your cells become endowed with their strengths. Nature developed each phyto-compound for a specific purpose, and Table 3-3 shows that nature's purpose translates into you in proven ways!

Besides Primary Immune Function, Table 3-3 reveals strong antioxidant activity for many phyto-compounds. As we shall see if coming chapters, antioxidants play an important role in immune defense systems and are an integral part of the Healing → Immune action plan described in Chapter 2.

POWER to the Functions

Eat a balanced meal of carbohydrates, proteins, fats and fibers, and you power all four adrenal functions and systems equally. Need to heal? Eat more protein, and fatty acids for cell membranes. You can help your adrenal gland and body with the job at hand. An extreme illustration is marathon running. Carbo-loading beforehand is already well known for such rigorous energy output,[200, 201] however, marathoners would do well to load up on fats too since distance running also involves maximum stress. The best fat to handle severe stress is found in salmon, as we will learn in Chapter 5.

Variety within each food type increases the POWER. Carbohydrates and your energy performance need variety not for *same old, same old* glucose, but (1) to nourish a healthy Primary Energy Function since adrenaline + carbohydrates = energy, while no adrenaline + carbohydrates = no energy; and (2) for insulin peace and tranquility, which is explained in Chapter 10. The best complex carbohydrates to meet these goals are presented in Chapter 4. Everywhere junk carbohydrates and empty calories tempt your health with their siren song. As much as possible, avoid them. For fats, variety and discipline are also paired, variety in good fats (fatty acids) and discipline in avoiding bad fats. Protein metabolism and healing require complete protein foods. Unfortunately, animal protein, while an easy complete solution, carries the double hazard of cholesterol and triglycerides. Fish and vegetable proteins are much healthier choices. Getting enough high quality low-risk complete protein is crucial to good repair and remaining young inside. Maximizing good protein and minimizing bad carbohydrates and fats are prime factors in determining body shape, *hourglass* or *pear shaped*. Finally, fiber and phyto-compound variety defend life almost exponentially. Table 3-3 phyto-compounds and Table 7-6 Immune herbs are frontline soldiers in this battle. If necessary, employ stranger and stranger phyto-compounds from around the world to empower defense. And always, variety builds health.

<u>Calorie restriction (CR)</u> is the most effective intervention for increasing lifespan in a number of animal species including mammals.[202] Calorie restriction does not require excessive leanness, but is clearly present when body fat falls within the normal range.[203] Too many calories are bad for health, and the reasons go beyond the obvious dangers of obesity. Calorie restriction reduces metabolic rate, oxidative stress and inflammation, and is the most potent, broadly acting cancer-prevention regimen in experimental models. Restricting calories maintains many physiological functions at more youthful levels, and prevents or delays the onset of diabetes and other age-related diseases.[202-206] Aging is characterized by protein degradation, an accumulation of altered proteins in the body. This leads to a gradual deterioration of cell functions. Metabolic turnover of proteins is basic to life; and calorie restriction and moderate exercise restore youthful protein activity and turnover in aged animals.[207, 208]

<u>Sulfur regenerates life</u>. Within the macronutrient category hides this secret healing ingredient. The power of sulfur-containing protein is evidenced in Table 3-2 where methionine, the lone sulfur essential amino acid, plays a critical role in gene transcription, cell membrane fluidity, skeletal muscle formation, liver cell proliferation and regeneration, and many other vital metabolic pathways. In Table 3-3, sulfhydryl Vitamin U of green cabbage juice heals stomach ulcers. From Chapter 7, sulfur-containing alpha-lipoic acid, the most powerful antioxidant known, destroys a wide variety of free radicals; recycles Vitamin C, Vitamin E and other antioxidants; helps coordinate the antioxidant defense network and rejuvenates stressed endocrine machinery. These are just a few examples of the power of sulfur to rebuild tissue, function and health.

An egg has the highest sulfur content of any food, and a complete chicken can develop from that small life source. Other sulfur-rich foods are fish and meat, milk and cheese, beans, wheat germ, Brussels sprouts, red hot peppers, horseradish, garlic and onions. When healing needs are greater than normal, use these foods extensively. Take sulfur supplements for major tissue repair; MSM (methylsulfonylmethane), a natural substance in plants and milk, is the best known. 1000 mg of MSM taken with a complete protein meal generates significant healing and tissue regeneration. An alternative sulfur supplement is one cooked onion, basically onion soup. Cooking changes onion's pungent sulfur nature, but sulfur can neither be created nor destroyed, and a cooked onion as part of a high protein meal delivers gentle, positive results. For normal repair, incorporating small amounts of sulfur foods into protein meals to duplicate an egg's sulfur-protein profile is an effective long-term strategy to stay young and full of life.

CAUTION ☛ Avoid indiscriminate or continuous high sulfur use because extra sulfur requires extra amino acids and many other synergistic healing raw materials to achieve therapeutic effect. Take sulfur supplements only when major tissue repair is the #1 assignment. And remember, scar tissue can never be healed; it is dead and part of the past. Internal balance must be your overall goal.

Improve Digestion. Pancreatic enzymes break down all four-food types, and therefore the exocrine pancreas and adrenal gland are linked metabolically in a direct and consequential way. Figure 3-A shows this link, with effects described below.

Adrenal Gland Template   *Exocrine Pancreas*

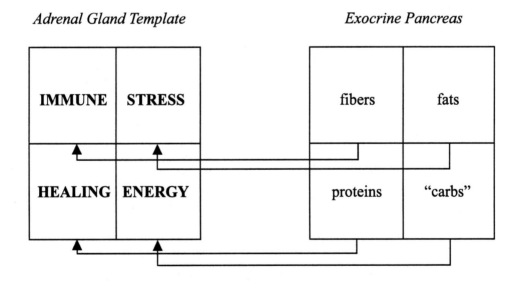

| IMMUNE | STRESS | | fibers | fats |
| HEALING | ENERGY | | proteins | "carbs" |

FIGURE 3-A. ADRENAL EXOCRINE-PANCREAS LINK.

Improve or just stimulate one or all of the exocrine pancreas functions and you improve (stimulate) the corresponding adrenal function(s). For instance, consider the protein → Primary Healing Function link. The trace metal molybdenum (Table 6-2) catalyzes all protein processes in the body. Accordingly, molybdenum is a raw material for healing in two ways, first improving protein digestion and then its metabolism. Other factors contributing to good digestion apply as well; for example stomach acid is crucial to protein digestion. Too little is negative, and too much can easily be made too little by antacids and thereby impact healing. Chapter 10 examines pancreatic digestion, stomach acid and stomach digestive aids, and Chapter 11 describes the importance of bile in fat digestion.

Nature's complexity in action. Food type, metal catalysts and other nutrient categories have their own Figure 2-B pattern and dynamics imprinted within them. Figure 2-B is the template for their actions. In other words, proteins must be in equilibrium with carbohydrates, or the adrenal medulla equilibrium of Healing ⇌ Energy will be affected. Similarly for Chapter 4-7 nutrients, different B vitamins, fatty acids, trace metals and herbs nourish different Figure 2-B functions. Positive nutrition of many types can then be implemented to satisfy needs exactly. The endocrine puzzle grows more complex, but it can be learned and put to good use.

Stored Food Energy is weight gain from eating more calories than your body needs for current tasks. The human body stores only carbohydrates and fats – NOT proteins and fibers. Nature designed us that way, and in fact storing proteins and fibers causes rare and often fatal diseases such as primary systemic amyloidosis (protein depositing in organs and tissues),[209] in which amyloid infiltration of the heart leads to arrhythmias and congestive heart failure.[210] On the other hand, stored reserves of carbohydrates and fats are normal and can easily be converted back into chemical energy to power Primary Energy and Stress Functions in the same way as if just eaten. Chapter 2 "Stamina" explains the conversion back. Nature provides this back-up system, a safety net, so your body can meet all the energy and stress demands imposed by life on this planet.

There are no reserves – NO SAFETY NET – for Healing (proteins) and Immune (fibers, phyto-compounds) systems. If these adrenal functions are in desperate need from healing or immune trauma, then body proteins from muscles and protein structures or fibers and phyto-compounds from connective tissue are broken down to power healing repair or immune defense, a very bad situation in which you grow old fast, right before your eyes. In such circumstances, you must step in and provide their back-up system, supplying vast and varied proteins, fatty acids and sulfurs or fibers and phyto-compounds.

***

4. B VITAMINS

Nutrition nourishes physiology, your glands and organs and their functions and activities. B vitamins are essential nutrition, one of the five raw materials your adrenal gland and endocrine system need to perform properly under all circumstances. B's supply the water-soluble building blocks for hormones, neurotransmitters, enzymes, coenzymes, cofactors and other end products of Energy, Healing, Stress and Immune functions and systems. Because B vitamins are water soluble and washed away by blood, these tasks can falter and fail if B nutrition is not supplied daily.

Only the adrenal gland, pancreas and liver utilize B vitamins. This chapter describes adrenal therapeutic action and effects. Chapters 10 and 11 explain pancreas and liver bile use, respectively.

In the Eye of the Beholder

B vitamins are the "jet fuel" for Energy, Healing, Stress and Immune action. Specifically, a direct and immediate relationship exists between each and every B and an important task. For example (from the Chapter 2 "Nutrition" introduction),

$$\text{pantothenic acid} \rightarrow \text{adrenaline} + \text{water.}$$
$$C_9H_{17}NO_5 \rightarrow C_9H_{13}NO_3 + 2H_2O$$

B vitamin adrenal and pancreatic roles are highlighted in Figure 4-A below, and each of these B's is explored in depth including review of its medical literature later in the "Supplementation" section of the chapter. There is an overriding reason for discussing individual B vitamins later, not sooner... and that is, complex interactions and equilibriums exist between all the B's within the Figure 4-A framework, for instance pantothenic acid with B2 and B6, separately with B1 and PABA, and probably with biotin and others. Such complexity demands natural management long term, NOT all-knowing human intervention and pills! Nature is the wisdom of the ages; nutritional science remains but a pale imitation.

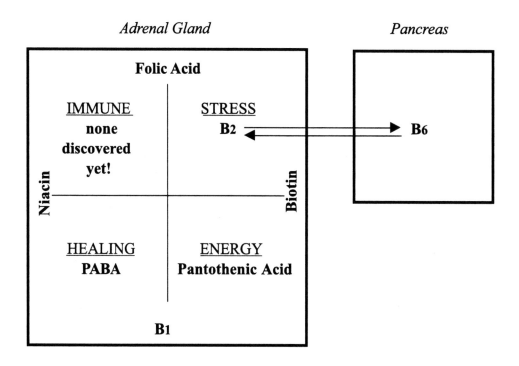

FIGURE 4-A. INDIVIDUAL B VITAMINS FOR THE ADRENAL GLAND AND PANCREAS.

"Primary B Vitamins" are in the center of each primary adrenal function, "Connecting B Vitamins" at the edges (function interfaces, e.g. B1 and biotin). B2 ⇌ B6 equilibrium must always be satisfied, even short term. Not shown: biotin also "connects" Energy and Stress with the endocrine pancreas.

Figure 4-A identifies two types of adrenal B vitamin metabolism: (1) "primary B vitamins" nourish the primary adrenal functions of Energy, Healing, Stress and Immune; and (2) "connecting B vitamins" aid, connect and facilitate the metabolic pathways between Healing ⇌ Energy, Immune ⇌ Stress, Energy → Stress and Healing → Immune. Pancreatic B vitamin metabolism also involves primary and connecting roles.

Complexity in practice. B vitamin raw materials impact metabolism quickly, in the case of pantothenic acid, energy from adrenaline. Yet, everyone has a different experience with B vitamins. When young and healthy, you can get along with or without their powerful therapeutic action – there's no noticeable difference. Here Definition (2) of "powers" adrenal functions from Chapter 3 "Adrenal Functioning and Metabolism" is at work. When age and B vitamin deprivation finally wear out Definition (2) healthy functioning, then large-dose multi-B supplements can bring palpable relief. Longer term, however, such supplementation seems to obey the law of diminishing returns. Still other people, taking single B's, find terrible side effects. To paraphrase Winston Churchill, B vitamins are a riddle wrapped in a mystery inside an enigma.

The author's experience includes most of the above, and one more hard-learned lesson that came after my health was *completely shot* and every raw material nutrient had to be supplied perfectly every day. That basic discovery is…

NATURAL MANAGEMENT

The best way to satisfy your daily B vitamin requirements is with nature's original goodness – wholesome, unrefined, unadulterated B vitamin-rich foods. And not with human-designed pills. Not single B vitamin supplements, not even the best modern multi-B formula can match nature's wisdom and design. Why?

Diminishing Returns. You may be able to take B vitamin supplements for months, perhaps even years with good results. Eventually however, for the two reasons explained below, adrenal functioning will start to go downhill, and then get worse and worse with more and more B vitamin supplementation. For the author, *eventually* comes in only three days! Just three tablets, one per day, of a modern, balanced, complete multi-B supplement and adrenal gland functioning is out of whack, and my health is falling apart.

The two reasons for the downturn in adrenal functioning and long-term negative effects of B vitamin supplements are:

(1) ALL B VITAMINS ARE INTERCONNECTED IN A COMPLICATED MATRIX.

B's perform their magic together, or eventually not at all. Even the best multi-B formula is not perfectly balanced to Mother Nature's standards. Each B must be in harmony (a correct ratio of amounts) with every other B – a complex, impossible puzzle that supplement formulators can only guess at. Months to years of being a little off in these ratios take its toll.

Another problem with B supplements—Each B vitamin is given in the same dose, day after day. Nature loves variety; variety builds health. *You can't get harmony when everybody keeps singing the same note.*

The third and biggest problem with B supplements—Not all B vitamins have been discovered, or ever will be! The B vitamin that nourishes Primary Immune Function is still unknown, as shown in Figure 4-A. More on this missing link ahead. Additionally, complex anti-stress and immune-boosting B factors exist within nutritional yeasts and leafy green vegetables. No one knows their chemical compositions, or how to put them in a bottle as well as they're put in their original containers. With all B vitamin supplements, you're overdosing on the B's in the formula and underdosing (zero) on the unknown, undiscovered B vitamins that are found in perfect balance ONLY in nature's wholesome foods.

Most B vitamins were identified less than 100 years ago. Niacin was first in the late 1880s, PABA (para-aminobenzoic acid) just before 1910, and B_1 and B_2 in the 1920s. Pantothenic acid (B_5), B_6 and biotin were discovered during the 1930s, and folic acid in 1941. Don't be lured in by incredible human discoveries; nature still hides more than she reveals. When discovered and undiscovered are interconnected in an unknowable way, yield to a higher authority – don't try to outthink Mother Nature.

(2) SOFT FUNCTIONING.

B vitamin supplements contain large, sometimes massive amounts of many B's – 50 mg, 100 mg. These amounts are far too much. Consider 100 mg of the B raw material pantothenic acid waiting at the adrenal medulla's "door" (beating down the door actually) to be made into adrenaline. This massive dose knocks adrenal functioning askew... EXCEPT when used in the treatment of mild to severe energy exhaustion (more on this therapy in the "Supplementation" section). Beyond and worse than askew however, massive B doses produce a separate phenomenon called "soft."

Too little of any B vitamin is bad, but so is too much! Too much B raw material produces soft functioning in the adrenal gland. This is functioning that cannot maintain performance, faltering badly and rapidly when the gland is worked. A good analogy, soft functioning is easily *"bent out of shape."* If you are healthy with a strong constitution and adrenal gland, you may not experience soft functioning, but be aware of the possibility. The phenomenon is most noticeable during stress. Massive amounts of B vitamins, designed to help you cope with stress, prove counterproductive and actually make the adrenal gland more susceptible to stress. A soft adrenal gland falls apart easily under stress, and so more B supplementation is needed to handle this stress, creating a vicious downward spiral. The answer is just the right amount of all B's, known and unknown, in perfect balance from natural B vitamin-rich foods. Less is more.

NOTE: Too much B vitamin jet fuel is also possible with B vitamin-rich foods. This occurs not from massive B amounts, but from too many doses. See "Therapeutic Action" ahead.

A big dose of just one B vitamin makes not only its corresponding adrenal function soft, but somehow affects the entire gland. Aspirin and some herbs also cause soft functioning. Taking aspirin to relieve a stress headache guarantees the next headache, unless little or no stress is incurred for 24 hours or more, until the adrenal gland function hardens up again. Twenty-four hours is the usual hardening time, but dosage and potency are factors. Soft functioning is an important adrenal and endocrine phenomenon, and reference to the definition here will be made many times in coming chapters.

The Solution: B vitamins naturally! Taking B vitamins the way Mother Nature intended builds strong, healthy Energy, Healing, Stress and Immune functions and systems. B vitamin-rich foods are the manna your body will thrive on today, tomorrow and for the rest of your life. Put supplement pills: single B's, multi-B's and B's with minerals on the shelf for now and see if you don't discover a better long-term answer.

Transition. If you're still getting positive results from B vitamin supplements, then an appropriate course is to s-l-o-w-l-y wean yourself from them before you hit the long-term wall of diminishing returns from the following: loss of internal balance particularly in immune functioning, lack of nutritional variety, deprivation of unknown missing B's and continuous soft functioning effects. Instead, incorporate the goodness of wholesome B vitamin-rich foods into your diet, and reduce the amount and frequency of supplementation. You'll find that you don't really need massive B's for energy or any other adrenal task. Unrefined, unadulterated, nutritious good food is superior to pills here.

And what of B vitamin supplementation? Its primetime role is short-term targeted use: (1) to fix adrenal exhaustions, (2) to correct adrenal imbalances, and (3) to overcome past B vitamin deprivation. These remedies are given later in the chapter, including the role of each individual B in adrenal well-being.

REAL FOOD… *life-giving, life-sustaining*

Table 4-1 presents the B vitamin-rich foods that your Energy, Healing, Stress and Immune functions and systems need to make all their hormones and other end products and to perform properly under all circumstances. Surprisingly, the adrenal medulla and adrenal cortex run on completely different nutrition. B vitamins from whole-grain cereals power medulla Energy and Healing, while nutritional yeasts and green vegetables fuel cortex Stress and Immune tasks. For all of these foods, organically grown is better than non-organic. 'Organic' means using natural farming methods: manure, compost and other natural recycled fertilizers with no pesticides or intensive methods. Actually, organic has two definitions in this book, the one above and a scientific term meaning 'carbon based,' as in organic chemistry vs. inorganic chemistry. Organic chemistry is the stuff of life.

TABLE 4-1. ADRENAL B VITAMIN FOODS.

ADRENAL CORTEX runs on...	1. <u>Nutritional Yeasts</u>
	2. <u>Green Vegetables, especially leafy greens</u>:
	   broccoli, spinach, kale, endive, escarole,
	   beet greens, romaine lettuce, Swiss
	   chard, collards, dandelion greens, etc.

ADRENAL MEDULLA runs on...	<u>Whole-Grain Cereals</u>: whole wheat: breads, breakfast cereals, wheat germ, kamut and spelt. brown rice: long grain, short grain, wild. rye millet barley oats (Energy/nerve Function only)

Adrenal Medulla

The adrenal medulla runs on whole-grain cereals. Nothing else supplies its B vitamin requirements properly or sufficiently. Variety is key. The more different types of whole grains you eat, the healthier your Energy and Healing functions will be and the equilibrium between them. All the cereals in Table 4-1 feed both medulla functions equally except oats, which nourishes Energy/nerves only. In fact, oats is the #1 nerve vitamin on the planet.

The term "whole grain" refers to unrefined cereal products, where the germ and bran of each grain seed are still present. Germ is the life center of the seed, that which sprouts when the seed is planted. Bran is the seed's surface layer, full of fiber and nutrients. Most of the nutritional goodness of cereals lies within the germ and bran, which sadly are milled of and thrown away with white bread, white rice and other "refined" products. Avoid these denatured cereals – they are empty calories, as you literally starve in the midst of plenty! "Enriched" white bread is no better. Enriched means the natural goodness is gone and a few B vitamin supplements are added back, with their perils as noted in the last section. At their core, enriched breakfast cereals are junk food. Furthermore, many so-called whole-wheat breads are just enriched white flour with a pinch of whole grain, molasses for color, and high-fructose corn syrup for sweetness. Read labels carefully. There still are a few real whole-wheat breakfast cereals in the vast supermarket wasteland, but very few. You can find good tasting, organically grown whole-wheat bread and breakfast cereals at the health food store. Bread was once the "Staff of Life." It can be again.

Wheat germ is 100% germ, in a sense a natural supplement. It is energy in a bottle and a good place to start improving nutrition if you need more energy. A rounded tablespoon twice a day supplies more energy, more goodness than any modern, advanced, *super* B vitamin tablet. Over time, add variety. Kamut and spelt are ancient wheats, not as productive as modern strains, therefore not grown by agribusiness. Whole wheat becomes tasty breads, cookies and other snacks. Oats are an unbeatable energy breakfast. Brown rice fuels Eastern cultures, China, Japan, India and Southeast Asia, as it has for millennia. Whole-grain rice contains unknown energy and healing factors found in no other grain. And it sticks to your ribs throughout the day. Rye, barley and millet add their own positive imprint to medulla health. Buckwheat, rich in the flavonoid rutin, is not cereal, but of the rhubarb family. However, whole-grain buckwheat, amaranth and quinoa provide reinforcing nourishment. Amaranth is from the Middle East, *gooey* and best added in small amounts to cereals and foods. Quinoa is South American, light and good in combination with any cereal.

Preparation time—Brown rice (long, short and wild) takes approximately one hour to cook in water after bringing them to a boil, then reducing heat and simmering. Sorry, five-minute rice is comparatively worthless. Amaranth and pearled barley, which is typically used in soups, also take about an hour. Barley flakes, millet and quinoa require a half-hour. Buckwheat cooks in only 5 to 10 minutes. Wheat germ and rolled oats can be instant cereals, although hot oatmeal warms the body and soul. Rye is easiest and best as rye bread.

Dr. Atkins and other proponents of low-carbohydrate diets rightly denunciate junk carbs, but they wrongly fail to point out the essential role of good carbs, that is, whole-grain cereals. Whole-grain cereals are nature's perfect energy food. As complex carbohydrates, they digest slowly and supply a steady stream of glucose to fuel body cells over many hours.[1, 2] Whole grains also provide the B raw materials to make Primary Energy Function hormones, adrenaline and others, thereby sparking Energy metabolism, as explained in Chapter 3. <u>There are three basic ways your body can get energy: whole-grain cereals build health and vitality throughout your life. The other two, refined sugar and caffeine, slowly wreck your health</u>. Simple sugars from the sugar bowl, sugarcoated enriched breakfast foods, sweets, candy, soft drinks containing high-fructose corn syrup, and the like gradually exhaust adrenal medulla hormones (no adrenaline means no energy, and the *sugar high* disappears) and wear out pancreatic insulin, bringing on hypoglycemia and diabetes. Meanwhile, caffeine and other nerve stimulants produce jangled, hyperactive nerves and hypoactive healing. Caffeine triggers adrenaline flow and energy, but all to soon induces mild energy exhaustion from inadequate real nutrition. Then, a caffeine fix is needed to generate any energy. And sub-par energy gives rise to a sub-par immune response, as revealed in Figure 12-A(1).

Whole-grain cereals are almost perfect for healing too. Their protein and B vitamins power Primary Healing Function and its metabolisms. However, cereals provide incomplete protein with different missing essential amino acids, for instance lysine in wheat,[3] isoleucine in rice,[4] and must be augmented with animal or fish complete protein, or other incomplete vegetable proteins to insure perfect participation by the body's entire amino-acid *construction crew*. Another important consideration, the gooiest portions of cooked whole-grain cereals contain special healing polysaccharides found nowhere else. These polysaccharides are plentiful in cooked brown rice and millet for example. Do not drain them away before serving.

Whole-grain cereals are one of nature's REAL FOODS and an important rite of passage to a new and healthy lifestyle. Of course, many more raw material nutrients from Chapters 3 and 5-7 contribute to adrenal medulla end products and performance.

Review of the Medical Literature

Refined vs. whole grain… Epidemiological studies consistently show that cardiovascular disease and Type II [adult onset] diabetes occur at higher rates in persons deriving more of their energy requirements from refined grains and simple carbohydrates than from whole grains.[5] Relatively high intakes of whole-grain cereals significantly decrease rates of coronary heart disease.[6] Whole grains generally have low glycemic indexes [resulting blood glucose profiles] and low insulin demand; and consumption is inversely associated with obesity biomarkers.[7] Refined cereal consumption increases the risk of stomach, large bowel and other digestive and non-digestive cancers.[8] Conversely, whole grains protect against cancers, particularly gastrointestinal cancers.[9] Whole grains also possess antioxidant activity, with buckwheat greater than (>) barley > oats > wheat = rye.[10]

Wheat... Wheat germ taken of 30 grams [1 oz] daily for four weeks markedly reduces total cholesterol in high blood cholesterol individuals, with VLDL cholesterol [V: very; LDL: low-density lipoproteins, so-called bad cholesterol] falling by 40%.[11] Whole wheat is safe and effective for cholesterol modification and weight reduction in moderately obese women.[12] Wheat and barley whole-grain cereals significantly improve the postprandial [after a meal] blood glucose profiles of diabetics.[2] Wheat bran protects against a range of cancers, especially colon and breast cancers, in both human and animal studies.[13] By scavenging nitrite free radicals [nitrites used in curing meats produce carcinogenic nitrosamines], a wheat bran serving equivalent to two pieces of whole-wheat bread can halve stomach nitrite concentrations.[14] A normal serving of whole-wheat breakfast cereal shows strong in vitro [in laboratory vessel] antioxidant activity.[15] In an animal study, whole-wheat flour, rich in both minerals and phytic acid [insoluble fiber component of plant cells, negatively impacts mineral absorption], does not adversely affect mineral absorption, but instead improves the bioavailability of some minerals.[16]

Rice... Special tocotrienols [Vitamin E is the general term for all tocopherols and tocotrienols; alpha-tocopherol is its most active biological form] in rice bran possess hypocholesterolemic, antioxidant and antitumor properties. These tocotrienols reduce total and LDL cholesterol in chickens, and demonstrate greater antioxidant activity and B16 melanoma suppression [B16: mouse melanoma model; melanoma is a skin tumor of pigment-producing cells] than alpha-tocopherol [Vitamin E by standard definition] and other known tocotrienols.[17] To reduce the risk of stroke, the following foods are recommended: fish, whole-grain rice, oats and corn, fiber-rich legumes, and fruit and vegetables high in Vitamins C and E.[18]

Rye... Whole-grain rye bread decreases total and LDL cholesterol in hypercholestrolemic men.[19] Rye bread reduces gastrointestinal compounds associated with colon cancer risk by altering bacterial metabolism, accelerating intestinal transit and increasing fecal output, thereby also improving bowel function.[20] High-fiber rye and to a lesser extent high-fiber wheat improve bowel health.[21]

Barley... is an especially useful cereal for diabetics. Barley has a low glycemic index [resulting blood glucose profile] and a high insulinemic index in Type II [adult onset] diabetics.[22] Barley cholesterol effects are given below.

Oats… reduce blood cholesterol, modulate glucose metabolism and improve gastrointestinal function.[23] When taken with a meal, oats or barley, both very high in beta-glucan soluble fiber, increase the viscosity of the meal mass in the small intestine and delay nutrient absorption. Diabetics can benefit from this action, as 10% beta-glucan in a cereal food achieves a 50% reduction in glycemic peak. Furthermore, three grams or more of beta-glucan daily significantly lowers LDL cholesterol levels.[24] Oat bran reduces LDL by up to 23%.[25] For celiac disease [digestive disease of the intestinal lining; inflammatory response to gluten, the elastic protein of dough], while it is generally accepted that oats, wheat, rye and barley must be excluded from the diet, a growing body of evidence indicates that moderate intake of oats can be consumed safely by many celiac adults. However, wheat contamination of commercial oat products remains a risk.[26, 27]

Adrenal Cortex

The adrenal cortex runs on two kinds of B vitamin-rich foods: nutritional yeasts and green vegetables, especially leafy greens. Broccoli and spinach are most important here, but again variety builds health. Therefore kale, endive, escarole, beet greens, romaine lettuce, Swiss chard, collards and dandelion greens all play a role in developing strong cortex functioning and equilibrium. By comparison, iceberg lettuce is of little nutritional value. Both nutritional yeasts and green vegetables contain anti-stress and immune-boosting factors that remain unidentified, not found on any B vitamin list. All nutritional yeasts and greens nourish Stress and Immune systems equally.

Yeasts are single-celled fungi, best known for the role in leavening breads and brewing alcoholic beverages. Nutritional yeasts, however, are not of these types, although the first nutritional yeast was called brewer's yeast and is still available. Nutritional yeasts are not alive, rather the remains of fungi reproduction on nutrient-rich hosts such as honey and molasses. During daughter-to-daughter reproduction, these fungi gather host nutrients into their cells in specific patterns and amounts. Yeasts grow rich in B vitamins, amino acids, trace metals and many other vital factors.

The original nutritional yeast, brewer's yeast, is bitter, hard to digest and for most people best avoided. Fortunately today, many good tasting easy-to-digest nutritional yeasts are on the market. Find at least two you like, grown on different substrates. Use plain yeasts with nothing added, such as a chromium supplement. First choice for anti-stress: TWINLAB® Natural Nutritional Yeast (brown label). A rounded tablespoon gives good effect and can be put in juice or milk.

Nutritional yeasts help you weather the storm and stress of life. They significantly enhance cortex functioning and, in fact, are so POWERFULLY GOOD that they should not be taken without also ingesting whole-grain cereals, either earlier in the day or at the same time, to nourish medulla functioning. This is to maintain normal adrenal execution or functional flow from medulla → cortex, as shown in Figure 2-B. Occasionally, yeast alone is OK if Stress and/or Immune improvement is obviously needed, but their repeated use without whole grains will cause homeostatic pituitary suppression and adrenal medulla distress. Green vegetables are subtler in their cortex action and can be taken alone without this concern.

The importance of nutritional yeasts to cortex functioning cannot be overemphasized. With them, you build strong, vigorous Stress and Immune functions and systems throughout your life. Without them, you slowly deplete these assets. The only nutrition more fundamental to cortex well being than nutritional yeasts is fish and seafood and their Omega 3 oils.

Nutritional yeasts <u>may</u> aggravate Candida, a fungus infection caused by immuno-suppression,[28, 29] i.e. exhaustion somewhere in the immune system. Chapter 12 gives exhaustion cures. Once your immune system is back to its young self, then nutritional yeasts can be added to the diet without complaint. Just as an Immune dysfunction in white blood cell activity can be made worse by nutritional yeasts, the same is true for a Stress dysfunction in red blood cell activity. If instead of a strong boost in stress ability when yeasts are added to the diet, the opposite occurs; then mild to severe anemia is probably present. See "Iron" and its medical literature in Chapter 6 for correction. Unlike leavening and brewing yeasts, very little is reported in the medical literature on nutritional yeasts.

Review of the Medical Literature

Nutritional yeasts... Adding fiber to the diet, particularly beta-glucan, is one way to reduce blood cholesterol and heart disease risk. Oats and yeast are rich sources of beta-glucan.[30, 31] Taken prior to surgery, supplements of immune-enhancing nutritional yeast, Omega 3 [fish] fatty acids and amino acid L-arginine improve the outlook for patients at high risk of infection.[32] Brewer's yeast contains an organic form of chromium that increases the effectiveness of insulin.[33]

Green vegetables... See folic acid, the known B vitamin of green vegetables, ahead and Table 3-3 regarding phyto-compound constituents.

THERAPEUTIC ACTION... how to take B vitamins, fatty acids, trace metals and herbs.

Figure 4-B shows the time-dependent therapeutic action of B vitamins, fatty acids, trace metals and herbs following ingestion. These Chapter 4-7 nutrients all act on adrenal functions and body systems in the same basic, positive way: raw materials contribute to/become end products. This fundamental performance sustains life.

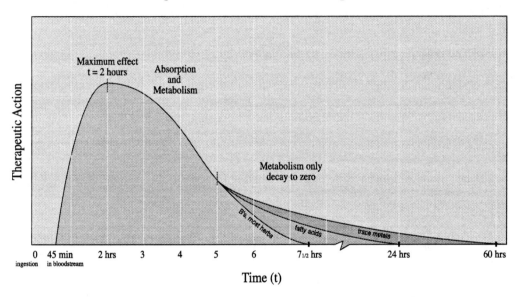

FIGURE 4-B. THERAPEUTIC ACTION OF B VITAMINS, FATTY ACIDS, TRACE METALS AND HERBS.

With ingestion at time t = 0, B vitamins, fatty acids, trace metals and herbs first reach the bloodstream and adrenal functions at t = 45 minutes from the earliest digested product. However, some nutrients are actually absorbed right through the stomach lining and have therapeutic effect earlier. For example, the B vitamin niacin reaches the bloodstream only 15 minutes after ingestion, or even faster with topical (on the skin) application. Vitamin B12 in sublingual (under the tongue) lozenge goes directly into the bloodstream.

Therapeutic action rises straight-line from none at t = 45 minutes to maximum effect at 2 hours (of course, adjust t = 2 hour maximum effect accordingly for niacin or sublingual B12). Beyond 2 hours, action drops off but remains strong until about 5 hours after ingestion, then decays to zero as indicated in Figure 4-B. Differences in therapeutic action between B vitamins, fatty acids, metals and herbs lie only in the decay-to-zero part of the curve. Whole-grain cereals, nutritional yeasts and green vegetables, as well as B vitamins in supplement form, decay to zero 7¹/₂ hours after ingestion. Like water-soluble B's, most herbs also decay to zero in 7¹/₂ hours, while fatty acids take 24 hours and trace metals approximately 60 hours (2¹/₂ days).

B vitamin therapeutic action nourishes adrenal functions for only 7¹/₂ hours before blood washes away the effect. Benefits, however, last much longer! Each time you eat whole-grain cereals for the adrenal medulla and nutritional yeasts and green vegetables for the cortex, your adrenal gland thrives and becomes healthier and healthier. And a healthy adrenal gland can function properly even without raw materials recently supplied; compare Definitions (1) and (2) of "powers" adrenal functions in Chapter 3. The same is true for fatty acid, trace metal and herb nutrients. Healthy functioning permits great flexibility in your nutrition program. Poor functioning, on the other hand, requires close adherence to the principles outlined here to achieve a health turnaround.

Multiple Dose Effects

In this book, one serving of B vitamins, for instance, a bowl of shredded whole-wheat cereal will be referred to as a "maintenance" therapeutic action, or maintenance serving or dose, producing a "rev" of the adrenal function(s). Before this first serving decays to zero at t = 7¹/₂ hours, ingesting a second similar serving, say brown rice, will create a combined therapeutic action – A MUCH STRONGER EFFECT. This combined, stronger action will be called "stimulation" therapeutic action, serving or dose, and stimulates adrenal function(s) into action. In like manner, a third serving before the first expires produces "harmful overstimulation" or OVERDOSE, and should be avoided. Here the term overdose does not mean toxicity to tissues, but rather a hyperactivity and forced functioning from too frequent use relative to need. Table 4-2 presents the shorthand terminology used throughout the rest of the book.

TABLE 4-2. SINGLE AND MULTIPLE THERAPEUTIC ACTIONS.

Description of serving or dose	Adrenal Effect	Number of doses	Symbol
Maintenance serving	"rev"	1X	▲
Stimulation servings	stimulate	2X	▲ ▲
Harmful Overstimulation servings	overdose	3X	▲ ▲ ▲

One B vitamin maintenance serving (1X) does as it says, "maintains health" for a normal lifestyle with no severe demands currently upon the mind and body. Stimulation servings (2X) are appropriate for physical labor and sports, and necessary in overcoming B vitamin deprivation and adrenal exhaustion (long-term deprivation). Continue 2X until your energy comes back and you can handle stress easily. Breakfast is the most important meal of the day and should include whole-grain cereals for energy and total medulla health. Add nutritional yeasts and green vegetables during the day for stress and total cortex health. Whole-grain cereals, nutritional yeasts and green vegetables each can be taken separately to 2X as needed, but not 3X. In the same way, adjust 1X maintenance and 2X stimulation and rebuilding of health for fatty acids, trace metals and herbs to meet Energy, Healing, Stress and Immune needs exactly.

B vitamins interact therapeutically with many herbs and trace metals, specifically those affecting the adrenal gland and pancreas. B's do not interact with fatty acids, one water-soluble and the other oil-soluble, except in terms of calories as carbohydrates and fats together can easily become weight gain. Adrenal and pancreas herbs should be taken at the same time as B vitamin-rich foods; their effects overlay the B effects and adjust adrenal and pancreatic performance as desired, yet with only maintenance (1X) therapeutic action. If taken separately (B first, herb second is better), the herb will produce stimulation (2X) where they overlap. This can be useful early in a good nutrition program, but not later.

B vitamins should not be taken with or soon after trace metals; their combined action is too strong and can create temporary adrenal hyperactivity and imbalances. Instead, take B's early in the day and save trace metals for the late afternoon or early evening.

Table 4-2 single and multiple therapeutic actions, descriptions and symbols accurately reflect what happens not only for B vitamins, fatty acids, trace metals and herbs, but also for every endocrine gland and function, not just those of the adrenal gland. The only exception is the pituitary gland (Chapter 8), where 2X is already a harmful overstimulation with respect to adrenal oversight. Again, 3X of anything with strong nutritional content is overdose. Caffeine is actually an herbal nutrient for the nervous system and can stimulate Energy/nerves and adrenaline flow – or at 3X (3 cups of coffee within $7^1/_2$ hours) every day, it will wreck your nerves!

The above use descriptions are meant as an outline and guide to possible effects in your body. If you are healthy and have a strong constitution, mostly likely you will only feel the immediate effects of 3X intake. The modest, positive 1X and 2X therapeutic actions of good nutrition only become apparent over time.

Rules, diagrams and complex interactions – it all sounds foreign and unnatural? Maybe at first when you're just beginning a healthy nutritional program, however, you have to jump in and learn to *swim* as you go. When nutritious, wholesome foods become habit and then integrated into lifestyle, you can forget all the rules and *go with the flow*. The closer you get to nature, the fewer the rules. A healthy nutritional program and lifestyle will give more years of life, and more life in those years.

B VITAMIN SUPPLEMENTATION

Good nutrition has consequences, and so does poor nutrition. An inadequate intake of nutrients accumulates a debt of dysfunctions and diseases, specifically adrenal exhaustions and imbalances in your Energy, Healing, Stress and Immune functions, which then cause chronic diseases of autoimmune (hyperactive Immune) and/or degenerative (hypoactive Healing) attack on dependent body systems, acute diseases and premature aging.

B vitamin supplements can: (1) fix adrenal exhaustions, (2) correct adrenal imbalances, and (3) overcome past B vitamin deprivation. Look again at Figure 4-A at the beginning of the chapter and the role that each known B vitamin plays in adrenal and pancreatic functioning. Employ these B's sparingly in a targeted effort to rebuild functional weak spots (nascent dysfunctions) or full-blown impairments.

Adrenal exhaustions and imbalances are permanent errors embedded in adrenal performance, either hypoactive or hyperactive functioning in Energy, Healing, Stress or Immune tasks. If you have no energy, if you can't handle the stress of life, or if fatigue is your daily companion, then these and other hypoactive exhaustions will make you old before your time, as will hyperactive-hypoactive imbalances within the medulla and cortex. Don't despair – your adrenal gland is amazingly resilient and lost or impaired functioning can be brought back to life and full health.

Hypoactive exhaustions can be mild (sub-par functioning) to severe (little or no functioning and output). Similarly, the hyperactive half of imbalances can be mild to severe. MILD exhaustions and imbalances need a steady diet of whole-grain cereals, nutritional yeasts and green vegetables – 2X usage at the start and later 1X – to restore function as much as possible and to *prime the pump* before targeted high-dose B vitamin supplement regimens, presented ahead in "Primary B Vitamins" and "Connecting B Vitamins," attempt to fix the embedded adrenal errors. In like manner, Chapter 6 trace metals taken naturally and followed by targeted metal supplementation provide strong nutrition to overcome mild dysfunctions. SEVERE exhaustions and imbalances require Chapter 12 remedies, which combine B vitamin and trace metal supplements in concerted action. Of course, all raw materials: macronutrients, B vitamins, fatty acids, trace metals and appropriate herbs contribute to the solution and must be liberally supplied.

CAUTION ☛ B vitamin supplementation has side effects, those diminishing returns as a result of loss of internal balance particularly in immune functioning, lack of nutritional variety, deprivation of unknown missing B's and continuous soft functioning effects. For best health, take at least five servings of natural B vitamin-rich foods before each adrenal exhaustion or imbalance cure given ahead. Trace metals and amino acids also form impossibly complex equilibriums and interactions, and their supplementation produces side effects too. On the other hand, Vitamin C and Vitamin E have no or simpler equilibrium interactions, and are scientifically proven to be needed in supplement form (higher amounts than found in food) for best health – and this can be accomplished with only positive effects, no negative side effects. These nutrients are examined in depth in upcoming chapters.

Commercially available multi-B vitamin supplements can be a temporary stopgap measure in two situations: (a) when age and past nutritional deprivation finally wear out adrenal performance, and (b) when trauma overwhelms you. Physiological trauma can take several forms. Stress trauma is the shock and ordeal of accident, death in the family, divorce, etc. Basically, upheaval in one's life becomes out-of-control extreme stress. Energy trauma is intense high-energy use or hyperactive nerves, emotions or mood swings, again personal upheaval, however, this time affecting the nervous system. Healing trauma overwhelms repair systems. Life-threatening burns or tissue damage, or sustained healing without result such as an aneurysm or harsh cosmetics reapplied daily soon exhaust all resources. Immune trauma is usually recurring hyperactivity; a pathogen strikes with ferocity, then hides and cannot be defeated by a weakened immune system. Raw material nutrient needs become extraordinary during traumas and, if not met quickly, can trigger severe adrenal exhaustions and imbalances, and dependent body system diseases such as arthritis, multiple sclerosis, lupus and fibromyalgia.

Commercial multi-B supplements bring palpable relief, renewing your energy and stress ability, but they must be a short-term fix because of diminishing returns. Nature's perfect long-term solution is REAL FOOD. Therefore, after the initial benefits of this *imperfect* B supplementation nutrition, transition s-l-o-w-l-y to whole-grain cereals, nutritional yeasts and green vegetables before diminishing returns leave you confused about B vitamin effectiveness and worse off than before you started the supplements. Buy only the best multi-B vitamin supplements at the health store – you get what you pay for! Alternate between two different formulations to prolong their effectiveness. Multi-B chelated-multi-metal supplements provide even stronger therapy in the breach (ala Chapter 12 remedies), but with even a shorter window of opportunity before side effects occur.

Primary B Vitamins

From Figure 4-A, the primary B vitamins are:

Energy Function	–	pantothenic acid (B5)	$C_9H_{17}NO_5$
Healing Function	–	PABA (para-aminobenzoic acid)	$C_7H_7NO_2$
Stress Function	–	B2 (riboflavin)	$C_{17}H_{20}N_4O_6$
Immune Function	–	**none discovered yet!**	–
Pancreas	–	B6 (pyridoxine)	$C_8H_{11}NO_3$

No known B vitamin nourishes Primary Immune Function and the immune system, a fact that further argues for lifetime use of nature's wholesome B vitamin-rich foods since all current supplements lack any direct immune B activity. This undiscovered B vitamin lies somewhere within nutritional yeasts. Connecting B vitamins folic acid and niacin only indirectly improve immune response.

Another important fact about primary B vitamins is that B2 (Primary Stress Function) and B6 (pancreas) must be in balance with each other, as indicated by the equilibrium arrows ($\rightleftharpoons$) in Figure 4-A. Taking B2 alone will injure your pancreas, bringing on pancreatitis or worse. B6 alone will injure your adrenal cortex and stress ability. Ingesting B2 and B6 together with no other B's present "revs" (1X) both cortex Stress and pancreas; however, it violates the normal Energy → Stress pathway and results in pituitary suppression. Pantothenic acid is also required with B2 and B6 for normal metabolism and functional flow! Table 4-3 reveals the delicate interaction of Energy, Stress and pancreas primary B's.

TABLE 4-3. PANTOTHENIC ACID, B2, B6 INTERACTIONS.

B Vitamin(s) taken	Resulting functioning of …			
	medulla Energy	cortex Stress	pancreas	pituitary
Pantothenic acid	↑			
B2		↑	↓	
B6		↓	↑	
1B2+1B6		↑	↑	↓
2Panto+1B2+1B6	↑	↑	↑	

Within the Table 4-3 framework, B2 and B6 can be adjusted to favor either Stress or pancreatic supplementation therapy. For instance, B6 can be reduced by one-half to spur B2 Stress revitalization while still protecting the pancreas from injury. After the desired result is obtained, adjust B2 and B6 again to achieve equal ($\rightleftharpoons$) functioning levels.

Mild Adrenal Exhaustion

Adrenal exhaustion is unresponsive nonfunctioning. Few or no adrenal hormones are produced regardless of raw material input. Mild to severe exhaustion can occur in any one of the four primary adrenal functions: Energy, Healing, Stress and Immune, or in any combination or within any subfunction. It often manifests in Energy and/or Stress after months to years of using more energy and coping with more stress than the adrenal gland can handle with the nutrition provided.

Constant tiredness and little or no energy are obviously Energy exhaustion. Other symptoms can include dizziness, lightheadedness, feeling of impending fainting and headaches that feel like concussion, especially when the head is shaken. Stress exhaustion is being easily worn out or fatigued, basically falling apart under stress. Frequent headaches and arthritis indicate a defeated Primary Stress Function. Table 4-3 suggests two therapies: (1) pantothenic acid alone to improve Energy exhaustion, and (2) the formula 2 pantothenic acid + 1B2 +1B6 for Energy-Stress exhaustion. For these regimens, purchase each B vitamin separately – and again, use the best brands from the health store.

A good starting point for Energy-Stress exhaustion is 100 mg of pantothenic acid and 50 mg each of B2 and B6, but remember adrenal functioning may be "soft" for the next 24 hours. Surprisingly, soft functioning is less of a problem with pantothenic acid alone than with any other B vitamin, particularly if the need is great. 100 mg (no more) of pantothenic acid can be taken each morning for months to try to restore Energy function and metabolism. This is the one and only exception to the five-to-one rule of natural B-food servings to supplementation, but there must be need or medulla imbalance develops. With need, disruption to adrenal equilibrium ($\rightleftharpoons$) is minimal since exhaustion has already created the imbalance, and the Table 4-3 regimens are attempts at correction. Use these therapies in conjunction with fatty acids, trace metals and appropriate herbs, as well as natural-B whole-grain cereals, nutritional yeasts and green vegetables – a complete nutritional approach and solution.

All the above recommendations won't do the job if the nutritional deficit has developed over many years. In that case, B vitamin amounts must be increased, possibly up to 2500 mg of pantothenic acid with corresponding higher B2 and B6 and softer functioning. Beyond 2500 mg pantothenic acid, benefits turn negative as such large doses quickly deplete unknown B factors found in only whole-grain cereals, nutritional yeasts and green vegetables, producing unpleasant and scary side effects including puffiness to rapid enlargement of facial parts and other surface tissues randomly. Cortisone therapy also causes such symptoms. Needless to say, employ these large doses infrequently, at least one week apart and preferably two weeks apart, with plenty of Table 2-1 complete nutrition in between to correct newly created imbalances and shortages. Trace metal supplements, taken separately, will also help overcome past deprivations. See Figure 6-A and follow Chapter 6 supplementation guidelines. If Energy or Energy-Stress exhaustion does not get better with two regimens of 2500 mg pantothenic acid plus B2 and B6 for Stress exhaustion and separate metal supplementations, then you have a severe adrenal exhaustion, which requires Chapter 12 solution.

PANTOTHENIC ACID

With less than twenty key articles, the medical literature of pantothenic acid (B5) is a work in progress, emerging and developing. Still, pantothenic acid's role in energy metabolism and the central nervous system is revealed.

Review of the Medical Literature

Energy... Pantothenic acid is involved in muscle cell energy metabolism.[34] Pantothenic acid deficiency impairs energy processes,[35] resulting in generalized malaise. Pantothenic acid is necessary for synthesis of CoA [Coenzyme A: involved in many metabolic pathways including ester oxidation], yet surprisingly tissue CoA levels are unaffected when the vitamin is deficient.[36] High doses of pantothenic acid generate statistically significant increases in glucocorticoid production.[37] Author's Note: The CoA metabolic pathway of ester oxidation is basically fat burning by cells, and fat burning defines stress (Chapter 3). Figure 2-B physiology offers an explanation: high-dose pantothenic acid stimulates adrenal medulla energy (adrenaline), and in turn medulla energy stimulates (→ via CoA) adrenal cortex stress (glucocorticoids including cortisol).

Nerves... Decreased availability or utilization of pantothenic acid causes central nervous system damage with ataxia [loss of muscle coordination, especially in extremities]. Other vitamin cofactors here are biotin and Vitamin E.[38]

Immune... Pantothenic acid deficiency reduces antibody response to antigens [any invader eliciting an antibody response].[39, 40] Conversely, 300-600 mg pantothenic acid daily produces immunomodulatory action, increasing immunoglobulins [antibody proteins that fight infection] and peripheral neutrophil [strong against bacteria] phagocytes [white blood cells that engulf/devour microorganisms and cell fragments] in Hepatitis A patients.[41] Note: Figure 12-A(1) shows that NO Energy = NO Immune, and provides a physiological explanation for these effects.

Healing... Pantothenic acid stimulates migration, proliferation and protein synthesis of human skin fibroblasts [cells giving rise to connective tissue; -blast: immature, undergoing development] into wounds.[42, 43] Topical use of pantothenic acid for epidermal wounds reduces erythema [abnormal redness, inflammation of the skin], and provides more elastic and solid tissue regeneration. As adjuvant skin care, pantothenic acid improves skin dryness, roughness, scaling, erythema, pruritus [itching], erosion and fissures.[44] Note: Healing is a complex process; Figure 4-C ahead reveals that pantothenic acid, PABA and B1 are all needed to create the proper conditions for healing.

Finally, pantothenic acid may be of benefit in treating acne,[45] as a cardiac protector,[46] and in weight loss, enabling fasting without hunger, weakness and ketosis [excessive ketones from excessive fat burning].[47]

VITAMIN B2 (Riboflavin)

Red blood cells power Primary Stress Function, just as white blood cells power Immune. Vitamin B2 protects red blood cells from oxidation by keeping their natural internal antioxidant, glutathione, recycled and working. This reduces oxidative stress in the blood and throughout the body. Review "Breakdown and Repair" in Chapter 2, which describes the general antioxidant anti-stress link.

> ## Review of the Medical Literature

Fundamental role... Vitamin B2 (riboflavin) is a cofactor in glutathione reductase [reductase: an enzyme that acts as reducing agent, -ase: suffix meaning 'enzyme'], keeping endogenous [arising from within the organism] glutathione in a reduced [non-oxidized] state.[48] Glutathione is a major internal antioxidant [within cell mitochondria, the main defense against free radicals].[49] Therefore, B2 can be considered an indirect antioxidant vitamin.[48] B2 is crucial to erythrocyte [red blood cell] glutathione reductase (EGR) activity. Both basal and stimulated EGR are significantly elevated in rheumatoid arthritis patients. B2 deficiency is associated with increased arthritic activity, suggesting that impaired EGR facilitates continuing inflammation.[50] In fact, B2 can mount significant protection against oxidant-mediated inflammatory injury,[51] whereas deficiency produces oxidative stress within tissues.[52] Exercise [more stress] increases B2 requirements,[53] as does age to some extent.[54] Author's Note: B2's role in rheumatoid arthritis, inflammation and oxidative stress can be explained using Figure 2-B, with B2 as the Stress vitamin.

Migraine... 400 mg of Vitamin B2 is superior to placebo in migraine prevention, reducing the frequency of attack and number of headache days.[55]

Iron metabolism... Vitamin B2 has a special relationship with iron,[56] and red blood cells. B2 enhances hematological response to iron, while deficiency may be factor in anemia.[57]

Chronic B2 deficiency... causes skin and mucous membrane lesions including glossitis [inflammation of the tongue],[58] and esophageal cancer.[59]

VITAMIN B6 (Pyridoxine)

B6, the primary pancreas B vitamin, is multi-faceted in character, interlinking pancreas, glucose metabolism, amino acid metabolism and nervous system neurotransmitters in complex ways.

Review of the Medical Literature

Glucose metabolism... Although Vitamin B6 (pyridoxine) plays an important role in amino acid metabolism, most of the body's B6 is found in muscles, associated with glycogen phosphorylase [catalyzes stored glycogen back to glucose for cell use] glucose metabolism.[60] Here B6 is involved in gluconeogenesis [new glucose from sources other than current digestion] as the coenzyme pyridoxal phosphate. B6 deficiency impairs muscle gluconeogenesis, resulting in abnormal glucose tolerance.[61] While B6 does not directly affect oral glucose tolerance and insulin response to glucose [as biotin does],[62, 63] the vitamin can improve oral glucose tolerance through amino acid metabolism. By restoring tryptophan [essential amino acid] metabolism, B6 normalizes internal xanthine (xanthurenic acid) [initial step in the protein excretion pathway; a very harmful substance, which can damage the pancreas, inducing pancreatitis and diabetes], thereby improving oral glucose tolerance in women with gestational diabetes,[64] and those using oral contraceptives.[65]

Diabetic retinopathy... Diabetics treated with Vitamin B6 over periods of eight months to twenty-eight years developed no diabetic retinopathy [degenerative eye disease]. This action appears to be monumental, and the basis for a new treatment protocol.[66] B6 derivative pyridoxamine inhibits formation of advanced glycation and lipoxidized end products, thus protecting the diabetic retina against pathological changes.[67]

Homocysteine... Hyperhomocysteinemia [high levels of homocysteine in the blood] can develop from deficiencies in Vitamin B6, folic acid or Vitamin B12. Present in about 5% of the general population, hyperhomocysteinemia significantly increases the risk for both arterial and venous thromboembolic [blood vessel blockage] disease.[68] B6 is a cofactor in mediating homocysteine [a sulfur-containing amino acid formed from the essential amino acid methionine] transformation to cystathionine, the initial step in urinary excretion of sulfur. B6 deficiency leads to elevated homocysteine, which is atherogenic [depositing plaque on artery walls],[69-71] and associated with cardiovascular disease,[60, 69-73] including heart attack and stroke.[71, 72] Homocysteine increases the risk of coronary heart disease in most studies, although recent results are less consistent.[74-76] Folic acid and B12 are cofactors in homocysteine metabolism,[77, 78] and other disturbances in sulfur amino acid metabolism such as inherited enzyme abnormalities can cause homocysteine accumulation.[68, 79] In addition, kidney impairment raises homocysteine levels,[68] as does insulin resistance.[80]

Pregnancy and infants, B2 ⇌ B6... Nausea affects 70 to 85% of women during early pregnancy. Vitamin B6 is effective in reducing the severity of this nausea.[81] Prenatal exposure to glucocorticoids [maternal use of cortisone, prednisone or other steroids] adversely affects fetal growth and may increase the offspring's risk of insulin resistance, hypertension [high blood pressure] and cardiovascular events throughout life.[82] B6 counteracts steroidal hormone activity,[60] a safe physiological antagonist of glucocortiocoids.[82] Author's Note: B6 antagonism to glucocorticoids (natural and unnatural adrenal cortex stress hormones) is stating B2 ⇌ B6 physiology at another level. One more B2-B6 tie-in... B6 is a cofactor in the biosynthesis of cysteine [an amino acid], the rate limiting precursor to glutathione [see B2 above].[49]

Fetal and infant nervous system... Vitamin B6 is a coenzyme in the synthesis of neurotransmitters GABA [gamma-aminobutyric acid: inhibitory neurotransmitter, helps prevent system overload], dopamine [movement and emotion] and serotonin [especially important in the brain; made from the amino acid tryptophan]. B6 is essential for normal perinatal [after the 20th week of gestation] central nervous system development.[83, 84] B6/pyridoxine-dependent seizures (PDS) in infants are due to impaired GABA metabolism.[85] PDS is an uncommon heredity disease with a variable clinical picture; prognosis is favorable with early diagnosis.[86] Typically seizures develop with illness but otherwise are controllable using pharmacologic doses of B6.[87]

Adult nervous system... Vitamin B6 has significant modulatory effect on GABA and serotonin production. These neurotransmitters influence pain perception, depression and anxiety.[84] In animal study, a diet totally lacking in B6 produces peripheral neuropathy [injury to the sensation nerves of arms and legs].[88]

Immune... Vitamin B6 deficiency causes atrophy in lymphoid organs, resulting in lower lymphocyte numbers and impaired antibody responses and IL-2 production [Interleukin 2: hormone-like substance released by T-lymphocytes; stimulates more T-cell production and other immune defenses].[89, 90] Epidemiological studies show an inverse relationship between B6 intake and colon cancer risk. Recent animal study suggests that B6 suppresses colon tumorigenesis by reducing cell proliferation, angiogenesis [new capillary blood vessels], NO [nitric oxide: released during macrophage inflammation], and oxidative stress.[91]

Carpal tunnel syndrome... Vitamin B6 deficiency induces carpal tunnel syndrome [ligament inflammation in the wrist disturbs median nerve function].[66, 92] B6 and Vitamin C together are most important in treatment of symptoms.[93]

Antihypertensive... Vitamin B6 supplementation lowers blood pressure in many animal hypertension models. Preliminary evidence suggests the same antihypertensive action in humans.[94]

Anemia... Vitamin B6 is involved in hemoglobin synthesis.[34] B6 is effective treatment for sideroblastic anemia [bone marrow produces abnormal red blood cells containing an internal ring of iron granules].[57]

Dialysis... For patients with chronic renal insufficiency and on maintenance dialysis, B6 supplementation remains unresolved, however, the most recent papers evidence benefit.[95-99]

Heal Thyself

Healing B vitamins, fatty acids, trace metals and herbs maintain or rebuild youthful vigor in repair and antioxidation systems, thereby slowing aging. These natural healers counter today's high energy and high stress lifestyles, and so help to preserve internal balance. Obtaining PABA from wholesome foods is essential.

PABA (Para-aminobenzoic acid)

PABA supplementation becomes necessary when the body has a significant healing task before it. The making of new tissue is controlled by cell DNA, which unzips its double helix permitting exact copies. PABA stimulates and improves DNA healing both inside and outside (skin). Use PABA cautiously – it is jet fuel for healing action! 100 mg daily is usually sufficient to this end, however, higher amounts, up to 500 mg, may be required for severe burns and other healing traumas. 100 mg of PABA does not cause soft functioning, although larger doses can negatively impact stress ability. Of course, stress should be avoided during any major body repair. An adrenal cortex at rest benefits all aspects of healing.

Increasing amounts of PABA require increasing amounts of healing conutrients before and with its supplementation. When repair needs are great, use PABA in combination with Chapter 3 protein and sulfur macronutrients, Chapter 4 whole-grain cereals except oats and their *gooey* polysaccharides, Chapter 5 essential fatty acids (EFAs) plus Vitamin E and beta-carotene, Chapter 6 sources of "trace metals naturally" and the healing metal zinc, and Chapter 7 herbs Aloe vera and specific healers. A cautionary note, too much healing proves counterproductive – too much is as bad as too little. The correct solution, while different in every case, is always just the right amount of healing.

PABA supplementation has the unique ability to dampen nervous system hyperactivity without affecting adrenaline and energy. PABA can ease caffeine nerves, substance addictions (all addictions lie in the nervous system), hives, hyperactive mood including anxiety, and serious nerve diseases such as multiple sclerosis (MS) and amyotrophic lateral sclerosis (Lou Gehrig's disease).

Combining PABA with Vitamin B1 forms one-half of the Healing-Energy equilibrium mechanism (see Figure 4-C ahead) and moves Healing ⇌ Energy toward even more healing, but with less adrenaline and energy.

PABA research is in its infancy, most still in bacteria and animal studies where medical research usually begins. Russian scientists initiated PABA studies and interest, and author many of the articles.

> ### Review of the Medical Literature

Healing... PABA participates in DNA repair controlled by recA+ recF+ alleles [two alleles for each gene trait] in Escherichia coli [E. coli].[100] PABA reduces mutations by modulating the error-prone DNA repair SOS response [SOS system: DNA molecules are repaired by incorporating a base error that permits correct replication],[101] thereby significantly improving repair effectiveness,[102] and recovery of genome integrity.[103] These bacteria model studies will strongly influence the still fledgling field of mammalian DNA repair.[104] For animal nerve regeneration, PABA acts on neural scar connective tissue, inducing growth and accelerating maturation of axons [transmit nerve impulses; each nerve cell has one axon that can be over a foot long; large axons are surrounded by myelin sheath] from the central to peripheral stump of the injured nerve.[105]

Antioxidant... In animal studies, PABA maintains catalase [enzyme that eliminates the free radical hydrogen peroxide] and prevents lipid peroxidation [lipids: fats and fat-related compounds] in the eye retina.[106] PABA shows anticoagulant and anti-thrombotic [thrombosis: blood clot] activity.[107] PABA may reduce DDP [leukemia cancer drug] toxic side effects including nephrotoxicity [nephro- 'kidney'] without compromising DDP's antitumor effect.[108] To date in humans, PABA is used as a sunscreen ingredient for ultraviolet light (UV) protection against photocarcinogenesis, but again supporting research is animal based.[109-114]

Immune... PABA is an immunomodulator, and induces endogenous [arising from within the organism] interferon [family of hormone-like glycoproteins that fight virus infection/multiplication].[115] PABA demonstrates efficacy in all eye diseases involving interferon dysfunctions.[116]

Connecting B Vitamins

Having examined the primary B vitamins and their direct roles in adrenal functioning, let's now turn to the connecting B vitamins. Figure 4-A shows four function-connecting B's:

Healing $\rightleftharpoons$ Energy Functions   –   B1 (thiamin) $C_{12}H_{17}ClN_4OS$

Immune $\rightleftharpoons$ Stress Functions   –   folic acid $C_{19}H_{19}N_7O_6$

Energy $\rightarrow$ Stress Functions   –   biotin $C_{10}H_{16}O_3N_2S$

Healing $\rightarrow$ Immune Functions   –   niacin (B3) $C_6H_5NO_2$

VITAMIN B1 (Thiamin)

Vitamin B1 aids, connects and facilitates Healing $\rightleftharpoons$ Energy equilibrium and the metabolic pathway between them. B1 is responsible for the healthy back-and-forth dynamic between primary medulla functions. Deficiency can develop with these possible symptoms:

- labored breathing,
- nerve damage,
- sensitivity to pain,
- loss of mental alertness,
- mood problems including depression,
- impaired carbohydrate digestion,
- sleeplessness,
- heart irregularities and cardiac damage.

Whole-grains cereals, nutritional yeasts, sunflower seeds, soybeans, milk, eggs, and organ meats such as liver are rich sources of Vitamin B1. Wheat germ is a quick, natural B1 deficiency fix. This vitamin is especially vulnerable to being washed away in water and destruction during cooking.

A 100 mg B1 supplementation strengthens Healing $\rightleftharpoons$ Energy equilibrium and corrects deficiency symptoms. Labored breathing is often the first sign of trouble. Labored breathing and the other symptoms listed above can also develop from raw material imbalances between pantothenic acid, PABA and B1, and medulla nutrition in general.

B1 buffers the effect of PABA and these two can be taken together in one-to-one ratio, 1 PABA : 1 B1. As such, PABA and B1 then form one-half of the equilibrium mechanism of Healing $\rightleftharpoons$ Energy. The other half of this equilibrium is pantothenic acid alone, with exact equilibrium diagramed in Figure 4-C.

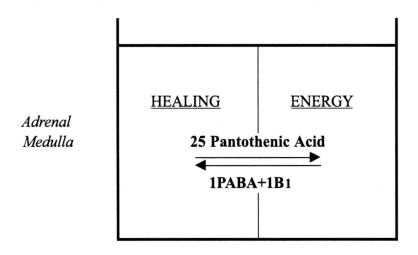

Adrenal
Medulla

FIGURE 4-C. ADRENAL MEDULLA B VITAMIN EQUILIBRIUM.

Pantothenic acid alone pushes medulla equilibrium toward Energy. Ratios of less than 25 pantothenic acid to 1 PABA + 1 B1 push the balance toward Healing. Imposing exact equilibrium (25:1:1) can help correct medulla imbalance and cure mild Energy and Healing Function exhaustion. A good supplementation starting point is 1250 mg pantothenic acid and 50 mg each of PABA and B1. As discussed earlier, 2500 mg pantothenic acid is maximum dosage with these considerations: soft functioning, limited use (two tries only, one to two weeks apart), and plenty of whole-grain cereals before, in between and after such therapy.

The medical literature of Vitamin B1 is large in comparison to that of pantothenic acid, B2, B6 and PABA. It deals mainly with B1 nerve diseases Wernicke-Korsakoff syndrome and beriberi.

Review of the Medical Literature

Nerves... In Western societies, Vitamin B1 (thiamine) deficiency usually manifests as Wernicke-Korsakoff syndrome (WKS). Commonly seen in alcoholic patients, but also in those with impaired nutrition from other causes, WKS pathology is characterized by central nervous system neuron loss, gliosis [dense, fibrous, growing, irregular support structure surrounding neurons near a degenerative lesion] and vascular damage surrounding heart ventricles and the cerebral aqueduct. B1 deficiency also causes beriberi [below], a cardiac and peripheral nerve disease.[117] B1 treatment is effective in the early stages of WKS and beriberi, but delay often results in permanent damage.[118]

B1 and the brain... Acute cerebral effects of Wernicke-Korsakoff syndrome (WKS) are Wernicke encephalopathy (WE) [encephalopathy: brain disease], which in most cases progresses to chronic Korsakoff syndrome.[119] WE diagnosis involves the triad of confusion, ataxia [loss of muscle coordination, especially in extremities], and ophthalmoplegia [paralysis of eye muscles].[120] Korsakoff syndrome is disproportionate memory impairment relative to other cognitive functions.[121] B1 deficiency causes neurotoxicity, which affects neurons, astrocytes [large star-shaped neuroglial cells in the brain and spinal cord; neuroglia: supporting, insulating cells surrounding neurons], microglia [removes waste from nerve tissue], and brain endothelial [lining] cells.[122] Oxidative stress exacerbates WKS brain lesions.[122-124] Chronic alcohol consumption produces B1 deficiency, WKS and other brain abnormalities.[125-127] Other causes of B1 WKS are gastrointestinal disease, AIDS,[108] and as a rare complication of kidney dialysis.[128] Recently, B1 deficiency has also been associated with pAD [probable Alzheimer's Disease].[129]

B1 and the heart... In the latter half of the 19th century, beriberi developed in large numbers of Dutch East Indies personnel. Eventually, this mysterious paralysis was associated with diet. Beriberi coincided with eating polished [refined] white rice, and could be prevented with unpolished whole-grain rice.[130] In its late stages, beriberi presents cardiac shock and acute heart failure. Chest x-rays show heart enlargement and pulmonary edema [abnormal accumulation of fluid, swelling]. Intravenous Vitamin B1 infusion can bring rapid clinical improvement.[131] So-called 'wet beriberi' is cardiac failure, while 'dry beriberi' involves peripheral polyneuropathy [injury to the sensation nerves of arms and legs].[132] Another B1-heart association, B1 deficiency may be factor in congestive heart failure [ineffective pumping of the heart causes fluid to accumulate in the lungs].[133]

Energy and mood... Vitamin B1 is essential for normal glucose metabolism.[134] While deficiency deranges glucose metabolism,[135] and can cause lactic acidosis [acidosis: acid blood, low pH], [134, 136] excess B1 has no effect.[135] In four double-blind studies, B1 improves mood.[137]

Side effect... In rare cases, high-dose injections of Vitamin B1 can cause anaphylaxis [allergic shock].[130, 139]

FOLIC ACID

Folic acid aids, connects and facilitates Immune ⇌ Stress equilibrium, and the back and forth *tango* between this cortex couple as they respond to the worst of life's difficulties. Folic acid plays the *music* for them just as B1 plays the *music* for Energy and Healing. Folic acid is the known B vitamin of green vegetables. Therefore, eat lots of greens (once again, mother was right) and get folic acid plus many related, undiscovered B factors in nature's perfect balance so Stress and Immune don't miss a *beat*, and forget about folic acid supplementation. Besides the Food and Drug Administration (FDA) limits folic acid in supplements to low levels. One extra-safety exception is supplementation during pregnancy, as explained in the literature review below.

Folic acid is well reported in the medical literature. It shares responsibility with Vitamin B6 and Vitamin B12 in two important tasks: red blood cell development and homocysteine control.

Review of the Medical Literature

Anemia and pregnancy... Folic acid (folate) is necessary for red blood cell development,[34] playing a crucial role in nucleic acid [DNA, RNA] synthesis. Folic acid depletion causes megaloblastic [large, immature, dysfunctional red blood cells] anemia by preventing normal proliferation of rapidly dividing bone marrow cells.[140-142] With pregnancy, consequences can very serious, including open neural tube defects,[143, 144] retarded fetal growth, preterm delivery and low birth weight. In addition, folic acid deficiency elevates plasma homocysteine; and high maternal homocysteine is linked to spontaneous abortion, placental abruption, preeclampsia [toxemia in late pregnancy, which can progress to eclampsia (convulsions and coma)], poor pregnancy outcome, and reduced gestational duration and birth weight.[145] Folic acid supplementation prevents 70% of neural tube defects,[146] and 50% of spina bifida.[147] A caution, vitamin profile blood tests do not identify women at risk for neural tube defects, therefore folic acid supplementation is the only certain course.[148] Deficiency during pregnancy can also cause hereditary and acquired disorders in offspring.[149] Note: See also iron deficiency anemia during pregnancy in Chapter 6.

Pregnancy drug cautions... Folic acid deficiency can develop during pregnancy with use of such common drugs as triamterene [mild diuretic], trimethoprim [often taken with sulphonamides], phenobarbital [sedative, also for convulsions], carbamazepine [convulsions, epilepsy, mania], phenytoin [epilepsy, seizure disorders], and primidone [convulsions, seizures]. Primidone may risk not only neural tube defects, but also oral cleft and cardiovascular and urinary tract defects.[150] Folic acid deficiency is common in oral contraceptive users.[151]

General cautions... Folic acid deficiency frequently develops in smokers, alcoholics and the elderly.[151] Folic acid supplementation can mask a serious Vitamin B12 deficiency.[152, 153]

Folic acid and adults... Folic acid deficiency causes DNA aberrations, resulting in spinal cord syndromes (similar to those of Vitamin B12 deficiency),[140] cognitive defects particularly with memory functioning late in life,[154] and mood disturbances,[140] including both phases of bipolar disorder, depression and mania.[155, 156] Folic acid deficiency is most tightly associated with depressive disorders, B12 deficiency with psychosis.[157] The neurotoxic effects of homocysteine also are a factor here.[79, 158] Recent studies implicate folic acid deficiency and resulting elevated plasma homocysteine in neurodegenerative disorders such as Alzheimer's disease.[159]

Homocysteine... Homocysteine raises both venous and arterial thrombosis [blood clot formation] risk, and even moderate increases are associated with deep venous thrombosis, myocardial infarction [heart attack], cerebral infarction [stroke] and peripheral vascular disease.[160] Folic acid alone, or in combination with Vitamins B6 and B12, reduces plasma homocysteine.[161] Folic acid is the key element of treatment, with daily doses of at least 0.4 mg effectively lowering homocysteine levels, even in non-folic-acid-deficient individuals. B6 and/or B12 can decrease homocysteine further in certain groups of patients.[68] Folic acid supplementation may be warranted for dialysis patients to control homocysteine,[162] although predated B6 dialysis studies are not homocysteine linked.[95-99]

Immune and white blood cells... Folic acid deficiency disrupts tissue barriers to infection, depresses cell-mediated immunity [T-lymphocyte system], inhibits humoral immunity antibody formation [secreted by B-lymphocytes circulating in the blood], impairs phagocytosis [white blood cell ingestion of bacteria, etc.],[39] and promotes carcinogenesis as evidenced in uterine cervix, lung, esophageal, stomach and most compellingly colorectal cancers.[163, 164] Carcinogenic mechanisms involve disrupted DNA integrity and repair, as well as altered DNA methylation, which changes the expression of critical tumor suppressor genes and proto-oncogenes [normal cell genes go 'onco,' that is, mutate into a tumor cell].[165, 166]

Eyes and hearing... Folic acid may be a factor in progressive bilateral optic nerve disease,[167] and age-related hearing problems.[168]

BIOTIN

Biotin connects medulla Energy to ($\rightarrow$) cortex Stress directly, and also through an intermediate step: Energy $\rightarrow$ endocrine pancreas $\rightarrow$ Stress. Unlike Healing $\rightarrow$ Immune action, Energy → Stress has an extra supporting gland in its metabolic pathway. Biotin, a coenzyme, assists in carbohydrate (glucose) and fat (ester) utilization.

There's plenty of biotin in whole grain cereals, no need for supplementation. The exception is diabetes. Then biotin stimulates insulin-producing beta islets and improves glycemic control, as reported in the following literature review. Daily biotin use requires balancing with occasional niacin supplementation (Figure 4-A).

Review of the Medical Literature

Glucose metabolism... Biotin deficiency impairs oral glucose tolerance.[134] Glucokinase (GK) [kinase: phophorylation, or an enzyme transfers a phosphate group] regulates glucose metabolism in pancreatic beta islet [insulin-producing] cells and hepatocytes [liver cells]. In response to elevated blood glucose, normal insulin secretion, postprandial [after a meal] hepatic glucose uptake, and temporary suppression of hepatic glucose output and gluconeogenesis all require GK action. In Type II [adult onset] diabetic patients, GK activity is subnormal in hepatocytes and may be reduced in beta islet cells. Biotin supplementation increases GK activity in beta islet cells and promotes GK gene transcription and translation in hepatocytes, while suppressing transcription of the rate-limiting enzyme for gluconeogenesis. In animal diabetic models, high-dose biotin improves glycemic control. Oral biotin supplement 3 mg t.i.d. [3 times per day, at each meal] significantly reduces fasting blood glucose in Type II diabetics, without side effects. Biotin should also improve Type I [juvenile diabetes] glycemic control.[169]

Ester metabolism... Biotin deficiency causes fatty acid abnormalities;[170] specifically biotin-dependent carboxylase [catalyzing enzyme] shortages disorder fatty acid synthesis, gluconeogenesis and amino acid catabolism, thereby contributing to disease pathogenesis. Of special importance, biotin deficiency reduces acetyl CoA carboxylase [Coenzyme A, see pantothenic acid earlier].[171-173]

Other effects... Biotin deficiency can cause lethargy, orificial [mouth and other openings] lesions, hypotonia [diminished resistance of muscles to passive stretching], alopecia [loss of hair],[174, 175] thymus [source of immune T-cells] injury,[176] and at its worst central nervous system damage with ataxia [loss of muscle coordination, especially in extremities].[38] Biotin status is impaired in both early and late pregnancy,[177] with significant but indirect evidence suggesting that this marginal biotin deficit can be teratogenic [causing birth defects].[178] Ingesting raw egg white will cause biotin deficiency.[179]

NIACIN (B3)

Niacin opens arteries and capillaries and is a natural part of the inflammation mechanism, common to both Healing and Immune responses. You can feel this opening of blood vessels or "flush" in the face, arms and legs if you ingest 100 mg or more of niacin. The warming of the skin is very pronounced. Never take more than 200 mg of niacin. Many B vitamin foods richly supply this vitamin, particularly nutritional yeasts, so there is no need to supplement it. Niacinamide, a non-flush niacin supplement, while permitting larger doses, defeats the Healing-Immune purpose of this vitamin.

Niacin deficiency causes the disease pellagra, and niacin's medical literature is largely concentrated there.

Review of the Medical Literature

Pellagra... first described in Spain in 1730,[180] is characterized by four classic symptoms usually referred to as the four Ds: dermatitis, diarrhea, dementia and death. Other nonspecific symptoms can manifest in dermatological, gastrointestinal and neuropsychiatric systems. Erythema [abnormal redness, inflammation of the skin] on sun-exposed areas is frequently reported. Neurologic deficits or unexplained confusional states may be pellagra dementia encephalopathy [brain disease]. Most pellagrins respond to niacin supplementation and a high-protein diet. Pellagra occurs with chronic alcoholism, malnutrition including anorexia nervosa, and amino acid imbalance.[181-183] Crohn's disease [an inflammatory bowel disease: thickening of the intestinal wall, frequent obstruction] and esophagitis often accompany pellagra.[184-186] Among tuberculosis patients on isoniazid [TB drug], pellagra encephalopathy can develop rapidly, followed by death in one to three months. The reason, isoniazid inhibits tryptophan [essential amino acid] conversion to niacin.[187] The tryptophan-niacin pathway is also impaired in alcoholic pellagra patients.[188] Niacin is easily synthesized from tryptophan, and with tryptophan normally present in abundance, this pathway is crucial to healthy niacin metabolism.[189]

Healing → Immune... Niacin and Vitamin E improve healing in burn patients, including better graft attachment.[190] Niacin deficiency disrupts tissue barriers to infection, inhibits humoral antibody formation [from B-lymphocytes circulating in the blood],[40] and decreases NAD [nicotinamide adenine dinucleotide, a coenzyme], which may increase carcinogenesis.[191] Niacin may be a secondary AIDS preventive in HIV patients.[192]

Inflammatory response and prostaglandins… Niacin causes flushing [capillaries open, with noticeable reddening and warming of the skin], apparently by stimulating prostaglandin (PG)E1 [prostaglandins: potent mediators of many conduction/transmitter functions regulating cellular activities, particularly inflammatory response]. In schizophrenics, larger niacin doses are required to produce flushing than in normal individuals, and this may be a simple biochemical test for a major schizophrenia group.[193] Niacin's role in prostaglandins and separately prostaglandins' role in schizophrenia are well confirmed.[194, 195] Note: Prostaglandins are studied in depth in Chapter 5.

Cardiovascular, blood profile… Niacin reduces blood triglycerides, low-density lipoprotein (LDL) cholesterol [so-called bad cholesterol], lipoprotein(a) [another bad lipoprotein], and apoprotein B [protein derivative], and strongly increases high-density lipoprotein (HDL) cholesterol [so-called good cholesterol]. Niacin is currently the most potent HDL agent available. These effects decrease cardiovascular disease risk. However, niacin cardiovascular therapy is problematic, requiring multidose regimens, which cause flushing [described above] and pruritus [itching] side effects.[196-198]

Secondary B Vitamin

VITAMIN B15 (Pangamic Acid, $C_4H_9NO_2$)

Healing function has a secondary B vitamin, which provides minor supportive nutrition. B15 facilitates oxygen going to cells (cellular respiration), and not cells going to oxidation (injury or death). Originally isolated from apricot kernels, B15 is sufficiently supplied by whole-grain cereals, rice especially. No need for supplementation. Vitamin B15 is a minor antioxidant and interest has waned with only one published article in the medical literature since the early 1990s. The existence of B15 hints that many more subtle B vitamins remain hidden in food.

Review of the Medical Literature

Antioxidant… Vitamin B15 (pangamic acid) reduces damage to subcellular hepatocyte [liver cell] structures; however, its combination with other nutrients is more conducive to intracellular repair and regeneration.[199] B15 lowers liver cholesterol levels,[200] and inhibits copper-dependent LDL [low-density lipoprotein, so-called bad cholesterol] oxidation [making LDL worse, more likely to deposit on artery walls].[201] At high concentrations, B15 increases cell oxygen uptake,[202] but does not significantly affect the short-term maximal treadmill performance of athletes.[203]

LAETRILE (amygdalin)

Besides Vitamin B15, apricot kernels also contain amygdalin. Sometimes called Vitamin B17, amygdalin is a bitter-tasting cyanogenic glycoside popularly referred to as Laetrile and touted as a cancer cure in the 1970s. Supporting evidence, if any, remains unpublished. The medical literature finds no benefit and possible severe cyanide toxicity. Apricot kernels themselves can be toxic, however, one per day is safe.

Laetrile generated tremendous *heat and smoke* in the late 1970s and early 1980s, but in the end no efficacy *fire*. It all started with a theory.

Review of the Medical Literature

Theory… In the 1920s, Dr. Ernst T. Krebs, Sr. theorized that amygdalin (Laetrile) could kill cancer cells. The theory proved inconsistent with biochemical facts and was modified at least twice by his son, Ernst T. Krebs, Jr. Animal studies in the 1970s failed to show any tumor killing action by Laetrile. Review of medical records of patients who claimed that Laetrile reduced or cured their cancers showed insufficient evidence to judge efficacy. In a 1982 clinical trial [below] with cancer patient volunteers, Laetrile did not shrink tumors, alleviate cancer symptoms, increase survival time, or enhance well-being. On the contrary, several reports in medical literature document serious, life-threatening Laetrile toxicity. Considering the complete lack of efficacy and demonstrated ability to harm, Laetrile should not be part of any cancer treatment.[204]

Clinical trial… One hundred seventy-eight cancer patients were treated with amygdalin (Laetrile) plus a metabolic program of diet, vitamins and enzymes. Most subjects were in good general condition before treatment, and one third had not received previous drug chemotherapy. The pharmaceutical amygdalin preparations, dosages and schedule were in agreement with standard Laetrile practice. No substantive benefit was observed in terms of cancer improvement or stabilization, symptom improvement, cure or life span extension. Several patients evidenced symptoms of cyanide toxicity or had blood cyanide levels approaching lethal range.[205]

Cyanide toxicity (not part of the clinical trial)… One emergency room Laetrile user, after recovery from coma, presented signs of Parkinson's syndrome, brainstem neuritis [nerve inflammation with pain, tenderness, paralysis] and sensory motor neuropathy [nerve disease].[206] Another patient developed neuromyopathy [myo- 'muscle'].[207] Laetrile at 1/2 gram three times per day produced significant blood cyanide concentrations.[208] Deep coma, hypotension [low blood pressure], acidosis [acid blood, low pH] and death occurred in one patient after ingestion of 3 grams of Laetrile.[209] Two studies showed that amygdalin/Laetrile kills normal and cancer cells at the same rate.[210, 211]

Vitamin B12, Choline and Inositol

Vitamin B12 is living under an assumed name, its chemical composition unlike any other B vitamin: $C_{63}H_{88}N_{14}O_{14}PCo$. In reality, B12 is a cobalt (Co) trace metal complex and will be discussed in Chapter 6. A preview look: B12 aids, connects and facilitates adrenal medulla Primary Energy Function, adrenal cortex Primary Stress Function and the endocrine pancreas in their common tasks.

Two additional genuine B vitamins are choline and inositol. Found abundantly in whole-grain cereals and nutritional yeasts, they are essential for proper formulation of liver bile and natural control of cholesterol. See Chapter 11.

OVERVIEW

Nutrition becomes more and more important as you grow older and your physiology functions less and less well. The earlier you start with a good nutritional program, the more gland and organ functioning you keep through the years. By taking care of the present, nutrition insures a good future!

B vitamins are central to a complete nutritional program. A direct and immediate relationship exists between each and every B and an important task, for example pantothenic acid → adrenaline. Complex interactions and equilibriums exist between all B's, those known and those still unknown. Such complexity demands natural management long term, not all-knowing human intervention and pills. Put away this mythology and get your needed B vitamins every day from REAL FOOD. Whole-grain cereals power adrenal medulla Energy and Healing, while adrenal cortex Stress and Immune run on nutritional yeasts and green vegetables (folic acid plus many related, undiscovered B factors). This is simple and flexible complete B vitamin nutrition for life. 1X usage maintains health for a normal lifestyle with no severe demands currently upon the mind and body. Take at 2X for physical labor and sports, and to overcome past B vitamin deprivation and adrenal exhaustion.

The hectic pace of modern life overuses and abuses adrenal Energy and Stress functions and systems. Energy comes from whole-grain cereals naturally. Whole grains keep pancreatic hormones insulin and glucagon quiescent, which puts you in the zone of peak energy performance. Two well-known shortcuts to energy are refined sugar and caffeine; however, these nutritionally bankrupt tempters slowly wreck your health. Stress has become a scourge, but amazingly complete nutrition can turn bad stress into good stress. Nutritional yeasts and green vegetables are part one of the everyday solution to stress; Omega 3 fish fatty acids of Chapter 5 are part two. Achieving the zone of peak stress performance also requires sufficient antioxidants to prevent oxidative stress and keeping by-product ketones at safe concentrations.

Beyond B vitamins naturally, the following short-term B-supplementation therapies can be useful and effective:

For Mild Energy and Stress Exhaustion, take pantothenic acid supplementation alone for Energy exhaustion or the formula 2 pantothenic acid + 1B2 + B6 for Energy-Stress exhaustion.

For Adrenal Medulla Equilibrium and Mild Energy and/or Healing Exhaustion, use the formula 1 PABA + 1B1 $\rightleftharpoons$ 25 pantothenic acid to restore medulla equilibrium and overcome medulla exhaustion.

When Healing needs are great, PABA supplementation along with other powerful healers can produce spectacular repair. PABA also has the unique ability to dampen nervous system hyperactivity without affecting adrenaline and energy.

B1 deficiencies can develop. Possible symptoms are labored breathing, nerve damage, sensitivity to pain loss of mental alertness, mood problems including depression, impaired carbohydrate digestion, sleeplessness, heart irregularities and cardiac damage.

Folic acid supplementation during pregnancy.

Biotin supplementation with diabetes.

***

5. FATTY ACIDS

Fatty acids are one of the five raw materials your adrenal gland and endocrine system need to perform properly under all circumstances. They supply the fat-soluble building blocks for hormones, neurotransmitters, enzymes, coenzymes, cofactors and other end products of Energy, Healing, Stress and Immune functions and systems. Crucial to gland maintenance, these good fats *lubricate* your endocrine parts, and cells and tissues in general. They are especially important to cell membranes, first becoming essential components and then protecting them from free radical attack and oxidative stress. Fatty acids should be taken often – once a day usually works best for building health.

Fatty acids are more complicated than just the well-known fat-soluble vitamins: Vitamins A, D, E and beta-carotene, as explained below.

FATS, OILS, FATTY ACIDS?

To begin *at the beginning*, what is fat? "I know it when I see it!" Fat tastes good, has lots of calories and too much is bad for you. Yes, all true, but not very helpful in understanding what fat is. Organic chemistry (here 'organic' is a scientific term meaning 'carbon-based') offers the best answer, although the following brief explanation is technical alone.

All fats are glycerol esters,
which form according to these two chemical reactions:

> **any acid + alcohol (C_2H_5OH) → ester**
> **any ester + glycerol ($C_3H_8O_3$) → fat**

Fats are part of life and life's chemistry, i.e. carbon based. All fats are made according to these two chemical reactions whether from vegetable, fish, animal or man-made sources. Vegetable and fish fats are usually called oils, since they are liquid at room temperature. Why are they in a liquid state, and not solid like butter? Because vegetable and fish fats are "unsaturated," meaning not saturated with hydrogen atoms. The carbon atoms in a fat molecule can have one, two or three hydrogen atoms bonded to them. Completely unsaturated fats have only one hydrogen atom per bonding carbon atom. Completely saturated fats are called triglycerides (tri = three hydrogen atoms per bonding carbon atom, the maximum possible). The more hydrogen in a fat's chemical composition, the more saturated and solid it is at room temperature.

Digestion breaks fats down into esters and glycerol, which the body then uses in various metabolisms. Another name for esters is fatty acids. However, as explained in Chapter 3, the term "fatty acids" is reserved in this book and generally to describe the esters of vegetable and fish oils and their vitamins, because these particular esters play a special role in human nutrition. That role is explored in depth in this chapter.

The human body cannot make these special fatty acids from their acid and alcohol precursors; therefore you must supply them from good food choices. Fortunately, the human body can make all needed vegetable fatty acids from a basic chemistry set called essential fatty acids (EFAs) or more formally Vitamin F, as shown in Table 5-1.

TABLE 5-1. ESSENTIAL FATTY ACIDS (EFAs, VITAMIN F).

NAME	CHEMICAL COMPOSITION	RICHEST SOURCE
linoleic acid	$C_{18}H_{32}O_2$	safflower and sunflower oils
linolenic acid	$C_{18}H_{30}O_2$	soy oil
arachidonic acid	$C_{20}H_{32}O_2$	phospholipids:[1-4] soy lecithin granules
Other good EFA sources: olive oil, peanut oil, walnut oil. Poorer EFA sources: corn oil, canola oil, palm oil		

Linoleic acid is the only truly *essential* vegetable fatty acid, although the human body has great difficulty manufacturing linolenic acid from linoleic acid. Therefore, obtaining these two EFAs from the sources listed in Table 5-1 is best nutrition. Arachidonic acid synthesis from linoleic acid requires only a healthy liver. With impaired liver function, phospholipid supplementation becomes necessary to generate arachidonic acid—more on this later. EFAs are essential for cell nucleus functioning, glandular activity including hormone synthesis, and oxygen transport from blood to cells. They also nourish cell membranes, nerves and skin. Dry skin is grossly lacking in EFAs and other fatty acids. Vitamin F was the fifth fat-soluble vitamin discovered after beta-carotene (carotene) in the 1860s, Vitamin A in 1913, and Vitamins D and E in the early 1920s.

When the world was designated animal, vegetable or mineral, EFAs were classified as vegetable oils and recognized as "good fats." With increasing evidence since the 1960s, animal fats have come to be "bad fats" because of their saturated/triglyceride nature and a half-fat called cholesterol ($C_{27}H_{46}O$), which can deposit on, narrow and then clog arteries. These deposits, known as atherosclerosis, cause cardiovascular disease and eventually heart attack or stroke. However, cholesterol is needed for normal body functions, being a component of most tissues, particularly the brain and nervous system, blood, liver and bile, and adrenal and sex hormones. Thus, cholesterol is really a matter of degree – TOO MUCH IS BAD! This declared public enemy is discussed in greater detail in Chapter 11 and ahead in the medical literature reviews of each good and bad fat. Triglycerides also aggravate atherosclerotic mechanisms, and saturated fats in general are a cancer risk.

Collectively, all vegetable oils, both rich and poor in EFAs, are known as Omega 6 oils. In the early 1980s, a new good fat came on the scene, <u>fish</u> fatty acids, also known as Omega 3 oils, and of course eating fish and seafood. Sometimes a new idea is an old idea recycled; cod liver oil was a ritual for many children of the 1930s, 1940s and 1950s. Recent evidence on the essential nature of fish, seafood and Omega 3 includes decreased blood cholesterol and triglyceride levels, increased HDL (high-density lipoprotein cholesterol carrier, so-called good cholesterol) to LDL (low-density lipoprotein, so-called bad cholesterol) ratio, improved cardiovascular function and reduced heart disease. Omega 3 also lowers blood pressure, eases arthritic pain and other inflammatory conditions, and protects against some common cancers, notably breast, colon and possibly prostate cancer.

In the 1990s, more good fat – a special form of EFA linolenic acid, gamma-linolenic acid (GLA), proved to be essential for diabetics and others with Energy malfunctions. GLA relieves diabetic neuropathy, improves skin diseases such as eczema, and provides anti-inflammatory pain relief. Richest sources of GLA are evening primrose oil, borage oil and black currant oil.

BAD FATS

How can one make good sense out of the plethora of terms: fats, oils, unsaturated, saturated, triglycerides, cholesterol, fatty acids, EFAs, Omega 6, Omega 3 and GLA? How about a simple plan – get as much good fat and as little bad fat as you can! The who, why, when and how much of good fats is presented in the next section. First though, the bad fats…

Animal Fats

What harm can too much cholesterol from animal fats do? And what of saturated fats and triglycerides? Let's see what the medical literature says.

Review of the Medical Literature

Cholesterol… Atherosclerotic lesions [plaque deposited on artery walls] are an accumulation of cholesterol esters. Excessive low-density lipoprotein (LDL) cholesterol in the blood is modified and denatured by oxidation or other reactions on the vascular wall, and then taken up by macrophages [long-living, large white blood cell; -phage: anything that devours] using their scavenger receptors. This results in formation of 'foam cells' of cholesterol esters on the vascular wall.[5] Controlling hypercholesterolemia [-emia: of the blood] and lowering LDL cholesterol reduce coronary artery disease, coronary events and mortality.[6-8]

Saturated fats, triglycerides… Triglycerides alter the blood lipoprotein distribution, decreasing HDL cholesterol [high-density lipoprotein cholesterol, so-called good cholesterol] and increasing small dense, more readily oxidizable LDL cholesterol [so-called bad cholesterol].[9] Macrophage binding and uptake of triglycerides may also contribute to the foam cells of atherosclerotic lesions.[10] Acute coronary syndromes including unstable angina [chest pain], myocardial infarction [heart attack] and sudden death are due to progressive atherosclerotic processes, culminating in the rupture of plaque and formation of thrombi [blood clots]. These acute events account for more than 250,000 US deaths yearly.[11]

Saturated fats and cancer... Lower saturated fat consumption significantly improves prostate cancer survival. Men in the upper one-third ranking of saturated fat consumption have three times the risk of dying from prostate cancer as those in the lower one-third ranking.[12-14] For breast cancer, saturated fats are moderately but directly related to cancer risk,[15] or there is a borderline statistical link,[16] or no link exists.[17, 18] More generally, body fat accumulation in adulthood correlates with colon, kidney, endometrium and postmenopausal breast cancers. Higher intake of meat and dairy products increases prostate cancer risk, while red meat consumption raises colon cancer risk.[19] Red meat, especially fried or well-done, is associated with lung cancer.[20] Overall, studies during the last 30 years show good correlation between dietary fat consumption and mortality from various cancers. High fat intake is also a major cause of obesity, hypertension [high blood pressure], diabetes and gallbladder disease.[21]

Meat. Serve lean cuts of meat, trim away visible fat, limit portion sizes and use low-fat cooking methods.[22] Except for pork tenderloin, most cuts of pork are high in saturated fats,[23] and should be strictly limited or completely avoided. Chicken and turkey are *lean* in bad fats and much better choices. Beef is in-between, OK for healthy persons in limited quantities. The worse the grease in the pan is in solidness and appearance after cooling to room temperature, the worse the bad fats are inside of you!

Meat does not contain any fatty acid nourishment; nevertheless meat plays an important role by providing complete protein and fat together, protein to power Healing Function and fat for Stress Function with its fat burning by cells, which yields 9 calories per gram. Jointly these two carry out breakdown and repair duties in the body easily. Review this concept in the Chapter 2 section on "Breakdown and Repair." Vegetarians have to work hard at nutrition to accomplish the same task, but then they have the benefits of no bad fats. A third, outstanding alternative is fish and seafood, again complete protein and fat together, and this is Omega 3 good fat. The more fish and seafood in your diet, the healthier you will be.

Milk and Dairy Products contain moderate levels of saturated fat and cholesterol. *Lean* milk (low fat, 2% or less) and its dairy products are usually no problem for healthy persons. Rich in protein and bioavailable calcium, these foods are still good for you and your bones if you can digest them. Lactose intolerance is the most common digestive disturbance among adults, but today the digestive enzyme lactase can be taken in supplement form to relieve this distress. Another solution, active-culture yogurt is milk predigested by lactobacillus and other friendly bacteria. Yogurt requires no further action by the human digestive system, and so even those that are lactose intolerant can partake of its many health benefits. Beyond milk's nourishing profile, yogurt controls bad breath and intestinal gas/flatulence, alleviates diarrhea and inhibits the growth of ingested strep, staph, salmonella, and other virulent bacteria. More on this gut saver in Chapter 10. Like meat and fish, milk and dairy products (except skim) provide complete protein and fat together in a convenient, natural food.

For growing children, milk and dairy products are essential for healthy bones and development.[24-28] Bone density and bone mineral content in young adults are directly related to calcium intake from milk and other diary products during childhood and adolescence.[26] Unfortunately, just when the need is greatest, most adolescents have diets extremely low in calcium, with teenage girls twice as likely to be deficient as teenage boys, 85% vs. 43%.[27] What's more, high calcium intake in later life may not offset the increased risk of osteoporosis resulting from inadequate calcium during the early formative years.[28]

Eggs. An egg contains six grams of complete protein and is the richest food source of sulfur, a rejuvenating nutrient. Eggs are complete protein and fat together, but cholesterol *heavy*.[29-33] One egg contains approximately 200 mg of cholesterol. The recommendation of not more than 300 mg cholesterol per day to prevent high blood cholesterol and cardiovascular disease is often used to justify restricting eggs to just three or four per week.[29] Still, one egg daily is unlikely to have a substantial impact on the risk of heart disease or stroke among healthy adults.[30] However, with high blood cholesterol levels or heart disease, limit eggs or fix your cholesterol problem. A natural solution is given in Chapter 11. Finally, on the general principle that *you get out of something only what you put in*, organic eggs from free-range chickens, as opposed to "factory eggs" in the supermarket, have more high-quality nutrients put into them.

Fried Foods

Heated animal fats, as with heated vegetable and fish oils, can become rancid. Rancidity is far more than unpleasant odor, its last manifestation; it is goodness destroyed, particularly the fat-soluble vitamins present in vegetable and fish oils. Furthermore, after digestion and absorption, rancid oils and fats go on to sweep up these same vitamins from the blood – *a double whammy*! And still, there is a bigger problem. Heated oils and fats become chemically altered, changing into trans-fatty acids (and esters), which are foreign to the human body and contribute to atherosclerosis, heart disease and possibly cancer. "Trans" and "cis" are two different arrangements of atoms for the same compound, technically called isomers. Nutritionally, the human body runs only on cis fatty acids, oils and fats. Cis is what's normally found in food.

Frying food in hot oil or grease causes unhealthy rancidity and the cis → trans isomer switch. The hotter the cooking temperature, the more bad actors there are. And some of that oil and grease becomes part of your food. The worst is fried food at restaurants: change the oil, or rancidity and trans fat? Which is cheaper??

> ## Review of the Medical Literature

Rancidity... As a class, lipids [fats and fat-related compounds] contribute desirable qualities to food such as texture, structure, mouth-feel, flavor and color. However, lipids are chemically unstable and readily undergo free radical chain reactions, which degrade their structure and that of nearby proteins, vitamins and pigments. Newly created cross-linked lipids become nonnutritive, while oxidized fragments are volatile and perceived as the off-flavor of rancidity.[34-36]

Trans-fatty acids... have a more straight-line structure than their cis counterparts, therefore properties more like saturated fatty acids. Dietary trans-fatty acids increase LDL [low-density lipoproteins, so-called bad cholesterol] in the blood, but to a lesser extent than saturated fatty acids. They also raise Lp(a) [another bad lipoprotein] and lower HDL [high-density lipoproteins, so-called good cholesterol]. Trans-fatty acids may compete with EFAs for elongating and desaturating enzymes, thereby interfering with the formation of eicosanoids [prostaglandins and other hormone-like mediators of conduction/transmitter functions regulating cellular activities]. These unfavorable effects can be expected to increase coronary heart disease risk. This is confirmed in some but not all epidemiological studies.[37-40] Trans-fatty acids are linked to colon cancers,[41] and breast cancers,[16, 41] or oppositely no major associations exist between trans-fatty acids and breast cancer risk and proliferative benign breast disease.[42, 43] Author's Note: The trans-fatty acid cancer map remains largely *terra incognito.*

Other fried effects… Frying creates heterocyclic aromatic amines (HAA), which are mutagenic and animal carcinogenic.[44, 45] Note: HAA could explain the fried red meat link to lung cancer noted earlier.[20]

Partially Hydrogenated Fats… include me out!

"Partially hydrogenated" means chemically adding hydrogen atoms to unsaturated fats, usually vegetable oils, to make them solid or semi-solid at room temperature, as in soft-spread margarines. Unfortunately, this process also flips isomers from cis to trans, creating trans-fatty acids with their unnatural risk and no reward. As much as possible, avoid partially hydrogenated fats.

Easier said than done! In the American supermarket, almost all processed foods containing fat are made using partially hydrogenated fats: all margarines, commercial-brand peanut butters, snack foods including potato chips and pretzels, breads and bakery goods, crackers, cookies, donuts, candies, chocolates, etc. Partially hydrogenated fats are everywhere and they're very bad for you – no joke. The commercial food industry isn't really concerned about your health, so you better be. To underscore this industry's total disregard for health, a new term is appearing that is free of the bad press of "partially hydrogenated." That new term is "fully hydrogenated," which means trans triglycerides! Read labels and ingredients lists carefully. Many good alternatives can be found at the health food store now. For the kids, there's old-fashioned peanut butter. You have to mix the peanut oil back in each time, but the original goodness is still in there and it tastes better. Good tasting breads and baked goods are at the health food store too. Instead of margarine, how about old-fashioned butter again, in moderation. The human body has had thousands of years of practice handling butter and its cis saturated fat and cholesterol, but only about 50 years with made-made trans, partially hydrogenated margarine.

The partially hydrogenated health risk is from trans-fatty acids alone. The medical literature reveals the shear magnitude and pervasiveness of this silent danger.

Review of the Medical Literature

Estimates of trans-fatty acids in the US food supply have been calculated from US Department of Agriculture-Economic Research Service (USDA-ERS) fats and oils production and food use data. Adipose tissue [animal, vegetable and man-made fats stored in human fatty tissue] isomer profiles indicate that 90-95% of trans-fatty acids in human tissues come from partially hydrogenated vegetable fats and oils. This represents a dietary trans-fatty acid intake of from 11 to 27 grams per person per day.[46] Similarly, partially hydrogenated vegetable oils appear to be the major source of trans-fatty acids in adipose tissue of Canadians.[47, 48]

New Designer Fats

New man-made fats such as Olestra, now invading snack foods, are so out of harmony with the human body that they are never digested, therefore never absorbed from the intestinal tract. This is OK in one sense; you get the taste of fat without calories, but not OK for optimal health because these new designer fats cause a dose-dependent decrease in the availability of fat-soluble vitamins,[49, 50] and individuals consuming large quantities may experience mild to moderate gastrointestinal symptoms of loose/soft stools, gas and/or nausea.[50]

GOOD FATS

Good fats are fatty acids of three types:

✓ Omega 6 vegetable oils rich in essential fatty acids (EFAs) and gamma-linolenic acid (GLA),
✓ Omega 3 fish oils and eating fish and seafood,
✓ The well-known fat-soluble vitamins: Vitamins A, D, E and beta-carotene, naturally occurring in and extracted from these vegetable and fish oils.

Table 5-2 presents the good fats that your Energy, Healing, Stress and Immune functions and systems need to make all their hormones and other end products and to perform properly under all circumstances. As with B vitamins (compare to Table 4-1), the adrenal medulla and adrenal cortex run on completely different fatty acids and vitamins.

TABLE 5-2. ADRENAL FATTY ACIDS AND VITAMINS.

ADRENAL CORTEX runs on…	— Fish oils (Omega 3) and eating fish and seafood, — Vitamin A (Immune, also eyes), — Vitamin D (Stress and especially its dependent body system, bones).
ADRENAL MEDULLA runs on…	— EFAs and GLA vegetable oils (Omega 6), — Vitamin E (antioxidant, healing), — Beta-carotene (healing).

In all things nutritional, variety is important, and so it is with fatty acids and their vitamins. Small amounts of different vegetable and fish oils and fish and seafood remain *in play* in the body long after digestion and metabolism and continue to uniquely benefit adrenal and endocrine functioning. Purity and wholesomeness are vital too. Use only Omega 6 and Omega 3 oils that have not been heated (rancidity) during their extraction process; these are called cold-pressed oils. Avoid chemical extraction as well; natural processing gives a more healthful product. After opening a newly purchased bottle of cold-pressed oil, pinprick a few Vitamin E capsules and add their contents to the bottle to preserve freshness and prevent oxidation/rancidity. For Vitamins A, D, E and beta-carotene, natural sources are superior in bioavailability, gentleness and effect to cheap synthetics such as synthetic Vitamin E acetate.[51-53] The ultimate in cheap synthetic antioxidants are food preservatives BHA (butylhydroxyanisole) and BHT (butylhydroxytoluene). BHA and BHT promote tumors, whereas Vitamin E is not carcinogenic.[54, 55]

Fatty acids and their vitamins have one big problem… CALORIES! One gram of fat yields 9 calories, more than twice that of carbohydrates or proteins. This is chemical energy for catabolic (stress and fat burning) and anabolic (new cells, tissues and hormones) processes, or unfortunately for the dreaded third possibility, stored food energy (weight gain) if metabolism has slowed down from age or couch. Cardiovascular exercise is one answer here. Another answer is not taking needed fatty acids – EFAs, GLA, Omega 3, Vitamins A, D, E and beta-carotene – at the same time as proteins and carbohydrates, particularly carbohydrates. By ingesting these fatty acids alone, washing them down with a little juice, or with fiber such as on salads, calories for that meal are kept low. Eating fish and seafood is not a weight concern, as their Omega 3 amounts are much less than in pure oils or supplement capsules.

Toxicity can occur with fatty acid vitamins. Unlike B vitamins that are water-soluble and wash away by blood, fat-soluble vitamins can accumulate in tissues to toxic levels. Vitamin D is the biggest concern, but 400-800 IU (International Units) per day are safe and healthful. Much less problematic are Vitamin A, Vitamin E, beta-carotene, Omega 3, GLA and EFAs. Details are given in the literature review of each fatty acid. Omega 3, GLA and EFAs suffer only hyperactivity *toxicity* from too much therapeutic action.

Therapeutic Action

Figure 5-A highlights the role of individual good fats. Omega 6 EFA oils feed both Primary Energy and Healing Functions and systems equally. Similarly, Omega 3 and eating fish and seafood nourish Stress and Immune equally. Other fatty acids in Figure 5-A act as indicated with specific effects noted parenthetically.

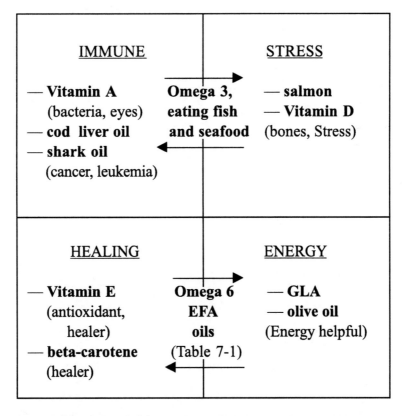

IMMUNE	Omega 3, eating fish and seafood	STRESS
— **Vitamin A** (bacteria, eyes) — **cod liver oil** — **shark oil** (cancer, leukemia)		— **salmon** — **Vitamin D** (bones, Stress)
HEALING	Omega 6 EFA oils (Table 7-1)	ENERGY
— **Vitamin E** (antioxidant, healer) — **beta-carotene** (healer)		— **GLA** — **olive oil** (Energy helpful)

FIGURE 5-A. ADRENAL FATTY ACID ROLES.

Omega 6 EFAs and Omega 3 fish fatty acids and vitamins produce therapeutic action as shown in Figure 4-B. Review terminology there including Table 4-2 multiple dose effects. Fatty acids first reach the bloodstream and adrenal gland at $t = 45$ minutes, normal digestion in progress. Maximum therapeutic effect occurs at $t = 2$ hours, then drops off, but remains strong until 5 hours. To this point, fatty acids, B vitamins, trace metals and most herbs behave exactly the same. Differences in therapeutic action always lie in the decay-to-zero part of the curve, with fatty acids decaying to zero in 24 hours. Thus, normal fatty acid therapeutic action guarantees availability to all tissues for 24 hours after any intake. After that, the liver must supply fatty acid needs from storage.

1X, 2X, 3X indicate the total number of doses ingested before the first dose decays to zero. Take fatty acids at 1X to maintain health, or at 2X to overcome past deprivation and rebuild fatty acid metabolism. Using Figure 5-A, adjust 1X maintenance and 2X stimulation and rebuilding of health to satisfy Energy, Healing, Stress and Immune needs exactly. Count Omega 6 and Omega 3 oils separately, each can be taken to 2X. Avoid 3X or overdose. Fatty acids are very tolerant of missed days and doses. Furthermore, they do not strongly interact with B vitamins, trace metals or herbs, all of which operate in the water medium.

Adrenal Medulla

The adrenal medulla runs on Omega 6 EFA and GLA vegetable oils, Vitamin E, beta-carotene and carotenes in general – and NO other fats. EFAs feed both sides of the medulla equally. Vitamin E and beta-carotene, as antioxidants and healers, operate within Primary Healing Function while GLA nourishes Primary Energy Function. Olive oil supplies Energy factors too. Cold-pressed extra-virgin olive oil is perfection in olive oil.

ESSENTIAL FATTY ACIDS (EFAs)

For salads, light cooking or just supplementation, use vegetable oils richest in EFAs as outlined in Table 5-1. Variety in linoleic and linolenic acids from their best sources – safflower, sunflower, soy, olive, peanut and walnut oils – is fundamental to good health. Regarding arachidonic acid, a healthy liver produces its phospholipid precursor from linoleic acid and omnipresent phosphorus. However, if and when age or injury slow down liver functioning, supplementing with phospholipid-rich soy lecithin granules may become necessary.

Arachi-phobia. Arachidonic acid has received a lot of negative press, being blamed for out-of-control inflammation. More to the truth, arachidonic acid as precursor to eicosanoids (general term), prostaglandins, thromboxanes and leukotrienes mediates inflammatory response. Yes, Omega 6 arachidonic acid forms more potent eicosanoids than Omega 3 fatty acids, but internal balance between these two fatty acid types is the proper homeostatic solution. Moreover, impairment in the metabolic pathway of EFA linoleic acid → phospholipids → arachidonic acid → eicosanoids can be the culprit in a number of immune dysfunctions and imbalances, including the faulty NK- and T-lymphocyte cellular immunity of chronic fatigue syndrome (CFS), as revealed in the medical literature review below. Soy lecithin supplementation restores normalcy to an impaired CFS arachidonic acid-eicosanoid system. Other possible causes of raging inflammation are Stress exhaustion, Immune subfunction imbalances, loss of vasoconstriction-vasodilatation homeostasis (Chapter 7), and zinc, manganese, nickel (Chapter 6), gamma-linolenic acid, Vitamin E and Omega 3 deficiencies. The herb Lobelia (Table 7-6) helps to restore general well being during any inflammatory distress.

EFA intake. Surprisingly, the daily human requirement for EFA oil rich in linoleic acid and linolenic acid is only about one-quarter teaspoon. And that can be consumed in one serving, a daily maintenance dose (1X). Although fatty acids are very tolerant of missed days and doses, rebuilding health demands more discipline. Overcoming past EFA and Omega 3 deprivation requires more oil more often, but not to 3X overdose. Large nutritional debts may need weeks with amounts of approximately one-half teaspoon EFAs, GLA, Vitamin E and Omega 3 twice daily (2X) to restore fatty acid function. Moderation over time succeeds, while ingestion of greater than one teaspoon at once, even alone, can produce weight gain in someone with sedentary metabolism.

Obtaining some EFAs in their *original containers* provides synergies not found in the extracted oils alone. Close to nature and the renewal of life, sunflower seeds and pumpkin seeds in particular contain many unknown vital/revitalizing nutritional factors. Almonds, cashews, chestnuts, filberts, peanuts, pecans, and walnuts are very good too. These are true snack foods.

Review of the Medical Literature

Discovery timeline and overview... As discovered in 1929, polyunsaturated fatty acids (PUFAs) [n-6 "Omega 6" EFAs and later n-3 "Omega 3" families] are necessary for life and health. With multiplicity of members, no two of which equivalent, PUFAs become structural components of cell membranes,[56] and precursors to prostaglandins and other eicosanoids [generic term], which are powerful regulators of cell and tissue functions including inflammatory response, white blood cell functions, platelet aggregation, vasoconstriction and vasodilatation, blood pressure, bronchial constriction and uterine contraction.[57] Eicosanoids derived from 20 carbon [see Table 5-1] EFA arachidonic acid are especially potent in their effects. Eicosanoid 'prostaglandins' were first found in human seminal plasma in the 1930s, and their chemical structures and synthesis biochemistry were determined by the early 1960s. More eicosanoids were identified in the 1970s including thromboxane A2, a potent platelet aggregating agent; prostacyclin, antagonist to thromboxane A2; and leukotrienes, a whole new class of eicosanoids. One key leukotriene action is bronchoconstriction in allergic response.[58]

Cell membranes, new tissue... As cell membrane structural elements, essential fatty acids (EFAs) are instrumental in the formation of all new tissue. The human body cannot synthesize primary EFAs; consequently we depend on dietary sources for an adequate supply.[59]

Pregnancy and infants... Fetal development requires high EFA amounts from maternal source.[59] At birth, EFA deficiency can cause blood platelet dysfunction, reduced prostaglandin synthesis and turnover, altered pulmonary surfactant [lung collapse possible],[60] and impaired development of the vision system.[61]

Brain development... Arachidonic acid and docosahexaenoic acid [DHA: Omega 3 type] are the major fatty acid structural components of the brain, and depend solely on dietary sources. Fatty acid-derived prostaglandins affect conduction and transmission functions in the brain with profound effects on sensory, motor, motivational, arousal, cognitive and social behavior.[62, 63] Inattentive, impulsive and hyperactive behavior in children characterizes attention-deficit hyperactivity disorder (ADHD). While ADHD causes are not known, they are thought to be biological and multifactorial. In several studies, some ADHD physical symptoms are similar to fatty acid deficient symptoms observed in humans and animals; and a subgroup of ADHD children with many coincident symptoms had significantly lower plasma arachidonic acid and DHA levels than ADHD subjects with few such symptoms or control subjects.[64] Regarding the severe brain dysfunction of schizophrenia, direct and indirect evidence points to defective prostaglandin (PG)E1 metabolism.[65]

Alzheimer's disease (AD)... The brains of those who die from AD show EFA deficits. One hypothesis [proposed, not proven] is that EFA-deprived brain cell membranes allow passage of an enzyme into the membrane bilayer, which cuts and releases beta-amyloid protein [thick protein deposit/plaque] into the extracellular space. Beta-amyloid protein appears to be the main constituent of senile AD brain plaques.[66] Additionally, PUFAs [Omega 6 and Omega 3] may maintain cognitive functions by preventing neurodegeneration.[67]

Nerve health, multiple sclerosis (MS)... Fatty acids are essential to central nervous system (CNS) myelinogenesis [myelin: insulating fatty acid sheath surrounding nerves; -genesis: suffix meaning 'origin, formation']. Linoleic acid deficit has been found in plasma and erythrocytes [red blood cells] of MS patients [MS cause: autoimmune/inflammatory destruction of the myelin sheath], suggesting the need for a diet of increased unsaturated fatty acids and reduced saturated fats. [61]

Cardiovascular... EFA linoleic and arachidonic acid deficiency relative to saturated fat correlates with coronary heart disease mortality.[68, 69] Dietary EFAs consistently reduce total cholesterol and low-density-lipoprotein cholesterol [LDL or bad cholesterol]. Epidemiological evidence suggests an inverse relationship between Omega 6 fatty acid consumption and blood pressure, although clinical findings are inconclusive.[69]

Liver... PUFA deficiencies occur with cholestasis [arrest of normal bile flow; bile emulsifies fats, permitting dissolution in blood], acute hepatitis and advanced cirrhosis. With cirrhosis, PUFA shortages are also due to impaired synthesis of metabolites in the liver.[70]

Skin... displays highly active PUFA metabolism, synthesizing, metabolizing and interconverting a variety of fatty acids.[71] Author's Note: Dry skin is an early warning sign of fatty acid deficiency.

Immune... Normal immune response requires EFA linoleic acid. EFA metabolite deficiencies impair T- and B-lymphocyte mediated responses.[69] Three clinical observations about viral infections are well known but poorly understood: (1) susceptibility of people with atopic eczema [inflammatory skin condition; redness, itching and oozing lesions] to viral infections, (2) viral infections precipitating an atopic syndrome, and (3) the development of a fatigue syndrome [chronic fatigue syndrome, below] following viral infections. A unifying hypothesis is interaction between viral infections and EFA metabolism.[72] Growing evidence suggests that the PGE group of prostaglandins is a negative feedback modulator of immune response, while eicosanoids derived from arachidonic acid are immuno-stimulatory.[73] As for cancer, PUFAs suppress ras [a frequently detected oncogene in animal and human cancers; oncogene: mutated version of a normal gene; can convert a normal cell to tumor cell] activity and inhibit tumor cell proliferation.[67] EFAs and their metabolites, particularly arachidonic acid and gamma-linolenic acid [GLA, ahead], as well as Omega 3 decosahexaenoic acid [DHA] and eicosapentaenoic acid [EPA], can induce apoptosis [gene-directed, programmed cell death] in tumor cells.[74]

Chronic fatigue syndrome (CFS)... presents hyper- and hypo-responses in immune functions, hypothalamus-pituitary (HP) axes and the sympathetic nervous system [originates in the thoracic and lumbar spinal cord and regulates involuntary actions], all related to impaired EFA metabolism.[75] CFS immunological deficits indicate decreased cellular immunity [T-lymphocyte system, NK (natural killer) cells, etc.].[76] EFA dietary changes can adjust the ratios of both cell membrane EFAs and EFA metabolites [arachidonic acid → immuno-stimulatory eicosanoids] and thereby correct CFS hypo-responsive functioning.[75] See also immune/viral infections above.[72, 73] A complete review of CFS medical literature is given in Chapter 12.

Other actions and roles... EFA deficiency or defective metabolism negatively impacts glucose regulation and transport, estrogen availability,[77] premenstrual syndrome [PMS] and premenstrual breast pain.[78] EFA deficient animals develop severe osteoporosis with arterial and kidney calcification. A similar clinical picture occurs in the elderly, with osteoporosis bone loss and ectopic [abnormally positioned within the body] calcification of tissues including arteries and kidneys.[79]

GAMMA-LINOLENIC ACID (GLA)

Gamma-linolenic acid is no problem if you are healthy. It is synthesized directly from EFA linoleic acid. However, supplementation becomes necessary with Energy or nerve dysfunctions including diabetic neuropathy, multiple sclerosis and skin disorders such as eczema. GLA is also anti-inflammatory. Richest sources are evening primrose oil and borage oil; black currant oil incorporates both GLA and Omega 3. Evening primrose oil contains estrogen factors that can be beneficial, but should be avoided with breast cancer risk. Complicated is this organic chemistry we all live with!

Review of the Medical Literature

GLA metabolism... Linoleic acid, the principal dietary essential fatty acid (EFA), must be metabolized to other fatty acids to be fully utilized by the body. The first step in this metabolic pathway is delta-6-desaturation to gamma-linolenic acid (GLA), which is slow and rate limiting in humans. If for any reason delta-6-desaturation is impaired, supply of further metabolites becomes inadequate. A direct supply of GLA is useful in these circumstances, as occurs with atopic eczema [inflammatory skin condition with redness, itching and oozing lesions] and diabetes, which are inherited and acquired examples of inadequate delta-6-desaturation.[80]

Skin... GLA administration improves atopic eczema with respect to these criteria: clinically assessed skin condition, objectively assessed skin roughness and elevated blood catecholamines [adrenaline, etc.] in most but not all studies.[81-83] GLA is beneficial in Sjogren's syndrome [immunologic destruction of exocrine glands such as sweat, tear and salivary glands; symptoms include dry eyes, dry mouth, persistent cough] and may help other dry eye conditions.[84] GLA from evening primrose oil produces positive results in both primary Sjogren's syndrome and systemic sclerosis [hardening of tissue].[85]

Anti-inflammatory... Dietary GLA increases its elongase product dihomo-gamma-linolenic acid (DGLA) in cell membranes without affecting immunostimulatory arachidonic acid. Upon inflammatory stimulation, DGLA is converted to 15-(S)-hydroxy-8,11,13-eicosatrienoic acid and prostaglandin E1, both of which are anti-inflammatory and antiproliferative,[86, 87] thereby giving evening primrose oil and borage oil clinical benefits in rheumatologic disorders [such as rheumatoid arthritis].[87]

Asthma... may arise from a biased Th2 [subset of helper/inducer T-lymphocytes] immune response, which increases cytokines [non-antibody protein/signaling molecules of the immune system] and leukotrienes [family of potent hormone-like eicosanoids produced by immune response to antigens; they contribute to defense, inflammation and hypersensitivity]. Gamma-linolenic acid and eicosapentaenoic acid [Omega 3 EPA] reduce the levels of inflammatory mediators associated with asthma.[88]

Diabetic neuropathy... Conversion of dietary linoleic acid to gamma-linolenic acid, dihomo-gamma-linolenic acid, arachidonic acid and other Omega 6 metabolites is inadequate in diabetic patients. This disturbs 1- and 2-series prostaglandins [potent mediators of many conduction/transmitter functions regulating cellular activities] derived from them, leading to a variety of microvascular abnormalities, reduced blood flow and neural hypoxia [inadequate oxygen to nerves]. ROS [reactive oxygen species/free radicals] generation and aggravation of neural capillary endothelial [lining] damage further escalates the hypoxia. Continuing endoneurial hypoxia then impairs axonal transport [axon: transmits nerve impulses; each nerve cell has one axon that can be over a foot long; large axons are surrounded by myelin sheath] and neural ATP-ase [enzyme catalyzing ATP, adenosine triphosphate, the primary energy source within all living cells], causing demyelination. EFA metabolite depletion contributes to abnormalities in myelin use and replacement, membrane-bound receptors and enzymes, and other axonal structures.[89]

Diabetic neuropathy in practice... GLA administration corrects faulty nerve function in animal models of diabetes. Diabetic neuropathy human trials evidence significant benefits over placebo in neurophysiological parameters, thermal thresholds and sensory evaluations.[90, 91] Impaired microcirculatory perfusion [getting blood to the tissues] plays an important role in both diabetic neuropathy and diabetic retinopathy. These disorders respond to high-dose antioxidants, GLA, Omega 3 fish oils, carnitine [amino acid compound: transports esters/fatty acids across the mitochondrial membrane; see Table 3-2], arginine [amino acid], chromium [Chapter 6], and ginkgolides [from the herb Ginkgo biloba, Chapter 8].[92] Unsaturated fatty acids are a major free radical target; and synergistic benefits occur between GLA and antioxidants.[93]

Multiple sclerosis (MS)... GLA from Borago officinalis [borage oil] strongly inhibits the clinical incidence and histological manifestations [study of tissue at the microscopic level] of acute EAE [experimental autoimmune encephalomyelitis (brain and spinal cord inflammation) is a widely accepted mouse model of human MS], as well as clinical relapse of chronic relapsing EAE.[94] See also demyelination above.[89]

Other actions and roles... GLA, arachidonic acid, and eicosapentaenoic acid [EPA Omega 3] have selective tumoricidal activity.[95] GLA is beneficial in breast pain management,[96] and may play a role in duodenal ulcers.[97]

Drug interactions... Do not use evening primrose oil or borage oil with anticonvulsant drugs. GLA may lower the seizure threshold.[98]

VITAMIN E

Vitamin E protects cell membranes and fatty acid tissue from oxidation, thereby slowing aging. It is the most powerful fat-soluble antioxidant. To work properly inside of your body, all other fatty acids require 'E' antioxidant protection. Vitamin E also aids in healing; this activity is most obvious with topical application to skin cuts, burns and surgical incisions.

Nature wants the best for you, however, in the grand scheme of things, she cares about individuals only to the extent that they fulfill their reproductive destiny. A balanced diet delivers approximately 30 IU (International Units) of Vitamin E daily. This is sufficient to get your genes to the next generation, but if you want to live a much longer and healthier life beyond the years in which nature has an interest, then Vitamin E and Vitamin C supplements are crucial. Here is one of the few nutritional areas where you can improve upon Mother Nature!

The naturally occurring Vitamin E present in all vegetable oils and many foods is insufficient to prevent free radical damage and oxidative stress in the human body. Supplementation is absolutely necessary. 200 to 400 IU of natural Vitamin E complex daily is about right for all adults, with correspondingly lower amounts for children according to body weight. 800 IU on very stressful days can be helpful, but never more than 800 IU as mild toxicity begins above that level. Vitamin E first thing in the morning before breakfast provides all-day protection. Combining 'E' with other needed fatty acids is an excellent idea.

The Recommended Daily Allowance (RDA) for Vitamin E is 15 IU daily for adults, 22 IU for pregnant and lactating women. The following medical literature tells a very different, true story! Do not decide nutritional needs according to RDA, which better stands for "Really Dumb Amounts."

The scientific literature below reveals Vitamin E's many miracles. This vitamin is always a positive in your life – NEVER NEGATIVE.

Review of the Medical Literature

Unequaled antioxidant... Vitamin E is a potent peroxyl [OO^{--} radical, also prefix denoting an extra oxygen atom] free radical scavenger, a chain-breaking antioxidant that prevents cell membrane damage.[99] As a universal participant in antioxidant defense reactions within biological membranes, Vitamin E protects during all stages of possible oxidative injury.[100]

Complex, unique action... Vitamin E, known since 1922 as an essential nutrient for reproduction, consists of tocopherols and tocotrienols, of which alpha-tocopherol provides the highest biological activity. Beyond antioxidant activity, alpha-tocopherol performs signaling functions in vascular smooth muscle cells [such as heart muscle walls] that other tocopherols cannot accomplish. The liver sorts out specific RRR-alpha-tocopherol from all incoming tocopherols to incorporate into blood lipoproteins [such as LDL, see cardiovascular disease below], thereby protecting lipoproteins from oxidation.[101] Gamma-tocopherol eliminates peroxynitrite [ONOO⁻] free radicals more effectively than alpha-tocopherol. Peroxynitrite forms when active oxygen reacts with nitric oxide released during macrophage [long-living, large white blood cell; -phage: anything that devours] inflammation.[102] Natural Vitamin E delivers approximately twice the bioavailable alpha-tocopherol to human plasma and tissues as synthetic Vitamin E.[53] Author's Note: These findings show that "natural Vitamin E complex" with all its naturally occurring tocopherol and tocotrienol forms and concentrations is your best 'E' supplement. Vitamin E by standard definition is just alpha-tocopherol.

Fatty acid protector... Vitamin E protects polyunsaturated fatty acids (PUFAs) [Omega 6 and Omega 3 families] against auto-oxidation [rancidity].[103] By the same mechanism, Vitamin E prevents oxidation of PUFAs in tissues. In animal experiments, increasing dietary fatty acid unsaturation [unsaturated vs. saturated] increases its peroxidizability and reduces the time necessary to develop symptoms of Vitamin E deficiency. Therefore, reducing total fat intake while increasing PUFA consumption requires additional Vitamin E protection. Extra Vitamin E may also be necessary with completely saturated triglyceride fats.[104]

Mitochondria and aging... Mitochondria [cell *organ* responsible for respiration and energy production] and particularly mitochondrial DNA (mtDNA) are major targets of free radical attack. Mitochondrial oxidative damage accumulates with aging, with mtDNA damage several times greater than nucleus DNA damage. As a consequence, in the brain and liver, mitochondrial size increases and mitochondrial membrane electrical potential decreases. Vitamin E and Vitamin C protect against this age-related oxidative mtDNA damage, as well as oxidation of mitochondrial glutathione [natural internal antioxidant: the main defense against oxidative stress within cell mitochondria]. Thus, Vitamin E and Vitamin C can prevent mitochondrial aging.[105]

Cardiovascular disease... Vitamin E has cardioprotective effects, inhibiting low-density lipoprotein [LDL, so-called bad cholesterol] oxidation, smooth muscle proliferation, and blood platelet aggregation and adhesion, while preserving normal coronary dilation.[106, 107] For platelets, Vitamin E may be effective through regulation of arachidonic acid [Table 5-1 EFA] metabolism.[108] In the US Nurses Health Study and the US Health Professionals

Follow-up Study, Vitamin E supplementation produced a 34% and 39% reduction respectively in cardiac event risk. The Iowa Women's Health Study reported a 47% decrease in cardiac mortality with Vitamin E supplementation. In the best known trial, the Cambridge Heart Antioxidant Study, 400 or 800 IU of Vitamin E daily resulted in a 47% drop in fatal and nonfatal myocardial infarction [heart attack] in patients with proven coronary atherosclerosis [deposited plaque on artery walls].[106] Current evidence suggests that coronary heart disease patients would benefit from supplementations of 400 IU Vitamin E and 500 to 1000 mg Vitamin C daily.[109] Vitamin E acts as the first risk discriminator in cardiovascular disease, Vitamin C as second risk discriminator. Optimal cardiac health requires Vitamins E and C, Vitamin A, carotenoids and vegetable conutrients.[110]

Cardiovascular theory and practice... Impressive in vitro [in laboratory vessel], cellular and animal studies leave no doubt that Vitamin E is the most important fat-soluble antioxidant. This vitamin protects animals against oxidative stress. Many studies in vitro, in animals and in humans support the hypothesis [proposed, not proven] that oxidation of low-density lipoprotein (LDL) initiates a complex sequence of events leading to atherosclerotic plaque. Some evidence shows that ex vivo [outside the body] oxidizability of a patient's LDL is predictive of future cardiac events. Vitamin E also protects against other medical conditions indicative of atherosclerosis, such as intermittent claudication [leg pain brought on by walking, similar in nature to angina].[111] 300 IU Vitamin E per day for three to six months improves blood flow and walking distances in patients with intermittent claudication.[112] 100 to 800 IU Vitamin E per day is safe. Nutrient variety is another factor; antioxidants act synergistically and Vitamin E combined with other antioxidants may be even more cardio-effective. The scientific community must recognize that the dose-effect curve of Vitamin E for all conditions and all possible combinations of helpful micronutrients will never be complete. At some point, the weight of scientific evidence should be judged adequate; clearly we are very close. In view of the low risk of reasonable Vitamin E supplementation, and the difficulty in obtaining more than 30 IU per day from a balanced diet, supplementation appears prudent now.[111]

Diabetes, platelet and cardiovascular complications... Premature atherosclerosis and other vascular disorders are serious complications of diabetes. LDL oxidation generates foam cells, fatty streaks and plaque formation on the arterial wall. Hyper-reactive blood platelets increase adhesion and aggregation.[108] Diabetes alters plasma coagulation and fibrinolysis [dissolution of fibrin, the insoluble protein in blood and the end product of coagulation]; of critical importance is greater plasminogen activator inhibitor (PAI-1) [stops the enzyme that breaks down fibrin and dissolves blood clots]. Atherosclerotic plaques formed in the presence of high PAI-1 may be more likely to rupture and result in thrombosis [blood clot]. These modifications in blood platelets, coagulation and fibrinolysis all contribute to the high rate of vascular events seen in diabetics.[113] Low Vitamin E levels in platelets increase their aggregation, and this tends to be exacerbated in diabetic patients. In several studies of Type I juvenile diabetes, and to some extent in Type II adult-onset diabetes, Vitamin E supplementation of several hundred IU significantly reduces lipid [e.g. blood cholesterol] peroxidation and platelet aggregation. Doses as low as 200 IU markedly decrease platelet adhesion and inhibit formation of protruding pseudopods [blunt-ended projection from the cells], typical of activated blood platelets.[108, 114] Another consideration, Vitamin E improves insulin activity by inhibiting oxidative stress during glucose transport. Vitamin C produces similar results.[115] Lastly, animal and clinical studies reveal that high doses of Vitamin E can apparently partially reverse diabetic injury to retinal and renal vessels.[116]

Other blood benefits... 800 IU Vitamin E daily improves blood parameters in patients with sickle-cell disease, G6PD deficiency [inherited glucose 6-phosphate dehydrogenase deficiency; causes anemia], and beta-thalassemia [serious blood disorder].[112]

Immune... Antioxidants play an important role in immune cell function, maintaining the integrity and functionality of membrane lipids, cell proteins and nucleic acids [DNA, RNA], and controlling gene expression and signal transduction [transmembrane signaling, which translates external stimulus from hormones, growth factors, etc. into changes in cell transport, metabolism, function, growth or gene expression]. Healthy immune response requires optimal antioxidant levels across all age groups,[117] with critical need in the elderly.[117, 118] Vitamin E deficiency results in increased infectious disease and tumor incidence. Supplementation brings various immune benefits; for example, high Vitamin E intake significantly improves cellular immunity [T-lymphocyte system, NK cells, etc.] in the elderly and those with AIDS.[119] Vitamin E has direct antiviral effect.[120]

AIDS... Apoptosis [gene-directed, programmed cell death involving activation of an intrinsic cell suicide program] is the main cause of CD4+ T-lymphocyte [helper T-cell, target of HIV] depletion in acquired immune deficiency syndrome (AIDS). Oxidative stress also causes apoptosis; hence an oxidation mechanism may be a factor in AIDS-related CD4+ T-cell apoptosis. This correlates with observed low antioxidant levels in AIDS patients.[121] Additionally, Vitamin E plays a key role in T-cell differentiation [maturation] in the thymus.[119]

Cancer... Despite numerous articles and several scientific reviews on the role of antioxidants, diet and lifestyle modifications in cancer prevention, these factors have been largely ignored in human cancer management. Extensive in vitro [in laboratory vessel] and limited in vivo [inside the living body] studies show that Vitamin E (alpha-tocopherol), Vitamin C, Vitamin A (retinoids) and carotenoids induce cell differentiation and to various degrees inhibit growth in rodent and human cancer cells.[122] Oxidative stress and reactive oxygen species (ROS) free radicals can trigger many carcinogenic processes.[123] Strong evidence exists for Vitamin E, selenium, soy proteins and reduced fat intake in prostate cancer prevention.[124] Vitamin E shows promise in lung,[125] oral and pharyngeal cancer prevention,[126] and may reduce colorectal cancer risk by quenching free radical mutagenic action.[127]

Radiation/Chemotherapy... Individually and in combination, antioxidant vitamins enhance the cancer inhibitory effects of chemotherapy, radiation, hyperthermia and tumor cell response modifiers, as evidenced for the most part in in-vitro studies. These vitamins also reduce the toxic effects of several standard chemotherapeutic agents on normal cells.[122]

Anti-inflammatory... Vitamin E inhibits inflammation.[107] Trauma and infection cause inflammatory stress. Consequences can include tissue damage, increased inflammatory mediators and suppressed lymphocyte function. Vitamin E and Vitamin C not only reduce tissue damage but also prevent increased cytokine [non-antibody protein/signaling molecule of the immune system] production.[128] Vitamin E and selenium supplementation strongly alleviate joint pain and morning stiffness in rheumatoid arthritis patients.[129] Vitamin E is beneficial in rheumatic diseases, principally through pain reduction.[130] 300-600 IU daily improves arthritis symptoms.[112] In acute pancreatitis, Vitamin E eases the severe inflammation.[131]

Exercise and free radicals... Several mechanisms may explain exercise-induced muscle damage; one is that free radicals are part of the inflammatory response.[132] While conflicting data exist, the preponderance of evidence shows that physical exercise promotes free radical generation.[133] Supplementing with 100-200 mg Vitamin E daily is recommended for all endurance athletes to prevent exercise-induced oxidative damage and achieve the full health benefits of exercise.[134]

Neuromuscular... Tardive dyskinesia (TD) [involuntary, irreversible neurological impairment of muscles; can include rolling of tongue, twitching of facial and other small muscles] may be due to neuron damage from free radical generation during increased neurotransmitter metabolism and turnover. Vitamin E, as a free radical scavenger, evidences positive effects in 12 of 18 TD clinical trials.[135] 400 IU or more of Vitamin E daily is beneficial.[136] Patients with TD for less than five years respond better than those with long-standing TD.[135]

Brain, Alzheimer's disease, etc.… In the brain, cell respiration generates partially reduced forms of oxygen. Brain insult accelerates this production. The most reactive oxygen forms such as hydroxyl radical [OH⁻] can oxidize proteins, lipids and nucleic acids. Oxidative stress is the difference between the rate of free radical generation and elimination. Oxidative injury, a threshold phenomenon involving overwhelmed antioxidant mechanisms is implicated in trauma, epilepsy, stroke and numerous degenerative diseases.[137] A large body of evidence indicates that oxidative stress plays an significant role in the pathogenesis of Alzheimer disease, Parkinson's disease and amyotrophic lateral sclerosis [ALS, Lou Gehrig's Disease]. Antioxidants, especially Vitamin E, prevent such neuron death in vitro.[138] In the brains of Alzheimer patients, beta-amyloid plaques [thick protein deposits] become toxic to neuron cell cultures through free radical mechanisms. Vitamin E prevents beta-amyloid damage in cell cultures and delays memory deficits in animal models. In a placebo-controlled clinical trial, Vitamin E appears to slow functional deterioration leading to nursing home placement in moderately advanced Alzheimer patients.[139-141] 'A beta' fragments [beta-amyloid peptides] accumulate in Alzheimer brain areas serving memory and information acquisition and processing. These fragments develop from abnormal proteolytic cleavage [splitting of proteins by hydrolysis] of their precursor, amyloid precursor protein (APP). Direct free radical scavengers such as Vitamin E and Vitamin C reduce 'A beta' toxicity with great efficacy.[142]

Pregnancy and infants… Vitamin E is useful in treating toxemia of pregnancy, intrauterine growth retardation (IUGR), and neonatal [the first four weeks after birth] jaundice.[143] Vitamin E reduces teratogenicity [birth defects] and oxidative lesions.[144] In newborns, Vitamin E can significantly retard onset of retinopathic eye damage during oxygen therapy, and may prevent intraventricular hemorrhages.[145] Despite extensive Vitamin E research and promising results in preventing retrolental fibroplasia (retinopathy of premature newborns), Vitamin E has not yet been incorporated into conventional care protocols.[146]

More on eyes: cataracts, AMD… Epidemiological studies show that antioxidants delay the onset of age-related vision disorders. While not yet possible to conclude that antioxidants prevent cataracts or AMD [age-related macular degeneration], epidemiological evidence suggests diets high in Vitamin E, Vitamin C and carotenoids, particularly xanthophylls [yellow-pigment fruits and vegetables], are insurance against developing these disorders.[147]

Wound healing… Antioxidants enhance healing of infected and non-infected wounds by reducing oxidative damage.[148] Blood antioxidant levels decrease following wounding, with

Vitamin E and Vitamin C falling 60-70%, and recovering completely only after 14 days.[149] Several nutritional factors may impair wound healing, in particular inadequate Vitamin E, Vitamin C, Vitamin A, zinc, protein and individual amino acids.[150]

Skin... possesses an elaborate antioxidant defense system to thwart ultraviolet light (UV)-induced oxidative stress. However, excessive UV exposure can overwhelm cutaneous antioxidant capacity, resulting in oxidative damage, immunosuppression, premature skin aging and skin cancer. One strategy for photo[sun]protection is supporting the endogenous [arising from within] antioxidant glutathione [within cell mitochondria, the main defense against oxidative stress; also immune modulator]. Vitamin E, Vitamin C and beta-carotene are very effective in photoprotection.[151]

Pollution, tobacco smoke... The hypothesis [proposed, not proven] that oxidative stress is an important, if not the sole, toxic mechanism behind air pollutants and tobacco smoke is compelling. The gas phase of cigarette smoke, NO_2 and O_3, oxidizes lung lipids [fat and fat-related lung tissue] by known biochemical mechanisms. Both Vitamin C and Vitamin E prevent this oxidation and protect human cells; Vitamin C is more effective against NO_2, Vitamin E more effective against O_3. Vitamin C also defends against air pollution in adults as measured by histamine challenge. Lastly, experimental animals from many species develop lung disease similar to human bronchitis and emphysema [chronic lung disease, difficulty breathing from enlargement and loss of elasticity of air sacs] after exposure to NO_2 and O_3.[152]

Male/female... Vitamin E is beneficial in treating male infertility.[153] For women, 300-600 IU per day improves premenstrual syndrome [PMS].[154] In postmenopausal women, Mayo Clinic recommends 800 IU per day of Vitamin E for mild 'hot flash' symptoms.[155]

Safety experience... Vitamin E toxicity is low. In animal studies, Vitamin E is not mutagenic, carcinogenic or teratogenic [causing birth defects]. In humans, double-blind protocols and large population studies show that Vitamin E supplementation has few side effects even at doses as high as 3200 mg per day (3200 IU per day).[156] During two large Alzheimer clinical trials, 2000 IU Vitamin E daily was relatively safe for periods up to two years.[136] Vitamin E intake at 100-300 mg daily is toxicologically harmless. However, high doses exacerbate the blood coagulation defect of Vitamin K [blood clotting vitamin, abundant in dark and green vegetables] deficiency,[157] specifically doses above 800 IU per day.[158] 100 to 800 IU Vitamin E daily is safe.[111] Finally, one patient who took megadoses of Vitamin E over a long period [dosage and duration not given] developed a necrotizing [necro- prefix meaning 'dead tissue'], nonprogressive myopathy [muscle disease].[159]

BETA-CAROTENE

Beta-carotene is the most powerful fat-soluble healer. Healer and antioxidant are two different facets of Primary Healing Function duties. Antioxidant protects cells and tissue from free radicals; healer repairs cells and tissue. Stiffness in joints and muscles, for instance, responds well to beta-carotene supplementation.

Beta-carotene (for healing) and Vitamin A (for immune) are NOT the same thing at all, although beta-carotene can be made into Vitamin A if you have a healthy liver, possibly and most easily as follows:

$$\text{beta-carotene} \; + \; \text{water} \; \rightarrow \; \text{Vitamin A}$$
$$C_{40}H_{56} \; + \; 2H_2O \; \rightarrow \; 2C_{20}H_{30}O$$

Often the liver's ability to change beta-carotene into Vitamin A is lost in adulthood. Accordingly, do not rely on beta-carotene for immune purposes. Instead take each of these fat-soluble vitamins separately, as needed.

If you are healthy and not recovering from surgery, severe burns or other tissue trauma – in other words, not in need of extraordinary healing – then beta-carotene and other carotenes/carotenoids from natural sources such as carrots, apricots, mangos, yams, squash, tomatoes, spinach, broccoli and beet greens provide sufficient raw material for healing. With vegetable neglect, a general carotenoid supplement can help meet this need.

For surgery, burns or other major reconstructions, your body and adrenal gland go strongly into healing mode, whereupon you can pitch in and improve overwhelmed mechanisms with 25,000 IU, occasionally up to 100,000 IU, of beta-carotene daily including topical application when appropriate. Extra Vitamin E and carotenoids also help, as do the good fats needed by the tissues in question. Even large doses of beta-carotene evidence little or no toxicity, particularly if they are being used up in the repair effort – see the safety citation in the medical literature review below. Getting the right amount of healing for each injury is vital, as too little and too much healing are both poor healing. Taking large beta-carotene doses when your body doesn't need them will knock medulla Healing $\rightleftharpoons$ Energy equilibrium out of whack, strongly toward healing and you'll wonder where your energy went. Beta-carotene levels below 5000 IU per day do not disturb medulla equilibrium.

NOTE: Beta-carotene and Vitamin A have higher International Units than Vitamin E. The large numbers for beta-carotene and Vitamin A do not indicate a relatively larger dose and effect, as 1 IU of dl-alpha-tocopherol = 1 milligram, while 1 IU of beta-carotene = 0.6 microgram or 0.0006 milligram! 1 IU of Vitamin A (retinol) = 0.3 microgram.

Beta-carotene supplementation is essential if your Primary Healing Function becomes hypoactive from permanent Healing exhaustion or hyperactive nerves. Beta-carotene will keep some fatty acid healing going until fundamental mechanisms can be fixed. Prime examples here are muscle and nerve diseases such as fibromyalgia and multiple sclerosis (MS). Of course, the damaged fatty acid myelin sheath of MS needs to be nourished with EFAs, GLA, Omega 3, Vitamin E and beta-carotene good fats – and no bad fats. Details in Chapter 12 "Correcting Dis-ease."

From time to time on a quiet day once every month or two, consider giving your body a rest and welcome "HEAL-IN" with 50,000 to 100,000 IU of beta-carotene taken alone. This "heal-in" also works well in the face of stress. Choose a stressful activity that is personally hard on your system, so beta-carotene can rejuvenate faulty glands and metabolic pathways as they are worked. Another good healing regimen for minor repairs is 5,000-10,000 IU of beta-carotene, 200-400 IU of Vitamin E and the good fats specific to the gland, metabolic pathway or tissue in question. This is perfect slow-and-easy fatty acid healing.

The medical literature of beta-carotene is incomplete, and in parts an unsolved mystery.

Review of the Medical Literature

Beta-carotene family tree... Carotenoids are plant pigments, with at least 600 different compositional members [see Table 3-3]. Approximately 50 carotenoids are present in human diet, with about 20 found in blood and tissues. Taken up by the liver and released into blood lipoproteins, carotenoids have provitamin A activity [provitamin: precursor that the body can convert into the vitamin] and are efficient free radicals scavengers, especially of reactive oxygen. Carotenoids protect LDL [low-density lipoproteins, so-called bad cholesterol] from free radical attack in vitro [in laboratory vessel]. However, in vivo [in the living body] results are inconsistent. Other carotenoid effects include gap junction [connections between cells, allowing passage of small molecules and electrical currents] enhancement, immune modulation and regulation of enzyme activity implicated in carcinogenesis [cancer origin/beginning].[160]

Carotenoids → Vitamin A... Most dietary Vitamin A comes from plant foods in the form of provitamin A carotenoids. This precursor role was first demonstrated in 1930. In vivo conversion of carotenes to Vitamin A varies from 20 to 80 percent efficiency depending on an individual's nutritional status; Vitamin A deficiency increases conversion, protein deficiency decreases it. While generally accepted that one mole [quantity equal to substance's molecular weight in grams] of beta-carotene produces one mole of Vitamin A, the conversion mechanism remains controversial. Obvious central cleavage of beta-carotene yields two molecules of Vitamin A, while excentric cleavage gives the observed one-to-one result.[161]

Overview... Beta-carotene and other carotenoids evidence antioxidant activity in vitro and in animal models. Mixtures of carotenoids and carotenoids combined with other antioxidants such as Vitamin E enhance activity against free radicals. Unfortunately, animal models are of limited value in studying carotenoids because most animals absorb and/or metabolize carotenoids differently than humans. Epidemiological studies reveal an inverse relationship between various cancers and dietary carotenoids or blood carotenoid levels. However, in three of four intervention trials [reported below], high dose beta-carotene supplementation did not protect against cancer or cardiovascular disease. Instead, in high-risk populations, specifically smokers and asbestos workers, these trials produced an increase in cancer and angina [chest pain]. Apparently, carotenoids, including beta-carotene, can promote health when taken in dietary amounts, but may have adverse effects at high dose in certain vulnerable populations.[162]

Cancer puzzle... The three large clinical trials testing beta-carotene on cancer were Alpha-Tocopherol Beta-Carotene Trial [ATBC] using male Finnish heavy smokers, Beta-Carotene and Retinol Efficacy Trial [CARET] with male asbestos workers and male and female heavy smokers, and Physician's Health Study of US male physician smokers. In all three trials, beta-carotene offered no protection against lung cancer. Unexpectedly, ATBC and CARET found greater lung cancer risk in subjects given beta-carotene compared to those given placebo. Certainly beta-carotene differs from the prototypical antioxidant Vitamin E. Most beta-carotene effects are probably not derived from antioxidant activity, but rather from biochemical action. However, the association between a diet rich in fruits and vegetables and reduced risk of disease remains solid. No evidence exists that consuming small amounts of beta-carotene from food or a multivitamin tablet is unwise for any population subgroup. High-dose supplementation is less clear for beta-carotene, carotenoids in general and other phytochemical antioxidants less well understood than Vitamin E. The ATBC and CARET results are a cautionary flag, pointing out the need for additional research.[163-165]

Cardiovascular disease... Epidemiological studies indicate an inverse relationship between blood and adipose [stored in human fatty tissue] beta-carotene levels and coronary heart disease [CHD] risk. Oppositely, randomized clinical trials show no benefit, and perhaps even a negative effect for beta-carotene supplementation. Confounding factors may help to explain these inconsistencies; for example, other carotenoids and plant-derived compounds are naturally present with epidemiological beta-carotene. Also, lipoprotein levels and the presence of inflammation, both CHD risk factors, affect the results.[166, 167]

Author's Note: Four factors may help explain the inconsistent and even negative beta-carotene effects in lung cancer and cardiovascular studies. FIRST, use of synthetic beta-carotene in the ATBC and CARET intervention trials. Dosage, regimen, smoking status, and antioxidant defense imbalances are other possible factors in their outcome.[168] SECOND, high-dose beta-carotene supplementation affects Figure 2-B equilibrium, specifically short-term use will benefit immune function, as Healing → (stimulates) Immune. Long term, however, abnormal homeostasis and dysfunction develops among the four primary adrenal functions in accordance with Figure 12-A(1), resulting in hyperactive Healing = hypoactive Immune! THIRD, beta-carotene → Vitamin A conversion can fail in damaged livers (likely in smokers and asbestos workers); consequently beta-carotene will produce no immune Vitamin A activity and more Figure 12-A(1) dysfunction. FOURTH, beta-carotene is only *a little bit* an antioxidant; it is mainly a healer, although research to date in this area consists of the following few articles.

Healing... Beta-carotene improves wound strength in animals.[169] For human fibroblasts [cells giving rise to connective tissue; -blast: immature, undergoing development], beta-carotene reverses growth factor resistance observed with high blood glucose levels. This can benefit wound healing of diabetic foot ulcers.[170] For duodenal ulcers, beta-carotene significantly reduces inflammatory and atrophic lesions, thereby enabling faster healing.[171] H. pylori [bacterium implicated in gastric ulcers and cancer] infection impairs Vitamin E, beta-carotene and Vitamin C protective effects in the stomach.[172]

Oral pre-cancer... Beta-carotene and Vitamin E reverse oral leukoplakia, a premalignant lesion to oral cancer, in eight clinical trials, five with beta-carotene alone, one with Vitamin E alone and two in combination.[173] Note: Healing may be key in pre-cancerous lesions.

Ultraviolet (UV) light... Skin possesses an elaborate antioxidant defense system to thwart UV-induced oxidative stress. Vitamin E, Vitamin C and beta-carotene are very effective in photo[sun]protection. Although treatments utilizing a single antioxidant are successful against many types of photodamage, balance in the skin antioxidants is important. In some studies, a single antioxidant can even cause deleterious effects,[151] specifically beta-carotene not only failed to protect against UV carcinogenesis, but produced significant exacerbation. This carcinogenic response could be due to instability of the carotenoid cation [positively charged ion], which likely depends upon other antioxidants for repair.[174] Note: Here beta-carotene could be the skin healer, while Vitamin E and Vitamin C stand antioxidant guard.

Cystic fibrosis (CF)... Cystic fibrosis [thick mucus clogs bronchi resulting in breathing difficulties, infection and lung fibrosis] patients have low plasma levels of antioxidant vitamins, especially beta-carotene. This may be due to fat malabsorption and chronic pulmonary inflammation. Beta-carotene supplementation decreases pulmonary exacerbations, which in turn reduces antibiotic use.[175] Adequate beta-carotene, fatty acids and selenium improve lung function in CF patients.[176]

Cognitive function... in elderly adults is helped by beta-carotene.[177]

Safety... Each year in the USA, approximately ten to fifteen cases of Vitamin A toxicity occur, usually at doses greater than 100,000 IU daily. No adverse effects are reported for beta-carotene.[178]

Adrenal Cortex

The adrenal cortex runs on Omega 3 fish oils, eating fish and seafood, Vitamin A and Vitamin D – and NO other fats. Of course, Primary Stress Function fat burning (9 calories per gram) uses any fat, but this is fat metabolism and not a fatty acid application.

Most fish oils and types of fish and seafood feed both sides of the cortex equally. The exceptions are salmon (Stress), cod liver oil (Immune, rich in Vitamin A) and shark oil (strongly Immune and anticancer). Sharks rarely get cancer and shark oil supplementation can significantly strengthen your cancer defense, especially against leukemia. However, moderation is necessary as straight shark oil is so potent that it can produce extreme Immune ←← Stress imbalance and severe headaches. With regard to Omega 3 vitamins, Vitamin A is necessary for resistance to and recovery from infection. Vitamin D acts on the Stress side of the cortex, though first and foremost 'D' aids the dependent body system of Stress, bones.

People in Western industrialized world are often woefully deficient in Omega 3 and its vitamins, typically ingesting 10:1 or even 25:1 ratio of Omega 6 vegetable oils to Omega 3 fish oils. This has lead to pandemic in stress and immune diseases. A balanced, healthy adrenal gland requires 2:1 ratio, minimum. Fish every day ensures healthy adrenal cortex functioning. This is the diet our species started with, and where we need to return.

OMEGA 3

Omega 3 oils are a little complicated in terms of "HOW" – how to get them and how much to take? First of all, eating fish and seafood offers hidden synergies not found in Omega 3 capsules alone. Fish and seafood supply small amounts of Omega 3, the equivalent of about eight to ten drops of oil per normal dinner serving. This is sufficient to maintain adrenal cortex health beautifully, perfectly… but not to rebuild broken health. Supplement capsules often complicate rebuilding goals; some are one inch long and yield over forty drops of Omega 3, far too much for a single serving. Oval-shaped capsules, ½ inch in length and containing approximately 500 mg of oil, are closer to daily human requirements. Cortex fatty acid health can be restored over several weeks by ingesting approximately fifteen to twenty drops of Omega 3 twice daily (2X) including goodly amounts of fish and seafood, then 1X maintenance thereafter. As always, slow and easy is the proper course; there are no magic pills in nature.

Omega 3 oils are composed of two major fatty acids: docosahexaenoic acid (DHA) and eicosapentaenoic acid (EPA). Exactly how DHA and EPA influence Primary Stress and Immune Functions is not known; no straightforward relationship exists. Strive for equilibrium in these Omega 3 types from their different sources, but not a strict one-to-one balance.

For vegetarians, not eating fish and seafood is a big obstacle to health. However, there is an alternative. Flax seed oil, rich the Omega 3 precursor alpha-linolenic acid, helps to satisfy Omega 3 needs, although in the final analysis, alpha-linolenic acid is a flawed substitute, as explained in the following literature review.

Review of the Medical Literature

Omega 3 need, effect... With solid evidence since the 1980s, Omega 3 fatty acids are essential nutrition and may favorably impact many diseases.[179] They rapidly incorporate into cell membranes and profoundly influence biological responses, including membrane stability and fluidity, cell mobility, gene expression, cell differentiation, receptor formation, binding of ligands [any binding molecule] to their receptors, and intracellular signaling directly and indirectly through eicosanoids [prostaglandins and other hormone-like mediators of conduction/transmitter functions regulating cellular activities]. Eicosanoids made from Omega 3 fatty acids are much less potent in their biological responses than those made from Omega 6 fatty acids, particularly in inflammatory response and stimulating cytokines [non-antibody proteins/signaling molecules of the immune system; include interleukins, lymphokines, interferons and TNF (tumor necrosis factor)]. In clinical studies, Omega 3 supplementation improves rheumatoid arthritis and inflammatory bowel disease [chronic disorder of ulcerative colitis and/or Crohn's disease with abdominal cramping and persistent diarrhea]; reduces cardiovascular disease, arrhythmias [abnormal heart beat: too slow, too rapid, too early, irregular] and hypertension [high blood pressure]; and protects against kidney disease and infection.[180] Omega 3 is both anti-inflammatory and anti-atherogenic [atherogenic: depositing plaque on artery walls].[181]

Omega 3 : Omega 6 ratio... For the earliest human beings, fats provided about 22% of energy requirements, with a ratio of polyunsaturated fatty acids (PUFA) to saturated fats estimated at 1:4 and Omega 6 to Omega 3 at 1:1. Human diets have changed dramatically over the last twenty thousand years, yet the Omega 6 to Omega 3 ratio remained constant until the 19th century. Today, fats provide nearly 40% of energy requirements for people in the developed world, with Omega 6 to Omega 3 ratio at 25:1 or even 50:1.[182] This high Omega 6 intake shifts the physiologic state to prothrombotic [thrombus: blood clot] and proaggregatory, with increased blood viscosity, vasoconstriction and vasospasm, and decreased bleeding time. Conversely, Omega 3 fatty acids are anti-inflammatory, anti-thrombotic, anti-arrhythmic, hypolipidemic [better blood fat profile] and vasodilatory. These benefits show up in the secondary prevention of coronary heart disease, hypertension [high blood pressure] and Type II [adult onset] diabetes. In some patients, Omega 3 fatty acids ease rheumatoid arthritis, ulcerative colitis, Crohn's disease [an inflammatory bowel disease: thickening of the intestinal wall, frequent obstruction], chronic obstructive pulmonary disease [wheezing, difficulty breathing and chronic cough, usually from smoking], and kidney disease.[183] Omega 3 to Omega 6 ratio also influences neurotransmission and prostaglandin formation, processes vital to maintaining normal brain function.[184]

Flax Omega 3... Most studies report on the fish oils eicosapentaenoic acid [EPA] and docosahexaenoic acid [DHA]. However, alpha-linolenic acid, which is found in leafy green vegetables, flaxseed, rapeseed and walnuts, desaturates and elongates into long-chain EPA and DHA.[183] Unfortunately, shorter chain alpha-linolenic acid does not convert easily to DHA in humans.[185] Only with very large amounts of flaxseed oil do the telltale effects of marine Omega fatty acids appear, e.g. lower blood triglycerides. Plant-derived Omega 3 fatty acids are not equivalent to the marine-based fatty acids in terms of lipoprotein metabolism and effects.[186]

Vitamin E synergy, immune interrelationships... Increased intake of Omega 3 fatty acids without adequate antioxidant protection can result in their free radical peroxidation, with accompanying losses in T-cell mediated function, NK cell activity [natural killer cells: active in spontaneous, non-specific immunity against cancer and viruses, first-line defense against cancer], and macrophage [long-living, large white blood cell; -phage: anything that devours] effectiveness. Simultaneous intake of Omega 3 and antioxidants such as Vitamin E minimize these risks without compromising benefits. Cytokines participate in normal immune response and mediate many biological functions through regulated production. Overproduction contributes to acute and chronic inflammatory, autoimmune and neoplastic [uncontrolled growth of abnormal tissue, i.e. tumor] diseases. In animal and human studies, dietary Omega 3 fatty acids reduce cytokine production,[187] whereas Omega 6 fatty acids increase it.[180]

Cancer... From epidemiological and experimental evidence, Omega 3 fatty acids are protective against breast, colon, and possibly prostate cancers. This chemopreventive activity involves inhibiting neoplastic transformation and cell growth, enhancing apoptosis [gene-directed, programmed cell death], and reducing angiogenicity [new capillary blood vessels]. A common feature here is decreased eicosanoid synthesis from Omega 6 precursors.[188, 189] Weight loss occurs with cancer despite adequate caloric intake; Omega 3 prevents such weight loss in animal models of cancer.[190]

Shark oil and cancer... Shark liver oil has been useful in treating leukemia, and more

recently in preventing radiation sickness from x-ray cancer therapy. Its special active ingredient is a group of ether-linked glycerols known as alkylglycerols. Natural endogenous
[arising from within the organism] alkylglycerols increase within tumor cells, apparently in
an attempt to stop cell growth. Alkylglycerols inhibit activation of protein kinase C [enzyme
for protein phophorylation], an essential step in cell proliferation. Alkylglycerols also stimulate macrophage defenses.[191]

Anti-inflammatory, allergic consequences... The increasing incidence of atopic [aller-
gic, inflammatory] diseases has been linked to dietary changes in polyunsaturated fatty acids
(PUFA). Western diets typically contain up to ten times more linoleic acid Omega 6 than
Omega 3. With linoleic acid metabolism dominating, resulting arachidonic acid-derived
eicosanoids shift the balance of T-helper cells to favor Immunoglobulin E [IgE antibody
proteins, associated with hypersensitivity reaction]. Omega 3 fatty acids will replace Omega
6 in cell membranes and modify this eicosanoid production, thereby favorably impacting
both specific and nonspecific immune responses. Careful dietary manipulation of Omega 3
and Omega 6 can play an important role in managing atopic disease inflammation.[192]
Author's Note: Omega 3's anti-inflammatory power also depends on the Immune ⇌ Stress
activity of each individual fish oil. Compare salmon oil vs. cod liver oil in Figure 5-A.

Asthma... From epidemiological evidence, Omega 3 and antioxidant deficiencies,
excess dietary Omega 6 and sodium, exposure to allergens and tobacco smoke, and lack of
breastfeeding are all factors in asthma.[193] Asthma may arise from a biased Th2 [subset of
helper/inducer T-lymphocytes] immune response. Eicosapentaenoic acid [Omega 3 EPA]
and gamma-linolenic acid [GLA] reduce the levels of inflammatory mediators associated
with asthma.[88]

Arthritis... Dietary Omega 3 supplements consistently reduce morning stiffness and the
number of tender joints in rheumatoid arthritis patients. Benefits do not become apparent
until Omega 3 is ingested for 12 weeks or more, with a daily minimum of 3 grams of eicosapentaenoic [EPA] and docosahexaenoic [DHA] acids. This dosage regimen significantly
decreases leukotriene B(4) [leukotrienes: family of potent hormone-like eicosanoids produced by immune response to antigens; they contribute to defense, inflammation and hypersensitivity; leukotriene B(4) metabolite stimulates cell nucleus function]. In several investigations, rheumatoid arthritis patients on Omega 3 supplements are able to reduce or discontinue use of NSAIDs [nonsteroidal anti-inflammatory drugs] and antirheumatic
drugs.[194, 195]

Gastrointestinal inflammation... Low rates of inflammatory bowel disease [chronic disorder of ulcerative colitis and/or Crohn's disease with abdominal cramping and persistent diarrhea] in Eskimos show epidemiologically the dietary importance of Omega 3 fatty acids on gastrointestinal health.[196]

Cardiovascular disease... Epidemiology reveals an inverse relationship between consumption of fish or other dietary Omega 3 fatty acids and cardiovascular events. In the Diet and Reinfarction Trial, two year overall mortality fell by 29% in survivors of a first myocardial infarction [heart attack] after they began eating fish at least twice a week. With Omega 3 integrated in the diet to resemble a traditional Mediterranean diet, five year cardiovascular mortality after a first myocardial infarction dropped by 70%.[197] Fish consumption does not correlate with coronary heart disease [CHD] mortality in low-risk populations; however, fish consumption of 40-60 grams [1½ to 2 oz.] daily strongly reduces CHD mortality in high-risk populations.[198]

Triglycerides, blood profile... Elevated blood triglycerides (TG), especially after a meal, increase coronary heart disease risk by: (1) generating atherogenic [depositing plaque on artery walls] chylomicrons [lipoprotein droplets, which convey fat from small intestine to blood and lymph], (2) forming low-density lipoproteins [LDL, so-called bad cholesterol] and reducing cardioprotective high-density lipoproteins [HDL or good cholesterol], and (3) activating coagulation factor. Omega 3 fatty acids lower both fasting and postprandial [after a meal] TG concentrations, thereby decreasing LDL formation. Omega 3 intake also enhances chylomicron clearance in arteries and blood vessels.[199] As for coagulation, saturated fats do not prevent cytokine-induced blood platelet adhesion, while fatty acid unsaturation using Omega 6 and, best of all, Omega 3 progressively inhibits platelet adhesion.[181]

Arrhythmia, tachycardia, fibrillation... Omega 3 fish oils reduce ischemic [insufficient blood supply]-induced ventricular tachycardia [rapid heartbeat, usually 150-200 beats per minute] and fibrillation [chaotic ventricle contraction, fatal unless treated immediately] in animal studies. In human studies, Omega 3 decreases the risk of sudden cardiac death. Some human trials suggest that fish oils can prevent ventricular arrhythmias [abnormal heart beat: too slow, too rapid, too early, irregular]. This effect may be independent of Omega 3 anti-atherogenic and anti-thrombotic [thrombosis: blood clot] actions,[200] in that fish fatty acids stabilize electrical activity in cardiac muscle cells by modulating sarcolemma [membrane sheath surrounding muscle fiber] ion channels, thus raising the electrical stimulus threshold and prolonging the refractory period before further stimulation is possible.[201]

DHA and the brain... Docosahexaenoic acid (DHA) is necessary for the growth and functional development of the infant brain. DHA intake improves learning ability and visual acuity, while deficiency is linked to learning deficits, attention deficit hyperactivity disorder, depression, aggressive hostility, fetal alcohol syndrome, cystic fibrosis, phenylketonuria [congenital disease involving impaired early neuron development], and adrenoleukodystrophy [demyelination of central and peripheral nervous system with adrenal insufficiency; subject of the movie "Lorenzo's Oil"]. Over the last half-century, many infants were fed formula totally devoid of DHA and other Omega 3 fatty acids. Meantime, DHA is abundant in mother's milk and in fatty fish such as salmon, tuna and mackerel. Taken up by the brain in preference to other fatty acids, DHA undergoes rapid use and turnover there. In adults, maintaining normal brain function requires DHA. Cognitive decline with aging and Alzheimer disease onset is associated with shortages of brain DHA.[202, 203]

Schizophrenia... Membrane phospholipid metabolism is abnormal in schizophrenic patients, with significant deficits in Omega 6 arachidonic acid and Omega 3 DHA in erythrocyte [red blood cell] membranes. Dietary supplementation to modify these membrane fatty acids improves schizophrenia and tardive dyskinesia (TD) [involuntary, irreversible neurological impairment of muscles; can include rolling of tongue, twitching of facial and other small muscles] symptoms. In general, schizophrenics who ingest more Omega 3 fatty acids have fewer severe symptoms.[204, 205]

Bipolar disorder... Substantial direct and indirect evidence now supports Omega 3 fatty acids in the treatment of bipolar disorder [periods of mania alternating with depression].[206]

VITAMIN A

Vitamin A is necessary for resistance to and recovery from infection. Vitamin A kills bacteria – an antibiotic that cannot be defeated! It also battles viruses and cancer, and generally improves immune and lymphatic responses. Supplementation with 10,000 IU per day will prevent infections from ever getting a foothold at their point of attack, the wet mucous linings of your body. Of course, each type of bacteria, virus or pathogen as well as each exposure has its own virulence; high exposures require much more Vitamin A. Eyes too need this vitamin to maintain their health. Night blindness is a common symptom of Vitamin A deficiency, and xerophthalmia (dry eye, no tears), the result of severe Vitamin A deprivation, is the major cause of blindness in children worldwide.

NOTE: As explained earlier in the beta-carotene section, Vitamin A
and beta-carotene and have higher International Units than Vitamin E.

These large numbers, however, do not indicate a relatively larger dose, as 1 IU of dl-alpha-tocopherol = 1 milligram, while 1 IU of Vitamin A (retinol) = 0.3 microgram or 0.0003 milligram. 10,000 IU of Vitamin A sounds like a huge scary amount, but actually it's only 3 mg!

Vitamin A toxicity is not a serious problem, only fear of it is. 100,000 IU daily can be taken for a month or longer, especially if *these troops are being lost in battle.* The lone safety exception is 10,000 to 30,000 IU Vitamin A maximum per day during pregnancy, as evidenced in the medical literature review below. Fear, that darkroom where negatives are developed, cannot withstand the light of the scientific medical literature. Each year in the United States, only ten to fifteen cases of Vitamin A toxicity are reported, usually at dosages greater than 100,000 IU. Possible symptoms include cracked lips at the corners of the mouth, dry itchy skin, tender bones, joint pain, hair loss, blurred vision and headaches. These symptoms quickly reverse when the vitamin is withdrawn.

A daily supplement of 10,000 IU Vitamin A is essential for adults against a host of silent invaders including pneumonia and meningitis, with correspondingly lesser amounts requisite for children against ear and other infections. Dry Vitamin A supplements, also known as "Allergy A," are gentler and easier to absorb than liquid capsules and appropriate for prevention. Moreover, they neither count as an Omega 3 dose nor influence Immune ⇌ Stress equilibrium. For aggressive intervention, take fish oil Vitamin A (liquid in a soft-gel capsule); it combines Omega 3 power with Immune ← Stress action. Overall, Vitamin A delivers inexpensive, natural defense with no side effects.

Review of the Medical Literature

Discovery timeline and overview... Vitamin A was discovered in 1913. In animal models and case reports, deficiency was soon associated with infection, stunted growth and ocular changes including xerophthalmia [dry eye, deficiency of tears], which leads to blindness. Eye consequences dominated clinical interest until the early 1980s, when a risk study uncovered a strong link between the severity of Vitamin A deficiency and respiratory and diarrhea infections and, most dramatically, death from infections. In Africa, hospital trials of Vitamin A in children with measles showed a consistent 50% drop in measles-associated mortality. Worldwide estimates are that Vitamin A supplementation could reduce childhood (1-5 years old) mortality in deficient populations by 35%, and prevent 1 to 3 million deaths annually.[207]

Natural Vitamin A activity... Naturally occurring retinoids, Vitamin A (retinol) and its active metabolites, are necessary for resistance to and recovery from infection, and for human reproduction and growth. Retinoids are also crucial to vision, hematopoiesis [formation of blood], bones, skin and controlling epithelial [surface tissue lining] cell differentiation [maturation] in the respiratory, digestive, nervous and immune systems. Retinoid activity begins in the human embryo soon after conception and continues throughout life. Many metabolites become ligands [molecules that bind to a receptor], which activate specific transcription factors and thereby gene expression.[208]

Dietary sources and metabolism... The two main dietary sources of Vitamin A/retinol are poorly bioavailable carotenoids from plant foods and easily absorbed retinyl palmitate from animal-based foods. Blood retinol concentrations are tightly regulated, probably through retinol-binding protein (RBP) [carrier responsible for retinol transport] synthesis in the liver, although infection and hormonal factors such as oral contraceptives can alter normal homeostasis. RBP-retinol complex efficiently delivers retinol to all tissues. This mechanism, however, can be bypassed with very high Vitamin A doses. In addition, some retinyl esters may reach tissues through chylomicrons [lipoprotein droplets, which convey fat from small intestine to blood and lymph]. High-dose Vitamin A therapy quickly corrects nutritional deficiency, but not without the possibility of toxic symptoms including teratogenicity [birth defects, see below].[209]

Measles and blindness... In children with measles [acute infection of morbillivirus], Vitamin A deficiency is strongly associated with increased morbidity [disease incidence] and mortality. Vitamin A supplementation reduces the severity of the illness, complications and mortality.[210, 211] Xerophthalmia [dry eye] is the major cause of blindness in children worldwide,[212] and responsible for 50% or more of all measles-associated blindness. Xerophthalmia is recognized now as a late manifestation of severe Vitamin A deficiency.[213]

Retinitis pigmentosa (RP)... is characterized by early onset of night blindness and progressive loss of visual field. Actually, RP is a group of hereditary retinol dystrophies [disorders due to defective or faulty nutrition], which affect rod photoreceptor cell function. Underlying defects develop in the daily renewal and shedding of photoreceptor outer segments, visual transduction mechanisms [converting a signal from one form to another, sensory cells convert light into nerve impulses], and/or retinol metabolism.[214, 215] Vitamin A supplementation is successful in treating common forms of retinitis pigmentosa,[216] and may increase the visual field. Another nutritional factor, lutein [a carotenoid, see Table 3-3] can bring short-term vision improvements in RP, especially for blue-eyed persons, and in AMD [age-related macular degeneration].[217]

Diabetes... Plasma Vitamin A/retinol and its carrier protein, retinol-binding protein (RBP), are abnormally low in insulin-dependent diabetics [Type I, often called juvenile diabetes], but not in non-insulin dependent diabetics [Type II, or adult onset]. Uncontrolled diabetes triggers this dysfunction in Vitamin A metabolism, which insulin treatment reverses.[218]

Infection prevention... Vitamin A is necessary for resistance to and recovery from infection.[208] Deficiency results in multiple derangements in the response to infection, notably altered antibody responses and greater epithelial [surface tissue lining/mucus surfaces] damage. Vitamin A-deficient epithelia may allow penetration of bacteria and other agents, bringing on infection.[219] Neutrophils [strong against bacteria] are the most prevalent white blood cell in circulation, and first line defense against invading microorganisms. Retinoids play a crucial role in neutrophil differentiation.[220] Overall, Vitamin A deficiency causes immunodeficiency through changes in mucus surfaces, impaired antibody responses to protein antigen [any invader eliciting an antibody response] challenges, and altered T- and B-cells and lymphocyte subpopulations. Vitamin A and its metabolites restore these immune subsystems and responses. Furthermore, this vitamin increases lymphocyte numbers against mitogens [promoting cell division, e.g. tumor] and inhibits healthy cell apoptosis [gene-directed, programmed cell death]. Epidemiological, immunological and molecular studies of the last decade evidence the central role of Vitamin A in immune defense. In at least 12 clinical trials where Vitamin A deficiency is endemic, supplementation in children reduces the severe morbidity and mortality of infectious diseases, particularly measles.[221-225]

Fetal development... All vertebrate embryos require Vitamin A/retinol to fulfill the developmental program encoded in their genome. In mammals, maternal homeostasis minimizes any variation in retinol concentrations reaching the embryo, as embryonic tissues are especially vulnerable to deficiency and excess, both of which cause abnormalities in many systems.[226, 227] Vitamin A metabolite retinoic acid regulates gene transcription through a class of nucleus receptors: retinoic acid receptors (RARs) and retinoid-X-receptors (RXRs). RARs play a fundamental role in early skeletal development. Improper RAR expression impedes chondrogenesis [cartilage formation], while promoting ectopic [abnormally positioned within the body] structures.[228] RXR alpha develops heart and eye structures.[226] Posterior hindbrain formation requires retinoids, as do associated structures and certain groups of neurons and neural crest cells [embryonic cells that become several different adult cell types].[229] Vitamin A is crucial in fetal lung development,[230] kidney vasculature development, and nephron [kidney filtering and excretion] endowment at birth. Fetal Vitamin A status may be largely responsible for the variations in nephron endowment present in the general population, and a major factor in adult chronic kidney disease and hypertension [high blood pressure].[231]

Vitamin A dosage during pregnancy… Excessive Vitamin A intake, like Vitamin A deficiency, remains an unresolved public health concern with respect to pregnancy and possible teratogenicity [birth defects]. For ethical reasons, human pregnancy intervention studies are not feasible. However, endogenous [arising from within the organism] plasma Vitamin A metabolites from one study of pregnant women with no fetal malformations were compared to trial data in non-pregnant women ingesting Vitamin A supplements of 4,000, 10,000 and 30,000 IU daily over three weeks. Even at 30,000 IU daily, peak plasma Vitamin A metabolites were in the range or slightly above the endogenous plasma levels found in the pregnant women with no fetal malformations. In another trial involving pregnant cynomolgus monkeys, NOAEL (no observed adverse effect level) was 7500 IU per kg of body weight, while LOAEL (lowest observed adverse effect level) was 20,000 IU per kg before developmental toxicity. Projecting these data, 30,000 IU per day should not be teratogenic in humans.[232] Still, in a single epidemiological study, supplementations greater than 10,000 IU per day were associated with birth malformations. In summary, no study finds adverse effects for Vitamin A supplementation at 10,000 IU daily, and 30,000 IU daily supports only very low risk.[233]

Synthetic Vitamin A toxicity… Synthetic retinoids [used in dermatology and cancer treatment, below] are Category X, strictly contraindicated during pregnancy because they are linked directly to human teratogenicity. Furthermore, owing to their long half-life elimination, synthetic retinoids require effective contraception for at least 2 years after treatment discontinuation. Common drug names are isotretinoin, etretinate, and etretin.[234] Half-life elimination is 10-20 hours for isotretinoin, 80-175 days for etretinate, and 2-4 days for trans-acitretin, though trans-acitretin partially decays to etretinate.[235]

Fetal alcohol syndrome… Interaction between ethanol and Vitamin A may be one mechanism behind fetal alcohol syndrome. This hypothesis [proposed, not proven] centers on these known facts: ethanol ingestion alters Vitamin A metabolism and its tissue distribution in adults; many similarities exist between fetal alcohol syndrome and birth defects from Vitamin A toxicity and deficiency; and retinoic acid mediates embryogenesis and differentiation.[236]

HIV transmission... Vitamin A deficiency, common among human immunodeficiency virus (HIV)-infected pregnant women, is associated with greater HIV-1 mother-to-child transmission and infant mortality. Vitamin A-deficient transmission may occur as a result of impaired mother and infant immune responses, placental and vaginal contamination, and increased HIV viral load in blood and breastmilk.[237] Breastfeeding is estimated to cause one-third to one-half of mother-to-child HIV-1 transmissions worldwide. HIV-1 DNA is found in over 50% of breast milk samples, and this is linked to Vitamin A deficiency and CD4 [helper T-cell; target of HIV] depletion.[238] HIV-infected individuals taking either very low or very high Vitamin A and beta-carotene (Vitamin A precursor) have higher rates of disease progression than those using intermediate intakes.[239]

Infants, breastfeeding... Deficiency or excess of Vitamin A in lactating women or their infants can adversely affect the health of both. Born with low Vitamin A stores, infants rely on maternal Vitamin A in breast milk to meet their needs.[240] For preterm and very low birth-weight infants, Vitamin A supplementation reduces morbidity and mortality, particularly the risk of developing chronic lung disease. Vitamin A maintains respiratory epithelial [surface tissue lining] cell integrity and enables normal lung growth.[241] Vitamin A also enhances B-cell function in immature immune systems,[242] and is an important factor in preventing and ameliorating diarrhea and growth failure in infants and children. [243]

Schizophrenia... Retinoid dysregulation may play a significant role in schizophrenia. Three independent lines of evidence support this hypothesis: (1) congenital anomalies resulting from retinoid dysfunction are similar to those found in schizophrenics and their relatives, (2) loci [gene positions on a chromosome] linked to schizophrenia are also the loci of retinoid cascade [series of reactions from one trigger] genes, and (3) retinoic acid regulates dopamine [neurotransmitter; helps to regulate movement and emotion] D2 receptor activation and numerous candidate schizophrenia genes.[244, 245]

Acne, psoriasis... Oral retinoids have transformed the treatment of acne, psoriasis and severe disorders of keratinization [keratin: tough, insoluble protein; the outmost layer of skin] now prevalent in children and adolescents.[246] Natural retinoids with the best therapeutic effects are Vitamin A [retinol], retinaldehyde, retinoic acid and all-trans-retinoic acid, which is the prototype for many synthetic Vitamin A derivatives.[247] Since their introduction in the 1970s, oral synthetic retinoids have proved effective in treating psoriasis.[248]

Skin and sun... Sun radiation causes dermatoheliosis [abnormal structural and functional changes within the skin], which manifests after age fifty when general regressive changes in the body overtake the skin. Vitamin A metabolites are crucial in keratin [the outmost layer of skin] cell growth and differentiation, as they possess hormone-like and morphogenetic [structural development/maturation] activity. By acting on epidermis, dermis and sebaceous [pertaining to or secreting fat] gland structures and systemic immunoreactivity, natural Vitamin A and its derivatives, along with several thousand synthetic products mimicking its chemical structure and biological effects, are effective for various skin disorders including dermatoheliosis.[249] Topical [applied to the skin] all-trans-retinoic acid can repair and possibly prevent skin sun-aging by modulating collagen [fibrous protein of connective tissue] synthesis in the dermis.[250]

Pre-cancers and cancers... Vitamin A is prophylactic [preventative] against various epithelial [surface tissue lining] cancers.[249] Vitamin A and other retinoids, beta-carotene, and possibly Vitamin E reduce oral pre-cancerous lesions. Retinoids also reduce pre-cancerous skin, lung and cervical lesions,[251] suppress oral and lung carcinogenesis in animal models, and prevent second primary tumor development in head, neck and lung cancer patients by changing the gene expression that regulates their cell growth and differentiation. Retinoic acid receptors (RARs: -alpha, -beta, and -gamma) and retinoid X receptors (RXRs: -alpha, -beta, and -gamma) mediate these effects on gene expression.[252, 253] In one study of synthetic retinoid 13-cis-retinoic acid (13cRA), second primary tumors of head and neck cell carcinoma developed in only 4% of 49 13cRA patients compared to 24% of 51 placebo patients.[254] Although the most studied chemopreventive drug against head and neck cancers, 13cRA unfortunately exhibits considerable toxicity.[255] Another synthetic Vitamin A analogue, acyclic retinoid, arrests second primary liver tumor development in cirrhosis patients.[256] Combining retinoids with cytokines [non-antibody proteins/signaling molecules of the immune system; include interleukins, lymphokines, interferons and TNF (tumor necrosis factor)] can significantly improve the efficiency of cancer therapy.[249]

Leukemia... Retinoids achieve high remission rates in acute promyelocytic [bone marrow] leukemia (APL) patients, but without cure. They rapidly improve the hemostatic profile, and with no aplastic [anemia] phase.[257] By combining all-trans-retinoic acid (ATRA) and chemotherapy, over 90% of APL patients achieve complete remission; 75% are cured.[258] Leukemia is a deregulated state of cell proliferation, differentiation and apoptosis induced by gene alterations including chromosomal translocations. ATRA is the first successful oncoprotein-directed therapy [onco- 'tumor forming'].[259]

Vascular disease... Retinoids favorably affect cell migration and proliferation, tissue remodeling, inflammation, fibrinolysis [dissolution of fibrin, the insoluble protein in blood and the end product of coagulation] and coagulation, and apoptosis, all of which are factors in vascular disease. Retinoids reduce experimental vessel wall narrowing from atherosclerosis, post-balloon angioplasty injury and bypass graft failure.[260]

Vitamin A and iron... Vitamin A favorably influences iron absorption, probably forming a Vitamin A-iron chelate.[261] Iron supplementation exacerbates existing infections, as bacteria also utilize iron in their metabolism and effectively compete for the iron in circulation. Accordingly, Vitamin A status must be adequate during iron supplementation.[262]

Parathyroid... Vitamin D [ahead] is an important regulator of parathyroid function and growth; however, retinoids also act on parathyroid cells.[263]

Bones... Excessive Vitamin A intake is associated with increased risk of hip fractures in humans.[264] Author's Note: Vitamin A and Vitamin D are natural antagonists within Immune ⇌ Stress equilibrium.

Safety experience... Each year in the USA, approximately ten to fifteen cases of Vitamin A toxicity occur, usually at doses greater than 100,000 IU daily.[178] Hepatotoxicity [hepato- prefix meaning 'liver'] has developed at Vitamin A doses greater than 50,000 IU daily, and 25,000 IU daily can elevate liver enzymes.[265] Synthetic Vitamin A derivatives, used principally in dermatology, evidence significant toxicity after long-term administration, including arthritis, bone abnormalities similar to seronegative spondyloarthropathy [arthritic inflammation of vertebrae without antibodies], diffuse idiopathic skeletal hyperostosis [excessive growth of bony tissue], myopathies [muscle diseases] and vasculitis [vessel inflammation].[266] See also earlier references,[232-235] regarding pregnancy or even its possibility.

VITAMIN D

Vitamin D is necessary for calcium absorption and healthy bone formation. Children especially need high calcium intakes for growing bones, and milk is the perfect answer, supplying calcium and 'D' together. 400 IU of Vitamin D daily prevents rickets (bow legs, its most recognizable sign) in young bones. For postmenopausal women susceptible to osteoporosis, calcium and Vitamin D (400-800 IU) supplements can maintain bone density and reduce the likelihood of hip fractures. The calcium source in these supplements should not be calcium oxide or calcium carbonate, which are poorly absorbed. Highly touted coral calcium is mostly ineffective calcium carbonate. Instead, use chelated calcium bound to an organic molecule, such as calcium citrate or an amino acid calcium complex.

Vitamin D nourishes Primary Stress Function too, not just its dependent body system of bones. This is evidenced in the following medical literature review by the vitamin's ability to reduce inflammation and immune overreactions and by the steroidal action of Vitamin D hormone. The strong link between Vitamin D and multiple sclerosis (MS) also suggests that the vitamin contributes to Primary Stress Function health. Basically, Vitamin D becomes anti-stress Vitamin D hormone and works with cortisol, aldosterone, and testosterone or estrogen hormones to maintain function in this part of the adrenal cortex.

Vitamin D is the most toxic of the fatty acid vitamins, with infants and children mainly at risk. The medical literature reports toxicity levels and effects. Symptoms can include weakness, nausea, headaches, diarrhea, vomiting, bone loss and calcification of soft tissues. Symptoms reverse when the vitamin is withdrawn.

Most people don't need extra Vitamin D. Sunshine is a good natural source; ultraviolet rays from the sun convert oils on the skin into this vitamin. Milk and dairy products are fortified with 'D' and fish oils contain it.

Vitamin D exists in three structural forms. Ultraviolet radiation synthesizes D1. D2, also known as calciferol, is found in fish oils and D3, cholecalciferol, in fish liver oils. These minor variations do not affect the vitamin's therapeutic effects. Also, Vitamin D is available as a dry non-fish "Allergy D" supplement, which aids calcium absorption without stronger Omega 3 'D' Immune → Stress action.

Review of the Medical Literature

Discovery and metabolism… The discovery of Vitamin D during 1919-1924 led to the elimination of rickets [below], a major medical problem at the time. In the 1960s, Vitamin D metabolism from vitamin to hormone was explained: Vitamin D is modified by 25-hydroxylation in the liver, after which the kidneys change 1 alpha-hydroxylation [1 alpha(OH) D3] into natural Vitamin D hormone 1 alpha,25-dihydroxyvitamin D3 [1,25-(OH)2D3]. This feedback-regulated metabolic pathway is the major endocrine system overseeing plasma calcium and phosphorus levels, and bone mass and health.[267] Natural Vitamin D hormone, also called calcitriol, controls parathyroid gland [Chapter 9] growth and suppresses parathyroid hormone (PTH) synthesis and secretion, which strongly promotes intestinal calcium absorption and bone formation.[268]

Meeting needs... Vitamin D fortification of milk and other dairy products has been successful in preventing rickets in children; however, its impact on adult health is less satisfactory. Unrecognized Vitamin D deficiency, common in the elderly, produces secondary hyperparathyroidism,[269] with high plasma PTH and resulting bone resorption [dissolution into blood],[270] particularly cortical [cortex: outer region] bone loss and increased hip fracture risk.[269]

Deficiency mechanisms... Three types of Vitamin D deficiency can occur: (1) primary deficiency of the parent compound, Vitamin D itself; (2) a deficiency of 1,25-(OH)2D3 [hormone] from faulty kidney production; and (3) resistance to 1,25-(OH)2D3 activity due to decreased responsiveness of target tissues. Each of these dysfunctions increases with age and has been implicated in intestinal calcium malabsorption, secondary hyperparathyroidism and osteoporosis.[270]

Correcting therapies... Two Vitamin D replacement therapies are effective: Vitamin D supplementation and active Vitamin D hormone [1,25-(OH)2D3] or analog [structural similar compound] therapy. 1000 IU of Vitamin D daily can correct a primary deficiency, while 1,25-(OH)2D3 deficiency or resistance often requires a Vitamin D analog [see psoriasis and postmenopausal osteoporosis, below] to rectify high plasma PTH and calcium malabsorption, and restore bone health.[270]

Pregnancy... Vitamin D safeguards mother and fetus from dysfunctions in calcium and phosphorus metabolism.[271] Supplementing 400 IU Vitamin D daily is recommended throughout pregnancy.[272] 800-1000 IU daily, the current recommendation in Europe, is probably too high if extra minerals are also provided. In very low birth-weight infants, bone disease is found with increasing frequency; notably radiological evidence of rickets is present in 55% of infants with births weights below 1000 grams [2.2 lbs] and in 23% of infants below 1500 grams, as well as bone fractures in 24% of infants below 1500 grams. Causes are inadequate calcium and phosphorus, Vitamin D deficiency, certain drugs and aluminum loading.[273]

Fetal brain, schizophrenia... Vitamin D acts on the central nervous system through its steroidal hormone action and various proteins such as nerve growth factor. Low maternal Vitamin D may adversely affect fetal brain development, increasing the risk of adult-onset schizophrenia in affected offspring. This hypothesis [proposed, not proven] explains schizophrenia associations with prenatal famine, winter births, higher incidence in urban births than in rural births, and dark-skinned immigrants to cold climates.[274] Lack of sunlight is directly linked to schizophrenia; an explanation is UV radiation on the skin synthesizes natural Vitamin D, which is then absorbed into the body.[267]

Rickets... Neonatal [the first four weeks after birth] rickets develops only in infants born to severe osteomalacia [softening of the bones with pain, weakness and bone fragility] mothers.[275] For infants eight months to two years old, the clinical features of emerging rickets are progressive leg bowing [its most recognized sign], poor linear growth, seizures and abnormal plasma calcium and phosphorus compounds. Beyond six months of age, breast milk may not contain enough Vitamin D to protect infants from rickets, especially those dark-skinned or living in cloudy northern climates.[276] While exposure to sunlight may maintain adequate Vitamin D stores, supplementation with 400 IU daily from birth to two years old is recommended in all breast-fed infants to insure against rickets.[277] Infants on vegetarian and macrobiotic [found in the region, usually vegetarianism] diets have a high incidence of rickets, and definitely need Vitamin D and calcium supplements. The Vitamin D requirement for term infants is between 100 and 400 IU daily.[278] A 400 IU supplement is safe and appropriate.[277] Note: Vitamin D has been added to commercial milk in the United States since the 1930s to prevent rickets.

Psoriasis... Vitamin D regulates cell growth and differentiation [maturation] in various tissues including the skin. In psoriasis lesions, inflammation triggers hyper-proliferation and impaired differentiation of epidermal keratinocytes [keratin: the outermost layer of skin]. Vitamin D and its analogs suppress this abnormal growth and stimulate terminal differentiation.[279] Most skin cells have a Vitamin D receptor. Vitamin D analogs have a higher therapeutic index and/or a greater degree of target selectivity than natural Vitamin D;[280] and employing natural Vitamin D hormone is not possible in most cases because of its potent calcemic activity [too much 'D' hormone suppresses PTH, which greatly increases calcium absorption, resulting in hypercalcemia, excessive calcium in the blood].[281] Over the last decade, topically-applied [on the skin] Vitamin D analogues have revolutionized psoriasis treatment by inhibiting cutaneous inflammation and epidermal proliferation, while enhancing normal keratinization.[282] Two FDA-approved drug analogues are calcipotriol for psoriasis and 19-nor-1,25(OH)2D2 for secondary hyperparathyroidism.[281]

Immune... Vitamin D plays a important role in the immune system, particularly T-cell mediated immunity.[283] Vitamin D hormone [1,25-(OH)2D3] is a natural internal immunoregulator. Through feedback signaling, macrophages [long-living, large white blood cells; -phage: anything that devours] can synthesize D-hormone and reduce immunological overreactions.[284] D-hormone supplementation also exerts this immunosuppressive activity.[285] In animal models, 1,25-(OH)2D3 prevents or markedly suppresses rheumatoid arthritis, lupus [systemic lupus erythematosus: autoimmune, inflammatory disease of connective tissue with skin eruptions, joint pain, kidney damage], experimental autoimmune encephalomyelitis [EAE, see multiple sclerosis below], inflammatory bowel disease [chronic disorder of ulcerative colitis and/or Crohn's disease with abdominal cramping and persistent diarrhea] and Type I diabetes.[283, 285] In humans, 1,25-(OH)2D3 exhibits immunomodulatory activity in scleroderma [hardening of the skin], antiproliferative activity in psoriasis, and antineoplastic [neoplastic: uncontrolled growth of abnormal tissue] activity in prostate cancer [next paragraph].[285] 1,25-(OH)2D3 complex immunoregulatory mechanisms involve inhibiting cytokines [non-antibody proteins/signaling molecules of the immune system], TNF-alpha [tumor necrosis factor alpha: a pro-inflammatory protein], IL-1 [Interleukin 1 activates/potentiates both B- and T-cells], IL-6 [stimulates B-cells], and importantly IL-12 [released by macrophages; initiator of cell-mediated immunity T-system]. At the cell level, 1,25-(OH)2D3 decreases Th1 helper cell [Th1 cells: subset of helper/inducer T-lymphocytes] expression directly or indirectly by inhibiting IL-12 from monocytes [precursor of macrophages, mediator of nonspecific immunity] and increases Th2 helper cells, which generate bone protective cytokines such as IL-4 and IL-10.[284]

Cancer... Prostate cancer is considered a male sex hormone dependent disease; however, many other hormones including 1,25-(OH)2D3 influence its growth and differentiation. Epidemiological evidence shows that 1,25-(OH)2D3 deficiency may be factor in prostate cancer genesis,[286] and in the development of other cancers. Specifically, the geographic distribution of colon cancer coincides with the historic distribution of rickets. Furthermore, colon cancer rates are inversely proportional to calcium intake. These findings suggest that 800 IU of Vitamin D daily and approximately 1,800 mg of calcium daily may prevent many colon cancers. Breast cancer death rates for white women rise with distance from the equator, as does rickets. 800 IU daily of Vitamin D may increase breast cancer survival rates.[287]

Multiple sclerosis (MS)... Intake of 1,25-(OH)2D3 completely prevents experimental autoimmune encephalomyelitis (EAE) [brain and spinal cord inflammation], a widely accepted mouse model of human multiple sclerosis. Besides these EAE data, circumstantial evidence is compelling that Vitamin D protects against MS. Vitamin D deficiency and MS have the same striking geographic distribution, nearly zero at the equator and increasing dramatically with latitude in both hemispheres, as well as two geographic anomalies, one in Switzerland with low MS rates at high altitudes and high MS rates at low altitudes, and one in Norway with low MS rates along the coast and high MS rates inland. In Switzerland, ultraviolet (UV) light intensity, greater at high altitudes, results in more Vitamin D synthesis on the skin, thereby accounting for lower MS rates. On the Norwegian coast, fish rich in

Vitamin D are consumed at high rates.[288]

Kidney failure and resulting hyperparathyroidism… Secondary hyperparathyroidism is a universal complication of chronic kidney failure [lack of Vitamin D hormone 1,25(OH)2D3 synthesis in the kidney]. Parathyroid gland hyperplasia [enlargement due to abnormal multiplication of cells] often occurs in these patients. Another factor, out-of-control phosphorus further increases plasma PTH and induces hyperplasia. Natural 1,25-(OH)2D3 hormone, calcium and phosphorus are all crucial in preventing secondary hyperparathyroidism and parathyroid hyperplasia.[289] Unfortunately in many cases, administration of 1,25(OH)2D3 causes hypercalcemia; however, several new analogs retain D-hormone's suppression of parathyroid activity, but with less calcemic action.[290]

Cardiovascular and hyperparathyroidism… Vitamin D and PTH affect cardiac and vascular functioning. With chronic kidney failure, resulting hyperparathyroidism and altered Vitamin D status contribute to increased cardiovascular disease and hypertension [high blood pressure] in these patients.[291] One mechanism here is calcification of atherosclerotic [depositing on artery walls] plaque lesions. Plaque calcification is an active homeostatic process similar to osteogenesis [bone forming].[292]

Osteoporosis… involves reduced bone mass, microarchitectural deterioration, and increased bone fragility and fractures. This disorder is widespread, especially in older men and women.[293] Diabetics show greater frequency of osteoporosis than age- and sex-matched healthy individuals,[294] and patients receiving glucocorticoid [cortisone, prednisone and other steroids] therapy are also at increased risk.[295] Beginning with menopause, women undergo accelerated bone loss,[293] with 40% of women over age fifty expected to experience osteoporosis.[296] Good nutrition, appropriate calcium and Vitamin D intakes, regular menstrual cycles and exercise are all key in achieving peak bone mass and preventing osteoporosis. Fracture risk factors include low body weight, a history of fractures, osteoporosis in the family, and smoking.[293] Osteoporosis hip, spine and wrist fractures, and the mortality resulting from hip fractures, justify prevention strategies. Optimal management requires maximizing peak bone mass in early adulthood and preventing rapid bone loss after the menopause.[296]

Osteoporosis treatment… Pharmacological and non-pharmacological interventions are effective in treating osteoporosis. Fluoride drugs stimulate bone formation.[297] Used in osteoporosis treatment for 30 years, fluoride salts possess anabolic action on structural bone, but safety and efficacy are still debated because of frequent side effects, particularly bone pain and dyspepsia [indigestion].[298] Calcium, Vitamin D and its metabolites including natural 1,25-(OH)2D3 hormone, bisphosphonates and estrogen hormone replacement therapy inhibit bone resorption [dissolution into blood].[297] Regardless of any prescription osteoporosis regimen, postmenopausal women should obtain 400 IU to 800 IU of Vitamin D and 1000 mg to 1500 mg of calcium daily, and perform weight-bearing exercise, for example walking every day for 20 to 30 minutes or one hour three times a week.[299]

Steroid use and bone loss... Corticosteroids/glucocortiocoids [cortisone, prednisone and other steroids] are widely prescribed for chronic inflammatory diseases.[300] Corticosteroids reduce intestinal calcium absorption and increase kidney calcium excretion, resulting in compensatory PTH release and bone loss. Corticosteroids also suppress D-hormone receptor expression, osteoblast [immature, bone-forming cell] function, and the favorable action of sex hormones and growth factors on bone formation.[284] Rapid bone loss occurs in the first one to two years of high-dose corticosteroid therapy. These patients need preventative treatment with active Vitamin D metabolites and/or bisphosphonates.[300]

Crohn's disease... Bone demineralization, usually osteoporosis, occurs in 20-60% of Crohn's disease [an inflammatory bowel disease: thickening of the intestinal wall, frequent obstruction] patients. Causes include corticosteroid therapy and reduced calcium and Vitamin D intake from loss of appetite, lactose intolerance and malabsorption.[301]

Toxicity... By accelerating intestinal calcium absorption, excessive Vitamin D produces marked and prolonged hypercalcemia. This toxic state continues for several months after withdrawal of Vitamin D, whereas hypercalcemia from 1 alpha(OH) D3 [precursor] or 1,25 (OH)2D3 [natural hormone] subsides after one week.[302] The maximum permissible Vitamin D dose for children is 800 IU daily. High doses are fraught with hypervitaminosis D danger,[303] specifically the possibility of Williams syndrome, which is idiopathic infantile hypercalcemia (IIH). An epidemic of mild IIH occurred in post-WWII Great Britain and Europe from excessive supplementation in government-supplied infant foods. Severe IIH causes mental deficiency, elfin face [elf like; dwarf], and supravalvular aortic stenosis [narrowing of aortic valve, obstructed blood flow].[304]

OVERVIEW

Fatty acids are a key element of a complete nutritional program. Medical science tells us that fatty acids are essential to cell membranes, becoming part of them, maintaining their fluidity and stability, and protecting them against free radicals and oxidative stress. These good fats also serve as cell fuel, and as precursors to biological active compounds such as prostaglandins. They are necessary for the formation of new tissue, for normal brain development and functioning, and in preventing schizophrenia and Alzheimer's disease. Fatty acids heal body tissues, most noticeably skin acne, eczema and psoriasis. They nourish and protect the nervous system especially its insulating myelin sheath, save bones from childhood rickets and osteoporosis in old age, and safeguard vision against childhood xerophthalmia, adult night blindness, cataracts, retinitis pigmentosa (RP), age-related macular degeneration (AMD) and diabetic retinopathy. Fatty acids kill bacteria, viruses, fungi and cancer, and alleviate the autoimmune/inflammatory attack of rheumatoid arthritis, multiple sclerosis, lupus, Crohn's disease and many other chronic disorders. Through various mechanisms including inhibiting LDL cholesterol oxidation, fatty acids improve atherosclerosis and cardiovascular disease. Truly a health prescription for life!

Fatty acids lubricate all endocrine parts, and cells and tissues in general. 1X usage maintains health for a normal lifestyle; 2X overcomes past deprivation and rebuilds fatty acid health. Using Figure 5-A, adjust 1X maintenance and 2X stimulation and rebuilding of health to satisfy Energy, Healing, Stress and Immune needs exactly. Count Omega 6 and Omega 3 oils separately, each can be taken to 2X. Avoid 3X or overdose. Fatty acids are very tolerant of missed days and doses, but rebuilding health demands more discipline.

A simple plan can significantly alter the course of your health and life for the better – get as much good fat and as little bad fat as you can! Ingest only life-sustaining natural fatty acids, not adulterated partially hydrogenated and trans-fatty acids. Vitamin E and other powerful antioxidants eliminate oxidative stress, thereby turning bad stress into good stress and slowing aging. Omega 6 EFAs engineer Energy and Healing, while Omega 3 powers Stress and Immune systems. Most Americans have a 10:1 to 25:1 Omega 6 to Omega 3 input ratio. Good health requires 2:1 ratio at a minimum. A prescription of Omega 3 fish and seafood every day would largely eliminate the current pandemic in stress and immune diseases.

***

6. TRACE METALS

Trace metals are one of the five raw materials that your Energy, Healing, Stress and Immune functions and systems need to make all their hormones and other end products and to perform properly under all circumstances. Unlike B vitamins and fatty acids, which require daily replenishment, take metals only occasionally and then in small or *trace* amounts to fill up metal reservoirs. These are storage reserves in the liver, bones, teeth and elsewhere, from which your body makes withdrawals as needed.

This chapter presents trace metals for the entire endocrine system, as they fit together beautifully into one mosaic. Metals facilitate endocrine tasks by becoming: (1) metalloenzymes in the functioning of a gland or organ; (2) catalysts, which are necessary to but not part of a chemical reaction; or (3) special messengers, complex organic molecules that travel between endocrine parts or to every cell.

As a further introduction, the following definition of terms is important.

Metal? All metals are elements and listed ahead in Table 6-1, "The Periodic Table of Elements." All elements, however, are not metals. Imperfectly defined, metal elements are solid, crystalline, ductile (can be worked into different shapes), conduct electricity and have a unique surface luster. Common examples include gold, silver, aluminum cans, steel (mostly the element iron), and brass (copper and zinc together). As you can see, combinations of metal elements are routinely called metals too, although technically alloys. But enough of strict definition, what's important is the role pure metal elements play in human nutrition. Nature chose many of them for specific tasks within the endocrine system, just as she chose strong roles for B vitamins and fatty acids.

Metal vs. Mineral—What's the difference? It is a distinction without a difference in terms of WHAT YOU WANT, metals inside of you doing their job. However, in terms of WHAT YOU GET, the difference is enormous. Most metals occur in nature as inorganic (not carbon-based) compounds, typically metals bound to oxygen such as metal oxides and carbonates, which we call minerals or, in their aggregate form, rocks. These are very stable compounds, and not easily digested and absorbed by humans. Instead, what your body needs are metals bound to organic (life's) molecules; such complex carbon-based metal compounds are readily absorbed and put to work. These employable metals are referred to as "chelated."

Unfortunately, in many metal/mineral supplements from the pharmaceutical industry and other producers, you still get inorganic metal oxides or carbonates that, while purer, are not very different from ground-up rock. When we were kids, we could eat rocks and maybe get 10% of the metals out of them. As adults, this absorption is near zero! Common usage of the terms "metal" and "mineral" remains fuzzy. The key point to remember is to look for and use only trace metals bound to organic molecules, i.e. chelated metals.

NATURAL MANAGEMENT

Like amino acids and B vitamins, trace metals act together in unison or not at all. They fulfill their tasks within the framework of impossibly complex equilibriums and interactions. Only nature fully understands these complexities. Therefore, nature must provide the answer here, NOT man with simple formulations that overdose you on the metals in the supplement and underdose (zero) on those not included. The solution for you and your body is a full spectrum of chelated metals from naturally complete and balanced sources. These perfect sources are metal-rich foods, herbs and other plant storehouses.

Unlike amino acids and B vitamins, however, metal equilibriums and interactions are not negatively impacted by short-term high-dose supplementation. Apparently metal storage reserves in the liver, bones, teeth and elsewhere can quickly and safely put away any excess. Thus, metal supplements can be an effective health maintenance strategy, particularly in meeting basic Energy, Healing, Stress and Immune needs, but they must be augmented with full-spectrum sources to insure perfect attendance by all metals during all body metabolisms.

Trace metal deficiencies are growing nutritional day- and nightmare in the modern world. As chronicled below, nature's perfect full-spectrum sources have withered during the last half of the twentieth century. Compounding this difficulty is the fact that severe stress or trauma depletes metal reserves quickly, resulting in major losses in metalloenzyme and catalytic activity. Such dysfunctions are a setup for acute and chronic diseases. Symptoms and signs of <u>multiple</u> trace metal deprivation include stiffness in the end of the fingers, sensitive teeth, sore tongue, gum abnormalities, open skin fissures, tender bones, frequent urination, sensitivity to allergens and inflammatory exacerbation, although each of these complaints can have other causes. Later in the chapter, the fundamental and essential role of each <u>individual</u> trace metal will be explored in a complete guide to supplementation, including individual deficiency symptoms and signs.

The best full-spectrum metal-rich foods, herbs and plant storehouses have the following characteristics: (1) natural source, (2) natural amounts – complete and balanced with nothing added, and (3) organically bound/chelated. These complete sources, presented next, can maintain health beautifully. Unfortunately, in the same way that natural B vitamin-rich foods of Chapter 4 cannot rebuild broken B vitamin health, natural metal-rich sources cannot rebuild damaged, deprived metal mechanisms. For that you need targeted high-dose supplementation. However, first and foremost, implement trace metals naturally. This is the answer even if some supplementation becomes necessary to deal with the stress and strain of modern life, or to correct a particular dysfunction. Put your metal/mineral pills on the shelf temporarily, and surrender to nature's superior knowledge and know-how about metal equilibriums, interactions and complexities.

"Trace metals naturally" is a term used throughout the rest of this book. It refers to the following full-spectrum sources.

Wholesome Food… from terra infirma

And immediately, there's a big problem. Commercially grown foods are for the most part raised on depleted soils, lacking in just about everything plants require. So farmers run around all growing season adding supplements to their fields – nitrogen for growth, minerals to put back what's not there, pesticides to protect unhealthy plants, and so on. Standard fertilizers contain only three ingredients: nitrogen (N), phosphorus (P) and potash, which is mostly potassium (K) carbonate. Since plants cannot practice alchemy or nuclear fusion to make the trace metals they need for good health, these metals must come from the soil, or not at all. N-P-K fertilizers are pretty much "not at all" for the plants and subsequently for you when you eat them!

Meanwhile back at the old-fashioned garden, organically grown plants, those utilizing manure, compost and other natural recycled fertilizers (that other definition of 'organic'), are healthier, less susceptible to pests and much richer in trace metals. An organic garden is an excellent source of complete, balanced, chelated trace metals – and goodness in general. The organic garden is nature's original and still best trace metal solution, but largely extinct in the modern world. The alternative is buying organic foods, which becomes very expensive and another obstacle in the quest to put *metal* in your performance.

If you are Amish or grow most of your own food in the old fashioned ways, or buy all organic foods, then stop reading this chapter. Full-spectrum trace metals are not a concern; you get enough to maintain good health. The rest of us need more sources, significant sources.

B Vitamin-Rich Foods

Chapter 4 whole-grain cereals, nutritional yeasts and green vegetables, the mother lode of B vitamins naturally, contain some trace metals too especially if organically grown. The best endowed are nutritional yeasts. While a welcome addition, these B-foods are not a significant metal source by themselves.

Herbs

Most herbs contain only small metal amounts – a minor source. However, a few herbs actually have the exact same therapeutic action as trace metal supplements, indicating they are rich in endocrine metals. Currently, only three such herbs are known and discussed below. When taking them, follow the usage guidelines given later in the chapter.

DANDELION ROOT

Dandelion Root is easily absorbed, excellent for sleep and effective in overcoming the symptoms and signs of multiple metal deprivations described earlier, particularly stiffness in the end of the fingers, sensitive teeth, sore tongue and frequent urination.

Loaded with myriad trace metals extracted from the earth by its deep roots, Dandelion Root should be part of everyone's health insurance. Take 1500 mg (maximum) in capsule form occasionally.

> The word "OCCASIONALLY" is the essence of ambiguity. Its meaning in this chapter is as follows: if wholesome organic food is not your daily fare, then get trace metals naturally from Dandelion Root or the other full-spectrum sources listed below on average once a week to keep metal reservoirs filled and endocrine functioning at its best. Variety is important in this once-a-week program. Many nutritional books recommend daily metal intake, but such dosing is more appropriate to overcoming disease than to general health maintenance and prevention.

BLACK CURRANTS

Take up to 4 oz of these raisin-like fruits occasionally. Black Currants supply trace metals to the pancreas, adrenal cortex, pituitary, and inadequately to the adrenal medulla. Taking Black Currants too often can cause medulla distress, yet another complication in satisfying metal requirements. Favorably, Black Currants can be combined with Blackstrap Molasses (next) to provide a full spectrum of trace metals. Black Currants are excellent for pancreatic health.

BLACKSTRAP MOLASSES

Blackstrap Molasses is the gooey remains of sugar extraction from sugar cane. As usual, the goodness is left behind when humans process and refine nature. Rich in iron, the stuff of hemoglobin, Blackstrap Molasses delivers a gentle, revitalizing iron boost to your system. Blackstrap Molasses also contains small amounts of copper, zinc and manganese.[1]

Even with its gentleness, take 1-2 tablespoons of Blackstrap Molasses at 1X dosing only–never 2X or more ('X' is defined ahead in "Therapeutic Action"), because iron mismanagement by your body can have serious consequences. The specifics of metal mismanagement and its relationship to antioxidant health are reported in the "Supplementation" section.

Avoid iron intake if you have an infection, as bacteria, viruses and other pathogens thrive and multiply on this new iron circulating in the bloodstream. Correcting iron-deficiency anemia (IDA) requires a bigger iron dose than that from Blackstrap Molasses. The best IDA solution is an amino acid chelated iron supplement, which is presented under "Iron" in the supplementation section. Anemia has many causes besides iron deficiency, so review the iron medical literature and anemia citation there.

Well Water, Spring Water

Getting necessary trace metals from well water, spring water and other groundwater sources is a great idea, except for the fact that these metals come mostly as mineral carbonates and are poorly absorbed by the adult digestive system. Furthermore, except for calcium, magnesium and silicon, the trace metals copper, zinc, chromium, cobalt, nickel and others analyze at less than 2 to 14 mcg (microgram: one-thousandth of a milligram) per liter in the two largest and best groundwater surveys.[2, 3] Iron is 47 mcg per liter.[2] These low concentrations provide little metal satisfaction.

Colloidal Minerals

Necessity is the mother of invention, and leave it to the health food industry to dig up (literally) another source of trace metals naturally. For want of a better term, these diggings are called "Colloidal Minerals," but they fulfill the requirements of (a) natural source, (b) natural amounts – complete and balanced with nothing added, and (c) organically bound/chelated trace metals.

"Colloidal" means particles in liquid suspension. Colloidal Minerals don't look natural, but they do act naturally. They contain seventy or more metals extracted from deposits of vegetation that lived long ago. Larger health food stores usually carry one or two good Colloidal Mineral supplements, and at least twice as many fake copies that do not meet the "natural source, natural amounts, organically-bound" test. Read labels carefully to be sure nothing is added. Human additives can be fool's gold here.

Changing Times

Since our grandparents left the farm, trace metals in the diet have gone from being no worry to missing in action. Today, the untold story in nutrition is the widespread trace metal deprivation in urban, suburban and even rural populations. The real consequences are unknown, probably unknowable. However, the "Supplementation" section ahead reveals just how crucial each trace metal is, and all of them working together in nature's perfect harmony are, to the enzyme and catalytic activities of your endocrine system and body.

Obtaining full-spectrum naturally complete and balanced trace metals is a serious problem with very few good answers. You just read about all the sources, at least all the significant sources: organic garden, Dandelion Root, Black Currants/Blackstrap Molasses and Colloidal Minerals. That's it. And how many of us incorporate even one of these into our diets? Getting a natural dose of all trace metals each week is vital to building health and preventing disease. Needless to say, the organic garden is the complete all-in-one solution. This past should be prologue.

Therapeutic Action

Figure 4-B shows trace metal therapeutic action. Review terminology there including Table 4-2 multiple dose effects. Like other nutrients, trace metals first reach the bloodstream and endocrine system at t = 45 minutes, normal digestion in progress. Maximum therapeutic effect occurs at t = 2 hours, then action drops off, but remains strong until 5 hours. All of these times are the same for B vitamins, fatty acids and trace metals, as well as for herbs. Differences lie only in the decay-to-zero part of the curve beyond 5 hours. Trace metals decay to zero in approximately 60 hours, while fatty acids take 24 hours and B vitamins and most herbs $7^{1}/_{2}$ hours.

Whether from natural source or by supplement, trace metals interact with B vitamins and herbs and should always be taken after them, at least 2 hours and preferably 5 hours afterward, unless for sure the metal and B vitamin or herb nourish different endocrine areas. Trace metal interactions with B vitamins and herbs can create temporary adrenal and endocrine hyperactivity and imbalances. Metals operate in the water medium and do not strongly interact with fatty acids. Early evening is a good time for "trace metals naturally."

Multiple dose effects 1X, 2X, 3X indicate the total number of doses taken before the first dose decays to zero therapeutic action. Repeated doses at 1X can be as often as every 60 hours ($2^{1}/_{2}$ days apart) for say, Dandelion Root and then subsequently another natural metal source such as Colloidal Minerals. Three days apart is preferable, but again "occasionally" should be at least once a week to maintain good metal health, with variety of source from week to week. 2X vanquishes the sluggish metabolism of multiple metal deprivations. 2X early in a nutritional program is good, but not later except to overcome trauma and other functional hyperactivity including inflammatory syndromes. As usual, 3X of anything with strong nutritional content is an overdose. Of course, organic garden foods can be eaten daily because metal concentrations are lower and not subject to Figure 4-B dynamics.

SUPPLEMENTATION

Metal supplements deliver powerful therapeutic action; a single dose is sufficient to fill a metal reservoir for weeks to months and rebuild health. In general, avoid 2X and 3X doses of the same metal except for specific dysfunctions and diseases, as detailed in Chapter 12. Metal supplements should be taken after all B vitamins, fatty acids and herbs of the day. Late afternoon, at least 5 hours before sleep and not early evening, is the last best time to ingest them because their strong effects may disturb adrenal equilibrium and sleep. Unlike B vitamin supplements, metal supplements do not cause soft functioning.

Nature Rules. The beauty of nature runs deep, a harmony both hidden and seen, although oftentimes only dimly seen through an imperfect prism. Nature has rules for this harmony, and we need to fit ourselves into her patterns and rhythms. The more we impose outside solutions, the more we need to understand and follow her laws. A good example is chelated trace metal usage, from wholesome organic foods to out-of-the-bottle supplementation.

Trace Metal Source	Nature's Rules to follow...
Organic foods	No rules.
B vitamin-rich foods	B vitamin therapeutic action.
Most herbs	Herb therapeutic action; the same time profile as B vitamins.
Dandelion Root, Black Currants, and Blackstrap Molasses	Trace metal therapeutic action.
Colloidal Minerals	Trace metal therapeutic action.
Out-of-the-bottle metal supplementation	(1) Trace metal therapeutic action, and (2) only one trace metal at a time!

One at a Time

Out-of-the-bottle supplementation is a far larger metal dose than that from Dandelion Root, Colloidal Minerals and the like. And here nature throws us a curve ball – another rule. To illustrate, a large dose of organically bound copper (for medulla Primary Energy Function) taken alone causes no problem; the copper reservoir is filled for weeks to months and your energy and nervous system improve. Similarly, a large dose of organically bound zinc (for Healing) alone – no problem. However, supplement copper and zinc together and you'll feel great the first day from hyperactive medulla stimulation. Unfortunately, the second day and for several more days, you'll feel drained out, *"something like the cat dragged in,"* because the entire adrenal medulla has gone on an orgy of functioning using up all the copper and zinc ingested and ending up in a functional wash out of temporary exhaustion. More copper and zinc on the second day can briefly overcome the wash out, but this will produce further trace metal and endocrine imbalances.

Accordingly, with out-of-the-bottle metal supplementation, take each trace metal separately. Never ingest two or more metals together even if they are for completely different glands or functional areas, as interactions occur. For unrelated trace metals or those of the same functional pathway, for example Energy → Stress, several hours between them is OK. For close relatives such as equilibrium (⇌) copper and zinc, one day apart is necessary. Throw out all trace metal supplements and multi-mineral supplements that contain two or more metals together – they are bad for your health. Instead, buy each trace metal separately and use as needed to nourish Energy, Healing, Stress or Immune tasks or to correct functional weak spots and exhaustions.

A BIG EXCEPTION to this one-at-a-time rule is combining trace metals with their corresponding B vitamins. For example, copper plus zinc (Figure 6-A ahead) with pantothenic acid plus PABA (Figure 4-A). Here metals and B's together create a hyperactive response, but this hyperactivity is more nutritionally complete and does not end up in a functional wash out. Such combinations are found in commercially available multi-B-vitamin chelated-multi-metal supplements. These can be powerfully good medicine. However, save their potency to overcome past nutritional deprivation or current trauma, as explained in Chapter 4 and ahead in this chapter. Multi-B-vitamin multi-metal combinations are a short-term fix. Long-term use brings side effects because human solutions are flawed compared to nature's perfect harmony. Chapter 12 explores B vitamin-metal combinations fully with targeted treatments for adrenal dysfunctions and resulting chronic diseases.

The Lineup

Table 6-1 shows the Periodic Table of Elements with the trace metals that the endocrine system needs to function properly shaded, at least those that for sure are endocrine protagonists. Table 6-2 reveals the specific role each metal plays.

TABLE 6-1. PERIODIC TABLE OF ELEMENTS.

Endocrine System Trace Metals "shaded".

(Shaded elements shown in bold.)

1	2	3	4	5	6	7	8	9	10	11	12	13	14	15	16	17	18
1 H																	2 He
3 Li	4 Be											5 B	6 C	7 N	8 O	9 H	10 Ne
11 Na	12 Mg											13 Al	14 Si	15 P	16 S	17 Cl	18 Ar
19 K	20 Ca	21 Sc	**22 Ti**	**23 V**	**24 Cr**	**25 Mn**	**26 Fe**	**27 Co**	**28 Ni**	**29 Cu**	**30 Zn**	31 Ga	**32 Ge**	33 As	**34 Se**	35 Br	36 Kr
37 Rb	38 Sr	39 Y	**40 Zr**	**41 Nb**	**42 Mo**	43 Tc	44 Ru	45 Rh	46 Pd	47 Ag	48 Cd	49 In	50 Sn	51 Sb	52 Te	53 I	54 Xe
55 Cs	56 Ba		72 Hf	**73 Ta**	**74 W**	75 Re	76 Os	77 Ir	78 Pt	79 Au	80 Hg	81 Tl	82 Pb	83 Bi	84 Po	85 At	86 Rn
87 Fr	88 Ra		104 Rf	105 Db	106 Sg	107 Bh	108 Hs	109 Mt	110 Ds								
			57 La	58 Ce	59 Pr	60 Nd	61 Pm	62 Sm	63 Eu	64 Gd	65 Tb	66 Dy	67 Ho	68 Er	69 Tm	70 Yb	71 Lu
			89 Ac	90 Th	91 Pa	92 U	93 Np	94 Pu	95 Am	96 Cm	97 Bk	98 Cf	99 Es	100 Fm	101 Md	102 No	103 Lw

TABLE 6-2. TRACE METAL ROLES.

Trace Metal	Symbol	Atomic Number	Role
Titanium	Ti	22	Glucose metabolism – pituitary.
Vanadium	V	23	Glucose metabolism and adrenal cortex Primary Stress Function.
Chromium	Cr	24	Glucose metabolism – Glucose Tolerance Factor (GTF) and other metabolites.
Manganese	Mn	25	Adrenal cortex Primary Immune Function.
Iron	Fe	26	Hemoglobin.
Cobalt	Co	27	Vitamin B12 aids, connects and facilitates adrenal medulla Primary Energy Function, adrenal cortex Primary Stress Function, and endocrine pancreas in their common tasks.
Nickel	Ni	28	Aids, connects and facilitates adrenal medulla Primary Healing Function and adrenal cortex Primary Immune Function in their common tasks, e.g. inflammation.
Copper	Cu	29	Adrenal medulla Primary Energy Function.
Zinc	Zn	30	Adrenal medulla Primary Healing Function.
Germanium	Ge	32	Pituitary energy-stress function.
Selenium	Se	34	Pituitary healing-immune function.
Zirconium	Zr	40	Catalyst for all fiber processes in the body.
Niobium	Nb	41	Catalyst for all catabolic fat processes in the body.
Molybdenum	Mo	42	Catalyst for all protein processes in the body.
Tantalum	Ta	73	Catalyst for all anabolic fat processes in the body.
Tungsten	W	74	Catalyst for all carbohydrate processes in the body.

Is Table 6-2 a complete list – the ultimate? Hardly. It does name and place all major endocrine players. However, a steady diet of just Table 6-2 metals will prove to be incomplete nutrition, negatively impacting various metabolisms, most noticeably immune and fatty acid health. Minor endocrine players not listed in Table 6-2 include lithium (Li, 3) for behavioral normality,[4] and boron (B, 5) for proper calcium and bone metabolism.[5-7] Possibly up to ten more Periodic Table metals have minor roles, not counting sodium (Na, 11) and potassium (K, 19) and their electrolyte Na ⇌ K equilibrium, which is part of aldosterone/fatigue function, and calcium (Ca, 20) and magnesium (Mg, 12) essential for healthy bones, cartilage and teeth, and their Ca ⇌ Mg equilibrium for muscle contraction and relaxation. Na ⇌ K and Ca ⇌ Mg are discussed in detail in Chapter 11.

Figure 6-A shows each Table 6-2 trace metal in its endocrine place. The symmetry of Figure 6-A is silent elegance. To every function there is a metal, and a purpose for every metal from atomic number 22, titanium, through atomic number 30, zinc. The high atomic numbers, 40 and above, are the catalysts zirconium, niobium, molybdenum, tantalum and tungsten, and align in the same columns with numbers 22 to 24 titanium, vanadium and chromium on the Periodic Table of Elements. Speculating on the theory that life arose out of the primordial soup of long ago, Mother Nature used almost every metal available! She skipped only inert metals such as silver (Ag, 47) and gold (Au, 79), metals rare in the earth's crust, and arsenic (As, 33) and other toxic elements. A recent Scientific American article explains that the ancient earth had an embarrassment of riches, with far greater diversity of molecules than life could possibly use. Minerals imposed order on the chaos by confining, concentrating, selecting and arranging these molecules. This may have jump-started the first self-replicating molecular system, which then began using up the resources in its environment. Through variants and eventually mutations, competition for limited resources led to a process of molecular natural selection.[8]

Complexity, perplexity. Because the unknown is always with us, let Mother Nature handle the unbelievable complexity of the Periodic Table of Elements long term with the organic garden, Dandelion Root, Black Currants/Blackstrap Molasses and Colloidal Minerals. Use Table 6-2 and Figure 6-A short-term to meet current Energy, Healing, Stress and Immune needs exactly, or to correct past trace metal deprivations, those causing MILD adrenal exhaustions and imbalances. Targeted metal supplementation in these cases and related B vitamin supplementation

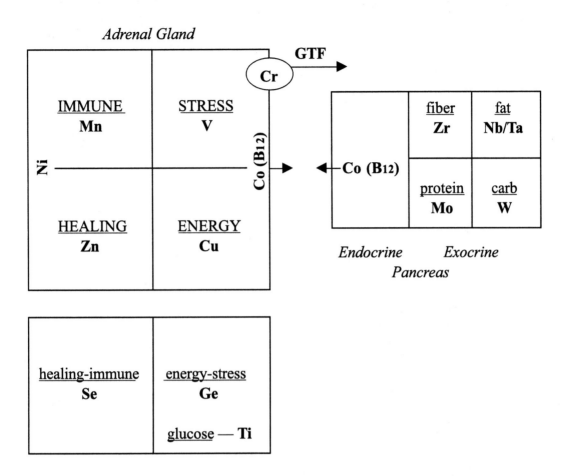

Adrenal Gland

Endocrine   Exocrine
Pancreas

Pituitary Gland

FIGURE 6-A. INDIVIDUAL TRACE METALS FOR THE ADRENAL GLAND, PANCREAS AND PITUITARY.

Nickel (Ni) and cobalt (Co) "connect" Healing-Immune and Energy-Stress-endocrine pancreas functioning, respectively.

separately (see Chapter 4) along with fatty acids and appropriate herbs can restore much of lost vigor and health. SEVERE adrenal and endocrine exhaustions, dysfunctions and diseases require Chapter 12 remedies of targeted metals and B vitamins taken together.

CAUTION ☛ Trace metal supplementation has side effects. These side effects produce only endocrine imbalance, not toxicity (poison to tissues). To redress imbalances, take at least two servings or doses of trace metals naturally such as Dandelion Root and Colloidal Minerals for each supplementation regimen or sequence that follows. With an organic garden diet, five to ten servings between supplementations are necessary. Unlike B vitamin supplementation, metal supplementation can be an effective health maintenance strategy to meet crucial needs, but it must be tempered with full-spectrum trace metals naturally to eliminate side effects. Metal supplementation is for the most part a non-toxic methodology; molecules are chelated (organic, close to nature) and dosage levels low relative to intoxication thresholds. However, two of Table 6-2 trace metals, nickel and niobium, require precautions in their use as detailed later in their profiles.

Correcting long-term metal deprivation may require supplementation of all Table 6-2 metals. This could be accomplished in one extended sequence regimen; for example, Day 1: supplement zinc and manganese (healing-immune action plan), Day 2: copper and vanadium (energy-stress action plan), Day 3: nickel and cobalt-B_{12} (connectors), Day 4: titanium and chromium, Day 5: molybdenum and zirconium, Day 6: tungsten and niobium/tantalum, Day 7: iron, Day 8: selenium, and Day 9: germanium. After this sequence, continue with trace metals naturally to achieve complete nutrition and metal health.

Metals for Glucose Metabolism

The endocrine pancreas regulates glucose (sugar) metabolism with two hormones, insulin and glucagon. Glucose regulation also requires three trace metals: titanium, vanadium and chromium, which act together or not at all. Weight lifters and body builders are familiar with vanadium and chromium supplements to maximize workouts. However, they and all of us need titanium too for proper glucose fueling of body cells. Titanium, vanadium or chromium deficiency especially aggravates diabetic and hypoglycemic tendencies and syndromes.

Remember, supplementation is for rebuilding health. Maintaining health is simple and easy with "trace metals naturally."

TITANIUM

Titanium is essential to pituitary control of glucose metabolism. Titanium metalloenzymes become part of pituitary energy-stress functioning, as indicated in

Figure 6-A. Titanium is needed least often of the three glucose metals, chromium most often, but repeated supplementation with vanadium and chromium will soon run you short of titanium, shutting down glucose fueling at its control point. Regrettably, no titanium supplement is on the market at this time. Therefore, you will have to make your own, and "how to" is explained in the last section of this chapter.

A single article in the medical literature reports on the nutritional role of titanium... Dietary titanium improves infant growth in animals.[9]

VANADIUM

Vanadium is a cofactor in the adrenal regulation of glucose metabolism through two cortex subfunctions: glucose tolerance factor (GTF) and gluconeogenesis. In actuality, vanadium metalloenzymes nourish the entire Primary Stress Function, not only GTF and gluconeogenesis, but also stress (cortisol), fatigue (aldosterone) and cortex sex. Vanadium deficiency causes glucose intolerance and contributes to stress exhaustion and its arthritis syndromes.

Vanadium must be in balance with chromium and titanium, and Immune manganese too. And still take each of these metals one at a time in a supplementation sequence. 5 mg of vanadyl sulfate is sufficient for minor problems; 10 mg (maximum) temporarily moves cortex Immune ⇌ Stress equilibrium toward Stress.

> ### Review of the Medical Literature

Nature... As an enzyme cofactor essential for energy metabolism,[10] vanadium possesses powerful insulin-mimetic [resembling in action] activity, producing antidiabetic and cardioprotective effects. Vanadium also lowers blood pressure. Organic [chelated] vanadium complexes are two to three times more insulin-mimetic potent than inorganic vanadium.[11]

Animal studies on diabetes... In a pioneering 1985 study, vanadium corrected elevated blood glucose levels to normal in streptozotocin (STZ) diabetic rats [model for Type I insulin-dependent juvenile diabetes; STZ: antibiotic that in high doses induces diabetes].[12] The antidiabetic action continued for months after vanadium treatment withdrawal with corrected STZ-rats showing normalized glucose and weight gain, and improved basal insulin.

Near-normal glucose tolerance occurred despite insignificant insulin response to elevated glucose.[13] Longer trials of up to one year found no vanadium toxicity in either STZ or control rats. Overall, vanadium reduced blood glucose, cholesterol and triglycerides in a number of animal diabetic models.[12]

Human diabetes... Vanadium improves glycemic control in human diabetics. Beyond direct insulin-mimetic activity, vanadium enhances insulin sensitivity and prolongs insulin action. These effects appear to be due to PTP inhibition [PTP: protein tyrosine phosphatase enzyme, negative regulator of the insulin signaling pathway]. While exact biochemical mechanisms are not fully understood, clearly vanadium acts differently than insulin, and bypasses defects in insulin activity. Vanadium is a potential pharmacological agent for insulin-resistant diseases.[14] Author's Note: Vanadium and herb Fenugreek (Chapter 10) in combination give even better diabetic control.

Weight training/muscle mass... Vanadium is a common supplement used by athletes to enhance weight training.[15] Contrarily, most studies show that chromium, vanadium and boron supplementation do not influence muscle development and fat-free weight gains during resistance training.[16, 17]

Sources... Food is the main dietary source of vanadium.[15] Vegetables and vegetable oils, grains, cereals, skim milk and lobster are good sources, while fruits, meats, butter, cheese, fish and beverages are poor sources.[18] In the United States, estimated daily vanadium intake is 10-60 mcg.[15] However, depending on air, water and food in the particular region, daily intake can vary from 10 mcg to 2 mg. Organic [chelated] vanadium forms are safer, more absorbable, and able to deliver up to 50% more therapeutic activity than inorganic forms.[18] In general, vanadium toxicity is low.[15]

Possible overdose toxicity... Excessive vanadium decreases erythrocyte [red blood cell] deformability, and causes oxidation of erythrocyte membranes and blood hemolysis [red blood cell breakdown], resulting in anemia.[19] Author's Note: Follow the dosage recommendations given above. Take extra antioxidants if you work in a vanadium environment.

CHROMIUM

Chromium forms Glucose Tolerance Factor (GTF) through adrenal cortex metabolism. GTF then partners with insulin in escorting glucose into every cell. In essence, both GTF and insulin are catalysts for glucose metabolism, controlling blood glucose levels and glucose fueling of cells. Insufficient chromium/GTF impacts diabetes much like insulin shortage. Insulin resistance and "brittle diabetes" are often due to chromium depletion. Hypoglycemia is similarly exacerbated.

The first indication of chromium deficiency is usually short-term memory losses. Your brain runs almost exclusively on glucose, consequently insufficient chromium impairs brain energy. You think you're getting Alzheimer's, but it's just *Sometimers*!

Diabetics need chromium supplementation and so do sugar lovers, who overuse pancreatic insulin and drain away significant amounts of chromium. Age brings reduced glucose tolerance, and chromium can reverse this downward trend. Avoid GTF supplements; they are an end product of chromium metabolism and can be very harsh on the adrenal gland. Instead, let the adrenal cortex synthesize GTF and other metabolites from elemental chromium bound to an organic molecule (chelated) such as chromium picolinate. Take up to 400 mcg of chromium as needed, typically not more than once a month. However, for diabetics once a week is a good starting point. See the medical literature below.

Sesame Seeds aid in chromium assimilation and buffer the metal's first metabolism in the adrenal cortex. This can benefit those with adrenal cortex dysfunctions. Buffering dosage is one to two teaspoons of sesame seeds spread out over several hours after chromium ingestion. An unidentified factor in sesame seeds plays an important role in chromium/adrenal cortex/glucose metabolism, but apparently is of help only during heavy chromium assimilation. Too many sesame seeds cause pituitary suppression (correct with Ginkgo biloba, see Figure 8-B), and that can occur quickly if there is no extra chromium to process.

Review of the Medical Literature

Overview... Chromium is an essential nutrient. Chromium deficiency is associated with glucose intolerance.[20] This landmark discovery was made in 1950s studies of total parenteral [other than by digestive tract] nutrition (TPN) patients. These patients developed severe diabetic symptoms including glucose intolerance, impaired energy, weight loss and brain and nerve disorders. However, when chromium was added to TPN fluids, diabetic symptoms were relieved and exogenous [outside, injected] insulin was no longer necessary.[21] Chromium is required to promote the action of insulin in all body tissues.[22] People consuming Westernized diets have suboptimal chromium intake. Physical trauma or other forms of severe stress can compromise their chromium status and health.[21]

Absorption and activity... Inorganic [non-chelated] chromium is poorly absorbed. Chromium is much more bioavailable in yeast, or as chromium picolinate.[20] Chromium circulates in the blood as free $Cr+3$ [its non-toxic valence state], $Cr+3$ bound to transferrin [protein carrier of iron], or $Cr+3$ complexes such as glucose tolerance factor (GTF).[23] Tentatively identified as a chromium-nicotinic acid complex,[24] GTF is naturally synthesized in the body from dietary chromium. GTF binds to insulin and increases its activity approximately three-fold.[25]

Intake and effects... The majority of people on Western diets obtain less than the estimated safe and adequate daily chromium requirement of 50-200 mcg, established by the US National Academy of Sciences.[26, 27] Insufficient chromium produces symptoms and signs similar to diabetes and cardiovascular disease. Doses above 50-200 mcg may be required to treat certain chronic disease states. In a Chinese study, 1000 mcg [1 mg] of chromium daily was effective in relieving many Type II [adult onset] diabetic symptoms, including correcting HbA1C [a hemoglobin]. Recent evidence finds little or no toxicity from chromium supplementation.[26]

Pancreatic hormones, mechanisms... Chromium improves blood glucose profiles and related variables in Type I [juvenile diabetes], Type II [adult-onset diabetes], and gestational and steroidal-induced diabetics,[28] as well as in hypoglycemic patients.[29] Chromium's beneficial effects on blood glucose, insulin resistance and lipids [fats and fat-related compounds] occur even in healthy individuals.[30] Chromium increases beta [insulin producing]-cell sensitivity, insulin binding, insulin receptor numbers and insulin receptor enzymes.[29]

Weight loss... Chromium supplementation may be helpful in weight loss and retaining a lean body mass.[26] Chromium is only a small part of the weight and body composition puzzle; exercise and a healthy diet are far more important.[31]

Athletes... Exercise may increase urinary chromium losses. Athletes who restrict food intake may compromise their chromium status.[32]

Immune system... Chromium improves immune responses, with positive effects on T- and B- lymphocytes, macrophages [relatively long-living, large white blood cells; -phage: anything that devours], cytokines [non-antibody proteins/signaling molecules of the immune system], and hypersensitivity reactions.[22]

Bones... Chromium picolinate supplementation decreases urinary excretion of calcium and hydroxyproline [related to collagen] in postmenopausal women.[33]

Aging... brings decline in glucose tolerance. Improving glucose-insulin metabolism may increase lifespan and reduce the chronic diseases of aging.[34] While plasma chromium in healthy elderly adults is similar to that of young adults, higher urinary excretion occurs in the elderly, suggesting altered metabolism and lower chromium stores. Diets of these healthy elderly adults often contain less than 30 mcg of chromium per day, which is probably insufficient during times of stress and illness.[35]

Dietary sources... Few data exist on the chromium content of foods, or on dietary intake in various populations. Staple foods are typically low in chromium, with little geographic variation. Food processing using stainless-steel equipment significantly increases dietary chromium intake. Meat grinding, homogenization and acidic fruit juices in steel cans are prime examples. Average intake varies considerably from country to country. Developing countries such as Brazil, Iran and Sudan have high intakes of 50-100 mcg daily, whereas the developed countries of United States, Sweden and Switzerland are at 50 mcg or less, below the estimated safe and adequate dietary requirement of 50-200 mcg per day.[36] In the US population, chromium deficiency is widespread, not only due to suboptimal intake, but also from high consumption of simple sugars, which increases chromium losses.[37]

MANGANESE

Manganese is essential for immune health. The mitochondria enzyme manganese superoxide dismutase (MnSOD) prevents superoxide (O_2^-) free radicals from causing cell damage, mutagenesis and many diseases. Tumor cells are always low in MnSOD!

Zinc lozenges have gained popularity for their immune-boosting, cold-fighting ability, but zinc actually works indirectly for the most part and requires 3X dosing or more to achieve efficacy. This overstimulates adrenal medulla Healing, which then stimulates Immune into action. Several days later, however, multiple doses of zinc leave the immune system suppressed, a natural consequence of pituitary-adrenal homeostasis. Manganese, on the other hand, provides direct and correct immune nutrition and therapeutic action. A 1X dose of manganese is sufficient to achieve effect. Zinc is directly tied to the immune system in one area though; deficiency causes thymus atrophy and impaired T-lymphocyte response. Therefore, ingesting zinc first and manganese later, both at 1X, can bring the healing-immune action plan (Chapter 2) to full expression. See "Zinc" for more on its immune role.

Manganese alleviates immune exhaustion, immune subfunction imbalances and connective tissue disorders. Manganese also plays a role in inflammation and vaso-constriction. Take 5 mg of manganese for minor problems; 10 mg (maximum) temporarily moves adrenal cortex Immune ⇌ Stress equilibrium toward Immune. Manganese must be in balance with its partner vanadium and sequenced with it after the immune system is back up to speed. Of course, take no manganese before or during the stress of the day, instead wait until only relaxation and rest lie ahead.

> ## Review of the Medical Literature

Roles… Manganese is an essential cofactor for three enzymes: superoxide dismutase [more below], hexokinase [catalyst in glucose metabolism] and xanthine oxidase [involved in the breakdown of nucleic acid purine to xanthine and uric acid; see molybdenum ahead].[38] Manganese deficiency impairs free radical defenses, insulin production, and lipoprotein and growth factor metabolisms. Deficiency during early development causes skeletal abnormalities and irreversible ataxia [loss of muscle coordination especially in extremities].[39]

Superoxide dismutase… Superoxide radicals (O_2^-) are a normal byproduct of oxygen metabolism. Superoxide dismutase enzymes (SODs) catalyze the destruction of superoxide to hydrogen peroxide (H_2O_2) and back to oxygen (O_2). Left free, superoxide causes cell injury, mutagenesis and many diseases. In all cases, SODs protect cells against such destructive action.[40]

MnSOD… Superoxide dismutases (SODs) exist in three forms: manganese superoxide dismutase (MnSOD), CuZnSOD [see copper and zinc], and extracellular SOD.[41] MnSOD protects mitochondria [cell *organ* responsible for respiration and energy production] from superoxide attack.[42]

Cancer… Free radicals both initiate and promote multistage carcinogenesis. Compared to normal cells, tumor cells are always deficient in MnSOD activity.[43]

Nerves... Manganese deficiency may be a factor in spinocerebellar degeneration.[44] Superoxide (O2$^-$) reacts with nitric oxide (NO) to produce the strong oxidant, peroxynitrite (ONOO$^-$).[45] MnSOD protects neurons from this nitric oxide-mediated neurotoxicity.[46] Note: Neurotoxicity occurs with both not enough and too much manganese, as follows.

Brain and not enough manganese (SOD)... Manganese is required for normal brain functioning.[47] Two major groups of dementia exist in old age: (1) multi-infarctual [dead or dying tissue from deprived blood supply] dementias as a result of cerebrovascular disorders and stroke, and (2) primary degenerative disorders such as Alzheimer's disease and Parkinson's disease. Free radicals are a significant factor in each of these injuries.[48] MnSOD protects brain mitochondria from superoxide (O2$^-$),[42] and neurons from peroxynitrite (ONOO$^-$).[45, 46]

Brain and too much manganese... Environmental manganese exposure results in neurotoxicity. This was first described in 1837 in Scottish workers exposed to high dust levels while grinding black manganese oxide. Resulting central nervous system [CNS] damage causes a Parkinson's-like syndrome, which is usually irreversible.[49] Symptoms include tremor, muscle weakness, bent posture, excess saliva and whispered speech. For many years, the similarity between manganese neurotoxicity and Parkinson's disease was neither recognized nor understood.[50] While neurological diseases such as Parkinson's disease, Alzheimer's disease and Huntington's disease [an inherited CNS disease involving adult-onset dementia and bizarre involuntary movements] are linked to iron mismanagement in the brain, particularly in striatum [striped gray and white matter] and basal ganglia [cerebral cortex area involved in movement] regions, manganese mismanagement and accumulation in brain appears to target these same areas.[47]

Cardiovascular... Anti-atherogenic [atherogenic: depositing plaque on artery walls] nutrients include antioxidants, fish oils and other unsaturated fatty acids (if protected from oxidation by antioxidants), fiber and trace metals manganese, copper, zinc and selenium.[51]

Exercise... Muscle exercise increases reactive oxygen species (ROS) and other free radical generation. Exercise-induced muscle redox [reducing/oxidizing] disturbances need the protective antioxidant enzymes superoxide dismutase (SOD), glutathione peroxidase (GPX) and catalase, which eliminate superoxide (O2$^-$), unstable hydrogen peroxide (H2O2) and other hydroperoxides, and H2O2, respectively. Regular endurance training, especially high-intensity exercise, increases SOD and GPX activity in worked muscles.[52]

Dietary sources, deficiency and toxicity... Manganese intake varies greatly depending on food choices, water source and supplement use. People consuming Western diets obtain from less than 1 mg to greater than 10 mg of manganese per day. Deficiency and intoxication levels are debatable, as the symptoms of both are non-specific. Early deficiency symptoms include reproductive failure, growth retardation and changes in blood glucose and HDL cholesterol [high-density lipoproteins, so-called good cholesterol]. Toxic symptoms can be anemia and growth retardation. Plasma manganese and lymphocyte [white blood cell] MnSOD activity are the preferred manganese status tests.[53] The estimated safe and adequate daily dietary intake (ESADDI) for adults is 2-5 mg of manganese.[54] Food is the most important source with daily intake ranging from 2-9 mg. Homeostasis [stability/equilibrium in a system through feedback] regulates gastrointestinal manganese absorption.[38]

IRON

Iron is essential to red blood cell transport of oxygen (O_2) to all cells. Each red blood cell contains millions of hemoglobin protein molecules, which carry oxygen safely and efficiently. The critical heme part of hemoglobin is $C_{34}H_{32}N_4O_4Fe$. Red blood cells form in bone marrow and are deactivated at the end of their life by the liver and spleen.

Anemia is not enough red blood cells and hemoglobin, therefore not enough oxygen delivered to cells. Symptoms can include weakness, pallor, little energy, inability to handle stress – frequently accompanied by a dull headache, rapid fatiguing and limited stamina. Preventing anemia is critically important in pregnant women and children, as explained in the following medical literature review. When caused by iron deficiency, anemia is best cured using an amino acid chelated iron supplement; take 25 mg of iron every three days (1X only, see cautions below) over several weeks to total 200-250 mg. Iron tablets from the pharmacy, usually inorganic ferrous sulfate, are very harsh in comparison, with side effects much more likely.

Adrenal cortex Primary Stress Function, with its high caloric metabolism and oxygen utilization, depends to a significant degree on red blood cells, just as cortex Immune relies on white blood cells. Consequently, anemia shows up first and foremost as a Stress dysfunction. Hyperactivity anywhere in the body is severe stress and uses up significant amounts of hemoglobin and iron.

CAUTIONS ☛ Take iron supplements at 1X dosing only, and add antioxidants during assimilation to protect against iron mismanagement including the possibility of free iron in the blood and iron-induced free radicals in the brain, which can cause Alzheimer's disease and Parkinson's disease. Iron must always be guarded by a panoply of antioxidants: Vitamin C and Vitamin E daily, MnSOD and CuZnSOD, and so on. In addition, avoid iron supplementation when battling infection, as bacteria, viruses and other pathogens thrive on this new iron circulating in the bloodstream. 10,000 IU of dry Allergy Vitamin A ingested with iron will defend against any undetected infection and improve iron absorption.

Review of the Medical Literature

Oxygen metabolism... Erythrocytes [red blood cells] have two main functions: oxygen transport and carbon dioxide elimination.[55] Healthy organ and body processes require sufficient oxygen (O_2) delivered to cells. Following uptake by the lungs, O_2 is bound to hemoglobin [oxygen-carrying protein in red blood cells, made up of iron-containing heme and globin protein], enabling dissolution in blood.[56] Oxygen depends on iron not only for transport (hemoglobin), but also for storage in myoglobin [oxygen store in muscle fibers], and for lung respiration using cytochromes [heme oxidation-reduction reactions].[57] Iron deficiency, the most common worldwide nutritional disorder, causes anemia [low red blood cell count], which most often occurs in pregnant women, infants and children.[58]

Iron metabolism... involves four major proteins: (1) transferrin, for blood transport of iron; (2) transferrin receptor, which controls iron-transferrin uptake; (3) ferritin, or iron storage; and (4) iron regulatory protein (IRP), which manages both iron intake and storage.[59, 60] Abnormalities in these proteins can lead to iron deficiency or overload; both conditions have damaging consequences.[59]

Anemia

Characterization... Iron deficiency produces perinatal [after the 20th week of gestation] morbidity [disease incidence], defects in infant psychomotor development, impaired school performance in children and diminished work capacity in adults. Few if any studies find these abnormalities in the absence of anemia. Therefore, adequate iron can be defined as normal blood erythrocytes and hemoglobin. However, optimal iron is sufficient ferritin storage to avoid iron deficient erythropoiesis [red blood cell production]. Eliminating this milder form of iron deficiency requires normal hemoglobin, ferritin and transferrin receptors.[61]

Diagnosis... Full-blown iron deficiency anemia (IDA) diagnosis is as follows: hemoglobin can screen for anemia, after which more specific laboratory tests are required to establish iron deficiency as the cause. Traditional iron deficient erythropoiesis measurements are ambiguous, being similarly affected by anemia from chronic disease [ahead]. Iron stores are virtually non-existent in uncomplicated IDA, thus low serum ferritin (below 20 mcg/L) usually confirms IDA when anemia is present. Unfortunately, serum ferritin can be falsely elevated to normal range in IDA patients with infection or chronic inflammation. However, serum transferrin receptor (TfR) is upregulated during iron deficiency; and IDA is easily identified by elevated serum TfR. Therefore, the optimal combination of laboratory IDA tests is hemoglobin, serum ferritin and serum TfR.[62]

Pregnancy... Two commonly occurring anemias during pregnancy are IDA (75%) and folic acid deficiency megaloblastic anemia [see Chapter 4]. Severe maternal anemia causes spontaneous abortion, fetal death, prematurity and low birth weight.[63] Pregnancy IDA results in significant mother and infant morbidity,[64] including preterm delivery, low birth weight and poor neonatal [first four weeks after birth] health.[65] In developing countries, IDA occurs in more than half of pregnant women. The adolescent growth spurt and start of menstruation increase iron needs dramatically. Women who become pregnant during or shortly after adolescence are likely to have either IDA or low to absent iron stores.[64] Among all fertile women, 20% show iron ferritin reserves greater than 500 mg, the minimum required during pregnancy, 40% show stores of 100-500 mg, and 40% have virtually no ferritin. The daily demand for iron increases from 0.8 mg early in pregnancy to 7.5 mg late in pregnancy. Daily dietary intake averages 9 mg, which is below the estimated 12-18 mg recommended allowance.[66] Iron supplementation is advisable throughout pregnancy.[65]

Infant and childhood anemia... Infants and children are one of the population groups at greatest IDA risk.[67] The majority of epidemiological studies link childhood IDA with poor cognitive and motor development, and behavioral problems.[68] The first two years of life are crucial because of a major growth spurt in the brain then. Lack of iron adversely affects brain cells, myelin [insulating fatty acid sheath surrounding nerves], and neurotransmitters.[69]

Adolescent anemia... The adolescent growth spurt and acquisition of adult characteristics dramatically increase iron needs in adolescent boys and girls. Girls are especially vulnerable, and unlikely to build iron stores during this period. Preadolescent daily iron requirements of 0.7-0.9 mg rise to as much as 2.2 mg, and even higher in heavily menstruating young women.[70] Approximately 10% of US adolescents are anemic, with pregnant teens and those involved in athletics at greatest risk.[71]

Sports anemia, endurance training... IDA causes rapid fatigue upon exercising.[72] Athletes frequently develop low blood hemoglobin, low hematocrit [relative blood volume occupied by red blood cells], and low ferritin levels.[73]

Physiological anemia/losing iron... IDA may develop with excessive menstruation, regular blood donation, or blood losses from hemorrhoids, gastrointestinal bleeding, and the like. Factors that increase iron utilization are female contraception and aspirin therapy.[74, 75] Celiac disease [digestive disease of the intestinal lining] and gastritis including from H. pylori [bacterium implicated in gastric ulcers and cancer] infection decrease intestinal iron absorption.[76]

Less common anemias... not due to iron deficiency include: (1) anemia of chronic disease, which is low red blood cell production as a result of an underlying condition elsewhere in the body. Ferritin is usually normal and iron supplementation ineffective. (2) Kidney disease anemia occurs when erythropoietin [kidney hormone that stimulates bone marrow to produce more red blood cells] deficiency decreases red blood cell production. (3) Thalassemia is a congenital abnormality in the globin portion of hemoglobin. Thalassemia symptoms resemble mild IDA, but iron supplementation and transfusions are ineffective. (4) Myelodysplastic anemia develops when erythrocyte components do not mature, and this can progress to acute nonlymphocytic leukemia.[77]

Beyond hemoglobin... Iron is essential for electron transport, gene expression, mitochondrial respiration [mitochondria: cell *organ* responsible for respiration and energy production], and cell proliferation and differentiation. Iron can also harm tissues by generating reactive oxygen species (ROS) free radicals, which attack normal cells and contribute to neurodegenerative processes, atherosclerosis and cancer.[78, 79] The specialized iron metabolisms of acquisition, transport (transferrin), and storage (ferritin) shield cells from direct exposure to iron.[79] Adversely, superoxide (O_2^-) free radicals can oxidize 4Fe-4S clusters and release free iron into the system,[45] resulting in concentrated ROS damage.[80] Superoxide is the silent partner of iron mismanagement.[45] Note: Manganese and copper-zinc enzymes protect against superoxide damage.

Brain and Parkinson's disease (PD)... Iron is required for normal brain functioning. However, iron mismanagement in the brain is associated with Parkinson's disease, Alzheimer's disease and Huntington's disease. Damage occurs especially in striatum [striped gray and white matter] and basal ganglia [cerebral cortex area involved in movement] regions.[47] While the exact cause of these neurodegenerative disorders is unresolved, recent human and animal model studies indicate iron misregulation induces oxidative stress and reactive oxygen species (ROS), leading to neuron injury and death. In support of this hypothesis [proposed, not proven] are: (1) iron concentrations increase in the PD brain selectively in the neuromelanin [nerve proteins] of substantia nigra [midbrain area containing dopamine-producing cells] neurons, (2) ROS and lipid peroxidation byproducts [lipids: fats and fat-related compounds] also increase, while (3) glutathione [natural internal antioxidant: cofactor in eliminating hydrogen peroxide; within cell mitochondria, the main defense against oxidative stress] and other antioxidants decrease in the PD brain, and (4) mitochondrial electron transport becomes impaired.[81]

Alzheimer's disease (AD)... Amyloid deposits [thick protein plaque, a.k.a. beta-amyloid] within the neocortical parenchyma [essential elements of the cerebral cortex] and cerebrovasculature characterize AD. Iron, copper and zinc have recently been found to be concentrated in amyloid plaque.[82] Aging, the most obvious AD risk factor, involves free radical mechanisms and neurons are extremely sensitive to free radical attack. Furthermore, AD brain lesions are typical of free radical damage, specifically DNA damage, protein and lipid peroxidation, and advanced glycosylation [adding sugar molecules to protein chains]. Iron, copper, zinc and aluminum mismanagement produce free radicals, and in the presence of free radicals, beta-amyloid generates more free radicals. Antioxidants can eliminate beta-amyloid toxicity.[83]

Friedreich ataxia... is the most common inherited neurodegenerative ataxia [loss of muscle coordination, especially in the extremities]. Mounting evidence suggests that Friedreich ataxia [early symptoms: unsteady gait, slurred speech, jerky eye movements] is due to iron accumulation in mitochondria, creating free radicals, cell damage and death.[84]

Immune vs. pathogen... Iron is crucial to both human and pathogen. Iron status must be sufficient to maintain optimal immune response, but insufficient to facilitate pathogen multiplication.[85] Iron supplementation exacerbates infection, as bacteria effectively compete for the iron in circulation. [86, 87] In HIV patients, iron accumulation and iron-mediated oxidative stress may be related to shorter survival. Viruses like HIV, which involve the DNA lifecycle, need iron for replication.[88] Cancer frequently causes anemia of chronic disease [as described above]; misdiagnosis as iron deficiency anemia (IDA) and subsequent iron loading can increase tumor proliferation.[89] Author's Note: From Chapter 5... Vitamin A is necessary for resistance to and recovery from infection.[90] Accordingly, Vitamin A status must be adequate during iron supplementation to prevent exacerbating any undetected infection.[87] Vitamin A also favorably influences iron absorption, probably by forming a Vitamin A-iron chelate.[91]

Dietary sources... Meat is high in iron.[92] Iron and Vitamin B12 are the two nutrients most likely to be missing from vegetarian diets.[93] However, a well-balanced plant-based diet can provide sufficient iron to avoid iron deficiency anemia (IDA), although iron stores may be low. Restrictive macrobiotic [found in the region] vegetarian diets are associated with increased IDA incidence. Plant constituents inhibit iron absorption, while Vitamin C, citric acid and other organic acids aid in absorption.[94] The interaction between absorption enhancers such as meat and organic acids, and inhibitors such as cereal bran, phytic acid [an insoluble fiber component of plant cells], soy products, egg yolk and calcium determines the amount of iron obtained from food.[95]

Toxicity... Large doses of iron can cause oxidative damage.[96] Adult ferrous sulfate supplements are the leading cause of accidental pediatric poisoning, despite child-resistant packaging.[97] In the United States, iron-related childhood injuries rose from 1200 annually in 1980-1985 to 3000 for1986-1996; fatalities peaked at 10 in 1991.[98]

COBALT (Vitamin B12)

The trace metal cobalt forms a complex organic molecule in nature known as Vitamin B12, chemical formula $C_{63}H_{88}N_{14}O_{14}PCo$. B12 aids, connects and facilitates adrenal medulla Primary Energy Function, adrenal cortex Primary Stress Function and the endocrine pancreas in their common tasks. As a special endocrine messenger, B12 regulates Energy → Stress functioning and thereby glucose and ester utilization. Insulin uses up B12, and B12 uses up folic acid and other green vegetable B vitamin factors. Folic acid supplementation can mask a serious B12 deficiency.

A Vitamin B12 deficiency may take five years or longer to develop into "pernicious anemia" with symptoms of weakness or soreness in arms and legs, difficulty in walking, jerking of the limbs, impaired reflex response and other manifestations of nervous system disorder. When symptoms appear, it's too late – irreversible spinal cord and nerve damage have already occurred. Therefore, prevention must be your goal.

If there's one trace metal supplement to take regularly, it's Vitamin B12! Supplementation is essential for vegetarians as dietary B12 is found almost exclusively in animal protein, particularly organ meats. Deficiency is common in diabetics and the elderly. Normal B12 absorption requires a gastric secretion called "intrinsic factor." As you get older, this gastric glycoprotein can be AWOL for no reason. B12 absorption from food or ingested tablet is impaired in most adults. The best way to ensure healthy Vitamin B12 status is with sublingual (under the tongue) lozenge; this B12 goes directly into the bloodstream. A dose of 2000 mcg sublingually once a month is adequate maintenance for adults, 4000 mcg maximum with prolonged deficiency or the special needs cited in the medical literature. 2000 mcg B12 taken twice, one hour apart, can jump-start sluggish glucose and ester metabolism.

Review of the Medical Literature

Overview... Vitamin B12 (cobalamin) is unique among vitamins, containing not only a complex organic molecule but also an essential metal, cobalt.[99] B12 deficiency syndrome has five distinct stages, the last of which results in irreversible neuropsychiatric injury.[100] There are four stages of negative B12 balance: (1) plasma depletion; (2) cell depletion, which is low red blood cell B12; (3) biochemical deficiency, with decreasing DNA synthesis and increasing blood homocysteine [harmful sulfur-containing amino acid] and methylmalonate [intermediate in protein and fat metabolism, hence little synthesis of end product]; and (4) clinical anemia [low red blood cell count],[101] namely macrocytic [abnormally large red blood cells, i.e. megaloblastic] anemia. (5) Irreversible subacute spinal cord degeneration [pernicious anemia] is eventually fatal.[102]

B12 and folic acid... Vitamin B12 and folic acid [Chapter 4] participate together in red blood cell development.[103] Folic acid deficiency produces anemia by impairing purine [parent compound of nucleic acids] and pyrimidine [another nucleic acid parent] synthesis. B12 deficiency causes an identical anemia by trapping folic acid in intracellular space.[104] B12 and folic acid are also essential for homocysteine-to-methionine methylation [add a methyl group; in cell chemistry, to esterify—more below] and S-adenosylmethionine [SAMe, see Table 3-2] synthesis. SAMe facilitates DNA, neurotransmitter, protein and phospholipid [phosphate fatty acids, abundant in cell membranes] methylation reactions. B12 and folic acid deficiencies generate similar neurologic and psychiatric disturbances including depression, dementia and spinal cord demyelination [myelin: insulating fatty acid sheath surrounding nerves].[105] B12 deficiency is most tightly associated with psychosis, folic acid deficiency with depressive disorders.[106] B12 should be suspected in all unexplained anemia or neuropsychiatric symptoms.[107]

B12 pernicious anemia (PA)... PA neurological disease was first described two hundred years ago. Although some biological effects remain unexplained, Vitamin B12 depletion causes subacute spinal cord degeneration, polyneuropathy [of peripheral nerves] and psychosis.[108] The probable mechanism is inadequate SAMe impairing CNS [central nervous system] methylation.[109] Psychiatric symptoms can include fatigue, mood disorder, violent behavior, paranoid psychoses and dementia.[110] PA may remain latent [no symptoms] while continuing to damage nerve cells, especially in diabetics and elderly adults.[111, 112]

Vegetarianism... if correctly followed, provides complete nutrition with the sole exception of Vitamin B12. Vegetarianism decreases the risk of coronary artery disease, hypertension [high blood pressure], colon cancer, diverticulosis, gallstones and various metabolic diseases.[113]

Pregnancy... Vitamin B12 and folic acid levels are low in women with neural tube defect (NTD) pregnancies.[114] Review of seventeen case-control studies shows a moderate association between low maternal B12 status and fetal NTD risk.[115] Maternal B12 deficiency can also cause hereditary and acquired disorders in offspring.[116] For example, infants from severe maternal B12 deficiency develop behavior abnormalities associated with the brain basal ganglia [cerebral cortex area involved in movement] and pyramidal tract [projecting neurons in the cerebral cortex].[117]

Diabetes... Latent pernicious anemia (PA) occurs more frequently in Type I juvenile diabetics (11 per 1000) compared to the general population (1.3 per 1000). Manifest PA in Type I diabetics has a rate 3.9 per 1000. Vitamin B12 screening of Type I diabetics is an important preventive measure.[111]

Diabetic neuropathy... Vitamin B12 supplementation produces statistical improvement in and regression of diabetic neuropathy symptoms and signs.[118] Leg symptoms of paresthesia [abnormal neurological sensations: numbness, tingling, prickling, burning or increased sensitivity], burning pain and heaviness improve with B12 administration. Benefits appear within the first week and last for several months to four years. B12 is a safe and effective treatment for diabetic neuropathy.[119]

Multiple sclerosis (MS)... has been linked to Vitamin B12 deficiency in some studies.[120] Long-term B12 deficiency causes demyelination [myelin: insulating fatty acid sheath surrounding nerves; MS is autoimmune/inflammatory destruction of the myelin sheath].[105]

HIV → AIDS... Deficiencies in Vitamin B12, Vitamin E, Vitamin A or beta-carotene accelerate the progression of HIV infection to AIDS.[121]

DNA damage and cancer... Deficiencies in Vitamins B12, B6, folic acid, niacin, C or E, or in metals iron or zinc can induce single- and double-strand DNA breaks and oxidative lesions, thereby contributing to carcinogenesis.[122] Epidemiological study finds a threshold plasma B12 level below which breast cancer risk increases among postmenopausal women.[123]

Homocysteine and vascular disease... Epidemiological, experimental and clinical observations reveal a strong correlation between hyperhomocysteinemia [high levels of homocysteine in the blood] and vascular disease. Homocysteine is independent risk factor for arterial occlusive disease and thrombosis [blood clot].[124] Men and older adults are at greatest homocysteine risk. Diabetes, obesity, hypertension, cigarette smoking and excessive coffee may be contributing factors.[125] Vitamin B12, B6 and folic acid deficiencies lead to increased plasma homocysteine and are associated with cardiovascular diseases.[126] Folic acid is the key element of treatment; B12 and/or B6 can decrease homocysteine further in certain groups of patients.[127]

Elderly... Vitamin B12 deficiency is common in elderly adults,[128, 129] affecting an estimated 10-15% of those over 60 years of age.[112] Symptoms and signs range from lethargy and weight loss to dementia.[130] However, these older adults often lack the classical symptoms of B12 deficiency such as megaloblastic anemia.[112] Even in the absence of manifest anemia, B12 deficiency continues to damage nerve cells.[131] Elderly adults are especially vulnerable from interaction between degenerative neuropsychiatric B12 syndrome [pernicious anemia], B12 homocysteine cerebro-cardio-vascular disease,[128] and homocysteine neurotoxic effects.[105]

Alzheimer's disease... B12 deficiency increases with age, particularly beyond 65, and is associated with Alzheimer's disease.[131] While low plasma Vitamin B12 can cause cognitive impairment and dementia, much controversy exists over this Alzheimer's link.[132] The link may be indirect through homocysteine,[105] as hyperhomocysteinemia has recently been shown to be a strong risk factor for both dementia and Alzheimer's disease.[133] Physicians should employ B12 therapy liberally as an Alzheimer's preventative. The window of opportunity may be as short as one year.[132]

Absorption problems... Four billion year old Vitamin B12 has the most complicated vitamin metabolism. Uptake from the intestine to blood distribution involves no fewer than five separate binding molecules, receptors and transporters.[134, 135] These include intrinsic factor [protein secreted by the stomach lining that binds to B12, enabling absorption], transcobalamin [transporting protein in blood, responsible for delivery of B12 to most tissues], and haptocorrin [storage protein].[135] In children, intrinsic factor dysfunction causes megaloblastic anemia, neuropathy, infections, proteinuria [protein in the urine], mild general malabsorption and failure to thrive. B12 injections bring remission.[136] Similarly, in older adults and in those with Alzheimer's disease, B12 deficiency is due to or most likely to do to malabsorption.[130, 137] Untreated celiac disease [digestive disease of the intestinal lining; inflamed response to gluten, the 'elastic' protein of dough] frequently produces B12 deficiency.[138]

Diagnosis and treatment... While Vitamin B12 deficiency is easily treated, diagnosis is complicated by ambiguous tests. Current state-of-the-art tests can be normal in B12-deficient patients.[100] Serum holotranscobalamin II, the metabolically active B12 fraction, and methylmalonic acid [intermediate in fat and protein metabolism] are more reliable than total serum B12.[129] Further complicating the clinical picture, folic acid supplementation can mask a serious B12 deficiency,[139, 140] and pernicious anemia may present wide ranging complaints or be entirely asymptomatic.[141] No 'gold standard' diagnostic procedure exists for establishing B12 deficiency.[142] Fortunately, B12 therapy is straightforward using monthly injections or intranasal gel [works by absorption through the skin], which are far better absorbed than oral supplements.[100] Also, sublingual B12 is convenient and efficacious.[143]

NICKEL

Nickel aids, connects and facilitates adrenal medulla Primary Healing Function and adrenal cortex Primary Immune Function in their common tasks. Nickel is necessary for normal inflammation and vasoconstriction. It improves healing and eases autoimmune attack, especially on muscles and protein structures, the dependent body system of Healing. There is no nickel supplement on the market at this time; how to make your own is discussed at the end of the chapter.

Of all Table 6-2 trace metals, nickel and niobium are the most likely cause mild tissue toxicity in supplement form. *CAUTION* ☞ Limit nickel supplementation to once a month maximum. The first time the author took nickel, results were so positive – skin healing improved dramatically – that I took it again the next day and apparently induced temporary nickel mismanagement, resulting in a minor and transient short-term memory loss. The episode lasted only a few hours, however, a clear lesson in the importance of taking essential trace metals carefully so as not to disturb metal balances.

Overview... Nickel is essential in several animal species. Nickel deficiency reduces growth and reproductive rates,[144] especially affecting fetal development and decreasing life expectancy in breeding female animals. A constituent of all organs, nickel performs many vital metabolic functions,[145] including stabilizing nucleic acids.[146] Deficiency alters blood glucose and lipid [cholesterol, LDL, HDL] profiles,[144] by impairing dehydrogenases [enzymes that oxide by transferring hydrogen], transaminases [enzymes that catalyze by transferring an amino group] and alpha-amylase [amylase: carbohydrate digestive enzyme]. This results in markedly reduced carbohydrate metabolism and energy from glucose, glycogen [glucose storage in the liver] and fat sources. Nickel deficiency suppresses calcium incorporation into the skeleton and iron resorption [dissolution back into blood], thereby contributing to anemia. Deficiency can also disturb zinc metabolism and produce a psoriasis-like skin disorder.[145]

Dietary sources... Food and drinking water are the main nickel sources, with the typical American diet providing approximately 300 mcg daily. Nickel compounds do not accumulate in the food chain.[144]

Toxicity... Toxic doses of many transition metals [metals of four 'Periodic Table of Elements' series, with atomic numbers 21-29, 39-47, 57-79 and 89-beyond] can disturb redox [reducing/oxidizing] reactions in cells, producing oxidative stress that can derange cell signaling and gene expression systems, and lead to a variety of toxic effects including carcinogenesis.[147] Nickel metal and inorganic nickel compounds are well-known carcinogens. Nickel can also cause allergic contact dermatitis.[122]

COPPER

Copper metalloenzymes become part of adrenal medulla Primary Energy Function and its subfunctions of energy (adrenaline), nerves, start of sex (nervous energy), and mood. Copper is the best electrical conductor of all the metals, and nerves are the electrical conductor in the body. A natural fit! While the tie-in is obvious, exactly how copper contributes to nerve functioning is very complicated and explored in the medical literature review below. Suffice it to say, copper will help overcome energy exhaustion and nerve dysfunctions and diseases. Defective copper metabolism is a major factor in amyotrophic lateral sclerosis (ALS, Lou Gehrig's disease), Alzheimer's disease, and Menkes and Wilson's diseases.

Copper must be in balance with zinc and sequenced with it, but these two must be taken at least one day apart. 1 mg of copper is sufficient for minor problems; 2 mg (maximum) temporarily moves the Healing ⇌ Energy equilibrium toward Energy. Functional equilibriums, for example Healing ⇌ Energy, necessitate nutrient equilibriums such as Zn ⇌ Cu. Medical science describes metal equilibriums as "antagonisms." Always maintain these antagonisms or equilibriums. To illustrate, copper partners with zinc to form copper-zinc superoxide dismutase (CuZnSOD) enzyme, which protects the cytosolic or fluid portion of cells from superoxide (O_2^-) free radicals. ALS is directly linked to CuZnSOD malfunction; genetic malfunction is documented in following medical literature, but functional exhaustion of CuZnSOD is also possible and would have the same effect.

CAUTION ☛ Supplement zinc before copper in their sequence regimen to safeguard Healing and antioxidation systems. Being antagonistic toward zinc and antioxidation, copper can unleash free radicals, resulting in sore muscles and stiffness unless cell antioxidant defenses and Healing mechanisms are performing well. With Healing dysfunction or injury, copper supplementation will remain problematic until youthful healing and antioxidation are restored.

Review of the Medical Literature

Need and transport... All living systems require copper. A unique class of proteins called 'copper chaperones' provide safe intracellular delivery and homeostasis of this essential, yet toxic trace metal.[148] To date, only a few copper chaperones have been identified, but their use is widespread across bacterial, plant and animal species.[149]

Nerves... Copper plays a fundamental role in the human nervous system and its development. Menkes disease and Wilson disease [both below] are inherited neurodegenerative disorders of copper metabolism, which dramatically reveal its essential nature and its toxicity.[150]

Menkes disease/Nature of copper deficiency... First described in 1962, Menkes disease of early infancy is an X-linked [sex chromosome] recessive defect in copper metabolism,[151] that prevents intestinal absorption, causing blood, liver and body cells to suffer copper deficit and impaired cuproenzyme activity.[152] Occurring in one in 200,000 births, Menkes disease produces severe neurologic degeneration, mental retardation, arterial degeneration, hair and skeletal abnormalities and death in early childhood.[152, 153] Current treatment is copper injections; however, if therapy is started after two months of age, neurologic degeneration does not improve. The clinical spectrum here is wide; milder Menkes forms do occur as a result of mutations in the Menkes gene. Males showing mental retardation and connective tissue disorders should be DNA evaluated for Menkes disease.[152]

Wilson's disease/Nature of copper toxicity... Wilson's disease is an inherited disorder of copper accumulation and toxicity, resulting from a defective enzyme in the copper biliary excretion pathway.[154] Accumulating in liver cells, copper generates reactive oxygen species (ROS) free radicals; and copper and ROS toxicity together kill off liver cells. The copper is then released to damage the urinary system, red blood cells, brain, heart, skin, bones and joints, pancreas and other endocrine glands.[155] Liver, neurologic and/or psychiatric symptoms usually manifest in older children and young adults. Among severe side effects, 20-25% of patients develop nephrotic syndrome [type of kidney inflammation characterized by edema, weight gain, high blood pressure and anorexia] and systemic lupus erythematosus [lupus: autoimmune, inflammatory disease of connective tissue with skin eruptions, joint pain, kidney damage].[156] Wilson's disease can be treated effectively, especially with early diagnosis. Penicillamine [in cases of metal poisoning, the drug penicillamine chelates to the metal enabling urinary excretion] was the first anti-copper treatment. Today, zinc administration successfully manages Wilson's disease.[154] Liver transplantation may be necessary in severe cases.[155]

Other possible defects in copper metabolism... Copper chaperone ceruloplasmin transports 95% of plasma copper. An inherited defect in this copper-protein dehydrogenase enzyme produces progressive neurodegeneration of the basal ganglia [cerebral cortex area involved in movement] and retina. Mutations in the copper-containing superoxide dismutase enzyme, which operates in the cytosolic or fluid portion of the cell, cause motor neuron [a neuron connected to muscle, gland or other effector] degeneration and amyotrophic lateral sclerosis [ALS, Lou Gehrig's disease]. Copper is also implicated in Alzheimer and prion [transmissible, fatal neurodegenerative infectious agent, e.g. 'Mad Cow'] encephalopathic [brain disease] neuron damage.[150]

Superoxide dismutase... Normal oxygen metabolites include superoxide (O_2^-), unstable hydrogen peroxide (H_2O_2) and hydroxyl (OH^-) free radicals, all of which can damage biological systems if not eliminated by antioxidants. The copper- and zinc-enzyme superoxide dismutase (CuZnSOD) attenuates cytosolic superoxide damage,[157, 158] by catalyzing superoxide back to hydrogen peroxide and oxygen [O2]. Selenium-enzyme glutathione peroxidase (GSHPx) then eliminates the hydrogen peroxide.[159] See also zinc and selenium medical literature reviews ahead.

ALS/Lou Gehrig's disease... Familial amyotrophic lateral sclerosis (FALS) is a progressive, fatal paralytic disease of motor neuron death in the brain cortex, brainstem and spinal cord.[158] Approximately 20% of FALS patients have mutations in the SOD1 gene encoding CuZnSOD.[160] Expression of this mutant human CuZnSOD gene reproduces the disease in transgenic mice. SOD1 mutation converts the superoxide (O_2^-)-protective antioxidant CuZnSOD into a destructive prooxidant, which catalyses H_2O_2 damage selectively in motor neurons.[158, 161] In the early stages of ALS, cytoplasmic [substance between cell membrane and nucleus] inclusions cause neurofilament accumulation and aggregation within motor neurons.[162] Copper chelation therapy, dietary antioxidants and other neuroprotective agents inhibit the oxidative damage and can delay FALS onset, but do not extend FALS duration.[158]

Copper-zinc antagonism, i.e. Cu $\rightleftharpoons$ Zn... Copper-zinc antagonism occurs because physicochemically similar trace metals compete for ligands [any molecules that bind to a receptor]. The risk of copper deficiency or zinc deficiency increases with high intake of the other.[163] Author's Note: Copper-zinc antagonism and molybdenum-tungsten antagonism ahead confirm the principle of functional equilibrium ($\rightleftharpoons$), with Figure 2-B providing the first physiological explanation for these scientific observations.

Copper-iron interplay... Copper and iron are key redox [reducing/oxidizing] metals, and in significant ways regulate each other's metabolism.[164] Copper is a catalyst for iron absorption and heme [iron part of hemoglobin] synthesis.[165]

Alzheimer's disease... Metal mismanagement may the common denominator underlying amyotrophic lateral sclerosis [ALS, above], Alzheimer's disease, Parkinson's disease, prion diseases, mitochondria [cell *organ* responsible for respiration and energy production] disorders, and cataracts. Abnormal redox [reducing/oxidizing] reactions of metals such as copper and iron can generate reactive oxygen species (ROS).[166] For example, reduction of Cu+2 [valence: net electrical charge] to Cu+1 produces hydroxyl (OH^-) free radicals, and contributes to Alzheimer's disease neurodegeneration.[161] Copper-mediated toxicity and cumulative oxidative stress may account for the age-related deterioration seen in these neurodegenerative diseases.[167]

Mad Cow... Prion diseases are transmissible, fatal neurodegenerative diseases such as

Creutzfeldt-Jakob disease [Mad Cow] in humans, BSE [bovine spongiform encephalopathy] in cattle, and scrapie in sheep. Prion, a hypothetical infectious agent, may be a neurotoxic copper glycoprotein on an infected cell's surface. The outbreak of Mad Cow disease in Great Britain was probably due to consumption of BSE-infected meat. There is no known treatment for prion diseases.[168]

SIDS... Brain neuron aging and degeneration are features of sudden infant death syndrome (SIDS), Down's syndrome and Alzheimer's disease. In SIDS studies, CuZnSOD and glutathione peroxidase (GSHPx) [H_2O_2-eliminating selenium enzyme]-protected neurons decline in the brain hippocampus [cerebral cortex area involved in long-term memory] and neocortex [six-layered, most highly-developed cortex part] during postnatal development of SIDS infants compared to normal infants. SOD, GSHPx, CAT [catalase: another H_2O_2-eliminating enzyme], and Vitamin E protect neurons from damaging free radicals. Zinc upgrades the gene expression of all these antioxidants.[169]

Immune... Copper performs several immune functions, although little is known about mechanisms. Copper deficiency reduces neutrophils [specialized white blood cells, strong against bacteria], Interleukin 2 [hormone-like substance released by T-cells; stimulates more T-cell production and other immune defenses; IL-2 decreases during HIV infection], and probably T-cell proliferation.[170] Copper and zinc together inhibit AIDS viruses.[171]

Rheumatoid arthritis (RA)... RA inflammation and injury involve activated phagocytes [white blood cells that engulf/devour microorganisms and cell fragments] and other lymphocytes within the synovial [viscous joint fluid] and periarticular [surrounding the joint] tissues. Reactive oxygen species (ROS) triggered by these phagocytes exacerbate rheumatoid damage. Copper-zinc superoxide dismutase (CuZnSOD) scavenges toxic oxygen from these tissues and, administration directly into the joint, can bring therapeutic RA remission.[172]

Cardiovascular... Copper deficiency contributes to arteriosclerosis [abnormal thickening, loss of elasticity in artery wall], high blood pressure, faulty blood clotting, inflammation and anemia.[173] Men and women consuming typical American diets can suffer copper-deficient changes in cholesterol, blood pressure, glucose metabolism and electrocardiogram.[174]

Dietary status... Adults need between 1.0 and 1.25 mg of copper daily for normal metabolic functions.[175] Copper-rich foods include nuts, seeds, legumes and mushrooms.[174] Soluble carbohydrates, proteins and organic acids, except ascorbic acid [Vitamin C], enhance copper bioavailability and absorption.[176] Water generally contains low levels; however, low-pH water and beverages passed through copper piping and well water can infuse significant copper concentrations. Scientific studies support the World Health Organization (WHO) safe standard for copper in drinking water of 2 mg per liter.[177] Diagnosing marginal copper deficiency is uncertain;[175] one early clinical sign is low neutrophils [Note: B vitamin pantothenic acid similarly affects neutrophils]. Copper deficiency can occur with high zinc intake, gastric resection, total parenteral [other than by digestive tract] nutrition or malnutrition.[178]

ZINC

Zinc becomes part of adrenal medulla Primary Healing Function and its subfunctions of healing, antioxidation, inflammation and vasoconstriction. Zinc is directly linked to the immune system too, as deficiency causes thymus atrophy and impaired T-lymphocyte response. In addition to improving these primary mechanisms, zinc benefits the dependent body system of Healing – muscles and protein structures – playing a fundamental role in DNA synthesis, cell division, protein synthesis, muscle cell formation and muscle function. Zinc slows aging and suppresses apoptosis (gene-directed, programmed cell death).

Zinc is called an antioxidant and in a broad sense correctly so because the antioxidation subfunction lies within its province (see metallothioneins in the literature review below), but also in a narrow sense as zinc metalloenzymes such as copper-zinc superoxide dismutase (CuZnSOD) protect distant tissues, just as antioxidants Vitamin C and Vitamin E serve throughout the body. However, zinc does not need daily supplementation to achieve these effects. Moreover, zinc is intimately tied to other metals, especially copper and iron, in complex equilibriums and achieves healthy therapeutic action only within these internal balances.

Healing and protein/muscle dysfunctions and diseases desperately need zinc! Deficiency is common in the elderly. Particularly vulnerable is the prostate gland, which contains the highest zinc concentration in the male body. Take 5-10 mg of zinc for minor problems, 20 mg (maximum) temporarily moves Healing $\rightleftharpoons$ Energy toward Healing. Zinc supplements must be sequenced and in balance with copper, but these two must be taken at least one day apart.

Need... Zinc is essential for gene expression, cell division and growth,[179] antioxidation,[180] and immune system functioning.[181] Unknown before 1963, zinc deficiency today is recognized as widespread in the United States and throughout the world. However, assessing zinc status remains difficult.[182]

Nature... Zinc retards oxidative processes. Its antioxidant mechanism can be divided into direct and indirect activity. Indirect activity involves long-term zinc exposure, which induces metallothioneins [special superfamily of antioxidants, more below] and other proactive substances to be the ultimate antioxidants against oxidative stress. Direct activity involves protecting protein sulfhydryls [metallothioneins] and preventing hydroxyl (OH^-) free radical formation from abnormal redox [reducing/oxidizing] reactions of transition metals such as copper and iron.[180]

Superoxide dismutase... Normal oxygen metabolites include superoxide (O_2^-), unstable hydrogen peroxide (H_2O_2) and hydroxyl (OH^-) free radicals, all of which can damage biological systems if not eliminated by antioxidants. The copper- and zinc-enzyme superoxide dismutase (CuZnSOD) attenuates cytosolic superoxide damage.[157, 158] See "Copper" for a complete discussion of CuZnSOD and its role in amyotrophic lateral sclerosis (ALS, Lou Gehrig's disease), sudden infant death syndrome (SIDS) and other diseases, as well as the need for copper-zinc equilibrium to prevent Alzheimer's disease, etc.

Metal antagonism/need for equilibrium (Zn $\rightleftharpoons$ Cu, Fe)... Zinc-copper antagonism occurs because physicochemically similar trace metals compete for ligands [any molecules that bind to a receptor]. The risk of zinc deficiency or copper deficiency increases with high intake of the other.[163] Regarding iron, zinc becomes a substitute metal substrate for ferrochelatase [enzyme catalyzing heme formation] during iron deficiency, resulting in increased zinc in hemoglobin and erythrocytes [red blood cells].[183] Balance between zinc, copper and iron prevents abnormal redox [reducing/oxidizing] metal reactions from generating toxic hydroxyl (OH^-) free radicals.[180, 166]

Metallothioneins (MTs)... are a zinc superfamily of sulfhydryl-rich metalloproteins. MTs scavenge oxyradicals. This antioxidant activity is due to sulfhydryl nucleophilicity [affinity for the cell nucleus, thereby protecting it] and formation of metal complexes, as follows. Binding of transition metals displaying Fenton reactivity [antagonism] reduces oxidative stress, whereas singular release of Fenton metals increases free radical damage.[184] MTs apparently regulate the zinc-copper biological pool, supply zinc enzymes and transcription factors, and protect DNA from oxidative stress.[185] Heavy metals, cytokines [non-antibody proteins/signaling molecules of the immune system] and prooxidants induce MT synthesis and expression.[184] MTs have a zinc-sulfur cluster structure.[186]

Heart and membrane structures... MTs protect against oxidative injury in pharmacologic and genetic studies, with zinc-MT activity in the heart studied extensively.[187] A component of cell membranes, zinc maintains membrane structure and function, and prevents derangements of the vascular endothelium [lining of the heart, blood vessels]. Zinc is anti-atherogenic [atherogenic: depositing plaque on artery walls] and also reduces postischemic [after an episode of insufficient blood supply, e.g. heart attack, stroke] injury, probably through copper antagonism.[180, 188] Zinc protects against many cell-destabilizing agents.[188]

Thymus/immune... Zinc deficiency causes rapid and marked atrophy of the thymus gland [at the base of the neck; synthesizes and releases T-cell lymphocytes].[189] thereby lowering T-cell and overall lymphocyte numbers, as well as Interleukin 2 [hormone-like substance released by T cells; stimulates more T-cell production and other immune defenses],[190] immune response to mitogens [substances that stimulate cell division, such as carcinogens], and antibody and spleen T-cell response following immunization.[189] Zinc reduces the relative risk of cancer.[191] Zinc is necessary for normal T-cell division, differentiation and maturation.[189] The thymus hormone thymulin, central to T-cell maturation, requires zinc.[190]

Infections... Zinc deficiency significantly impairs immune system defenses, and can cause opportunistic infections and increased mortality, as shown in children with diarrhea, elderly adults, chronic gastrointestinal disorders, HIV/AIDS patients, kidney disease, sickle cell disease and acrodermatitis enteropathica [genetic disorder of zinc deficiency, symptoms: dermatitis, diarrhea, balding, delayed wound healing and immune deficiency].[192] In addition to thymus activity, zinc affects infection-fighting Vitamin A absorption, transport and utilization.[193] Zinc and copper together inhibit AIDS viruses.[171]

Common cold... Summarizing seven randomized controlled trials, zinc gluconate lozenges have therapeutic efficacy against the common cold, reducing symptoms and duration, but with side effects of nausea and bad taste. Also, the following protocol requirements must be met: minimum dose of 13 mg zinc per lozenge, therapy begins within 24 to 48 hours of onset of symptoms, and lozenges every 2 hours during the day for the duration of the cold.[194] In one study, the average time to resolve cold symptoms dropped from 7.6 days in the placebo group to 4.4 days in the zinc group.[195]

Healing... Zinc deficiency retards wound healing.[196] Matrix metalloproteinases (MMPs) are a family of at least fourteen zinc-dependent enzymes, which act as effectors of tissue remodeling and modulators of inflammation.[197, 198] These extracellular matrix remodeling proteases play an important roles in normal development, angiogenesis [new capillary blood vessels], wound repair and numerous neuroinflammatory disorders including multiple sclerosis (MS), cerebral ischemia [insufficient blood supply], meningitis [inflammation of the brain and spinal cord membranes, most often caused by bacterial or viral infection], encephalitis [inflammation of the brain], brain tumors, and Guillain-Barre syndrome [an uncommon, self-limiting polyneuritis causing loss of muscle strength].[199] Zinc ameliorates hypercatabolism [catabolism involves breaking down compounds, cells and tissues] in patients with severe head trauma,[200] and protects skin against UV radiation.[191] In conditions of primary zinc deficiency, supplementing zinc can improve acne vulgaris, alopecia areata [patchy baldness], and leg ulcers.[201]

Protein and muscles... Zinc is necessary for DNA synthesis, cell division and protein synthesis. Approximately 300 enzymes incorporate zinc; many of these are zinc-nucleoproteins involved in the gene expression of various proteins.[190] These 'zinc-finger proteins' [DNA binding proteins] are essential for muscle cell formation and maintenance. Zinc-finger proteins regulate muscle development,[202] including growth factors and steroid receptors.[190]

Gene expression... Zinc-finger proteins code up to 1% of the human genome.[203] Zinc-regulated genes are involved in growth and energy utilization, redox and stress responses, and signal transduction [transmembrane signaling, which translates external stimulus from hormones, growth factors, etc. into changes in cell transport, metabolism, function, growth or gene expression], especially affecting immune response.[204] Zinc regulates the machinery of gene expression, including gene transcription, chromatin [forms chromosomes during cell division], and RNA polymerases [catalytic enzymes]. As a result, zinc controls both the types of mRNA [single-stranded ribonucleic acid, important in protein synthesis] transcripts and their transcription rate. Defects in this process may account for zinc-deficit teratology [birth defects].[205] Specific zinc-finger proteins can be manipulated experimentally, enabling genome engineering, i.e. gene therapy.[206]

Preventing cell death... Apoptosis is gene-directed, programmed cell death, involving activation of an intrinsic cell suicide program. Oxidized lipids [fats and fat-related structures, as in cell membranes], inflammatory cytokines such as tumor necrosis factor (TNF), toxins and disease can induce apoptosis.[207, 208] Zinc suppresses apoptosis,[209] as subcellular pools of zinc maintain structural and functional cell integrity. Zinc also inhibits TNF production, a contributor to AIDS cachexia [general ill heath with emaciation] and wasting.[189] Cirrhosis patients often have zinc deficiency.[210] Overall, relatively nontoxic zinc can reduce the high rates of apoptosis found in many degenerative disorders.[208]

Nerves in the brain... As a neurosecretory cofactor released during neuron activity, zinc is highly concentrated in synaptic vesicles [membrane-bound compartments that contain neurotransmitters molecules] of forebrain neurons. These zinc-containing neurons form complex networks that interconnect most cerebral cortex and limbic structures of hypothalamus, hippocampus [long-term memory], olfactory/smell bulbs, and temporal-lobe amygdala [hearing and receptive areas], in essence, a 'private line' of cerebral cortex communication.[203] Zinc moderates brain neuron death from transient ischaemia [insufficient blood supply] or sustained seizures.[211]

Pregnancy, infants and children... Mild zinc deficiency during pregnancy is associated with higher maternal morbidity [disease incidence], impaired taste sensation, prolonged gestation, poor labor, atonic [muscular weakness] bleeding, and increased fetal risk.[212] Brain neuron aging and degeneration are features Down's syndrome and sudden infant death syndrome (SIDS). SIDS studies found decline in copper-zinc superoxide dismutase (CuZnSOD)-protected neurons in the brain hippocampus [long-term memory] and neocortex [six-layered, most highly-developed cortex part] during postnatal development compared to normal infants.[169] Early zinc supplementation in low birth weight or small-for-gestational-age infants is effective in improving growth.[213] Infant zinc requirements can be met exclusively by breastfeeding through age 5-6 months;[214] however, beyond 6 months, higher meat intake by breastfed infants may be needed to satisfy zinc and iron requirements.[215] In young children, zinc deficiency limits growth.[213] Diarrhea induces zinc losses in children; and growth retardation is closely related to childhood diarrheal diseases.[216] Zinc supplementation should be employed in cases of persistent diarrhea, severe stunting or low plasma zinc.[217]

Male/Female... During periods of growth and development, zinc deficiency causes growth failure, lack of gonad development in males,[190] and impaired ovarian development, estrous cycle, and pituitary LH [luteinizing hormone for sexual maturation] and FSH [follicle-stimulating hormone] in females.[218]

Prostate gland... has the highest zinc concentration of any organ.[218] Benign prostatic hyperplasia [BHP: nonmalignant enlargement of the prostate gland] and prostate adenocarcinoma [tumor involving cells of wall linings] are age-related. Prostate cancer is the most common malignancy in US men. High fat intake increases prostate cancer risk, while zinc, selenium and Vitamin E decrease risk.[219]

Elderly… Zinc deficiency is common in older adults.[220] With aging, thymus and peripheral immune functions show progressive decline. Zinc supplementation can restores these systems.[221] Zinc is a factor in retina health, and may improve age-related macular degeneration (AMD).[222] Elderly adults especially need the recommended daily allowance (RDA) of 15 mg zinc.[223]

Dietary status… Mild zinc deficiency is difficult to detect due to the lack of definitive indicators of zinc status.[224] No universally accepted single measure of zinc status in humans currently exists. With zinc deficiency, clinical signs and measures of zinc concentrations in a variety of tissues such as plasma and hair may uniformly confirm depleted body stores. However, the relative insensitivity and imprecision of these measurements make assessment of marginal zinc status problematic.[225] Zinc RDA is 15 mg for all adults.[226] Vegetarian diets generally contain less zinc than omnivore diets.[227] Zinc bioavailability from high phytate [an insoluble fiber component of plant cells] foods is less than 15% compared to 40% from animal protein.[228] However, some animal proteins such as cheese inhibit zinc absorption. Organic acids favor absorption and are utilized in chelated zinc supplements.[229]

Supplementation… Supplements of zinc oxide and zinc carbonate are insoluble and poorly absorbed by the human digestive system.[217] Iron, when taken with zinc, has negative effect on zinc absorption.[229] Oral zinc supplements are relatively nontoxic, except in extremely high doses. Zinc toxicity manifests as nausea, stomach pain, vomiting, lethargy and fatigue. Zinc-induced copper deficiency causes anemia, neutropenia [low neutrophils], and higher LDL [low-density lipoproteins, so-called bad cholesterol] to HDL cholesterol ratio. Both copper and iron metabolisms are adversely affected by excess zinc.[230]

Drug interactions… Zinc should not be taken with immunosuppressants such as corticosteroids and cyclosporine [anti-rejection drug after transplant surgery].[231]

GERMANIUM

Germanium metalloenzymes become part of pituitary gland functioning, specifically pituitary energy-stress, which regulates the adrenal energy-stress action plan. Obtain germanium naturally from Dandelion Root, Colloidal Minerals and other full-spectrum sources.

Supplement germanium to overcome faulty energy-stress action from long-term metal deprivation or pituitary suppression and atrophy as a result of cortisone therapy or other drug interventions. Germanium must be in balance with selenium, but they must be taken at least one day apart. NEVER take these two metals together.

Germanium most often comes in white powder. Only an extremely small dose is appropriate. A few specks of this powder, equivalent in volume to four or five grains of common table sugar or salt, are sufficient to achieve all possible benefits. Taking too much germanium or germanium at 2X dosing generates pituitary hyperactivity, which forces subordinate glands and most of the endocrine system into sustained hyperactivity – a very harmful result.

The medical literature on germanium is limited and unsettled.

Review of the Medical Literature

Two views... Germanium is a trace metal found in all living plants and animals. Therapeutic benefits include cell oxygen enrichment, free radical elimination, pain relief, detoxification of heavy metals and improvement in antiviral and immune parameters. Germanium promotes interferon [family of hormone-like glycoproteins that fight virus infection/multiplication], macrophage [relatively long-living, large white blood cell; -phage: anything that devours], NK cell [natural killer lymphocyte: active in spontaneous, non-specific immunity against cancer and viruses, first-line defense against cancer], and T-suppressor cell [set of T-cells capable of suppressing B-cell antibody formation] activity. In clinical trials and private practice, germanium demonstrates efficacy against cancer, arthritis and osteoporosis. Germanium is rapidly and safely absorbed and eliminated from the body.[232] Or a different view, germanium is not an essential metal. Germanium became popular in 1970s Japan and later elsewhere as an elixir for cancer and AIDS. While acute toxicity is low, 31 human cases of prolonged germanium supplementation, with total intake of 15 to 300 grams over 2 to 36 months, resulted in kidney failure and in some cases death. Kidney function recovery was slow and uncertain. Other adverse effects can include muscle weakness, anemia and peripheral neuropathy [injury to the sensation nerves of arms and legs].[233]

Anticancer... Between the sixteenth and nineteenth centuries, metals and metal-based compounds were used in treating cancer and leukemia. Renewed interest came in the 1960s, when an inorganic platinum complex demonstrated antitumor action. Subsequently, other metals and metal compounds showed effectiveness against malignancies in humans and animals.[234] Active metals such as germanium+4 [valence: net electrical charge], selenium+4, gallium+3, arsenic+5 and silicon as silica can concentrate within human cells, and may improve DNA electrical properties and gene expression, accounting for their preventative role in carcinogenesis.[235]

SELENIUM

Selenium metalloenzymes become part of pituitary healing-immune functioning, which regulates the adrenal healing-immune action plan. Selenium is generally known as an antioxidant and works through both pituitary oversight and the seleno-proteins described in the literature review below.

Selenium comes in capsule form, typically 250 mcg. This dose is far too high and generates hyperactivity in subordinate glands and systems. A proper supplementation is about 25 mcg of selenium. One exception is reported in the literature; high selenium doses fight cancer!

Absent cancer, selenium must be in balance with germanium, but they must be taken at least one day apart. NEVER take these two metals together. As with all pituitary nutrition, the goal is to maintain pituitary healing-immune ⇌ energy-stress equilibrium. In general, supplement selenium to overcome faulty healing-immune action from long-term metal deprivation or pituitary suppression and atrophy as a result of cortisone therapy or other drug interventions. Review Chapter 8 regarding supplementation cautions, and then interfere as little as possible with pituitary oversight of the endocrine system.

> ## Review of the Medical Literature

Nature… Selenium's essential role in animals was discovered in the 1950s, and in humans in 1973.[236] Antioxidation, cell growth, eicosanoid synthesis [eicosanoids: prostaglandins and other hormone-like substances derived from fatty acids], and thyroid regulation are major selenium functions.[237] Deficiency causes immune deficits, increased cancer and cardiovascular disease risk, congestive cardiomyopathy [heart muscle disease of obscure cause], skeletal myopathy, anemia, hair and nail changes, and abnormal thyroid metabolism.[238] The range between essential and toxic selenium concentrations is very close.[239]

Antioxidant... Selenium protects against oxidative stress. The selenium enzyme glutathione peroxidase (GSHPx) eliminates hydrogen peroxide (H_2O_2), other hydroperoxides and cytosolic [fluid portion of cells] peroxynitrite ($ONOO^-$) from within cells.[240, 159] This enzyme, however, does not completely explain the oxidative effects of selenium deficiency. Recently, identification of other selenoproteins has broaden selenium's role and activities.[240]

Selenoproteins... are selenocysteine enzyme antioxidants. Eleven selenoproteins have been identified to date: cellular glutathione peroxidase (GSHPx), extracellular or plasma glutathione peroxidase, phospholipid hydroperoxide glutathione peroxidase, gastrointestinal glutathione peroxidase, thioredoxin reductase (TrxR), selenoprotein W, selenoprotein P, selenophosphate synthetase and Types 1, 2, and 3 iodothyronine deiodinase. The various glutathione peroxidases prevent internal damage from peroxides. Cellular and plasma glutathione peroxidase are used to assess selenium status.[241] Thioredoxin reductase, confirmed in two forms: TrxRs and TrxR1/TrxR2, defends against oxidative stress, recycles Vitamin C and contributes to cell growth and transformation.[242] Selenoprotein W may be involved in muscle metabolism.[241] Selenoprotein P, an extracellular protein, contains most of the selenium found in plasma. It has antioxidant and transport functions, probably distributing selenium from the liver to peripheral tissues.[243] Thyroid deiodinases are catalysts in the formation and regulation of thyroid hormones.[241]

GSHPx and neurons... Brain neuron aging and degeneration are features of sudden infant death syndrome (SIDS), Down's syndrome and Alzheimer's disease. In SIDS studies, glutathione peroxidase (GSHPx) and copper-zinc superoxide dismutase (CuZnSOD)-protected neurons decline in the brain hippocampus [cerebral cortex area involved in long-term memory] and neocortex [six-layered, most highly-developed cortex part] during postnatal development of SIDS infants compared to normal infants. GSHPx, SOD, CAT [catalase: another H_2O_2-eliminating enzyme], and Vitamin E protect neurons from free radicals.[169] In animal studies, selenium deficiency impairs the enzyme activity necessary for brain development and function.[244] See copper, zinc and manganese for more on SODs and GSHPx and their antioxidant role in disease prevention, especially neurodegenerative diseases. See also cretinism/SIDS/selenium link in Chapter 9.

Mood... Five studies find that low selenium intake is associated with poor mood.[245] Chronic alcohol consumption adversely affects selenium status. The effects of alcohol on mood, behavior and cognitive function may be due in part to selenium deficiency.[246]

GSHPx and TrxRs/Immune... Phagocytes [white blood cells that engulf/devour microorganisms and cell fragments, e.g. macrophages] generate reactive oxygen species (ROS) during defense against infection.[247] As macrophage activation and phagocytosis give off this ROS 'respiratory burst', antioxidant enzymes such as selenium GSHPx and TrxRs simultaneously increase expression to protect nearby cells and tissue.[248] In general, immune functions depend on cell-to-cell communication, and require antioxidant protection. Oxidative damage to these signaling systems impairs immune response.[247]

Rheumatoid arthritis (RA)/Immune... RA inflammation and injury involve activated phagocytes and other lymphocytes within the synovial [viscous joint fluid] and periarticular [surrounding the joint] tissues. The ROS burst triggered by the phagocytes exacerbate rheumatoid damage. Selenium and Vitamin E supplementation strongly alleviate joint pain and morning stiffness in RA patients.[172]

Extra selenium = cancer fighter... Selenium increases natural killer (NK) cells [active in spontaneous, non-specific immunity against cancer and viruses, first-line defense against cancer] and lymphocyte differentiation into cytotoxic cancer-killing cells. Selenium supplementation significantly boosts tumor cytotoxicity, and appears to overcome age-related lymphocyte deficits.[249] For individuals with low or deficient dietary selenium, supplementation improves antioxidant protection through selenoproteins. However, at supplementation levels substantially greater than necessary for maximal selenoprotein expression, selenium goes on to inhibit tumorigenesis through enhanced immune system response, cell cycle regulation and apoptosis [gene-directed, programmed cell death; see selenium toxicity below], as well as altered carcinogen metabolism .[250] Selenium has efficacy against prostate, lung and colon cancers.[251]

Prostate cancer... A common disease of older men in Western societies, prostate cancer is associated with high fat, meat and dairy intake. Increased consumption of fruits, tomatoes, selenium and Vitamin E reduces prostate cancer risk.[252, 253]

Breast cancer... is largely absent in societies with diets containing less than 10% fat content. Dietary fat, alcohol and estrogenic food additives are associated with increased breast cancer risk, whereas fiber, flavonols, Vitamin C, selenium, Vitamin E and beta-carotene are associated with decreased risk.[254] Selenium may act with iodine in preventing breast cancer, but rigorous confirming studies are needed.[255]

Thyroid... Iodine is the principal component of thyroid hormones thyroxine (T_4) and triiodothyronine (T_3). Selenium enzyme iodothyronine deiodinase regulates T_3 synthesis and deactivation.[256] The thyroid gland has the highest selenium concentration of all organs.

In animal models, selenium depletion causes thyroid tissue fibrosis [forming fibrous tissue] and necrosis [death] following high iodide loading. Low selenium strongly correlates with thyroid carcinoma [malignant tumor that begins in the thyroid epithelium or lining] and the development of other tumors.[257]

Male/Female... Selenium, zinc and copper all play a role in male and female reproduction. The selenium content of male gonads increases during puberty,[218] and selenium improves sperm count and mobility.[258] In females, selenium deficiency causes infertility, abortion and placenta retention. Selenium losses through placenta and breast milk increase requirements in pregnant and lactating mothers.[218]

Cardiovascular... Selenium deficiency exacerbates atherosclerosis [depositing plaque on artery walls], ischemic [insufficient blood supply] heart disease, and cardiomyopathy [heart muscle disease of obscure cause].[259] In 1979, Chinese scientists linked selenium to Keshan disease, a juvenile cardiomyopathy endemic to Keshan Province, China. However, an infectious virus and interacting nutritional deficiencies of selenium, Vitamin E and fatty acids all may be factors.[260]

Selenium interactions... Selenium and Vitamin E act synergistically within the myocardium [heart muscle], providing antioxidant defense against iron overload.[261] Selenium promotes delivery of zinc from MTs [metallothioneins, see zinc medical literature earlier] to derivatives enzymes, thereby coordinating zinc and sulfur activity.[262] Selenium counteracts the heavy metal toxicity of mercury, cadmium, thallium and to some extent silver.[263]

Recommended amounts... For adult males and females, minimum daily selenium requirements are 21 and 16 mcg respectively to prevent Keshan cardiomyopathy, or 40 and 30 mcg respectively to achieve two-thirds of peak plasma glutathione peroxidase activity.[264] Or, the recommended daily selenium intake is estimated at 50 to 200 mcg.[265]

Sources and dangers... For the general population, food is the primary selenium source.[266] Protein foods such as meat and fish are high in selenium;[267] and selenoamino acids provide the highest bioavailable selenium.[268] Cereals and vegetables contain selenocysteine and selenomethionine.[266] Toxic selenium concentrations are only twice the nutritional requirements,[269] with the liver being the major target of toxicity.[270] Fossil fuel wastes and agricultural irrigation of arid, selenium-rich soils increase environmental selenium and have poisoned fish and wildlife.[269]

Selenium toxicity… At supranutritional levels, selenium compounds become toxic prooxidants [instead of antioxidants], producing superoxide (O_2^-), hydrogen peroxide (H_2O_2), and possibly other cascading oxyradicals. For instance, selenium oxidation of glutathione [natural internal antioxidant; within cell mitochondria, the main defense against oxidative stress] generates superoxide. This toxicity is countered by overall antioxidant defense and methylation reactions [creating non-toxic methylselenides]. Carcinostasis [-stasis: state of equilibrium, therefore no tumor development] correlates with selenium toxicity, [271] and selenium prooxidant activities may explain cancer cell apoptosis [gene-directed, programmed cell death],[270] i.e. a kind of targeted chemotherapy.

Catalysts

Catalysts are necessary to but not part of a chemical reaction. Nevertheless, supplementing catalysts raises body metabolism because chemical reactions dependent on those catalysts are more likely to proceed. Accordingly, take the five metal catalysts – zirconium (fiber), niobium (catabolic fat), molybdenum (protein), tantalum (anabolic fat) and tungsten (carbohydrate) – with great care and never at 2X dosing or more. Supplement only to overcome specific carbohydrate, protein, fat and fiber-related dysfunctions and diseases. Overall, you can maintain catalytic health with trace metals naturally from Dandelion Root, Colloidal Minerals and the like. Variety in these natural sources is particularly important in this application.

Zirconium, niobium, molybdenum, tantalum and tungsten participate in most body processes. They work together during digestion, aiding the stomach, pancreas and liver in carbohydrate, protein, fat and phyto-compound fiber breakdown. Catalysts then go on to serve the many internal metabolisms of these digested products. A few examples: muscles require the protein catalyst molybdenum for repair, but actually muscles also consist of fatty acid cell membranes and modest fiber and carbohydrate substructures. Therefore, all metal catalysts may be needed to cure muscle diseases. Weight loss involves withdrawal of stored carbohydrates and fats from body tissues and cannot happen if their catalysts are in short supply. Immune defense depends on fiber metabolism, which depends on zirconium. Understand the fundamental mechanisms and root causes behind a dysfunction or disease and you can trace back to find missing raw materials, be they metal catalysts or other key nutrients.

Hyperactivity in any endocrine process depletes the associated metal catalyst(s). On the other hand, normal functioning has no affect on catalyst concentrations in the body. Severe stress from a car accident, death in the family, or other trauma can use up the fat catalysts niobium and tantalum at a rapid rate, creating deficiencies and impairing future fat processes such as fatty acid healing. Multiple sclerosis (MS) involves destruction of the fatty acid myelin sheath surrounding and insulating nerves, and may have a severe stress/trauma trigger and catalytic depletion component. Chapter 12 has more on MS and other disease mechanisms.

The five metal catalysts sit together as a block on the Periodic Table of Elements, Table 6-1. Rotate that block 90 degrees clockwise and look at the mirror image, and you have something close to Figure 2-B. In practice, molybdenum (protein) moves adrenal medulla Healing ⇌ Energy equilibrium toward Healing, while tungsten (carbohydrate) moves Healing ⇌ Energy toward Energy; and zirconium (fiber) and niobium/tantalum (fat) similarly impact adrenal cortex Immune ⇌ Stress. However, do not attempt to correct imbedded adrenal imbalances using catalysts. Unintended side effects develop because such correction is at least two tiers, molybdenum → protein → medulla Healing, removed from the usual causes of adrenal imbalance. These five metal catalysts must be supplemented in a manner that preserves adrenal equilibrium.

Take each catalyst one at a time and sequence them for adrenal equilibrium. The lone exception to this one-at-a-time rule is niobium and tantalum, which must be taken together because they are the two halves, catabolism and anabolism, of fat metabolism. Why nature divided catalytic fat metabolism is unknown, but interestingly Column 5 of the Periodic Table of Elements: vanadium, niobium and tantalum are all fat-related.

Exception to Supplement Sequencing—Small doses of just one catalyst can be taken individually to correct a minor problem, then sequenced and balanced with just full-spectrum sources of trace metals naturally. For most people and in the absence of serious disease, molybdenum and protein processes are likely to be that minor problem. Why is explained ahead.

ZIRCONIUM

Zirconium is the catalyst for all fiber processes in the body. Zirconium is critical to immune health as fiber and phyto-compound foods power the immune system. Connective tissue diseases may suffer from zirconium deficit too.

Zirconium must be in balance with fat catalysts niobium/tantalum so that no adrenal cortex imbalance develops. Additionally, zirconium should be in balance with molybdenum and tungsten for complete adrenal and exocrine pancreas harmony, but this overall rebalancing is less important and necessary only after a second zirconium supplementation. No commercial zirconium supplement exists at this time; how to make your own is given at the end of the chapter – or based on the medical literature, supplementation is never needed, although the status of chelated bioactive zirconium is unknown in this circumstance.

> ## Review of the Medical Literature

Nature… Zirconium activity in biological systems is enigmatic. Ubiquitous and present in higher amounts than other trace metals, zirconium is not yet associated with any specific metabolism. Daily human uptake can be as high as 125 mg. Initial retention is in soft tissues, and later in bone. Toxicity is low, with nonspecific effects at high concentrations. Zirconium crosses the blood-brain barrier, and can accumulate in brain tissues. Zirconium's +3 valence [net electrical charge] and the high stability of its compounds are reminiscent of aluminum+3, which is linked to Alzheimer's disease.[272]

Lysosomes/storage within each cell… Certain metals concentrate within cell lysosomes [an enzyme-containing cell *organ* that breaks down protein and other large molecules into usable sizes for the cell]. Electron probe X-ray microanalysis evidences selective lysosome concentration of twenty-one of the ninety-two Periodic Table elements, six in association with sulfur and fifteen with phosphorus. Sulfur-bound metals are Column 10 nickel, palladium, platinum and Column 11 copper, silver and gold. Phosphorus-bound metals include chromium and niobium, Column 4 zirconium and hafnium, Column 13 aluminum, gallium and indium, and rare-earth elements lanthanum, cerium, samarium, gadolinium, thulium, thorium and uranium.[273]

NIOBIUM

Niobium is the catalyst for all catabolic fat processes in the body. Niobium must be taken with its fraternal twin tantalum, the anabolic fat catalyst, and niobium/tantalum supplementation must be sequenced and balanced with zirconium so that no adrenal cortex imbalance develops. Balancing with molybdenum and tungsten becomes necessary after a second niobium/tantalum supplementation. No niobium supplement is on the market; you'll have to produce your own.

Niobium enables efficient fat burning, and therefore is needed to handle stress and for weight loss. Poor stress ability from niobium deficiency can manifest as a dull headache. A similar headache occurs with iron deficiency anemia. Niobium also improves the catabolic parts of 'breakdown and repair' fatty acid healing and fat digestion. As mentioned in the catalyst introduction, stress trauma can use up vast quantities of niobium and tantalum, impairing future catabolic and anabolic fat and fatty acid processes.

Niobium shows no toxicity when supplemented just once. However, a second supplementation too soon after the first can induce prolonged catabolic fat/fatty acid hyperactivity, necessitating liberal use of most other adrenal cortex stress nutrients and WITHDRAWAL from all niobium sources including those providing trace metals naturally until the hyperactivity is broken (similar to caffeine withdrawal in Chapter 7). Usually one niobium supplementation is enough to correct any catalytic fat/fatty acid dysfunction. After that, metal maintenance can continue the positive outcome.

CAUTIONS ☞ (1) Limit niobium supplementation to once a month maximum, and (2) do not ingest any sources of trace metals naturally or cortex stress herbs that will therapeutically interact with a niobium supplementation.

There is very little medical literature on the micronutrient role of niobium; see zirconium above regarding lysosomes.

MOLYBDENUM

Molybdenum is the catalyst for all protein processes in the body. Muscles, tendons, glands and organs, all protein structures require it for their catabolic and anabolic metabolisms. Protein is the most plentiful substance in the body after water, and therefore molybdenum is needed more than any other catalyst and is usually the first to show signs of deficiency. One early sign is altered protein metabolism in the following nitrogen excretion pathway:

$$\text{purine} \xrightarrow{\text{Mo}} \text{xanthine} \xrightarrow{\text{Mo}} \text{uric acid} \longrightarrow \text{urea}$$
$$C_5H_4N_4 \qquad\qquad C_5H_4N_4O_2 \qquad\qquad C_5H_4N_4O_3 \qquad\qquad CH_4N_2O$$

Normally with molybdenum present, purine, the parent compound of nucleic acids, transforms easily to xanthine (xanthurenic acid), uric acid and then to urea, which the kidneys excrete. With insufficient molybdenum, this pathway stops at xanthine, a very harmful substance that damages the pancreas and can cause diabetes. However, the first symptom of xanthine poisoning is pancreatitis, inflammation of the pancreas. Here lack of molybdenum is characterized by mild discomfort or pain in the pancreas after digesting a big protein meal. Nitrogen waste excretion can also be interrupted at the uric acid → urea step. Buildup of uric acid in the blood leads to deposition of crystals in small joints, especially the big toe, resulting in gout. Gout may be partly catalytic in origin, but its catalyst remains unknown.

Molybdenum is the one catalyst available in commercial supplement form. 50 mcg is sufficient to fix a shortage problem such as xanthine in the blood. 150 mcg (maximum) fills the molybdenum reservoir for weeks to months, but should be balanced with tungsten, and after a second such supplementation, with zirconium and niobium/tantalum.

> ## Review of the Medical Literature

Nature... Molybdoenzymes play an essential role in biology,[274] catalyzing the basic metabolic reactions of the nitrogen, sulfur and carbon cycles. Molybdenum is incorporated into proteins as molybdenum cofactor (MoCo), typically a molybdenum atom coordinated to sulfur atoms of a pterin [protein enzyme] derivative.[275] MoCo is required to form molybdoenzymes xanthine oxidase [manganese is also a cofactor[38]], sulfite oxidase and aldehyde oxidase.[276] Tungsten metabolizes in a similar manner.[275]

Catalytic enzymes... Nitrogen cycle xanthine oxidase converts hypoxanthine [base purine] to xanthine and finally to uric acid. In animal studies, xanthine oxidase is widely distributed in the small and large intestines, liver, lungs, kidneys and other tissues.[276] With abnormal metabolism, xanthine and xanthine oxidase can generate free radicals such as superoxide (O_2^-) and induce pancreatitis.[277] Sulfur cycle sulfite oxidase is the terminal enzyme in the sulfur-amino acid oxidation pathway. Sulfite oxidase activity occurs mainly in the liver, heart and kidneys, but this enzyme is also present in mitochondria [cell *organ* responsible for respiration and energy production]. Carbon cycle aldehyde oxidase activity is greater in herbivores that in carnivores.[276]

Hereditary xanthinuria... is a rare genetic disorder of defective nitrogen cycle xanthine oxidase. Kidney stones develop from the large amounts of xanthine excreted in urine. Low purine food [limit meat], high fluid intake and alkalinization of urine are helpful therapies.[278, 279]

Molybdenum cofactor (MoCo) deficiency... another rare genetic disorder, causes neonatal [the first four weeks after birth] seizures, other severe neurological symptoms, high urinary xanthine and sulfite excretion, and early childhood death. No effective treatment exists.[280, 278]

Mo $\rightleftharpoons$ W equilibrium... Several molybdenum- and tungsten-containing enzymes catalyze hydroxylation and oxygen transfer reactions. Pterin groups with different active-site oxo and/or sulfido terminuses coordinate molybdenum and tungsten chemistry.[281] In rats, a tungsten-supplemented diet depletes molybdoenzyme xanthine oxidase.[282]

Dietary status... Food is the major source of molybdenum for the general population. Daily dietary intake averages 100 to 500 mcg. Molybdenum is relatively nontoxic,[283] however, copper deficiency increases the risk of molybdenum toxicity.[284]

Overdose toxicity... The only known case of acute molybdenum poisoning occurred from supplementation loading of 300 to 800 mcg per day over 18 days, for a total dose 13.5 mg beyond dietary intake. This adult male in his late thirties developed acute psychosis with visual/auditory hallucinations, petit mal seizures and one severe grand mal attack. One year later, toxic encephalopathy [brain disease] continued with cognitive deficits, learning disability, depression and post-traumatic stress disorder.[285]

TANTALUM

Tantalum is the catalyst for all anabolic fat processes in the body, necessary for the anabolic parts of 'breakdown and repair' fatty acid healing and the synthesis of fat-based hormones and enzymes. Overall efficiency of ester metabolism requires both tantalum and niobium catalysts. See "Niobium" regarding usage. There is no commercially available tantalum supplement, therefore manufacture your own.

The medical literature on the micronutrient role of tantalum: none.

TUNGSTEN

Tungsten is the catalyst for all carbohydrate processes in the body including carbohydrate to glucose digestion, glucose fueling of cells, carbohydrate body structures and carbohydrate weight loss. Excessive energy use or nervous system trauma can deplete tungsten reserves. This impairs future catabolic and anabolic energy and nerve processes, and is analogous to stress trauma and its niobium/tantalum deprivation consequences. Tungsten shortage may be a factor in amyotrophic lateral sclerosis (ALS, Lou Gehrig's disease) and other nervous system disorders.

Tungsten must be in balance with molybdenum and generally, secondarily with zirconium and niobium/tantalum. No tungsten supplement exists; making your own is presented next.

> Review of the Medical Literature

Nature… Tungsten (atomic number 74) is chemically very similar to molybdenum (atomic number 42). Tungstoenzymes form from pterin [protein enzyme] in a manner similar to molybdoenzymes. While molybdenum's essential role in biology has been understood for decades, tungsten's role was first characterized in hyperthermophilic [surviving at boiling water temperatures and above] archaea [microorganisms/bacteria that thrive in an oxygen-poor environment].[274]

Mo ⇌ W equilibrium… Several molybdenum- and tungsten-containing enzymes catalyze hydroxylation and oxygen transfer reactions. Pterin groups with different active-site oxo and/or sulfido terminuses coordinate molybdenum and tungsten chemistry.[281] In rats, a tungsten-supplemented diet depletes molybdoenzyme xanthine oxidase.[282]

MAKE YOUR OWN SUPPLEMENT

Metals contain *billions and billions* of atoms lined up in crystalline form, like tennis balls stacked in neat rows inside a giant box. The goal in preparing a metal sample and creating a supplement dose is to peel off some of the surface atoms and chemically bind them to organic molecules (chelate them). The best organic molecule to bind to is hot lemon juice from real lemons with the juice and metal sample together in a Pyrex dish, then heated using boiling water or steam from below.

Most metal samples first need to be oxidized, that is, have an oxide coating put on their surfaces. This metal oxide layer reacts more easily and completely with hot lemon juice than the metal itself. Creating the surface oxide usually requires an electric stove, eye protection and gloves, and something to hold the sample, metal tongs or perhaps a fork.

Thin metal sheet is easiest to work with; 0.01 inch (0.25 mm) is ideal thickness. It can be cut to size with a scissors and held between fork prongs. A good 'standard sample size' is a square 1/2-inch long on each side. Of course, the bigger the sample size and surface area, the bigger the eventual metal dose ingested.

The following Table 6-2 trace metals are not available in commercial supplement form: titanium, nickel, zirconium, niobium, tantalum and tungsten. All of these can be purchased as thin metal sheet on the Internet. Some of these metals are found in the home too, or are hidden parts of well-known products.

Sample Preparation. To oxidize metal sheet, use an electric stove with a burner set on high (red hot coils). Place a metal sample directly above and about 1/8 inch from one of the coils until hot and oxidizing, and the sample turns color. Each metal forms a different colored oxide, for example titanium oxide is blue, niobium oxide dull to dark gray. Nickel forms two oxides, one black and one blue, both are OK.

After the sample turns color and the oxide coating is well formed over the entire surface, immediately quench the sample in cold water. Quenching creates a high-energy unstable surface layer, which is easier for the hot lemon juice to peel off.

Turn the sample over and repeat the heating and quenching cycle. Some metals may require slightly different preparation. For example, nickel surfaces will often oxidize in water at room temperature in about a month, or within hours in boiling water, and the resulting nickel oxide coating is not tightly bound to the metal surface, thus no need for heating and quenching.

Supplement Preparation. Place the oxidized sample in hot lemon juice for 5 minutes, then cool and drink the lemon juice, which looks unaffected but actually contains many, many chelated metal atoms. EUREKA, your own homemade supplement!

Reusing the Same Sample. One big problem with obtaining subsequent supplement doses from an already oxidized sample is that any new oxide coating added during a second sample preparation does not form on the sample surface, but instead at the metal-oxide interface underneath the already metal-depleted old oxide layer. Consequently, old oxide coatings must be ground off or scrapped away with a sharp knife before sample preparation begins anew.

OVERVIEW

Age is not a state of mind; it is a state of body. Aging is not linear; it only seems so by standard human measures. Actually, aging is closer to geometric in its progression – little occurs when you're young and all body systems are working well, but later as these systems struggle and accumulate failure, aging accelerates dramatically. Two destructive forces will prove foremost in your demise: (1) loss of one or more antioxidant defenses. A specific antioxidant failure leads to serious disease. General decline in the antioxidant defense network turns you into a heap of scar tissue, both inside and out, from oxidative stress. And (2) running out of metals. Metals impose order on body chaos. Fundamental adrenal and endocrine chemical processes grind to a halt without metalloenzymes and metal catalysts. You don't feel good; nothing works right! You literally become a hollow shell of what you can be.

It is hard to view the importance of trace metals clearly. Who would believe that the hidden affects so profoundly? Individual trace metal roles as described in the medical literature tell the metal nutrient story best. You absolutely need small amounts of all these metals in perfect balance for vibrant health and long life. Take nature's full-spectrum metal sources of Dandelion Root, Colloidal Minerals, Black Currants/Blackstrap Molasses and, best of all, the organic garden to maintain health. Collectively, these are called "trace metals naturally" in this book. Chelated supplementation can be an effective health maintenance strategy too, particularly in meeting current Energy, Healing, Stress and Immune needs exactly, but it must be augmented with the full-spectrum sources to insure perfect attendance by all metals during all body metabolisms. In times of severe stress or trauma, even healthy metal reserves in liver, bones, teeth and elsewhere become depleted, triggering dysfunction and disease. Then extensive supplementation is required to overcome the deprivation and return to normal.

***

7. HERBS

Herbs are one of the five raw materials that your Energy, Healing, Stress and Immune functions and systems need to make all their hormones and other end products and to perform properly under all circumstances. They are essential for good health because like B vitamins, fatty acids and trace metals, herbs are vitamins too! Or more precisely, they contain vitamin/nutritional factors. Herbs supply key nutrients to optimize adrenal and endocrine performance. However, they are needed only in very small amounts; therefore a term such as "micronutrient" is appropriate to distinguish herbs and indicate dosage. Another good definition of herb is: critical nutrition, sometimes very potent nutrition, for a specific adrenal or endocrine spot, as opposed to B vitamin and fatty acid foods, which operate over a bigger domain and require larger servings. Because of strong therapeutic effect, continuous use of the same herb can turn a fine-tuning vitamin factor into a counterproductive, overdose abuser of functioning. Accordingly, use herbs cautiously. Provide for your needs, but don't overwhelm your system with a good thing.

This chapter describes adrenal herbs, though many of these have other endocrine duties as well. Herbs for the pituitary, pancreas and liver are presented in Chapters 8, 10 and 11, respectively. All herbs are capitalized throughout the book to make recognition easier. The following general introduction explains the nature and proper use of herbs.

Therapeutic Action

The therapeutic action timeline of most herbs is exactly like that of B vitamins, with maximum effect at 2 hours after ingestion and decay to zero in 7½ hours (see Figure 4-B). Herbs act on adrenal and endocrine functioning in three possible ways, as shown in Table 7-1. Many herbs "rev" adrenal functioning, or more precisely some specific part of adrenal functioning. This action is exactly maintenance dose

(1X, ↑) therapeutic action as described in Table 4-2. A second dose of the same herb before the first dose decays to zero at t = 7½ hours produces a much stronger effect. Stimulation (2X, ↑↑) can be helpful in restoring function, but always avoid 3X harmful overstimulation, or overdose. Taking an adrenal herb with B vitamin whole-grain cereals, nutritional yeasts or green vegetables can gently adjust and fine-tune functioning while still maintaining 1X. This is an excellent way to build health over time.

TABLE 7-1. HERBAL ACTION ON ADRENAL AND ENDOCRINE FUNCTIONING.

Nature of Action	Symbol
"rev"	↑
"get things running right"	()
suppression	↓

The following new terms and therapeutic actions are specific to herbs alone. Some herbs "get things running right" (()). These rebalance adrenal functioning, bringing back equilibrium and normal activity between or within affected primary functions. Take "get things running right" herbs at 1X dosing only; 2X proves counterproductive. A few herbs "suppress" (↓) one specific part of the adrenal gland, usually within the medulla. 1X only here too, as 2X transfers the suppression to the pituitary gland.

Herbs are the ultimate fine-tuners of the adrenal gland and endocrine system. Their targeted nutrition and potent vitamin nature revitalizes functions and rebalances metabolisms with an assortment of therapeutic actions from rev (↑, 1X) and stimulation (↑↑, 2X) to "get things running right" ((), 1X) and suppression (↓, 1X). Herbs can correct past nutritional deficits and restore health to your crucial Energy, Healing, Stress and Immune functions and systems.

Occasional Use

"Occasionally" describes proper herb usage. This modifier has a slightly different meaning for herbs than for trace metals. For any herb, "once a week" is the maximum use necessary to maintain health, although much less often is usually sufficient. Remember, herbs are <u>micro</u>nutrients and required only in very small concentrations. Caffeine is actually an herbal factor and potent nerve micronutrient – that's its problem! Too much, too often (3X or more) produces toxic overdose nerve and energy side effects. All overused, abused herbs will similarly vex their area of influence. Of course, many herbs can be taken at 2X for one day to jolt lazy, faulty functioning back to normal, or at 1X over several days to the same effect. Some nutritional books recommend daily intake of this or that particular herb for extended periods. Such employment, however, is more suitable to overcoming dysfunction and disease than prevention, and effective only with very abnormal adrenal functioning. With normal or near-normal functioning, continuous use of any herb generates severe imbalances, and eventually dysfunction. Think of herbs as exotic foods. A different herb each day provides outstanding nutritional variety.

Combining Herbs

Chinese herbal tradition involves ingesting several to many herbs at the same time. It is hard to argue with their long and storied history, their knowledge of hundreds of herbs (the author certainly learned much), and their success... BUT (always a "but") combinations can produce a result different from and worse than the sum of each herb separately. Much depends on the function being helped; the adrenal medulla is especially vulnerable to overstimulating interactions. Many useful herb synergies do exist and are indicated in the coming pages. Many more positive interactions await discovery. Each herb *tweaks* the millions of interconnected functions of the human body in a specific pattern; one can think of it as a symphony that cannot be heard except for the dominant theme. Putting two symphonies together can generate cacophony.

One example of cacophony is Oats and Nettle together. Oats are very good alone as a whole-grain cereal and the #1 nerve vitamin on the planet. Nettle alone is good for fatigue and nerves. Together, they are an aphrodisiac in folklore, and in fact the resulting nervous energy is intense. Unfortunately, it is also a serious, harmful overstimulation of the nervous system, far beyond 3X. The author's nerves were *in orbit* for a week after this combination, with another week exacted to fix all the damage to nerve/Energy function.

Guidelines on Herbal Combinations

Adrenal Medulla Herbs...........As a rule, take no more than one medulla herb per day. Combining medulla herbs whether they nourish energy, nerves or healing produces medulla hyperactivity, with a few notable exceptions such as Peppermint and Spearmint. Antioxidation herbs (Healing subfunction) act independently, and they can be taken without consideration of other medulla herbs or herbs in general.

Adrenal Cortex Herbs ....Alone is OK, and many cortex herb combinations work well. However, putting the strongest actors for the same functional purpose together can cause overstimulation, and should be avoided.

"Get Things Running
Right" (◊) Herbs...................Always take these herbs separately. Combining them with other herbs upsets their special therapeutic effect. And two "get things running right" herbs almost always clash.

Suppression (↓) Herbs............Always alone.

Pancreas Herbs.......................Same as adrenal cortex herbs.

Liver Herbs.............................All liver herbs can be taken together.

Pituitary Herbs ....No pituitary herbs together. Each must be taken separately to avoid harmful interactions and pituitary overstimulations.

When in doubt........................Play safe. Stick with combinations recommended by traditional practitioners: Chinese and Ayurvedic herbalists. Most modern combinations do not pass the test of time – thousands of years of trial and error!

Capsule, Tea and Tincture

Capsule, tea and tincture are the three most common ways to take herbs. Many herbs perform well in capsule form. Ground into a fine powder for easy assimilation, they have a known, specific dosage. Some herbs in capsule are too strong or have different or incorrect action; these should be taken as tea. Making tea is very easy: boil water, remove from the heat, add one to two teaspoons of the herb, steep for five to ten minutes, strain and serve. Teas are very soothing in their effect. Tincture dissolves the powdered herb in alcohol solution. More goodness goes into tincture than tea; tincture stores well for long periods; and all herbs can be taken as tincture. A standardized, concentrated tincture is called a fluidextract and contains one gram of the herb per cubic centimeter. Ingest only one or two drops of a fluidextract.

Quality

Quality is getting harder and harder to come by. There are over one hundred herbal providers in this industry, however, considerably fewer manufacturers. Product is sold and resold. Standards are often non-existent. Standardized extracts, originally introduced in Europe for herbs such as Ginkgo biloba, are now twisted to meet the standard for one or two ingredients, but otherwise bear little resemblance to nature's original goodness. Recently, the author found a grievous example of extract exploitation at the local pharmacy. The pharmacy brand Saw Palmetto Extract was labeled in a way that made it impossible to determine its Saw Palmetto content. The capsules contained a white powder, yet dried Saw Palmetto Berries are black in color. This brought to mind "The Three Stooges" short film on their restaurant misadventures. A customer ordered chicken soup from Moe. In the kitchen, Shemp prepared it by taking a chicken out of the icebox and pouring hot water though it! Don't buy herbs by price, advertising or company size. In fact, these are probably contraindicators. The best herbs companies/sources are Nature's Way® and Nature's Answer®. Beyond that, "Self" Magazine (350 Madison Avenue, New York, NY 10017 - http://www.self.com) rates herbal companies for quality (including quality assurance by outside laboratory), reliability and service. Choose from its 'A+' and 'A' lists.

Reference Books

What follows is herbal use to achieve complete nutrition and internal balance of functions, without reference to history or traditional uses. Many excellent resource books cover these subjects; inclusion here would be redundant and massive in size. If you want background on and some grounding in herbs, the following four books are excellent guides:

"Back to Eden" by Jethro Kloss
"The Herb Book" by John Lust
"The Little Herb Encyclopedia" by Jack Ritchason
"The Healing Power of Herbs" by Michael Murray

Adrenal Herbs

The list of adrenal herbs is huge, over 100 active participants. However, only about ten of these herbs are essential nutrition, and a few more satisfy special needs. The rest provide strong, corrective therapeutic action for functional weak spots, imbalances and exhaustions. A brief orientation to the major chapter sections ahead will help you to see *the big picture.*

Internal balance is the determining factor in sickness and health. Adrenal herbs can play a major role in building internal balance in two ways: (1) by "getting things running right" (◖) between and within your primary Energy, Healing, Stress and Immune functions; and (2) by delivering targeted, corrective nutrition to specific functions and subfunctions.

> "Adrenal Balance" (immediately below) examines the herbs Scullcap, Damiana, Angelica, Suma, Devil's Claw and Goldenseal Root, and shows how these six equilibrium specialists "get things running right" throughout the adrenal gland, thereby restoring harmony to your internal life. The solution to arthritis is outlined there.

The rest of the chapter focuses on building optimal health within each primary function and its supporting subfunctions:

> "Adrenal Medulla Energy/Nerve Herbs" (summarized in one place, Table 7-3) describe healthy ways to boost adrenaline and flagging energy, essential nerve nutrition with Oats and Valerian, St. John's Wort for mild depression and *the blues*, Kava to ease anxiety, and so

forth. How to maintain and rebuild function is explored, and in the case of coffee/caffeine, an overdose abuser of nerves, how to correct this forced hyperactivity and unnatural need that becomes caffeine fix syndrome. All addictions lie in the nervous system.

"Adrenal Medulla Healing Herbs" (Table 7-4) discuss the following herbs and functional systems. Aloe vera is excellent not only for burns, but for all types of external and internal repair. Some herbs empower specific healing; for example Alfalfa Seed Tea helps to heal the adrenal gland, pancreas and nervous system. "Fountain of youth" special factors glucosamine, DMAE and alpha-lipoic acid can actually reverse aging. Antioxidation is a key subfunction, and principal water-soluble antioxidants Vitamin C, Pine Bark Extract and Grape Seed Extract protect cells and tissues from free radical attack and oxidative stress. Lastly, vasoconstriction and vasodilation are Healing and Immune subfunctions, and here herbs can restore blood vessel homeostasis, which is corrective for blood pressure, varicose veins and bluing of small blood vessels, inflammatory '-itis' diseases such as arthritis, edema and related fatigue headaches, and possibly migraine with its uncontrollable dilation of blood vessels in the brain.

"Adrenal Cortex Stress/Fatigue Herbs" (Table 7-5) deliver powerful nutrition to nourish your cortisol and aldosterone hormones. All cortex herbs are anti-inflammatory and much gentler than NSAIDs (nonsteroidal anti-inflammatory drugs) or steroids. Raw Garlic prevents fatigue, while Guarana relieves fatigue. Sarsaparilla and American Ginseng improve the cortex sex subfunction, with help from male herbs Saw Palmetto Berries, Pygeum and Nettle Root for BPH (benign prostatic hyperplasia) or female herbs Black Cohosh for menopause and hormone replacement, and Chaste Berries for premenstrual syndrome (PMS) and menopause.

"Adrenal Cortex Immune Herbs" (Table 7-6) provide 24/7 life insurance against disease. Essential immune system herbs are Goldenseal Root (emergencies only), Blue-Green Algae, Vitamin C plus bioflavonoids, Echinacea, Astragalus and Green Tea. Twenty-seven more aides-de-camp help rebuild defenses and fight bacteria, viruses, fungi, allergies, cancer and leukemia. Life is not a rehearsal; preserve it the first time around!

Herbs are powerful medicine. Essential herbs are very nutritious and for the most part very gentle. Corrective herbs act in a manner similar to Western allopathic drugs, but generally without side effects because they are still of nature. Herbs have also con-tributed significantly to Western drugs. The opium poppy gives us morphine, an indis-pensable analgesic. Foxglove, botanical name digitalis purpurea, furnishes the heart stimulant digitalis. In 1897, Bayer added an acetyl radical to the salicylic acid of White Willow Bark, an American Indian herb for headache, to create acetylsalicylic acid aspirin. Science has examined approximately one-half of one percent of the higher plants for pharmaceutical potential, yet these have yielded 25% of the allopathic drugs on the pharmacist's shelf.[1] Because both herbs and drugs possess strong therapeutic action, adverse interactions between them are common. Herb-drug interactions are reported fully in the pages ahead. For more science on any herb or any medical topic, go to National Institute of Health (NIH) "National Library Of Medicine" Internet site where you will find the abstracts of all 15 million articles in the medical literature.

This chapter is filled with details. Most of these details concern corrective herbs for dysfunctions and diseases. Herbs are nature's pharmacy. Even with no government or drug company money to support research efforts, many herbs demonstrate efficacy in the scientific medical literature. Start your herb adventure simply though by under-standing "Adrenal Balance" below, then incorporating the essential herbs of Tables 7-3 to 7-6 into your diet.

ADRENAL BALANCE

Balance in your life is fundamental to good health. And so it is with adrenal bal-ance. Correcting minor adrenal imbalances can restore youthful vigor and your body's own life-giving chemistry. Table 7-2 and Figure 7-A below reveal four herbs that will help rebuild homeostatic equilibrium ($\rightleftharpoons$) and balance ($\rightarrow$) between and within the four primary adrenal functions by "getting things running right" ($\circlearrowleft$). Use Scullcap, Damiana, Angelica, and Suma to tweak and gently push imbalances out of your system.

TABLE 7-2. ADRENAL BALANCE HERBS.

Herb	"gets things running right" (↻) between...
Scullcap	Adrenal Medulla Healing ⇌ Energy
Damiana	Adrenal Medulla Energy → Adrenal Cortex Stress
Angelica	Adrenal Medulla Healing → Adrenal Cortex Immune
Suma	Adrenal Cortex Immune ⇌ Stress

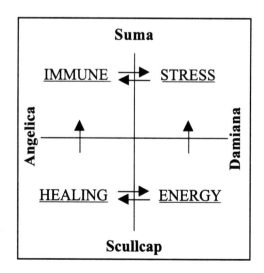

FIGURE 7-A. ADRENAL BALANCE HERBS "GET THINGS RUNNING RIGHT" BETWEEN FUNCTIONS.

SCULLCAP

Scullcap helps to rebuild adrenal medulla equilibrium ($\rightleftharpoons$) between Healing and Energy and their subfunctions. Regrettably, this herb is not all-powerful and cannot overcome severe medulla imbalances. However, it helps – an important tool in restoring medulla health.

Medulla equilibrium is a very *wishy-washy* mechanism. Every medulla herb, as well as every medulla B vitamin, fatty acid and trace metal, pushes this equilibrium a little one way or the other. Thus, Healing $\rightleftharpoons$ Energy is in a continuous state of flux, and Scullcap tries to re-center any imbalance. To maintain healing/antioxidation $\rightleftharpoons$ energy/nerve health or to rebuild this equilibrium requires a constant balancing act of raw materials. Re-centering is not an instant one-time fix; nature never works by instant pills! Instead, re-centering involves selecting appropriate energy, nerve, healing and antioxidation nutrients to satisfy needs and relieve deficiencies, and using Scullcap first and last in the push toward healthy equilibrium.

Scullcap usage: Take 500 mg (maximum) in capsule form as needed. 1X only. Using Scullcap too often, more than once a week, causes it to lose effectiveness and become harsh. By rebalancing the adrenal medulla, Scullcap promotes sleep.

Substitute: Gotu Kola also "gets things running right" ($\circlearrowleft$) within the adrenal medulla, but with mild nerve suppressant ($\frac{1}{2}$ $\downarrow$) action. Gotu Kola is most useful in correcting imbalances caused by caffeine and other nerve stimulants. See Table 7-3 and its profile in the text there.

> Review of the Medical Literature

Three species of genus Scutellaria: S. lateriflora, S. baicalensis and S. galericulata are known collectively as Scullcap.[2] Note: Common American usage and that described in this book is Scutellaria lateriflora. All meaningful studies in the medical literature have been done on the similar-acting Chinese herb, Scutellaria baicalensis, which should be used for any of the critical applications listed below.

Antioxidant... Scullcap (Scutellaria baicalensis) and constituent flavonoids such as baicalein reduce oxidative stress by inhibiting lipid peroxidation [lipids: fats and fat-related compounds] and by scavenging superoxide [O_2^-], hydrogen peroxide [H_2O_2], and hydroxyl [OH^-] free radicals.[3, 4] In animal studies, another flavonoid of Scullcap, baicalin, is both antioxidant and biological response modifier, improving cellular repair of damaged DNA.[5]

Antioxidant/Energy... Scullcap protects animal mitochondria [cell *organ* responsible for respiration and energy production] membranes and prevents energy loss during hypoxia [inadequate oxygen].[6]

Emotions... Scullcap reduces psychoemotional stress, by stimulating and normalizing erythropoiesis [red blood cell production].[7]

Stomach ulcers... Scullcap evidences strong antiulcer activity.[8]

Anti-inflammatory... Scullcap flavonoid baicalein exerts anti-inflammatory and antioxidant effects, and is a well-known inhibitor of 12-lipoxygenase [catalyzing enzyme for arachidonic acid conversion to leukotrienes, part of the immune/inflammatory response].[9, 10] Baicalein lessens inflammatory-induced cell death of brain microglia [removes waste from nerve tissue] by suppressing cytotoxic NO [nitric oxide] production.[9]

Bacteria, viruses and fungi... Scullcap possesses antibacterial and antiviral activity.[11] Baicalin inhibits HIV-1 infection and replication.[12] Against Candida albicans [common fungus infection], Scullcap shows the highest activity of 56 widely used Chinese medical plants.[13]

Anticancer... Scullcap demonstrates strong dose-dependent growth inhibition of common human cancers, including squamous [scaly, platelike] cell carcinoma (SCC-25, KB), breast cancer (MCF-7), hepatocellular carcinoma (HepG2), prostate carcinoma (PC-3 and LNCaP), and colon cancer (KM-12 and HCT-15). Scullcap inhibits prostaglandin (PG)E2 [potent mediator of conduction/transmitter functions regulating cellular activities] production, which may account for the suppression of tumor cell growth.[14] Scullcap improves macrophage [long-living, large white blood cell; -phage: anything that devours] function and inhibits in vivo [inside the living body] tumor growth.[11] Flavonoids baicalein and baicalin strongly inhibit angiogenesis [new capillary blood vessels].[15]

Chemotherapy helper... In lung cancer patients, reduced T-lymphocytes during chemotherapy can be offset by incorporating Scullcap in the therapeutic regimen. Scullcap increases Immunoglobulin A [IgA: antibody proteins in tears, saliva, respiratory, gastroin-testinal, urinary and reproductive tracts protect mucous linings from infection] while main-taining Immunoglobulin G [IgG: circulate in the blood giving long-term immunity against previously encountered bacteria, viruses and other pathogens].[16]

DAMIANA

Damiana restores Energy → Stress balance. While no equilibrium arrows (⇌) exist between medulla energy and cortex stress, there still must be a *kind of balance* between these tasks. This is a balance of equal functioning levels or strength. To illus-trate, Primary Stress can become functionally stronger than Primary Energy if nutri-tional yeasts are consumed over an extended period without also taking whole-grain cereals (see Chapter 4). This functional strength imbalance causes a pituitary sup-pression as a normal homeostatic consequence. Damiana corrects all Energy → Stress imbalances, no matter the cause. Damiana strengthens your body's energy-stress action plan. It "gets things running right" between medulla and cortex, so challeng-ing tasks can change from energy (cells burn glucose) to stress (cells burn esters/fats) efficiently. Since sex lies within both these functions, Damiana also improves sexual balance. Take 500 mg (maximum) in capsule form, or as a tea. 1X only, as needed.

Medical literature review... Damiana (Turnera diffusa) is a sexual stimulant.[17] Damiana decreases the hyperglycemic peak in diabetic animals.[18]

ANGELICA

Angelica restores functional balance to Healing → Immune in the same way that Damiana works on Energy and Stress. Zinc lozenges have become popular for treat-ing colds and flu. They do work, but for the most part indirectly and only at 3X or more. Such dosing produces healing overstimulation, then immune stimulation, and several days later immune suppression! Homeostatic feedback causes this response. When a medulla function dominants (here from overstimulation), suppression even-tually develops in the next-in-line cortex function. When a cortex function dominates, the suppression ends up in the pituitary. Angelica corrects all Healing → Immune imbalances, no matter the cause. Angelica strengthens your body's healing-immune action plan. 500 mg (maximum) in capsule form, or as a tea. 1X only, as needed.

Botanically, Angelica has four major species. Angelica atropurpurea (American) is described here. Angelica atropurpurea and Angelica archangelica (European) have similar medicinal properties. Angelica sinensis (Chinese), also known as Dong Quai, generates very different therapeutic effects and is profiled in Table 7-5 and associated text. Angelica acutiloba (Japanese) behaves much like Chinese Angelica sinensis. No meaningful medical literature exists on the micronutrient role of American Angelica; most investigations have studied Dong Quai.

SUMA

Suma helps to rebuild cortex equilibrium between Immune ⇌ Stress and their subfunctions. Like Scullcap, Suma is not all-powerful in this endeavor. Rather, it is an important tool to be used <u>first</u> and <u>last</u> in correcting imbalances. The herb also improves pituitary oversight of cortex functions. Suma causes soft functioning, and therefore should be taken in the evening after the stress of the day is over. 1000 mg (maximum) from capsule as needed, 1X only.

Medical literature review… Suma (Pfaffia paniculata), like Damiana, is a sexual stimulant.[17] Suma improves the hydration and rheological [blood flow] properties of sickle cells [hemoglobin defect; sickled cells become trapped in capillaries causing severe anemia] including deformability, Na+ content and mean corpuscular volume.[19]

<u>Adrenal cortex equilibrium is not a wishy-washy mechanism like that of the medulla. IT IS ROCK SOLID</u>! When "in equilibrium," the cortex stays in equilibrium and is hard to knock off center. When "out of equilibrium" with arthritis for example, the cortex is hard to re-center and cure of this dependent-body-system disease. However, two herbs Devil's Claw and Goldenseal Root can restore Immune ⇌ Stress equilibrium beautifully, resetting the balance in new *concrete*.

How to reset cortex equilibrium—Take Devil's Claw and Goldenseal Root only after implementing the following steps: (1) for several weeks, liberally supply all cortex raw materials: Chapter 4 nutritional yeasts and green vegetables, Chapter 5 Omega 3 fatty acids, Chapter 6 trace metals, and cortex herbs from Tables 7-5 and 7-6 ahead. This will satisfy current needs, fill empty nutrient reserves and ease the nutritional debt. (2) Fix any adrenal cortex exhaustions, mild or severe. For mild cortex exhaustion, see Chapter 4 for appropriate B vitamin supplementations and

Chapter 6 for trace metal supplementations. Severe exhaustion requires Chapter 12 remedy. Then, (3) re-center cortex equilibrium using Figure 7-B below. These three steps together can cure arthritis!

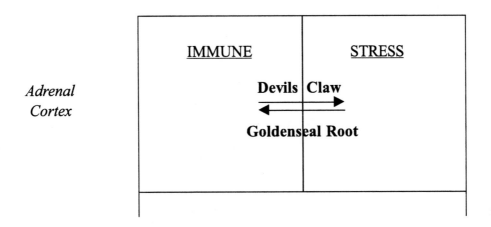

FIGURE 7-B. DEVIL'S CLAW AND GOLDENSEAL ROOT.
(Compare with Figure 4-C)

DEVIL'S CLAW

Figure 7-B shows that Devil's Claw moves Immune ⇌ Stress equilibrium toward Stress, which will for example ease the root cause and thereby the symptoms of arthritis. Of course, arthritis' root cause is first unsatisfied nutritional needs, second functional exhaustion, and only third correcting cortex imbalance. So third, move cortex equilibrium slowly one way (Devil's Claw) or the other (Goldenseal Root). At the start, 1000 mg of Devil's Claw once per day is appropriate, soon 500 mg, and then final adjustments with 250 mg per day. Don't look for total arthritic symptom relief at this point, as that may require healing and Primary Healing Function improvements too, especially with osteoarthritis. Instead, look for the hypoactive immune, hyperactive stress functioning of mild Cushing's syndrome (symptoms described in Chapter 2 "Drugs, Hormones and Gland Extracts"), indicating you have moved Immune ⇌ Stress too far to the Stress side. Don't worry, however, this is not a problem as Goldenseal Root can correct any overshoot. In fact, overshoot initially is good. A little back and forth final adjustment with Devil's Claw and Goldenseal Root adds micronutrient synergy.

Anti-inflammatory, rheumatism... Devil's Claw (Harpagophytum procumbens) has anti-inflammatory and analgesic action. It alleviates painful degenerative rheumatism, improving motility [spontaneous movement] and relieving pain.[20-22] Or oppositely, Devil's Claw lacks anti-inflammatory effect.[23, 24] This contradiction may be due to stomach acidity, as excess acid inhibits Devil's Claw activity while antacids protect its active ingredients.[21, 25]

Low back pain... Devil's Claw is effective in reducing acutely exacerbated low back pain.[26]

Heart... Devil's Claw decreases heart rate and arterial blood pressure, and protects against arrhythmia [abnormal heart beat: too slow, too rapid, too early, irregular] in animal studies.[27, 28]

Drug interaction... Devil's Claw may interact with warfarin [prescription drug, inhibitor of blood clotting].[29]

GOLDENSEAL ROOT

Goldenseal Root moves Immune ⇌ Stress equilibrium toward Immune, and will fix hypoactive immune functioning and help cure Cushing's syndrome. As with Devil's Claw, 1000 mg of Goldenseal Root once per day at the start (unless correcting Devil's Claw overshoot), soon 500 mg, and then final adjustments with 250 mg. Never take Devil's Claw and Goldenseal Root on the same day. Once reset in new *concrete*, cortex equilibrium will never move again if you provide all necessary raw material nutrients. Yes, temporarily out of balance will occur, but this is normal and non-arthritic.

Goldenseal Root can be useful short term in emergency situations to help your immune system fight off infection, cold, flu, pneumonia or worse. Goldenseal supercharges all immune defense systems and lymphocytes! Table 7-6 "Immune Herbs" explains this defense application. When the fight is won, however, rebalance cortex equilibrium with like dosage of Devil's Claw.

From time to time, employing Goldenseal Root, then readjusting with Devil's Claw a day or two later will strengthening both Stress and Immune functions. This invigorating therapy is also health checkup to be sure cortex equilibrium is perfect.

Finally, after completing any adjustments with Devil's Claw and Goldenseal Root, take Suma to "get things running right" (**Ɔ**) again <u>within</u> the entire cortex and all subfunctions.

Review of the Medical Literature

Immune... Goldenseal Root (Hydrastis canadensis) increases primary IgM response [Immunoglobulin M: typically the first antibodies in an immune response].[30] Plant alkaloid berberine is one active constituent. Berberine shows significant antimicrobial activity against bacteria, viruses, fungi, chlamydia [common sexually-transmitted bacterial infection], protozoans and parasitic worms. Berberine clinical uses include bacterial diarrhea, intestinal parasite infections and ocular trachoma [chronic infectious disease of the cornea].[31] Berberine also has antitumor activity,[32] and efficacy against multiple-drug-resistant mycobacterium tuberculosis.[33]

ADRENAL MEDULLA ENERGY/NERVE

Many herbs nourish the adrenal medulla, and a considerable number of these are nerve herbs. In general, medulla herbs have broad effects, that is, almost all medulla herbs (nerve or otherwise) improve both Energy and Healing functions to some extent. Just four medulla herbs are 100% Energy/nerve function in their activity: Oats, Valerian, Lavender and St. John's Wort. Likewise few medulla herbs are 100% Healing. In the tables ahead, medulla herbs are listed according to their dominant effect only, under specific subfunctions of Energy in Table 7-3 and Healing in Table 7-4. Some herbs like Sage possess equalizing medulla action and are listed in both tables.

Table 7-3 presents all adrenal medulla Primary Energy Function herbs. Details on how to use these energy, nerve, mood, start of sex (nervous energy), and energy/nerve suppression nutrients follow the table.

TABLE 7-3. ADRENAL MEDULLA ENERGY/NERVE HERBS.

Subheadings (underlined) specify use. Numbering of nerve herbs (#1 to #15) indicates "need for," not potency.

Herb	Comments
ENERGY	
American Ginseng	Activates the energy-stress action plan. See also stress (Table 7-5).
Fo-Ti	Essential for high-energy tasks.
Alfalfa Seed Tea	Also healing (Table 7-4).
Bee Pollen	Possible allergic reaction, test first (see text).
NERVES – MAINTAIN HEALTH, i.e. ESSENTIAL (in order of importance)	
#1 Oats	100% Energy/nerve, 0% Healing. Also a whole-grain cereal (Table 4-1). Not with Nettle.
#2 Valerian	100% nerve, 0% Healing. Excellent for sleep.
NERVES – REBUILD HEALTH (approximate order of importance)	
#3 Chamomile	Sleep.
#4 Wood Betony	Also pituitary-energy/nerve (Figure 8-B).
#5 Nettle	Also adrenal cortex fatigue (Table 7-5). Not with Oats.
#6 Hops	Herb or occasional beer.
#7 Buchu	Also endocrine pancreas (Table 10-1).
#8 Peppermint and Spearmint	Good together, or separately. Also immune (Table 7-6) and stomach digestion.
#9 Sage	Also healing (Table 7-4); nourishes the entire medulla.
#10 Bilberry	Also healing (Table 7-4) and endocrine pancreas (Table 10-1)
#11 Strawberry, Raspberry and Blackberry Leaves	Good together, or separately. Also endocrine pancreas (Table 10-1).

#12 Lavender	100% nerve, 0% Healing. Topical application only (#1 in potency). Ingestion pushes medulla equilibrium strongly toward nerves, but two stigmas (max.) ingested with Oats can correct severe Healing ← ← Energy/nerve imbalance.
#13 Blue Vervain	
#14 Black Walnut Hulls	Skin problems.
#15 caffeine	It's everywhere; no need to seek it out. #2 in potency. Too much causes Energy/nerve dysfunction. See "Rebuilding Nerve Health" text ahead.

FEELING DOWN, THE BLUES, MILD DEPRESSION

| St. John's Wort | 100% mood, 0% Healing. MAO inhibitor and much more. Can be taken daily. |

ANXIETY

Kava Kava	Natural, mild tranquilizer.
Valerian	Also nerves, above.
Licorice	Also adrenal cortex gluconeogenesis (Table 7-5). See text there.

START OF SEX (nervous energy)

| Oats | "Sow your wild oats!" |
| Yohimbe | Sexual/nerve dysfunction, see text. |

ENERGY/NERVE SUPRESSION (↓)

Kudzu	Strong nerve suppressant.
Gotu Kola	Nerve suppressant ($1/2$↓), plus adrenal medulla () and pituitary-medulla () (Figure 8-B).
Oregon Grape	Energy/nerve ↓, Healing ↑.

Energy

Adrenaline and other energy hormones come from the building block nutrients of complex carbohydrates, natural B vitamin whole-grain cereals, essential fatty acids (EFAs) and trace metals. Herbs enhance and fine-tune the action of these Chapter 3-6 nutrients. The four energy herbs listed in Table 7-3 – American Ginseng, Fo-Ti, Alfalfa Seed Tea and Bee Pollen – add long-lastingness (if that's a word) to your energy output.

AMERICAN GINSENG

American Ginseng activates and invigorates your body's energy-stress action plan, getting you ready for the activities of the day. Ginseng energizes you, strengthens stress ability and "gets things running right" (◊) between and within these two crucial functions and the entire adrenal gland.

American Ginseng is the best of several ginsengs. Korean/Asiatic Ginseng is not as potent, Siberian Ginseng a completely different plant. Wild ginseng is preferred over cultivated, and older roots and rhizomes over younger ones. Take American Ginseng at 1X dosing only, and not with other herbs, so as not to disrupt its ◊ corrective action. However, the natural B vitamin-rich foods of whole-grain cereals, nutritional yeasts and green vegetables "synergize" well with American Ginseng. 500 to 1000 mg once or twice a week in the morning is very effective.

CAUTION ☛ Some women may experience breast tenderness when taking American Ginseng. In such case, reduce dosage (a little bit still helps a lot) or substitute Korean Ginseng to alleviate this estrogenic effect. See the female medical literature citation below.

Review of the Medical Literature

Antioxidant, cardiovascular effects... American Ginseng (Panax quinquefolius) and other genus Panax have been used as revitalizing agents for millenia.[34] American Ginseng possesses strong antioxidant activity in both water and lipid [fat-based] mediums,[35] including protecting low-density lipoproteins [LDL, so-called bad cholesterol] from oxidation.[36] Ginseng further benefits cardiovascular health by inhibiting thrombin [catalytic enzyme, the last step in the blood clotting process], and may assist in hemodynamic balance of the vascular endothelium [lining of the heart and blood vessels].[37]

Memory and brain neurotransmitters... American Ginseng improves memory and learning in animals.[38] By facilitating acetylcholine [neurotransmitter, nervous system stimulant, vasodilator, cardiac depressant] release,[39] and GABA [inhibitory neurotransmitter; helps prevent system overload] neurotransmission,[40] American Ginseng modulates brain function.[41]

Antidiabetic... American Ginseng reduces postprandial [after a meal] blood glucose levels in non-diabetic and Type II [adult onset] diabetic patients.[42]

Immune... American Ginseng inhibits HIV-1 multiplication and shows antifungal activity.[43] Both Panax ginseng and Echinacea purpurea significantly boost NK [natural killer lymphocytes: active in spontaneous, non-specific immunity against cancer and viruses, first-line defense against cancer] function in all human population subgroups, from normal subjects to patients with chronic fatigue syndrome (CFS) [symptoms include weakness, fatigue, muscle pain, lymph node swelling] and AIDS.[44]

Female/Male... American Ginseng exerts estrogen-like effects,[45] and may relieve menopause symptoms. Concurrent use with breast cancer drugs synergistically inhibits cancer cell growth for most drugs evaluated.[46] Both American and Asian forms of ginseng enhance libido and copulatory performance. These effects may not be due to hormone secretion, but rather to direct ginsenoside [active compound] effects on the central nervous system and gonadal tissues. In males, ginsenosides facilitate penile erection through vasodilatation and relaxation of penile corpus cavernosum. Only the American form of ginseng affects the hypothalamic catecholamines [sympathetic nervous system effectors such as dopamine and epinephrine] involved in copulatory behavior and associated hormone secretion.[47]

Drug interactions... Ginseng may affect blood clotting, and should not be concomitant with warfarin [prescription drug, inhibitor of blood clotting]. In patients on phenelzine sulfate [strong MAO inhibitor, for depression and anxiety], Ginseng may cause trembling, headache and manic episodes. Because of possible additive effects, avoid Ginseng with estrogens or corticosteroids. Ginseng may interfere with digoxin [digitalis derivative for congestive heart failure with a small margin between therapeutic and toxic dose].[48]

FO-TI

Fo-Ti is essential for high-energy tasks such as physical labor and sports. Just a little of this Chinese herb Ho Shou Wu, 50 to 100 mg, builds energy endurance and performance.

> ## Review of the Medical Literature

Heart… Fo-Ti (Polygonum multiflorum) protects against myocardial [heart muscle] injury in rats by preserving glutathione [natural internal antioxidant: within cell mitochondria, the main defense against oxidative stress].[49] The traditional Chinese 'Dang-Gui Decoction for Enriching the Blood' of Angelica sinensis [Dong Quai, Table 7-5] and Astragalus [Tables 7-5 and 7-6] stimulates red blood cell production and improves cardiovascular function. Adding Fo-Ti to the formulation gives more potent and complete myocardial protection.[50]

Memory… Fo-Ti improves learning and memory ability and reduces pathological changes in the brains of mice.[51]

Immune… Fo-Ti is immunosuppressive and vasorelaxant.[52] Fo-Ti reduces tumor incidence in rats exposed to environmental mutagens and carcinogens.[53]

ALFALFA SEED TEA

Alfalfa seeds are the pituitary herb for exocrine pancreas carbohydrate digestion (Figure 10-A). Ingestion of just a few seeds fills this pituitary need for weeks to months and improves amylase enzyme breakdown of carbohydrates in the digestive tract. On the other hand, ingestion of NO seeds… instead making a tea out of thousands of alfalfa seeds gives some improvement in carbohydrate digestion with attendant Energy rev, but also generates both an immediate boost and a fundamental, long-lasting improvement within adrenal medulla Energy and Healing functions. Pituitary oversight improves too. The healing surge spills over to rejuvenate the entire adrenal gland, nervous system and pancreas (above and beyond carbohydrate digestion). Amazing little seeds!

To make Alfalfa Seed Tea, soak ¼ cup of seeds in water for several hours, or skip the soak, and heat in a pan slowly until the first signs of a rolling boil, then remove from the stove, steep for five to ten minutes, strain out the seeds, cool and serve. Good tasting in juice or milk. Be sure the seeds are for sprouting, not commercial seeds. Choose a quality brand, as there is some variability in therapeutic action from brand to brand. Organic seeds and those darker in color perform better. Take this tea only occasionally, once a week maximum, as other nutrients are used up in the healing surge and must be replenished through good nutrition.

No significant medical literature exists on the nutrient role of Alfalfa Seed Tea.

BEE POLLEN

Bee pollen is flower pollen rolled up into small round grains by bees. The preferred fuel of honeybees during their high-energy summers, bee pollen contains many life-sustaining factors. However, if you have pollen allergies, avoid it. If unsure, start by ingesting a single tiny grain and work your way up to a normal dose: a rounded teaspoon once a week to once a month. Try to find a local supplier, as most national brands now contain inferior Chinese product.

Review of the Medical Literature

Antioxidant/anti-aging... Bee pollen significantly reduces lipofuscin [brown pigment characteristic of aging, due to peroxidation of unsaturated fatty acids] in cardiac muscle, liver, brain and adrenal tissues of aging mice.[54] Bee pollen maintains liver glutathione [natural internal antioxidant: within cell mitochondria, the main defense against oxidative stress; in the liver, detoxifies free radicals, toxic oxygen radicals, and reduces disulfide groups] in mice after x-irradiation.[55] In human stroke patients, bee pollen and bee propolis [resinous hive building material made from tree buds] improve antioxidant defenses and brain blood supply, enabling more rapid and complete recovery.[56]

Chronic prostatitis... In preliminary studies, bee pollen shows promise for this common prostate condition.[57]

Immune... Bee pollen stimulates humoral immunity in rabbits, specifically Immunoglobulin M [IgM: typically the first antibodies in an immune response] and Immunoglobulin G [IgG: circulates in the blood giving long-term immunity against previously encountered bacteria, viruses and other pathogens].[58]

Possible allergic reaction… Although relatively rare, bee pollen allergy can be a life-threatening medical emergency. Conventional anaphylaxis [allergic inflammatory reaction, histamine release] treatment is usually effective.[59] Bee pollen allergic reaction can be immediate, or slow developing and subtle. Acute anaphylactic symptoms include sore throat, facial swelling and itching, difficulty breathing and stridor [harsh sound heard on breathing in], followed by respiratory distress.[60] Slow developing symptoms and signs can be malaise, decreased memory, headache, nausea, diarrhea with abdominal pain, itching and hypereosinophilia [abnormal accumulation of white-blood-cell eosinophils, which release histamines and are part of the inflammatory process].[61]

Nerves

Energy and nerves are tied together within adrenal medulla Primary Energy Function almost as equals. Each depends on the other for its well-being. More interdependency exists within the entire medulla as Energy/nerves depends upon Healing and a good equilibrium ($\rightleftharpoons$) between them. Complicated – yet simple, in that the medulla rises and falls as a unit.

Maintaining nerve function health is easy; rebuilding is a much more difficult assignment and quest. Just two herbs are needed for nerve maintenance, Oats and Valerian. This is simple, straightforward prevention. On the other hand, rebuilding nerve function may require taking all Table 7-3 nerve herbs, #1 to #15 and all Table 7-4 healing herbs, as explained ahead in assignment "Rebuilding."

OATS

Oats are essential for healthy nerve function. Oats are both the #1 nerve vitamin and a whole-grain cereal, which nourishes only the Primary Energy Function. As 100% Energy/nerve, 0% Healing, you can use Oats to push adrenal medulla equilibrium toward more Energy. Oats too often can become Healing too little, but this is rare except in horses. Of course, variety in whole-grain cereals forges strong medulla equilibrium.

Oats can relieve an adrenaline/energy headache. This is a headache feels like a concussion, especially when the head is shaken. Other possible symptoms are dizziness, lightheadedness and feeling of impending fainting. A real concussion feels as it does because healing (of the brain) strongly dominates over energy. A real concussion needs lots of healing nutrition immediately and throughout recovery.

Medical literature on Oats… See Chapter 4, however, nothing significant there on its key nerve role.

VALERIAN

Valerian is the #2 nerve vitamin and essential for youthful function. Valerian calms, soothes and relaxes every nerve in your body. It is excellent not only for halcyon days, but also for sleep. Use capsules, as this herb root stinks like unwashed socks. Take 500 mg once a week to once a month, more often with insomnia. Valerian works well with all whole-grain cereals except Oats.

Valerian is soothing medicine; do not interfere with its therapeutic action by taking it with other herbs. Valerian improves nerve function only. Nerve healing, fixing any physical damage, lies in the domain of Alfalfa Seed Tea and other healers.

Review of the Medical Literature

Mild sedative/tranquillizer… A traditional medicine of many cultures, Valerian (Valeriana officinalis) is used as a mild sedative and tranquillizer, and a sleep aid. It has official pharmacopoeia status in Europe. Valerian reduces the intensity of brain processes by inhibiting GABA [neurotransmitter; helps prevent system overload] breakdown.[62] Genus Valeriana decreases spontaneous and caffeine-induced motor activity, produces mild muscle relaxation, reduces animal aggressiveness, prolongs barbiturate action, and provides anticonvulsant and antihypoxic [hypoxia: inadequate oxygen] effects.[63]

Sleep… Valerian improves sleep structure and perception in insomnia patients,[64] increasing slow-wave sleep (SWS) and the density of K-complexes, while decreasing Stage 1 sleep. Valerian has no effect on sleep onset time, awake time following sleep onset, REM [rapid eye movement] sleep and self-rated sleep quality.[65] Or in another study, Valerian has good effect on poor sleep with 89% of participants reporting improved sleep and 44% perfect sleep, without side effects.[66] 600 mg of Valerian in the evening causes no effect on morning-after reaction time, alertness and concentration.[67] 600 mg per day of Valerian is at least as efficacious as 10 mg per day of oxazepam [prescription sedative and anxiety drug] in the treatment of non-organic [not caused by physical change or impairment] insomnia.[68]

Anxiety… In a preliminary study, Valerian shows anxiolytic [reduces anxiety, tension or agitation] effect on the psychic symptoms of anxiety, including a significant reduction in the psychic factor of the Hamilton Rating Scale for Anxiety.[69]

Overuse… of Valerian can produce headaches, chest tightness, hand and feet tremors, abdominal pain, mydriasis [excessive dilatation of eye pupils] and nephrotoxicity [nephro- prefix meaning 'kidney'].[70]

Drug interaction… Valerian should not be concomitant with barbiturates, as excessive sedation can occur.[48]

Rebuilding Nerve Function Health

How do nerves get out of whack and plague health? The most common way is overdosing on a nerve micronutrient. Whether from coffee (caffeine), beer (Hops, alcohol) or something else, the process and final result of hyperactivity in the nervous system are the same. For coffee, one cup is 1X, a micronutrient dose and rev of the nervous system. Two cups within 7½ hours are 2X and nerve stimulation, which triggers adrenaline flow. On to 3X harmful overstimulation, 4X and more, and eventually into caffeine fix syndrome (below). Beer too often can end up in the exact same place as coffee too often, with jangled nerves and needing a beer fix. Beer also adds a more potent addiction, alcoholism. All addictions lie in the nervous system.

When nerves are overstimulated to 3X and beyond, in other words "hyper," other nerve nutrients present in reserve amounts are consumed by the nervous system at accelerated rates, which soon leads to deficiencies. And what do these deficiencies cause? Surprisingly, overstimulation of the nervous system too! Too much or too little of a raw material nutrient is equally bad, and acts with the same vengeance – HYPERACTIVITY.

"Low little" hyperactivity is a common endocrine phenomenon. For instance, slight deprivation or injury to the insulin-producing cells of the pancreas causes not the expected hypoinsulinism, but instead overstimulated hyperinsulinism and consequent hypoglycemia (low blood sugar). Only great injury brings on hypoinsulinism and the familiar hyperglycemia diabetes. In like fashion, slight injury to nerve cells from nutrient deprivation produces hyperactivity. The good news, the damage is not severe and can be fixed. Severe nerve damage occurs with multiple sclerosis (MS), amyotrophic lateral sclerosis (Lou Gehrig's disease) and pernicious anemia.

So, hyperactive nerves can come from too much or too little of a good thing, nerve nutrients. Hyper nerves can also come from emotional turmoil and trauma, and from neurotoxins such as latex gloves, DDT and other insecticides. All these deplete nerve nutrition by the same hyperactive dynamic. Whatever the cause, nervous system hyperactivity usually manifests as tingling and numbness in the arms and legs. Now from these general principles, back to the specifics of coffee...

Caffeine Fix Syndrome

First, nerves go hyperactive from overdosing on caffeine. You hardly notice except for disturbed sleep. Sleep requires a gentle, natural shift in adrenal medulla equilibrium away from Energy tasks and toward Healing during the night. This circadian rhythm produces healthy restful sleep. Unfortunately, caffeine is harshly on the wrong side of sleep.

Second, "too much" toxicity develops. Here nerves stay hyperactive from developing deficiencies in all other nerve nutrients, as explained above. You notice faulty energy functioning, perhaps some immune deficits and more sleep sensitivity. Caffeine sensitivity increases too – 2X becomes an overdose.

Third, the caffeine fix is in! You <u>need</u> caffeine every morning just to fix jangled nerves and force an impaired energy function back to life. A little of any nerve nutrient, even the culprit, eases the deprivation and temporarily brings nerve peace. And coffee generates adrenaline. This is not the right way to get energy, but it does work. Want a better way to get adrenaline flow and energy? Try two small doses (swallows) of oatmeal one hour apart (2X). Oat nutrition builds energy and nerve health, whereas coffee uses its caffeine *boot* to kick tired, worn-out nerve and energy mechanisms.

Correcting Caffeine Fix Syndrome

Caffeine fix is an abnormal need, and WITHDRAWAL becomes necessary to regain health. Withdrawal stages for caffeine, beer, alcohol or any addicting substance proceed as follows: (1) too-much toxicity creates nerve hyperactivity; (2) with complete abstinence, near normalcy develops as the concentration of this needed/desired substance in the body falls; (3) then, too little of the substance occurs, a hyperactive condition too. Time for another fix or continue on with withdrawal? (4)

deprivation of the substance, the end stage of withdrawal with peak symptoms including intense craving and increasing hyperactivity; (5) finally abnormal functioning is broken, withdrawal is complete and true normalcy returns except for hypoactivity in energy, not nerves. With a neurotoxin cause, no craving or addiction to the culprit exists because neurotoxins do not provide nutrient satisfaction and relief. Otherwise, everything is the same.

During withdrawal, follow these steps and nutritional guidelines:

First, stop taking the culprit. Evidence on alcohol and more addicting substances strongly suggests quitting forever due to permanent sensitivity. With latex gloves and neurotoxins in general, definitely forever as sensitivity to these toxins, once established, never abates. The liver is involved here.

Second, rebuild nerve function health. Add back all depleted Chapter 3-6 Energy/nerve nutrients, and Chapter 7 nerve herbs one at a time. Follow the list in Table 7-3, #1 to #15, and stop when you're better. Of course, taking only nerve nutrition will push the *wishy-washy* Healing ⇌ Energy/nerve equilibrium strongly toward Energy/nerve and perpetuate hyperactive nerves. Therefore, you must balance nerve nutrients with Chapter 3-6 Healing nutrients and Table 7-4 Healing herbs. This also forges strong medulla equilibrium as you rebuild nerve function.

Impaired nerve function invariably leads to impaired adrenaline, and so the energy subfunction will have to be rebuilt. Will the fun never end? Your energy comes principally from Chapter 3-6 nutrition, and only secondarily from Table 7-3 energy herbs. Taking stimulating 2X doses of all energy raw materials for several weeks may do the job unless mild to severe energy exhaustion developed during the nerve abuse. Curing mild energy exhaustion requires supplementing Chapter 4 B vitamin pantothenic acid and separately Chapter 6 trace metals, notably copper. See Chapter 12 for severe exhaustion.

Third, healthy nerve function is restored. A little caffeine may be OK again. Maintain your nervous system with just Oats and Valerian, and probably Chamomile and Wood Betony to ensure tranquility and normalcy. Needless to say, an ounce of prevention is worth a pound of cure.

Feeling Down, The Blues, Mild Depression

Mood depends to a significant degree on Energy/nerve function. When you have lots of energy, you feel good – alive! Lack of energy is limiting, in a sense a loss. Depression is mourning losses, or it can be much more complex with severe depression or manic-depressive bipolar disorder. Complex causes require professional help. In its simplest characterization, however, depression is not enough energy and mania is too much energy. Nerves are key as they are directly tied to emotions, feelings and mood. Therefore, a reasonable first step toward good mood and mental health is a strong adrenal medulla and all that that entails including rebuilding Energy and nerve function, if necessary. The synergy of healthy internal function and professional help seems obvious.

ST. JOHN'S WORT

St. John's Wort has proven efficacy for mild to moderate depression. In Europe, St. John's Wort is prescribed more than Prozac and all other antidepressant drugs combined – with no side effects! Take this herb as an addition to and not a substitute for other good adrenal medulla nutrition. St. John's Wort works in a manner similar to many pharmaceutical antidepressant drugs, by modulating brain chemistry and neurotransmitters, and by inhibiting MAO (monoamine oxidase). MAO is a compound normally found in the body, however, if it gets out of control and blood concentrations become excessive, mood suffers and depression develops. St. John's Wort nourishes your mood subfunction perfectly. It also boosts energy.

St. John's Wort is a 100% "direct hit" on mood function. Like all functions in the body, mood function is a real entity, although its exact physical location or locations remain an unsolved mystery of anatomy. An analogy is the uncertain location of electrons in atoms. Our ability to describe nature precisely is limited.

When needed, St. John's Wort is one of the few herbs that can and should be taken every day, as in part it lowers MAO in the body to safe levels. Do not use St. John's Wort with antidepressant pharmaceuticals. Consult your physician. Take as directed or as needed, 100 mg to 500 mg per dose, up to 1000 mg daily, to reduce MAO, improve brain chemistry and mood, and send mild to moderate depression and *the blues* away.

Review of the Medical Literature

Overview… St John's Wort (Hypericum perforatum) is now successfully competing for status as a standard antidepressant therapy.[71] St John's Wort is efficacious for short-term treatment of mild to moderately severe depression in 27 clinical trials involving 2291 patients. St John's Wort is significantly superior to placebo and similarly effective to standard drug antidepressants, but with fewer patient side effects.[72]

St. John's Wort vs. imipramine and fluoxetine… For moderate depression, 350 mg of St. John's Wort three times daily is more effective than placebo and at least as effective as 100 mg daily of imipramine [tricyclic antidepressant prescription drug]. St. John's Wort is safe, and improves quality of life.[73] No difference in efficacy exists between St. John's Wort and fluoxetine [antidepressant prescription drug, the first serotonin uptake inhibitor],[74] however, the safety profile of St. John's Wort is substantially superior to that of fluoxetine, with adverse events at 8% for St. John's Wort. vs. 23% for fluoxetine. The most common side effects for St. John's Wort are GI [gastrointestinal] disturbances (5%) and all other adverse events less than 2%, whereas for fluoxetine: agitation (8%), GI disturbances (6%), retching (4%), dizziness (4%), tiredness, anxiety/nervousness and erectile dysfunction (each 3%).[75]

Safety profile… St. John's Wort was approved in Germany and Austria for treatment of mild and moderate depression in 1998. Effective dosage is 600 to 900 mg per day.[76] Side effects of approximately 3% are substantially less than with any current FDA-approved anti-depressant medication.[76, 77] Synthetic tricyclic antidepressants and monoamine oxidase (MAO) inhibitors [MAO: enzyme that chemically breaks down brain and other endocrine neurotransmitters including serotonin, dopamine, epinephrine and norepinephrine] can cause serious cardiac side effects including tachycardia [rapid heartbeat, usually 150-200 beats per minute] and postural hypotension [low blood pressure when standing], as well as unwanted anticholinergic [choline becomes neurotransmitter acetylcholine] side effects such as dry mouth and constipation. St. John's Wort is free of these cardiac and anticholinergic side effects.[77] St. John's Wort is safe and effective,[77, 78] and should be considered first-line treatment for mild to moderate depression.[78]

Mechanisms… underlying the antidepressant action of St. John's Wort are not fully resolved.[79] St. John's Wort shows only weak activity related to the mechanisms of synthetic antidepressants, that is, inhibiting MAO and reuptake of serotonin [central nervous system neurotransmitter/hormone and vasoconstrictor] and norepinephrine [adrenal medulla neuro-transmitter/hormone; as a hormone, constricts blood vessels and dilates bronchial tubes].

Clinical efficacy can be attributed to a confluence of mechanisms,[80] including hyperforin [a major St. John's Wort active constituent] inhibition of neuron uptake of serotonin, dopamine [neurotransmitter; helps to regulate movement and emotion], glutamate [fast, excitatory central nervous system neurotransmitter], GABA [inhibitory neurotransmitter; helps prevent system overload] and norepinephrine. No other antidepressant compound evidences such broad uptake inhibition.[81] Hyperforin is also the first antidepressant compound to inhibit serotonin uptake by elevating free intracellular sodium.[82] St John's Wort downregulates beta-adrenergic receptors, upregulates serotonin 5-HT(2) receptors and changes neurotransmitter concentrations in brain areas implicated in depression.[71] Other factors, St. John's Wort increases plasma GH [pituitary growth hormone] and decreases PRL [pituitary prolactin hormone: for breast development and milk production] while cortisol remains normal, suggesting that St. John's Wort mimics some aspects of human brain dopamine function.[83]

Seasonal affective disorder (SAD)... SAD major depression is characterized by regular autumn/winter symptoms, with full remission or hypomania in spring/summer. Light therapy and antidepressants have shown efficacy, with St John's Wort effective in two studies. [84]

Tranquilizer... St John's Wort may be an alternative to benzodiazepines [minor tranquilizers: central nervous system depressants, e.g. Valium] in cases of early depression.[85]

Depression plus anxiety... The comorbidity of depressive and anxiety disorders is a frequent diagnostic and therapeutic problem. Improvement occurs more quickly with a combination therapy of St John's Wort and Valerian than with St John's Wort alone. This therapy is well tolerated with no significant side effects.[86]

Female... St John's Wort eases premenstrual syndrome (PMS).[87] 300 mg of St John's Wort three times daily substantial improves psychological and psychosomatic menopausal symptoms with complaints falling 76% and 79% in patient and physicians evaluations, respectively. St John's Wort also improves sexual well being.[88]

Alcoholism... St John's Wort, as well as standard antidepressants, may reduce alcohol craving in a subgroup of patients.[89]

Side effects... St John's Wort has a good safety profile. The most common side effects are gastrointestinal disturbances, tiredness/sedation and dizziness/confusion. One potentially serious adverse event is photosensitization [itching skin lesions in light-exposed areas], but this is extremely rare and generally without clinical relevance at recommended dosages.[90, 76]

Drug interactions... Concomitant use of St John's Wort with standard antidepressant MAO inhibitors and serotonin reuptake inhibitors is ill-advised.[48] St John's Wort can lower blood concentrations of simultaneously administered drugs, including oral contraceptives, warfarin [inhibitor of blood clotting], theophylline [relieves bronchial spasms], fenprocoumon, digoxin [digitalis derivative; used in congestive heart failure with a small margin between therapeutic and toxic dose], indinavir [HIV protease inhibitor] and cyclosporin [anti-rejection drug after transplant surgery]. Discontinuing St John's Wort after extended use may lead to higher blood concentrations of simultaneously administered drugs.[91]

Anxiety

KAVA KAVA

Kava Kava eases anxiety, muscle tension, nervousness, excessive fear and worry, and phobias. A mild natural tranquilizer, Kava quiets the mind, usually without side effects. For mild anxiety and sleep problems, take 500 mg as needed. Clinical anxiety requires larger doses and prolonged use, and here consider the "Side Effects" listed below.

> ### Review of the Medical Literature

Overview... Kava Kava (Piper methysticum) is an integral part of the cultural life of the South Pacific islands, enhancing social interaction, relaxation and sleep.[92] Its active ingredients, known as kava lactones, exert significant analgesic and anesthetic activity through non-opiate pathways. Kava is a natural anxiolytic [reduces anxiety, tension or agitation], and in several studies compares favorably to prescription medications including benzodiazepines [minor tranquilizers: central nervous system depressants, e.g. Valium].[93] Kava is well tolerated and does not cause drowsiness or dependence.[94]

Anxiety/tranquilizer... Kava Kava is superior to placebo as a daily tranquilizer for nervous anxiety, tension and agitation with significant score reductions in the Hamilton Rating Scale for Anxiety.[95] Roughly equivalent in effect to 15 mg daily of oxazepam [prescription sedative and anxiety drug] or 9 mg daily of bromazepam [benzodiazepine prescription drug],[96] Kava is a safe and effective alternative to antidepressants and tranquilizers for anxiety disorder, without the side effects of benzodiazepines.[97] Kava is well tolerated and as effective as buspirone [prescription anxiety drug] and opipramol [tricyclic antidepressant] in the acute out-patient treatment of generalized anxiety disorder.[98] In total, eleven randomized, controlled trials with a total of 645 participants evidence that Kava is an effective symptomatic treatment option for anxiety. Adverse events are mild, transient and infrequent.[99] Anxiety of non-psychotic origin can include generalized anxiety disorder, adjustment disorder with anxiety, agoraphobia [abnormal, excessive fear of crowds, public places or open areas] and other specific phobias.[100]

Mechanisms... Kava Kava blocks norepinephrine [adrenal medulla neurotransmitter/ hormone; as a hormone, constricts blood vessels and dilates bronchial tubes] uptake,[93] and acts as a reversible MAO-B [MAO, monoamine oxidase: enzyme that chemically breaks down brain and other endocrine neurotransmitters including serotonin, dopamine, epinephrine and norepinephrine] inhibitor.[92] Kava shows modest anticonvulsant activity. In addition, Kava may possess GABA [inhibitory neurotransmitter; helps prevent system overload]-receptor binding capacity, but studies are conflicted on this point.[93] Kava in no way resembles benzodiazepines or tricyclic antidepressants in neurophysiological activity.[101]

Emotions... Kava Kava modulates emotional processes and promotes sleep without sedation. These effects result from action in limbic structures [hypothalamus, hippocampus, which is involved in long-term memory, olfactory/smell bulbs, and amygdala, the receptive areas and hearing].[101]

Menopause... Kava Kava demonstrates efficacy in psychosomatic dysfunctions of human menopause.[102]

Side effects... Heavy usage can cause a scaly skin rash called 'kava dermopathy' [first described by members of Captain James Cook's Pacific expeditions].[93] In toxicological and clinical studies, Kava Kava is virtually free of toxic effects, with the rare exception of hepatotoxicity in a few susceptible individuals.[103] In Europe between 1990 and 2002, Kava caused thirty-six adverse hepatic reactions of hepatic necrosis [death] or cholestatic [arrest of normal bile flow] hepatitis. Nine patients developed fulminant liver failure [a severe and rapid form of hepatitis and liver failure]; eight underwent liver transplantation and three died. In all other patients, complete recovery followed Kava withdrawal. The cumulative dose and latency period before hepatotoxic reaction were highly variable, [104] however, almost 80% of the patients took kavapyrones [standardized extract of kava lactones] in overdose (up to 480 mg per day) and/or for a prolonged time, more than three months and up to two years. An additional risk factor was co-medication with other potential hepatotoxic chemical or herbal drugs. Preventive measures should include doses of 120-210 mg kavapyrones per day for 1 month, maximally 2 months, as well as physician consultation.[105] Author's Note: 120-210 mg kavapyrones equals approximately 1500-2500 mg dried Kava rhizome. Generally, kavapyrones comprise 3-20% of the rootstock.

Drug interactions… Kava Kava potentates barbiturates and Xanax.[93] Kava concomitant with alprazolam [prescription drug for anxiety, central nervous system depressant] can produce coma.[48]

VALERIAN

Valerian acts as a mild sedative, tranquillizer and sleep aid. Valerian reduces anxiety, tension and agitation. See its medical literature review earlier.

LICORICE

Licorice eases anxiety and apprehension, but dosage must be kept low, 100 mg maximum. The details on Licorice effects and usage are given in the "Gluconeogenesis" Stress subfunction ahead.

Medulla Sex

Sex begins in the adrenal medulla Primary Energy Function with nervous energy – excitement, arousal – your nervous system runneth over! Oats is the best medulla sex herb; the old adage "sow your wild oats" attests to its prowess down the centuries. By way of example, Oats taken at 2X (stimulation dosing) one hour apart delivers a volcano of healthy nervous energy (except if you have functional exhaustion of Energy). However, Oats is the best only because it is the #1 nerve vitamin. All nerve and energy raw materials contribute here.

YOHIMBE

Yohimbe is for male and female sexual dysfunction from lack of nerve stimulation such as erectile dysfunction (ED) or orgasmic difficulties… or, in larger doses and at the other end of the spectrum, for anyone with too much nervous sexual energy and too much blood flow to sexual parts, usually the male. However, take too much Yohimbe and wait until tomorrow!

Norepinephrine is an adrenal medulla neurotransmitter and hormone similar to epinephrine (adrenaline), but with limited action as a hormone, only constricting blood vessels and dilating bronchial tubes. A natural equilibrium ($\rightleftharpoons$) exists between norepinephrine and epinephrine within Primary Energy Function. Yohimbe stimulates nor-epinephrine secretion and adjusts this equilibrium. At low doses, Yohimbe increases <u>neurotransmitter</u> norepinephrine producing nerve stimulation, while at high doses <u>hormone</u> norepinephrine spills over into the bloodstream causing vasoconstriction and a decrease in adrenaline. Only you can determine your correct Yohimbe dosage.

Review of the Medical Literature

Erectile dysfunction... Historically known as aphrodisiac,[106] yohimbine (bark of the African tree Pausinystalia yohimbe) is superior to placebo in the treatment of erectile dysfunction in seven clinical trials of satisfactory methodology. Serious side effects are infrequent and reversible.[107] Side effects from standard drug antidepressants can include orgasmic and ejaculation difficulties, and altered libido, arousal and erectile function. Yohimbine is one possible antidote.[108]

Mechanisms and side effects... Yohimbine pharmacological activity is principally as an alpha 2-adrenoreceptor antagonist.[106] Yohimbine increases sympathetic nerve activity [sympathetic nervous system regulates involuntary actions: breathing rate, heart rate, cardiac output, and blood pressure] and norepinephrine [adrenal medulla neurotransmitter/hormone; as a hormone, constricts blood vessels and dilates bronchial tubes] spillover from adrenergic nerve terminals, which raises blood pressure. Patients with autonomic [self-controlling, functionally independent] system failure are hypersensitive to yohimbine.[109] As an alpha 2 antagonist, yohimbine can induce panic attacks. Selective serotonin reuptake inhibitors (SSRI) suppress panic attacks, suggesting that serotonin [central nervous system neurotransmitter/hormone and vasoconstrictor] plays a role in panic attacks and yohimbine activity.[110]

Drug interaction... Combining yohimbine with tricyclic antidepressants increases hypertension [high blood pressure] risk.[111]

Energy/Nerve Suppression ($\downarrow$)

Energy/nerve suppressors are helpful in correcting caffeine fix syndrome and other hyperactivity within the nervous system and Primary Energy Function. Hyperactivity mainly affects nerves here, as nerve and energy functions split in opposite directions during dysfunction. Specifically, nerves go hyperactive and energy usually goes hypoactive. Only with mania does energy ever go hyperactive. Chapter 12 examines this subfunction imbalance in depth.

Kudzu, Gotu Kola and Oregon Grape can bring nerves *out of orbit* and back to earth, easing nerve nutrient losses from hyperactivity and reducing the need for the next caffeine fix, beer fix, alcohol fix, etc. Unfortunately, nerve suppression is only a short-term answer. The best solution lies in correcting the underlying cause, as explained earlier in "Rebuilding Nerve Function Health."

KUDZU (↓)

Kudzu is the most powerful medulla nerve suppressant and especially useful in treating alcoholism. Take 150 mg to 300 mg 1X only, two days in a row only, and not with any other suppressant. Using the herb more often than this transfers the suppression to the pituitary, which is effective but hard to reverse later and restore endocrine system homeostasis. Instead, the B vitamin PABA can continue nerve suppression gently until nerve function health is rebuilt.

Review of the Medical Literature

Alcoholism… Kudzu root (Pueraria lobata) possesses antidipsotropic (anti-alcohol abuse) action. Kudzu has been used in China to treat alcoholism safely and effectively for more than a thousand years.[112] Major constituent isoflavonoids puerarin, daidzin and daidzein suppress voluntary alcohol consumption in alcohol-preferring rats. Daidzin and daidzein shorten alcohol-induced sleep time,[113, 112] and Kudzu diadzein and genistein strongly inhibit human alcohol dehydrogenases (ADH) [metabolizing enzymes].[114] Or oppositely, the lone Kudzu human study is unsupportive, finding no statistically significance difference in craving and sobriety between Kudzu and placebo patients.[115]

GOTU KOLA (½↓)

Gotu Kola has about one-half the nerve suppressant strength of Kudzu. However, Gotu Kola also "gets things running right" (◊) within Primary Energy Function and the entire adrenal medulla, and within their pituitary oversight mechanisms. Valued in traditional Ayurvedic medicine, Gotu Kola is an important medulla-balancing herb (see Scullcap earlier). Take 500 to 1000 mg 1X only, two days in a row only, and not with any other suppressant. The venous health applications reported below require longer periods of use.

Review of the Medical Literature

Venous health... Gotu Kola (Centella asiatica), a medicinal plant since prehistoric times, is effective in treating chronic venous insufficiency [inadequate blood flow, most often manifesting in the legs with swelling, pain and muscle cramps; can lead to venous thrombosis] and striae gravidarum [stretch marks].[116] Gotu Kola improves venous hypertension [high blood pressure], capillary filtration rate, and venous edema, particularly ankle edema, by protecting the venous endothelium [vein lining] and reversing any alterations caused by chronic venous hypertensive microangiopathy [angiopathy: blood vessel disease].[117-119] Active in connective tissue modulation, Gotu Kola stimulates the synthesis and remodeling of collagen and other tissue proteins in and around the vein wall by modulating fibroblast [cell giving rise to connective tissue; -blast: undergoing development] activity.[117] Loss of vascular integrity can lead to varicose veins and hemorrhoids, and Gotu Kola may prevent their complications.[120] Gotu Kola is safe and well tolerated.[117] Its active ingredients include pentacyclic triterpene derivatives.[116]

Diabetes... Gotu Kola is helpful in diabetic microangiopathy [such as diabetic retinopathy], increasing blood microcirculation and decreasing capillary permeability.[121]

Wound healing... Gotu Kola can correct disturbances in wound healing.[116]

Antioxidant/cognitive... Gotu Kola possesses antioxidant and cognitive-enhancing properties in animal studies.[122, 123]

OREGON GRAPE (↓Energy/nerve, ↑Healing)

Oregon Grape is invaluable in correcting the combined dysfunction of hyperactive Energy/nerve and hypoactive Healing exhaustion. Take as a tea or 500 mg in capsule 1X only, two days in a row only, and not with any other suppressant.

ADRENAL MEDULLA HEALING

Table 7-4 gives Primary Healing Function herbs with subheadings indicating specific use. Again, most medulla herbs nourish both Energy/nerve and Healing functions to some degree, but usually with unequal strength. Therefore, Table 7-4 herbs are predominantly Healing in nature. Only three herbs, Aloe vera, Green Cabbage and Saffron are 100% Healing-0% Energy/nerve, although each of these contains some Immune phyto-compounds. Of course, antioxidation herbs belong to a special, separate subfunction and their actions lie solely within the Healing province.

TABLE 7-4. ADRENAL MEDULLA HEALING HERBS.

Subheadings (underlined) specify use. Numbering of healing herbs indicates "need for," not potency.

Herb	Comments
HEALING – MAINTAIN HEALTH, i.e. ESSENTIAL	
#1 Aloe vera	100% Healing, 0% Energy/nerve. Topically good for burns, internally Aloe vera heals EVERYTHING! Also Immune (Table 7-6) and pituitary-healing (Figure 8-B).
HEALING – REBUILD HEALTH (approximate order of importance)	
#2 Blessed Thistle	Also immune (Table 7-6) and pituitary-healing (Figure 8-B).
#3 Passion Flower	
#4 Siberian Ginseng	Also immune (Table 7-6).
#5 Sage	Also nerves (Table 7-3); nourishes the entire medulla.
#6 Comfrey	Also for stomach pepsin (protein digestion), see Chapter 10.
#7 Raw Garlic	Also cortex fatigue (Table7-5 and text there) and immune (Table 7-6).
#8 Saffron	#1 in potency; 100% Healing-Immune, 0% Energy-Stress. Take only as tea using 4-8 stigmas maximum. Not before or during any stress. Can correct severe Healing →→ Energy imbalance.
#9 Oregon Grape	Healing↑, Energy/nerves↓. See Table 7-3 and text there.
FATTY ACID METABOLISM	
Hydrangea	Catalyst for fatty acid activity here and for fat burning by cells (Table 7-5). Also pituitary-stress (Figure 8-B).

SPECIFIC HEALERS

Alfalfa Seed Tea	Helps to heal adrenal gland, nervous system and pancreas (Table 10-1). Also for energy (Table 7-3). Seeds for pituitary exocrine pancreas function (Chapter 8, Figure 10-A)
Bilberry	Helps to heal microvascular structures throughout the body. Essential for the pancreas (Table 10-1) and for eyes as you get older. Also nerves (Table 7-3).
Green Cabbage	Helps to heal gastrointestinal tract including stomach ulcers and chronic pancreatitis. 100% Healing, 0% Energy/nerve. Slippery Elm also soothes and heals the GI tract.
Horsetail	Helps to heal bones, hair, fingernails and connective tissue.

SPECIAL FACTORS... fountains of youth!

glucosamine	For major connective tissue matrix repair. Also for cortex gluconeogenesis and arthritis relief (Table 7-5).
DMAE	For major neuron/nervous system repair and general repair.
alpha-lipoic acid	Heals free radical/oxidative stress damage, rejuvenates endocrine machinery. Most powerful antioxidant known.

ESSENTIAL ANTIOXIDANTS (water-soluble)

Vitamin C and Bioflavonoids	Synergy when taken together. 500-1000 mg of Vitamin C daily provides essential antioxidant protection. Also for immune (Table 7-6) and liver (Table 11-1).
Pine Bark Extract	Variable use – to overcome severe stress, out-of-control free radicals.
Grape Seed Extract	Variable like pine bark.

VASOCONSTRICTION

Shepherd's Purse and Woundwort	Take together. Also for cortex fatigue (Table 7-5).

Herb	Comments
Heather	Also for fatigue (Table 7-5) and immune (Table 7-6).
Hawthorn Berries 2X	Also fatigue (Table 7-5 and text there).
SUPPRESSION (↓)	
Yellow Dock	

Maintaining and Rebuilding Healing Health

Maintaining Primary Healing Function health can be accomplished with just one herb – Aloe vera. And, of course, with the more basic healing nutrients of complete protein, whole-grain cereals especially *gooey* polysaccharides, essential fatty acids (EFAs) and Vitamin E, and trace metals. Interestingly, very nutritious dark-colored foods such as black cherries and figs contribute to Healing too. In fact, these foods benefit all four primary functions in non-quantifiable ways.

Rebuilding Healing function, like rebuilding nerve function, is a much more diffi-cult assignment. Rebuilding must involve the entire adrenal medulla because Healing ⇌ Energy is a *wishy-washy* equilibrium and can easily become imbalanced. First, take the basic Chapter 3-6 healing nutrients mentioned above for several weeks, 2X usage at the start, then 1X. Second, input most of the healing herbs, #1 up to #9, during this period, and other appropriate Table 7-4 herbs for your symptoms. Balance healing nutrition with the best energy and nerve basic nutrients and Table 7-3 herbs to preserve and strengthen Healing ⇌ Energy equilibrium throughout the rebuilding process. Third, fix any Healing exhaustion. Cure mild exhaustion with Chapter 4 B vitamin supplementation of pantothenic acid, PABA and B1, and separately Chapter 6 trace metal supplementation, notably zinc. Follow Chapter 12 guidelines for severe exhaus-tion. These rebuilding regimens are not easy, but absolutely necessary to restore health. Primary Healing Function is fundamental to youthful repair and long life.

ALOE VERA

Aloe vera is well known for healing burns. A personal story, the author once picked up the wrong end of a hot soldering iron. Result: a severe burn on the thumb right where the fingerprint is. I broke open an aloe leaf, wrapped the thumb in it juice-side in, with a bandage over that. Next morning, a completely healed normal thumb. Internally, the news is even better – Aloe vera heals everything! As evidenced in the medical literature below, it is essential to keep this micronutrient factor well supplied to all tissues.

For best effect, use aloe fresh from the plant, NOT bottled product, which loses potency over time. Outdoor varieties are therapeutically stronger than the common indoor plant. Still, the indoor variety is sufficient. Keep at least one plant in the house for skin problems including burns (topical use) and for general health maintenance (internal use).

Internal dosage is as follows. Remove the green skin; the opaque gel within contains the active ingredients. Ingest a gel amount equal in volume to about half the size of a green pea. Not much, however, this tiny volume is enough to significantly improve healing for several weeks to a month. Very strange nourishment, but nature works in such ways. The unusual taste of Aloe vera can easily be disguised in food. Take Aloe more often if your Healing function is working overtime on major reconstruction such as severe burns or tissue trauma.

Review of the Medical Literature

Healing mechanism... The body's fundamental response to all tissue injuries is 'wound healing', which restores tissue integrity. Wound healing is achieved through synthesis of a connective tissue matrix.[124] A provisional matrix or foundation of GAGs [glycosaminoglycans: special amino-sugar polysaccharides, start of linking and matrix] and proteoglycans (PGs) [protein GAG conjugates] is laid down in the early stage of wound healing, followed by granulation tissue of collagen [major fibrous protein of connective tissue] and elastin [elastic protein of connective tissue].[125] Collagen provides wound strength.[124] Both topical and oral Aloe vera treatment positively influences GAGs and wound healing.[125] Aloe vera also increases the collagen content of granulation tissue and its degree of crosslinking.[124]

Anti-inflammatory... An important part of healing is treating inflammation, and Aloe vera addresses many of its constituent processes,[126] including inhibiting the potent arachidonic acid [essential fatty acid] inflammatory pathway.[127] Aloe compounds acemannan, aloemannan and neutral polysaccharides possess anti-inflammatory activity.[128]

Diabetic wounds... Aloe vera enhances wound healing in diabetic rats, improving fibro-plasia [-plasia: growth, multiplication], collagen synthesis and maturation, inflammation and wound contraction.[129] Aloe also reduces blood glucose levels.[130]

Burns... Aloe vera heals burns and frostbite in animals.[131-133] In human study, topical Aloe-treated burn wounds heal in 12 days vs. 18 days for Vaseline gauze-treated wounds.[134] Aloe compounds aloesin, aloemannan and verectin have therapeutic effect on burns, wounds and inflammation.[128]

Skin... Topical Aloe vera is more effective than placebo for psoriasis, with no side effects. Aloe is a safe, alternative treatment for psoriasis.[135] In the management of occupational dry skin and contact dermatitis, use of Aloe-coated gloves improves skin integrity and decreases erythema [abnormal redness, inflammation of the skin] and wrinkling.[136] Skin exposure to ultraviolet radiation alters immune cell function in the skin, suppressing T-cell response and promoting cytokine [non-antibody protein/signaling molecule of the immune system; includes interleukins] release. Aloe reduces IL-10 [Interleukin 10: coregulator of mast cell growth; mast cells are involved in histamine release and allergic reaction],[137] and restores ultraviolet B (UVB)-suppressed immune cell function.[138] Aloe is effective in treating human radiation ulcers,[131] and may aid in healing chronic venous leg ulcers.[139] Aloe vera demonstrates efficacy in both topical and oral administrations.[140, 124]

Candida... Aloe vera possesses antibacterial and antifungal activity.[131] Macrophages [relatively long-living, large white blood cells; -phage: anything that devours] exposed to Aloe acemannan for one hour kill 98% of Candida albicans yeast compared to 0.5% for controls.[141]

Cancer... Aloe vera exhibits cytotoxicity against human tumor cell lines.[142] Aloe compounds acemannan, aloemannan and neutral polysaccharides have antitumor activity.[128] Aloe is antimutagenic and antileukemic.[142] In rats, Aloe protects against chemical hepatocarcinogenesis [liver cancer generated by chemicals].[143] Aloe contains manganese and copper-zinc superoxide dismutase [MnSOD and CuZnSOD; see Chapter 6] comparable to spinach leaves.[144]

Fatty Acid Metabolism

HYDRANGEA

Protein is the most important raw material for healing, but fatty acids are also essential because every cell in the body has fatty acids in its cell membrane. As a catalyst for fatty acid metabolism, Hydrangea facilitates proper and efficient healing. This herb becomes critical to repair efforts during severe injury, because hyperactivity anywhere in the body depletes the associated, necessary catalysts. See Table 7-5 and text there for more on Hydrangea.

Specific Healers

Specific healers have special healing ingredients for a particular gland, metabolic pathway or system. Table 7-4 presents four such herbs. Undoubtedly many more specific healers exist and are waiting to be discovered or have their benefits widely disseminated. Apply these specific healers in conjunction with Chapter 3-6 general healing nutrients and Table 7-4 healing herbs of Aloe vera and others related to the task. Specific healers are most effective after all interfering adrenal exhaustions and imbalances have been fixed.

ALFALFA SEED TEA

Alfalfa Seed Tea helps to heal the adrenal gland, pancreas, nervous system and many more metabolic pathways in unexpected ways. Functioning improves and dysfunctions ease their destructive grip. Take Alfalfa Seed Tea no more than once a week, as it synergizes with and thus requires the presence (previous input) of other nutrients to achieve therapeutic effect. Review Table 7-3 and text there for a complete discussion of this extraordinary energy and healing tea including how to prepare it.

BILBERRY

Bilberry and its special anthocyanin flavonoids help to heal microvascular structures throughout the body, notably those of the pancreas, eyes, kidneys, thyroid gland and nervous system. Bilberry is essential nutrition for pancreas; see Table 10-1 and related text. Bilberry also safeguards retinal capillaries as you get older. The medical literature below reveals the power of Bilberry to prevent the worst microvascular injures including capillary aneurysms, leaks and hemorrhages and to preserve vessel linings and improve blood flow. 40 mg of standardized 25%-anthocyanin Bilberry extract is a good maintenance dose. Rebuilding microvascular structures may require up to 400 mg in concerted action with other healers, as described in Chapter 12 "Heal the damage, as much as possible." A good brand choice here: NATURE'S HERBS® Bilberry Power Standardized Extract

Review of the Medical Literature

Diabetic retinopathy... Bilberry (Vaccinium myrtillus), rich in special anthocyanin/antho-cyanoside flavonoids [see Table 3-3 regarding flavonoids in general], reduces capillary leaks and hemorrhages in retinal vessels, particularly those caused by diabetic retinopathy.[145] Microvascular damage to the retina from diabetic glucose levels produces microaneurysms [aneurysm: permanent dilation of blood vessel wall at a weak point], hemorrhages and exudate [escaped fluid and cells from blood vessels] deposits such as 'cotton-wool spots' in the visual field. Subsequent neovascularization [new vessel growth] can trigger severe hemorrhage, scar-ring and permanent visual loss.[146] Anthocyanins help to prevent these malfunctions in connec-tive tissue synthesis, thereby easing diabetic retinopathy and decreasing the risk of blindness.[147]

More microvascular effects... Bilberry anthocyanins lessen microvascular damage from ischaemia-reperfusion injury [ischaemia: insufficient blood supply; reperfusion: restoration of blood flow] in animals, preserving the endothelium [vessel lining], reducing leukocyte [white blood cell] adhesion and improving capillary perfusion.[148] These special flavonoids also promote and enhance rhythmic arterial diameter changes, which redistribute microvascular blood flows and interstitial fluids.[149] Anthocyanins demonstrate significant vasoprotective and anti-edema activity in animals, with effects more lasting than rutin [a flavonoid] and twice as powerful.[150]

General vision... Anthocyanins and Vitamin E in combination can achieve therapeutic results in progressive myopia [nearsightedness].[151] In young male adults with good vision, Bilberry had no effect on night visual acuity and night contrast sensitivity.[152, 153] However, epi-demiological investigations [a wider population sample] find that anthocyanin products are asso-ciated with improved visual functions and reduced risk of cardiovascular disease.[154]

LDL (bad) cholesterol... Low-density lipoprotein (LDL) oxidation is one of the major caus-es of atherogenesis [depositing plaque on artery walls]. Bilberry evidences potent antioxidant protective activity on LDL cholesterol.[155]

Cancer... Anthocyanins protect against cancer.[154] Among ten edible berries, Bilberry is most effective in inhibiting the growth of HCT116 human colon carcinoma cells and HL60 human leukemia cells in vitro.[156]

Stomach ulcers... Bilberry shows promising antiulcer activity, probably by potentiating gas-trointestinal mucosa [mucous membrane] defenses.[157]

GREEN CABBAGE

Green Cabbage helps to heal stomach and duodenal ulcers, chronic pancreatitis and other gastrointestinal inflammations and sores. As the richest natural source of Vitamin U – so named for its ability to heal gastrointestinal ulcers, Green Cabbage was standard medical practice until the 1950s when along came pharmaceutical companies and their detail men (salesmen) to make big bucks selling modern medicine, with modern side effects too. Green Cabbage has no side effects if you can digest it.

In some people Green Cabbage causes digestive disturbance, usually flatulence. This can be avoided by taking fresh cabbage juice, which also increases the herb's effectiveness. Use a vegetable juicer to make a powerful therapeutic, or grind the cabbage in a blender with a little water until completely liquid, then strain through a tea strainer and serve. For best results, take cabbage juice on an empty stomach. Make fresh juice for each use as the active ingredient Vitamin U decays away in this state.

Other herbs evidencing antiulcer activity in the medical literature are Scullcap, Bilberry, Ginger, Green Tea against H. pylori infection, and Vitamin C. Aloe vera improves all healing.

> ## Review of the Medical Literature

Green Cabbage itself... Green Cabbage (Brassica oleracea) lowers the ulcer index and raises hexosamine [derivative of glucosamine, see its citation ahead] levels, indicating gastric mucous membrane protection in rats with aspirin-induced gastric ulcers.[158]

Vitamin U... Vitamin U [MMSC: methylmethioninesulfonium chloride] sulfhydryl compounds stimulate gastrointestinal mucus formation, increase protein synthesis and mucin [albuminoid protein substance found in mucus] secretion, and eliminate oxygen free radicals that cause tissue damage.[159, 160] In three double-blind human studies, Vitamin U: (1) stimulates duodenal ulcer healing and protects against recurrence,[161] (2) stimulates healing of erosive gastritis induced by NSAIDs [nonsteroidal anti-inflammatory drugs] and protects against bleeding complications,[162] and (3) protects against ulcerative colitis.[163]

Nephrotic syndrome... Vitamin U improves nephrotic syndrome [a type of kidney inflammation characterized by edema, weight gain, high blood pressure, protein in the urine, and anorexia] by increasing urinary volume and decreasing protein excretion and hyperlipidemia [high fat levels in the blood].[164]

HORSETAIL (Shavegrass)

Horsetail contains bioavailable silica, which strengthens and heals bones, hair, fingernails and connective tissue in general. Take as a tea if capsules cause side effects.

Review of the Medical Literature

Medical literature on Horsetail (Equisetum arvense) – very little. Horsetail displays antioxidant and vasorelaxant activity,[165, 166] and is useful in preventing and treating kidney stones.[167] Possible allergic side effect: seborrhea dermatitis, an inflammatory skin rash involving the sebaceous [pertaining to or secreting fat] glands.[168, 169]

Special Factors

When normal healing mechanisms are inadequate, three special factors can boost repair to extraordinary levels. These factors are: (1) glucosamine for major wound healing and connective tissue matrix repair, (2) DMAE for major neuron/nervous system repair and general repair, and (3) alpha-lipoic acid to heal free radical and oxidative stress damage.

Good nutrition slows aging. Nourish every cell and every task and you significantly retard the sands of time. Special factors go beyond slowing aging to actually reversing it! Ponce de Leon once searched for the "Fountain of Youth" in Florida; instead he should have looked for these powerful nutritional treasures.

GLUCOSAMINE

Glucosamine is a general precursor of glycosaminoglycans (GAGs), an essential element in tissue repair. While best known for its efficacy in repairing the degenerative joint cartilage of osteoarthritis, glucosamine is effective in any wound healing involving a connective tissue matrix. Take 500 mg (maximum) per dose, as needed, usually once a day, sometimes twice. GAGs work together with complete protein, sulfur supplementation and whole-grain cereal polysaccharides to achieve matrix formation. If possible, add the animal connective tissue protein (collagen and elastin) from the same body part that is to be healed, for example chondroitin for osteoarthritis. Using glucosamine sulfate and chondroitin sulfate supplies the necessary sulfur. See "Gluconeogenesis" Stress subfunction ahead for more on glucosamine's osteoarthritis application.

Review of the Medical Literature

Healing mechanism... The body's fundamental response to all tissue injuries is 'wound healing', which restores tissue integrity. Wound healing is achieved through synthesis of a connective tissue matrix.[124] A provisional matrix or foundation of GAGs [glycosaminoglycans: special amino-sugar polysaccharides, start of linking and matrix] and proteoglycans (PGs) [protein GAG conjugates] is laid down in the early stage of wound healing, followed by granulation tissue of collagen [major fibrous protein of connective tissue] and elastin [elastic protein of connective tissue].[125] Glucosamine is a general, multifunctional precursor of glycosaminoglycans [GAGs].[170]

DMAE

DMAE (dimethylaminoethanol) is an amazing healing vitamin for damaged neurons. By boosting cell membrane repair with on-site antioxidation and DNA synthesis, DMAE can permanently improve neuron function and nervous system health. A naturally occurring substance found in anchovies and sardines, DMAE retards the aging of neuron membranes and produces some reversal, i.e. heals injured cells. It improves memory, concentration and sleep. In essence, you become younger.

DMAE also benefits general repair. A prime example, topical use of DMAE makes skin younger. Direct application to the face gives a gentle, natural facelift!

The secret to DMAE is not to overdose, as it uses up PABA, polysaccharides, trace metals and other healing ingredients quickly, causing deficiency in these and precluding any further good. Take DMAE internally in amounts and frequency as though you eating the seafood itself. Of course, even a little DMAE is a lot of anchovies and sardines, but think in those terms. The right internal dose is just 10-15 mg (one-tenth to one-sixth of a typical DMAE capsule). Too much DMAE generates too much healing, and too much healing or too little healing yields the same result –

poor healing. Infrequent DMAE supplementation, not more often than once a week to once every few weeks, produces the best outcomes. Superior nutrition in between DMAE therapy is needed to replenish conutrient reserves.

CAUTION ☛ Too much DMAE or DMAE combined with excesses of other powerful healing ingredients causes severe adrenal medulla imbalance. Regarding adverse interactions, do not take DMAE with Valerian, Fenugreek or other hormone or neurotransmitter stimulators; overstimulation can injure delicate mechanisms.

Review of the Medical Literature

Neuron anti-aging… Protein replacement in biological systems occurs mostly as a result of continuous damage (cross-linking) from hydroxyl [OH $^-$] free radicals. DMAE scavenges hydroxyl radicals, and is incorporated in brain neuron cell membranes as phosphatidyl-DMAE, a phospholipid precursor [phospholipids: phosphate fatty acids, most abundant lipids in cell membranes], thereby protecting membrane components on site and slowing age-dependent deterioration.[171-173]

General repair… DMAE stimulates DNA synthesis in plasma-starved fibroblasts [cells giving rise to connective tissue; -blast: immature, undergoing development] and even enhances normally modest insulin-induced DNA synthesis, suggesting that DMAE may have growth regulatory functions independent of its phosphatidyl role.[173] DMAE provides significant protection against cell death from kinase [phophorylation, or an enzyme transfers a phosphate group] overexpression.[174]

Interferon… DMAE boosts human and animal interferon [fights virus infection and multiplication].[175, 176]

DMAE in practice… DMAE improves symbol recognition and memory test results in adults,[177] and may help children with learning and behavioral disorders.[178] DMAE has a positive effect on Meige's syndrome [involuntary facial movements, eyelid spasm].[179] A case of essential tremor [tremor associated with purposeful movement] was successfully treated for 10 years using DMAE, but with dyskinesia [neurological impairment of voluntary movements] side effects in mouth, face and respiratory musculature.[180] DMAE either improves dyskinesia and chorea [progressive loss of neuron functioning],[181, 182] or contributes to them as a acetylcholine neurotransmitter inhibitor.[183, 184] High DMAE doses can also cause mood alternations.[185]

ALPHA-LIPOIC ACID

Alpha-lipoic acid is the most powerful antioxidant known, with a unique set of therapeutic actions. First, this natural internal sulfur-containing antioxidant destroys a wide variety of free radicals including many of the nastiest. Second, it recycles other antioxidants – Vitamin C, Vitamin E and glutathione – and helps coordinate the body's antioxidant defense network. Third, alpha-lipoic acid rejuvenates stressed and diseased endocrine machinery. Supplementation provides unmatched stress relief, while at the same time forging a younger endocrine system. Alpha-lipoic acid heals free radical/oxidative stress damage. Of course, scar tissue is dead and beyond help.

With all this good comes a *CAUTION* ☛ Misuse or overuse of alpha-lipoic acid causes severe Primary Energy Function exhaustion and collapse of adrenaline production. As a natural internal antioxidant present in all cells, alpha-lipoic acid supplementation forces functioning of your entire antioxidation defense network. This drains away significant adrenal medulla resources from Primary Energy Function and can easily become extreme Healing ←← Energy imbalance and adrenaline exhaustion. The best way to use this hazardous "fountain of youth" antioxidant is in a very small dose; 10-15 mg of alpha-lipoic acid gives only good results over time. By combining low-dose alpha-lipoic acid with targeted healing nutrients and essential nutrition for the injured cells and tissue in question, particularly B vitamins, fatty acids and "trace metals naturally" (individual metal supplementations are too strong here; take them beforehand), you can regenerate endocrine and body functions in ways not possible by any other means. Infrequent alpha-lipoic acid supplementation, not more often than once a week to once every few weeks, produces the best outcomes. Superior nutrition in between alpha-lipoic acid therapy is needed to replenish conutrient reserves.

Review of the Medical Literature

Multi-faceted antioxidant... Alpha-lipoic acid (thioctic acid) plays a fundamental role in cell metabolism. Naturally occurring within mitochondria [cell *organ* responsible for respiration and energy production],[186] alpha-lipoic acid and its reduced form, dihydrolipoic acid, scavenges hydroxyl [OH^-], superoxide [O_2^-], peroxyl [OO^{--}], peroxynitrite [$ONOO^-$], hypochlorous acid [$HClO$] and singlet oxygen [O_2, energized but uncharged form of oxygen generated during a metabolic burst of leucocytes] free radicals. Alpha-lipoic acid also recycles other antioxidants, specifically Vitamin C, glutathione [natural internal antioxidant: cofactor in eliminating hydrogen peroxide (H_2O_2); within cell mitochondria, the main defense against oxidative stress; in the liver, detoxifies toxic oxygen radicals and reduces disulfide groups], and thioredoxin [intercellular disulphide reducing enzyme], which in turn regenerate Vitamin E.[187]

Alpha-lipoic acid is a thiol… Thiols are organic sulfur derivatives, mercaptans [RSH where R = radical] with sulfhydryl residues. Thiols play a central role in coordinating the antioxidant defense network,[188] by (1) quenching free radicals, (2) chelating metals, (3) recycling other antioxidants, and (4) buffering thiol/disulfide redox [reducing/oxidizing reactions]. Thiol redox status in intracellular and extracellular space regulates enzyme activity, protein structures and transcription factor [a protein required in RNA sequencing of DNA] activity and binding. High thiol levels reduce oxidative stress, and in some cases can prevent or treat human diseases.[189]

Possible thiol toxicity… Large increases in circulating free thiols produce toxic effects, probably from the destabilizing action of elevated blood thiol/disulfide ratios and changes in the thiol redox gradient across cells affecting transport and signaling processes, which are dependent on the forming and breaking of disulfide linkages in membrane proteins.[189] In that case, alpha-lipoic acid and dihydrolipoic acid may exert prooxidant activity and generate superoxide.[190]

Oxidative stress… Alpha-lipoic acid reduces oxidative stress in study models of neurodegeneration, diabetes and prevention of glycation reactions [sugars reacting with proteins, particularly critical proteins of long-living nerve cells], cataract formation, ischaemia-reperfusion injury [ischaemia: insufficient blood supply; reperfusion: restoration of blood flow], radiation damage and HIV activation.[191] Adequate glutathione is crucial in protecting against exercise-induced oxidative stress,[188] and alpha-lipoic acid recycles glutathione.[187]

Diabetic neuropathy… Alpha-lipoic acid significantly reduces the symptoms of diabetic pathologies, including diabetic neuropathy [polyneuropathy of peripheral nerves], vascular damage and cataract formation in clinical and experimental studies.[187, 192] With diabetes, reactive oxygen species (ROS) increase as a result of metabolic changes, autoxidation and advanced glycation. Diabetes also compromises protective glutathione and its redox cycle. Short term, ROS reduce nerve blood flow, causing endoneurial [endo- prefix meaning 'within, internal'] hypoxia [inadequate oxygen] and nerve conduction deficits. Antioxidants correct blood flow deficits and endoneurial oxygenation. Long term, ROS exposure damages neurons and Schwann cells [wrap around the nerve axon (long fiber), providing electrical insulation and forming the myelin sheath].[193] Alpha-lipoic acid is especially effective in preventing and treating reactive oxygen and nitrogen species diabetic complications. Alpha-lipoic acid also increases glucose uptake into cells through a mechanism it shares with insulin.[187]

Alzheimer's and Huntington's disease... Oxidative stress is a hallmark of Alzheimer's disease,[194] with advanced glycation and lipid peroxidation end products [lipids: fats and fat related compounds] accumulating in beta-amyloid plaques. Alpha-lipoic acid can reduce the formation of these end products;[195] and in a preliminary study, alpha-lipoic acid stabilized cognitive functions, as measured in neuropsychological tests.[194] In mouse models of Huntington's disease [inherited central nervous system disease of adult-onset dementia and bizarre involuntary movements], alpha-lipoic acid improves survival.[196]

Atherosclerosis... Alpha-lipoic acid inhibits the initiating mechanism of atherogenesis [depositing plaque on artery walls], which is endothelial [lining of the heart and blood vessels] activation and monocyte [type of white blood cell, precursor of macrophage] adhesion.[197]

Heart... Alpha-lipoic acid lessens mitochondrial-induced oxidative stress in aged rat hearts. Notably, cardiac myocytes [muscle cells] of old, alpha-lipoic-acid-supplemented rats have significantly lower oxidant output, and not markedly different from myocytes of unsupplemented young rats. Alpha-lipoic acid also reduces DNA damage and restores myocardial Vitamin C concentrations.[198] Alpha lipoic acid and Vitamin E protect aged rat hearts from ischaemia-reperfusion-induced ROS lipid peroxidation. Importantly, cardiac performance improves during reperfusion.[199]

Liver... Alpha-lipoic acid mitigates alcohol-induced damage, metal intoxication and mushroom and carbon tetrachloride poisoning of the liver.[186] Alpha-lipoic acid reverses age-related declines in rat liver glutathione levels, and age-related increases in oxidative stress vulnerability.[200]

Antioxidants (water-soluble)

Whenever you feel *under the weather*, for no good reason or for a good reason, one cause for sure is free radicals overwhelming your system. Antioxidants protect against free radicals by destroying them at their point of attack, cell membranes and within cell *organs* such as mitochondria, or through search and destroy in the bloodstream. By whichever mechanism a particular antioxidant works, the result is the same – less damage to cells and therefore less aging.

<u>You can actually feel free radical buildup in your system; it is identical to stress buildup</u>! Free radicals are the principal manifestation of stress. When young and healthy, stress doesn't bother you because your endocrine system is very efficient in keeping free radicals under control. With aging, however, these bad actors get out of control, run amuck and attack endocrine machinery. The harder a cell is working, the more vulnerable it is and likely that free radical attack can be successful. You need to preserve these key cells from this oxidative stress.

While you can feel stress build-up, unfortunately you cannot feel cell oxidation (except in the extreme, such as sore muscles) and aging (only in pictures over the years). Consequently, use antioxidants to manage stress, the initiator and primary indicator of bad things happening inside of you. Antioxidants restore endocrine balance too, decreasing not only hyperactive stress, but hyperactivity anywhere in the body. For example, antioxidants reduce autoimmune inflammation, which further improves Stress ability.

Vitamin E is the most powerful <u>fat-soluble</u> antioxidant; supplementation with 200-400 IU daily should be a constant in your nutritional program to preserve cell membranes and other fatty acid structures (review Chapter 5). Another constant is Vitamin C. Taking 500-1000 mg daily along with bioflavonoids provides base-line protection for your <u>water-soluble</u> tissues. Natural Vitamin C-bioflavonoid sources such as rose hips and acerola cherries are your best supplementation route, except with an acid-sensitive stomach. Then, use non-acidic Ester-C. Add more protection with the multitude of less well-known antioxidants present in fruits and vegetables: citrus, spinach, broccoli, lettuce greens, tomatoes, carrots, and so forth (Table 3-3). Finally, variables in your antioxidant arsenal are Pine Bark Extract and Grape Seed Extract. These powerful free radical destroyers eliminate severe stress and recycle Vitamin C and Vitamin E, thus reducing the threat to both water-soluble and fat-soluble tissues.

VITAMIN C and BIOFLAVONOIDS

Though technically not an herb, Vitamin C comes from herbal sources. Vitamin C fulfills three roles simultaneously: (1) antioxidant against many free radical types, (2) frontline immune soldier, and (3) system-wide detoxifier. This vitamin destroys not only free radicals, but also viruses, bacteria and cancer. And 'C' neutralizes all manner of harmful substances in the blood: allergens, food preservatives, pesticide residue, pollution, gasoline vapors and other toxic chemicals. The medical literature below explores Vitamin C's essential antioxidant role. Table 7-6 and associated text reveal its immune capabilities and Chapter 11 its "detox" action, with medical literature specific to those roles reported there.

Bioflavonoids synergize Vitamin C in its antioxidation, immune and detoxification activities. Also known as Vitamin P, bioflavonoids are water-soluble phytocompounds such as rutin, citrin, hesperidin, flavones and flavonals, and commonly found in rose hips, acerola cherries, citric pulp and some other fruits. Bioflavonoids improve capillary wall elasticity and connective tissue health. Easy bruising and black-and-blue marks indicate bioflavonoid deficiency. For a complete profile, see Table 3-3 medical literature.

Human beings are one of the few mammals not to manufacture their own Vitamin C internally. We have a genetic defect in this mechanism, which apparently did not matter at the birth of our species. Now however, diets are much different and in some important ways inferior, and extra Vitamin C has become crucial to antioxidant, immune and liver defense. A daily supplement of 500 to 1000 mg will make up for our genetic imperfection.

Review of the Medical Literature

Antioxidant nature... Cells continuously produce free radicals as part of their metabolic processes. These free radicals are neutralized by elaborate antioxidant defense systems consisting of enzyme and non-enzymatic antioxidants. Non-enzymatic antioxidants include Vitamin C (ascorbic acid), Vitamin E and flavonoids. A negative imbalance between free radicals and antioxidants is referred to as oxidative stress.[201] Vitamin C is a potent antioxidant, an electron donor, and this accounts for all its known functions and properties.[202] Vitamin C is a primary water-soluble antioxidant in both cells and blood, and can donate electrons to the alpha-tocopheroxyl radical [Vitamin E]. This recycling of Vitamin E helps protect cell membrane lipids [fats and fat related compounds] from oxidation. [203]

Mitochondria and aging... Mitochondria [cell *organ* responsible for respiration and energy production] and particularly mitochondrial DNA (mtDNA) are major targets of free radical attack. Mitochondrial oxidative damage accumulates with aging, with mtDNA damage several times greater than nucleus DNA damage. As a consequence, in the brain and liver, mito-chondrial size increases and mitochondrial membrane electrical potential decreases. Vitamin C and Vitamin E protect against this age-related oxidative mtDNA damage, as well as oxida-tion of mitochondrial glutathione [natural internal antioxidant: the main defense against oxida-tive stress within cell mitochondria]. Thus, Vitamin C and Vitamin E can prevent mitochon-drial aging.[204]

Brain and nervous system… The brain and central nervous system [CNS] accumulate and maintain relatively high Vitamin C concentrations.[205] Vitamin C is both neuroprotective and neuromodulating.[203] Neurons employ Vitamin C in many chemical and enzymatic reactions and for interneuron communication. Its release into the brain extracellular fluid regulates dopamine [neurotransmitter; helps to regulate movement and emotion] and glutamate [fast, excitatory CNS neurotransmitter] transmission.[205]

ALS/Lou Gehrig's Disease… Amyotrophic lateral sclerosis is a progressive, fatal neu-rodegenerative disease in which upper and lower CNS motor neurons [neurons connected to muscles, glands and other effectors] become damaged and then die. Patient death usually occurs from respiratory failure. The following evidence supports a Vitamin C-ALS link: (1) CNS motor activity is associated with Vitamin C release; (2) a close relationship exists between CNS Vitamin C levels and injury tolerance; (3) Vitamin C blood and cell levels decline with age, especially in males; (4) the scorbutic [diseased with scurvy] guinea pig is an animal model for ALS; and (5) Vitamin C eliminates superoxide [O_2^-] free radicals, as does superoxide dismutase [SOD metalloenzyme; CuZnSOD malfunction can cause ALS, see Chapter 6].[206] SOD catalyzes the destruction of superoxide (O_2^-) to hydrogen peroxide (H_2O_2) and back to oxygen (O_2).[207] Vitamin C also eliminates hydrogen peroxide.[208]

Alzheimer's disease… 'A beta' fragments [beta-amyloid peptides, thick protein plaque] accumulate in Alzheimer brain areas serving memory and information acquisition and pro-cessing. These fragments develop from abnormal proteolytic cleavage [splitting of polypep-tide proteins by hydrolysis] of their precursor, amyloid precursor protein (APP). Direct free radical scavengers such as Vitamin C and Vitamin E reduce 'A beta' toxicity with great effi-cacy.[209]

Vascular protection… Oxidative stress is a significant causative factor in atherosclerosis [depositing plaque on artery walls] and vascular dysfunction. Antioxidants play multi-faceted preventative roles. Lipid-soluble antioxidants such as Vitamin E present in low-density lipoproteins [LDL, so-called bad cholesterol] and water-soluble antioxidants such as Vitamin C present in extracellular fluid of the arterial wall inhibit LDL oxidation and atherogenesis.

Meanwhile, antioxidants within the cells of the vascular wall prevent endothelial [lining of the heart and blood vessels] activation and expression of monocytes [type of white blood cell, precursor of macrophage] and other adhesion molecules, and improve endothelium-derived nitric oxide (EDNO) activity.[210] EDNO is pivotal in regulating vascular tone through vascular smooth muscle cell relaxation and vasodilation.[211] Vitamin C ameliorates defective ENDO vasodilation.[212] EDNO activity is also anti-atherogenic, inhibiting monocyte-endothelial interactions, smooth muscle cell proliferation and blood platelet aggregation.[211] Furthermore, Vitamin C markedly decreases LDL-induced arterial smooth muscle cell apoptosis [gene-directed, programmed cell death].[213] Vitamin C is necessary for collagen [fibrous protein of connective tissue] synthesis, critical to maintaining vascular integrity;[214] and Vitamin C reduces blood histamine levels [allergic reaction] that can cause vascular endothelial cell separation.[215] Overall, Vitamin C improves endothelial vasodilator dysfunction resulting from coronary artery disease, hypercholesterolemia [high blood cholesterol], hyperhomocysteinemia [homocysteine: harmful sulfur-containing amino acid], diabetes, high blood pressure, smoking and aging.[211, 212]

Cardiovascular in practice... Vitamin C protects against coronary heart disease, total circulatory disease, high blood pressure and stroke.[216, 217] Current evidence suggests that coronary heart disease patients would benefit from supplementations of 400 IU Vitamin E and 500 to 1000 mg Vitamin C daily.[218] Vitamin E acts as the first risk discriminator in cardiovascular disease, Vitamin C as second risk discriminator. Optimal cardiac health requires Vitamins E and C, Vitamin A, carotenoids and vegetable conutrients.[219]

Diabetes... Insulin promotes cellular Vitamin C uptake, whereas hyperglycemia [high blood sugar] inhibits it.[220] Hyperglycemia also increases free radical concentrations, and the resulting oxidative stress can cause numerous diabetic complications.[221] Hyperglycemia-related tissue scurvy is common in Type I [juvenile] diabetes,[220] and induces atherosclerosis. Acute scurvy also results in microvascular complications such as capillary hemorrhaging [of diabetic retinopathy].[214] Excessive glycosylation [adding sugar molecules to protein chains] of protein structures is another diabetic concern. Vitamin C reduces nonenzymatic glycation.[222] Dietary intervention with 200-600 mg of Vitamin C daily is advantageous in Type I diabetes.[223]

Eyes... Age-related macular degeneration (AMD) is the leading cause of blindness in the United States and other developed countries, while age-related cataracts are the leading cause of visual disability. Epidemiological evidence suggests diets high in Vitamin E, Vitamin C and carotenoids, particularly xanthophylls [yellow-pigment fruits and vegetables], are insurance against developing these disorders. [224] Vitamin C protects against age-related cataracts by preventing oxidative damage in the lens.[225]

Wound healing... Antioxidants enhance healing of infected and non-infected wounds by reducing oxidative damage.[226] Blood antioxidant levels decrease following wounding, with Vitamin C and Vitamin E falling 60-70%, and recovering completely only after 14 days.[227] Several nutritional factors may impair wound healing, in particular inadequate Vitamin C, Vitamin E, Vitamin A, zinc, protein and individual amino acids.[228]

Bones and cartilage... Epidemiological studies find a positive association between Vitamin C intake and bone density.[229] Vitamin C is important to the development, mainte-nance, repair and remodeling of cartilage.[230]

Scurvy... Most mammals make their own Vitamin C internally, however, humans require an external source. Scurvy develops only after many weeks of severe deficits in Vitamin C intake. The earliest symptom is fatigue. The skin can show ecchymoses [black and blue marks], xerosis [dry, hard, scaly skin], follicle hyperkeratosis [thickening overgrowth], leg edema [abnormal accumulation of fluid, swelling], and poor wound healing. Gum abnormal-ities can include bleeding, swelling and purplish discoloration. Back and joint pain is common, sometimes involving hemorrhage. Anemia occurs frequently, and leukopenia [low white blood cell count] occasionally. Syncope [fainting, temporary unconsciousness due to insufficient blood supply to the brain] and sudden death are possible. Vitamin C administration produces rapid to dramatic improvement in scurvy and its symptoms.[231] Although scurvy is rare in the United States, two populations at great risk are alcoholics and the institutionalized elderly.[232]

Genetic defect/intake need... Most plant and animal species synthesize Vitamin C, but human beings cannot because of a gene mutation approximately 45 million years ago in cod-ing gulonolactone oxidase (GLO), the terminal step of Vitamin C synthesis from glucose.[233, 234] Consequently, Vitamin C must be an essential component of the human diet. Available evi-dence indicates that 200 mg of Vitamin C intake per day saturates tissues. However, optimal Vitamin C status awaits clearer definition.[233] A daily intake of at least 150-200 mg insures immune response, lung function and iron absorption. Vitamin C requirements for smokers are at least 60 mg and up to 140 mg higher per day than for nonsmokers. High Vitamin C intakes are safe,[235] with 2-4 g daily well tolerated in healthy individuals.[236] Gastrointestinal upset can sometimes occur with intakes above 2 g.[237]

Pollution, tobacco smoke... The hypothesis [proposed, not proven] that oxidative stress is an important, if not the sole, toxic mechanism behind air pollutants and tobacco smoke is com-pelling. The gas phase of cigarette smoke, NO_2 and O_3, oxidizes lung lipids [fat and fat-related lung tissue] by known biochemical mechanisms. Both Vitamin C and Vitamin E prevent this oxidation and protect human cells; Vitamin C is more effective against NO_2, Vitamin E more effective against O_3. Vitamin C also defends against air pollution in adults as measured by histamine challenge. Lastly, experimental animals from many species develop lung disease similar to human bronchitis and emphysema [chronic lung disease, difficulty breathing from enlargement and loss of elasticity of air sacs] after exposure to NO_2 and O_3.[238] Cigarette smoking decreases blood levels of Vitamin C and beta-carotene, indicating that smoking-related chronic inflammatory response is due to an imbalance in oxidant/antioxidant homeostasis.[239] In nonsmoking individuals, passive smoke quickly breaks down antioxidant defenses, accelerating lipid peroxidation including LDL accumulation. Vitamin C protects nonsmokers from the harmful effects of secondhand smoke.[240] Author's Note: Vitamin C detoxification of many more harmful substances is reported in Chapter 11.

Iron absorption... Vitamin C improves dietary iron absorption.[241] Of concern, Vitamin C can interact with catalytically active 'free iron' and cause oxidative damage by producing hydroxyl [OH^-] and alkoxyl [alkyl: C_nH_{2n+1}, such as methyl and ethyl] free radicals. However, Vitamin C maintains its antioxidant protection with or without iron cosupplementation.[242] Overall, iron uptake and storage is effectively controlled by internal regulatory mechanisms, and high Vitamin C intake does not induce iron mismanagement in healthy individuals.[243]

PINE BARK EXTRACT

When severe stress is overwhelming you, employ Pine Bark Extract and Grape Seed Extract to sweep free radicals from your system. Pine Bark Extract is generally more powerful than Grape Seed Extract, but only because it is more reliable. Considerable variation in effectiveness exists from product to product for both of these extracts. For pine bark, use only extract that is light brown in color and has a sharp pine taste. Pine Bark Extract is also known by the proprietary name, "Pycnogenol."

Take 30 to 50 mg (maximum) of Pine Bark Extract as needed to neutralize severe stress. Without need, however, such dosage is too strong and produces Healing ← Energy imbalance, which compromises adrenaline production. With need, the extract is used up in the free radical wars. Extreme stress such as trauma may require 3X dosing or more, and this proves not to be an overdose if *these troops* are lost in saving you. Pine Bark Extract also recycles Vitamin C, Vitamin E and the natural internal antioxidant glutathione.

On days of low to moderate stress, little or no pine bark is needed to protect your cells. Vitamin C and bioflavonoids, Vitamin E, and fruit and vegetable antioxidants can handle this free radical load.

Review of the Medical Literature

Antioxidant nature... Pycnogenol (standardized bark extract of Pinus maritima) contains flavonoids, mostly procyandins and phenolic acids, which are powerful free radical scavengers against reactive oxygen and nitrogen species. Pycnogenol also contributes to the overall antioxidant defense network through Vitamin C regeneration and protection of Vitamin E and glutathione [natural internal antioxidant: within cell mitochondria, the main defense against oxidative stress]. Pycnogenol improves nitric oxide metabolism in activated macrophages [relatively long-living, large white blood cells; -phage: anything that devours] by eliminating free radical interference. This benefits immune disorders, and neurodegenerative and vascular diseases.[244]

Cell respiration... Pycnogenol reversibly reduces [donates electrons to] cytochrome c [heme oxidation-reduction reaction, i.e. cell respiration] and prevents mitochondrial [cell *organ* responsible for respiration and energy production] and submitochondrial oxidation.[245]

Asthma... is a chronic inflammatory process. With strong antioxidant and anti-inflammatory properties, pycnogenol reduces asthmatic symptoms and blood leukotrienes [family of potent hormone-like eicosanoids produced by immune response to antigens; they contribute to defense, inflammation and hypersensitivity] in a preliminary study.[246] Pycnogenol inhibits histamine release from mast cells [resident white blood cells of connective tissue] in rats.[247]

Maintaining youthful tissue... Pycnogenol binds to elastin [elastic protein of connective tissue] and slows its rate of degradation.[248] Pycnogenol binds to many proteins and alters their structure, thereby modulating key enzyme activities and protein pathways.[203] Pycnogenol inhibits adipose tissue [animal, vegetable and man-man fats stored in human fatty tissue] accumulation.[249]

Neurological diseases... Antioxidant therapy benefits neurological diseases. Oxidative stress causes glutathione depletion, which induces glutamate [fast, excitatory central nervous system neurotransmitter] neuron cytotoxicity. Pine bark extract and Vitamin E significantly improve antioxidant defenses against glutamate neuron cytotoxicity.[250, 251]

Alzheimer's disease... is characterized by senile beta-amyloid plaques [thick protein deposits], neurofibrillary tangles, selective neuron loss and cerebrovascular beta-amyloidosis, in which beta-amyloid generates reactive oxygen species (ROS) that cause vascular endothelial [lining of blood vessels] cell damage. Pycnogenol scavenges beta-amyloid ROS.[252]

Vascular protection... Antioxidant therapy protects against cerebral ischaemia [insufficient blood supply, as in a stroke].[250] Pycnogenol reduces atherogenesis [depositing plaque on artery walls] and thrombus [blood clot] by inhibiting low-density lipoprotein [LDL, so-called bad cholesterol] oxidation and by preserving nitric oxide (NO), which decreases platelet aggregation and adhesion.[253] Reactive nitrogen species (RNS) decrease glutathione levels in endothelial cells; pine bark extract markedly improves RNS defenses.[251] Pycnogenol further benefits cardiovascular health through vasorelaxant activity, inhibiting angiotensin-converting enzyme (ACE) [contracts vascular smooth muscle, thereby raising blood pressure and stimulating aldosterone release] and increasing microcirculation.[203]

Diabetic retinopathy... characterized by capillary lesions with exudate [escaped fluid and cells from blood vessels] deposits and hemorrhages, causes vision loss. Pycnogenol improves capillary resistance and reduces leakage into the retina. Pycnogenol inhibits the progression of retinopathy and recovers some visual acuity.[254]

Cancer... The second leading cause of cancer deaths in US women is breast cancer. Pycnogenol produces significantly more apoptosis [gene-directed, programmed cell death] in human breast cancer cells (MCF-7) compared to untreated cancer cells. Pycnogenol does not affect normal human mammary cells (MCF-10).[255] Tobacco-related nitrosamine is a potent carcinogen. In rats, pycnogenol strongly inhibits liver and lung nitrosamine toxicity.[256] In addition, pycnogenol decreases smoking-induced platelet aggregation.[257]

GRAPE SEED EXTRACT

Grape Seed Extract and Pine Bark Extract relieve severe stress. Alternating between these two extracts is especially powerful in quenching free radicals and oxidative stress. Take 30 to 50 mg (maximum) of Grape Seed Extract as needed. Effectiveness varies greatly among Grape Seed Extracts; the only sure way to find a good brand is to taste and compare it with crushed grape seeds (*yuck*).

Red seedless grapes are a rich antioxidant harvest too. Their skins provide the antioxidants found in red wine, while the soft, undeveloped seeds contain some of the goodness and power of Grape Seed Extract. Result: gentle antioxidation throughout the body plus natural healing factors.

Review of the Medical Literature

Antioxidant nature… Proanthocyanidins, naturally occurring antioxidants found in fruits, vegetables, seeds, nuts, bark and flowers, exert powerful biological and pharmacological activities against oxidative stress. Grape seed proanthocyanidin extract (GSPE) provides greater protection than Vitamin C and Vitamin E against free radicals, DNA damage and lipid peroxidation.[258] GSPE potently eliminates superoxide [O_2^-] and hydroxyl [OH^-] radicals, 78-81% in vitro [in laboratory vessel] compared to 12-19% for Vitamin C and 36-44% for Vitamin E.[259]

Wound healing… Angiogenesis [new capillary blood vessels] plays a fundamental role in wound healing. Among many known growth factors, vascular endothelial growth factor (VEGF) is believed to be most important in stimulating wound angiogenesis. GSPE strongly upregulates VEGF expression in human keratinocytes [outermost layer of skin cells], and is able to drive VEGF transcription. In mice, topical GSPE application accelerates dermal wound contraction and closure, producing a more well-defined epithelial [surface tissue lining] region, higher cell density and connective tissue deposition, and better histological architecture.[260]

Chronic pancreatitis… GSPE eases human chronic pancreatitis.[258]

Cardiovascular… GSPE promotes cardiovascular health through a number of mechanisms. In hypercholesterolemic patients, GSPE significantly decreases oxidized LDL [low-density lipoproteins, so-called bad cholesterol], a biomarker for cardiovascular disease. GSPE improves post-ischemic [ischemic: insufficient blood supply] cardiac function including left ventricular function and reduces myocardial infarct size [localized tissue death due to lack of oxygen], ventricular fibrillation [chaotic ventricle contraction; fatal unless treated immediately], tachycardia [rapid heartbeat, usually 150-200 beats per minute] and cardiomyocyte apoptosis [cell death].[261] In rats, GSPE protects against myocardial infarction [heart attack] and heart muscle ischaemia-reperfusion injury [reperfusion: restoration of blood flow].[258]

Liver protection… GSPE pre-exposure reduces mouse liver necrosis [death] and animal lethality from acetaminophen [nonprescription NSAID pain medication] toxicity. [262] Highly bioavailable, GSPE can be an effective therapeutic tool in protecting multiple target organs from diverse drug- and chemical-induced toxicity.[263]

Cancer… GSPE is cytotoxic to human breast and lung cancer cells, and to gastric adenocarcinoma [tumor involving cells of the wall lining] while simultaneously improving the viability and growth of normal gastric mucous membrane cells. GSPE upregulates the normal bcl(2) gene [inhibits apoptosis, gene-directed, programmed cell death] and downregulates oncogene c-myc [oncogene = mutated version of a normal gene; can convert normal cell to tumor cell; c = proto-oncogene or DNA fragment, and it is the switch for growth and repair; myc = generally lung, breast and cervical carcinomas]. GSPE is significantly more protective than Vitamin C and Vitamin E against tobacco-induced oxidative stress and necrosis in human oral keratinocytes. Topical GSPE application enhances sun protection in humans.[258, 264]

Vasoconstriction/Vasodilation

Vasoconstriction and vasodilation nutrition maintains blood vessel homeostasis and the inflammation mechanism common to both healing and immune systems. Hyperactivity anywhere in the body rapidly depletes vasoconstriction nutrients. Vasoconstrictor herbs, which narrow blood vessels and temporarily raise blood pressure, can resupply this missing nutrition and restore vascular and microvascular health. Vasoconstrictors are corrective for blood pressure, varicose veins and bluing of small blood vessels, inflammatory '-itis' diseases such as arthritis, edema and related fatigue headaches, and possibly migraine with its uncontrollable dilation of blood vessels in the brain.

Vasoconstriction and vasodilation must be in equilibrium so the body can adjust blood flow to tissues as needed. This can be accomplished most easily as follows:

> **vasoconstriction ⇌ vasodilation**
>
> Shepherd's Purse/Woundwort ⇌ niacin (Vitamin B3)
> and Heather (alternate use)

Vasodilator niacin is amply supplied in Chapter 4 B vitamin-rich foods. Not so for vasoconstrictors, which while present in many foods are not richly found anywhere. Alternating use of Shepherd's Purse/Woundwort and Heather will correct vasoconstrictor deficiency. Hawthorn Berries at 2X dosing (Table 7-5) also gives modest constrictor effect, as do astringents Bistort (strongest known astringent herb), Rosemary (Table 7-6) and Alum Root. Use these constrictor and astringent herbs to build strong blood vessel and capillary homeostasis. The trace metal nickel is necessary for healthy vasoconstriction too. Meanwhile, niacin from whole-grain cereals and nutritional yeasts, along with blood-pressure-lowering vasodilation herbs of Raw Garlic and Hawthorn Berries at 1X, and Vitamin C and Omega 3 fish oils provide counterbalance. See also venous insufficiency in the index.

Migraine headaches. The solution to migraines lies, at least in part, in restoring vasoconstrictor ⇌ vasodilator equilibrium. Severe to extreme Stress exhaustion also underlies migraine headaches, and this requires Chapter 12 cure using Vitamin B2, which is superior to placebo in migraine prevention, reducing the frequency of attack and number of headache days.[265] The herb Feverfew shows efficacy against migraines,[266, 267] but it injuries adrenal tissues with high levels of camphor and terpenes. Juniper Berries contain camphor and terpene derivatives. If at all possible, avoid these two harsh herbs.

SHEPHERD'S PURSE and WOUNDWORT

Shepherd's Purse is a strong vasoconstriction herb. Adversely, it has the side effect of causing a queasy stomach. Combining Shepherd's Purse with Woundwort in equal amounts prevents this problem and adds micronutrient variety. A tea of these herbs can improve vascular and inflammatory mechanisms, and edema, fatigue and stamina as described in Table 7-5 and the text there.

Medical literature—There is nothing significant on the micronutrient role of Shepherd's Purse. Woundwort shows efficacy against viruses including herpes, hepatitis B and HIV.

Review of the Medical Literature

Nature… Woundwort (Prunella vulgaris) is traditionally used for wound healing and to alleviate fevers and sore throat pain. Woundwort contains antioxidant and immunomodulatory rosmarinic acid, immunomodulatory polysaccharide prunelline, and anti-inflammatory and anti-allergic triterpenes. It is strongly antiviral and moderately antimutagenic.[268-271] Woundwort reduces lipid peroxidation [lipids: fats and fat related compounds] and hemolysis [breaking down of red blood cells].[272] Rosmarinic acid modulates IL-2 [Interleukin 2: hormone-like substance released by T lymphocytes; stimulates more T-cell production and other immune defenses] following T-lymphocyte activation.[271]

Viruses... Of 472 medicinal herbs tested, Woundwort is one of the ten most effective against herpes simplex virus type 1.[273] It also demonstrates activity against herpes simplex type 2.[274] Of 300 herbs tested, Woundwort is one of the ten most effective against HbsAg, a surface marker on the hepatitis B virus.[275]

HIV/AIDS... Woundwort shows anti-HIV activity during the virus' adsorption and reverse transcription stages,[276] inhibiting HIV-1 attachment to the CD4 receptor [protein structure on the surface of T-cells and other cells that enables HIV attachment and entry].[277] Prunelline is the active anti-HIV Woundwort compound.[278] Of 204 herbs in common use in Japan, Woundwort spike [elongated flower cluster] and Lithospermum erythrorhizon root [Shikon, an Oriental herb] have the strongest anti-HIV-1 activity.[279]

HEATHER

A tea made from Heather's flowering shoots produces powerful vasoconstriction. To prevent queasy stomach, Heather may require buffering with Woundwort or 100 mg of niacin. Heather and Shepherd's Purse/Woundwort work toward the same goal in slightly different ways; alternating between them is complementary and corrects many vascular problems. From the medical literature, Heather is anti-inflammatory and anti-leukemic. Heather also benefits edema, fatigue and stamina.

Review of the Medical Literature

Anti-inflammatory... Heather (Calluna vulgaris) powerfully inhibits cyclooxygenase [enzyme found in most tissues, part of the normal inflammatory process].[280] Heather's cyclooxygenase and lipoxygenase inhibition and its ursolic acid constituent produce strong anti-inflammatory action.[281]

Leukemia... Heather, a specific inhibitor of arachidonate 5-lipoxygenase [catalyzing enzyme for arachidonic acid conversion to leukotrienes, part of the immune/inflammatory response], exhibits potent antiproliferative effects on human leukemia HL60 cells. This result suggests that arachidonate 5-lipoxygenase metabolites and/or leukotrienes [family of potent hormone-like eicosanoids produced by immune response to antigens; they contribute to defense, inflammation and hypersensitivity] may play a fundamental role in leukemia cell functions.[282] Ursolic acid inhibits arachidonate metabolism in HL60 cells.[281]

ADRENAL CORTEX STRESS

Adrenal cortex herbs are very different from medulla herbs. Most medulla herbs affect both Energy/nerves and Healing to some extent, whereas few cortex herbs impact both Stress and Immune functions. The notable exceptions are Astragalus, which strongly improves stress ability and immune response, and Yucca with rebalancing action. Generally cortex herbs perform specific roles within Stress or Immune subfunctions.

Table 7-5 presents Primary Stress Function herbs with subheadings indicating specific use within the subfunctions of stress (cortisol), fatigue (aldosterone), conclusion of sex (involving stress and fatigue and connected to the testes or ovaries), and gluconeogenesis. All Primary Stress Function herbs improve the autoimmune syndromes of arthritis and other '-itis' diseases. Autoimmune is basically Immune hyperactivity, and Stress herbs work to offset this cortex imbalance. A hyperactive immune system triggers inflammation; therefore all Primary Stress Function herbs are also anti-inflammatory.

TABLE 7-5. ADRENAL CORTEX STRESS/FATIGUE HERBS.

Subheadings (underlined) specify use. Numbering of fatigue herbs indicates potency and "need for."

Herb	Comments
<u>STRESS</u>	
Antioxidants	Antioxidation up = stress down!
American Ginseng	Activates energy-stress action plan. See energy (Table 7-3) and text there.
Astragalus	Essential during high stress. Also immune (Table 7-6). Not for fatigue.
Hawthorn Berries	General tonic, good for an ailing heart.
Hydrangea	Fat/fatty acid metabolism. Catalyst for fat-burning here and fatty acid activity (Table 7-4). Also pituitary-stress (Figure 8-B).

| Dong Quai | Stress/blood tonic of the Angelica species. Also mild balancing female herb. |
| Aspirin (derived from White Willow Bark) | Relief from stress/fatigue headache, but NSAID and soft functioning side effects are possible. |

FATIGUE – MAINTAIN HEALTH, i.e. **ESSENTIAL**

| #1 Raw Garlic | PREVENTS FATIGUE! Also healing (Table 7-4) and immune (Table 7-6). |

FATIGUE – REBUILD HEALTH (in order of importance)

#2 Guarana	RELIEFS FATIGUE! Contains caffeine too (Table 7-3).
#3 Nettle	Also nerves (Table 7-3). Not with Oats.
#4 Cayenne	Adrenal thermoregulation. Also immune (Table 7-6). Too much can be neurotoxic.
#5 Ginger	Fatigue-stomach digestion link. Can cure sour-stomach headache. Horseradish helps too. Ginger is also an immune herb (Table 7-6).
#6 Shepherd's Purse and Woundwort	Anti-edema vasoconstriction (Table 7-4 and text there).
#7 Heather	Powerful anti-inflammatory. Also anti-edema vasoconstriction (Table 7-4 and text there) and immune (Table 7-6)
#8 Hawthorn Berries at 2X	See stress above and its text. 2X dosing gives modest vasoconstriction (Table 7-4).

CORTEX SEX (see Table 7-3 for MEDULLA SEX)

Sarsaparilla	Excellent sexual tonic.
American Ginseng	Also stress (above) and energy (Table 7-3).
Nettle	Also fatigue (above) and nerves (Table 7-3). Not with Oats.

♂ MALE

| Saw Palmetto Berries and Pygeum | Good together. Male tonic, especially for the prostate. |

Herb	Comments
Nettle Root (not the standard leaf)	Prostate.
♀ FEMALE	
Black Cohosh	Proven efficacy for menopause and hormone replacement, alternative to estrogen therapy.
Chaste Berries	PMS and menopausal symptoms
Dong Quai	Also stress.
Wild Yam	
GLUCONEOGENESIS (adrenal cortex raises blood glucose levels)	
Yucca	Also immune (Table 7-6)
Licorice	Also anxiety (Table 7-3). Side effects possible.
glucosamine	Arthritis relief, not a cure. Also Special Factor (Table 7-4).

Stress Ability

Maintaining your ability to handle stress is a relatively simple matter. Cortisol and other stress-related hormones derive from the basic adrenal cortex nutrition of nutritional yeasts and green vegetables, Omega 3 fatty acids and modest Vitamin D, and trace metals. Where do stress herbs fit in? They boost functioning to a higher, more efficient level by supplying micronutrient anti-stress factors. Furthermore, stress herbs act as blood and heart tonics, improving red blood cell parameters. Red blood cells are to stress what white blood cells are to immune.

Rebuilding stress functioning is a much more difficult undertaking, requiring the following four steps. First, take the above Chapter 4-6 cortex nutrition for several weeks, 2X usage at the start, then 1X. Second, input all Table 7-5 stress herbs during this period except aspirin, plus other appropriate herbs for your symptoms. Third, fix any stress exhaustion. Arthritis and autoimmune complaints indicate permanent hypoactive functioning. Curing mild stress exhaustion requires supplementation of

Chapter 4 B vitamins pantothenic acid, B2 and B6, and separately Chapter 6 trace metals, notably vanadium. Chapter 12 solves severe stress exhaustion and resulting dependent body system diseases such as osteoarthritis and rheumatoid arthritis. Fatigue exhaustion can develop before stress exhaustion and may need attention first. This is explained ahead in "Fatigue." Finally fourth, reset Immune ⇌ Stress in perfect equilibrium using Devil's Claw and Goldenseal Root of Figure 7-B.

ANTIOXIDANTS

One basic rule is true all the time: antioxidation up = stress down! By eliminating free radicals, antioxidants reduce oxidative stress. The fundamental importance of Vitamin C, Vitamin E, metal enzyme antioxidants and phyto-compound antioxidants to well being cannot be overemphasized. Oxidative stress is bad stress, and will make you old before your time.

AMERICAN GINSENG

American Ginseng nourishes and balances Energy and Stress functioning. It can be the *cavalry* to the rescue when stress surrounds you. See Table 7-3 and text there including the review of medical literature.

ASTRAGALUS

Astragalus is essential in a high stress environment, boosting your ability to cope with the daily pressures and demands of modern life. This herb keeps functioning up and going strong. In fact, Astragalus is so powerful in its cortex boost that IT MUST NOT BE TAKEN AT THE SAME TIME as B vitamin-rich nutritional yeasts EXCEPT to cure severe exhaustion, as detailed in Chapter 12. In the absence of exhaustion (hypoactivity), ingesting Astragalus with nutritional yeasts generates severe cortex hyperactivity and worse, as this severe overstimulation uses up other necessary cortex raw materials to the point of depletion, thereby bringing on exhaustion! Astragalus taken two hours or more before or after nutritional yeasts creates little interaction, and no problem.

Chapter 12 discusses mild and severe stress exhaustion cures fully. Suffice it to say, combining Astragalus with nutritional yeasts requires not only need, but also priming the nutritional pump. In other words, this potent nutrient combination will injure the cortex if other supporting raw materials, particularly Omega 3 fatty acids, are not abundantly supplied beforehand over several weeks.

Astragalus improves all Stress and Immune functions, except fatigue where it has no effect. Take up to 1500 mg and 2X dose, as needed, at most twice a week, although more often with immune disorder. Astragalus stress-related medical literature is presented below; its immune review is given in the text following Table 7-6.

Review of the Medical Literature

Heart disease... Astragalus membranaceus markedly relieves angina pectoris [chest pain with the feeling of suffocation from total lack of oxygen in the heart muscle] and improves EKG performance in patients with ischemic [insufficient blood supply] heart disease.[283] For angina pectoris, Astragalus increases cardiac output without inhibiting adenosine triphosphatase [ATP: primary energy source within all living cells] activity, unlike conventional digitalis [heart stimulant drug] treatment.[284] Astragalus improves left ventricular modeling and ejection in congestive heart failure.[285] Astragalus may strengthen left ventricular function during myocardial infarction [heart attack] by reducing pre-ejection period/left ventricular ejection time (PEP/LVET) and free radical activity.[286] See also Dong Quai ahead regarding Dong Quai/Astragalus combination, a traditional Chinese formulation, which stimulates red blood cell production and enhances cardiovascular function.

Male infertility... A major cause of male infertility is poor sperm motility [spontaneous movement]. Astragalus significantly stimulates human sperm motility.[287]

Memory... In mice, Astragalus reduces alcohol-induced deficits in memory retrieval.[288]

HAWTHORN BERRIES

Hawthorn Berries are not specifically for stress, rather they rev every function in the body, and stress generally needs revving *first-est* with the *most-est*. Hawthorn is traditionally used for damaged, weakened hearts, another vulnerable stress point since the heart muscle never rests. The limited medical literature below cites this application.

Hawthorn Berries in combination with other adrenal nutrients can overstimulate functions and metabolisms; therefore take it alone at 500 to 1000 mg once a week to once a month to tone up stress ability and the entire body. With heart problems of any type, use Hawthorn Berries more often, up to once a day and possibly twice a day with these considerations: 2X dosing generates mild vasoconstriction, which while therapeutic against fatigue may be contraindicated for atherosclerosis where artery walls are already narrowed. On the other hand, the medical literature indicates its potential use for ischaemia, or insufficient blood supply.

Review of the Medical Literature

Heart tonic... Hawthorn Berries (Crataegus oxycantha) are of therapeutic benefit in the treatment of cardiovascular disease. Current uses are for angina [chest pain], hypertension [high blood pressure], arrhythmias [abnormal heart beat: too slow, too rapid, too early, irregular] and congestive heart failure [ineffective pumping of the heart causing fluid to accumulate in the lungs].[289] For congestive heart failure patients, Hawthorn Berries significantly improve exercise parameters before dyspnea [shortness of breath, labored breathing] and fatigue occur.[290] Animal studies indicate anti-ischemic [ischemic: insufficient blood supply] and anti-cholesterol activity.[289]

HYDRANGEA

Hydrangea root contains a vitamin factor that facilitates ester/fatty acid metabolism and its pituitary regulation. In effect, Hydrangea is as a catalyst for fat burning by cells (its use here) and for fatty acid healing (Table 7-4). Take Hydrangea as needed, usually once a month or less often, to maintain these metabolisms at peak performance.

Stress hyperactivity, especially stress trauma, depletes this Hydrangea micronutrient, as does the constant stress disease diabetes. Stress exhaustion and poor healing may also indicate deficiency. Symptoms can include labored breathing, upper respiratory congestion and infection, and small red spots under the skin, easiest seen on the back of the hand. Take Hydrangea at 1X dosing with mild deficiency or at 2X one hour apart to correct severely impaired ester/fatty acid metabolism. 2X generates pituitary stimulation, which washes away any pituitary suppression and atrophy, but such strong therapeutic action will temporarily increase the need for all fatty acids. Besides Hydrangea, deficiencies in Table 3-2 amino acid carnitine and Chapter 6 trace metal catalysts niobium and tantalum can similarly short-circuit ester/fatty acid metabolism.

Very little in medical literature exists on Hydrangea, nothing on its fatty acid/ester activity.

DONG QUAI

Dong Quai is a general stress and blood tonic for both sexes, and a mild female herb helping to balance her hormones and organs. Take as a tea or 500 mg (maximum) in capsule form, as needed. In the medical literature below, Dong Quai plus Astragalus is a traditional Chinese formula for blood and cardiovascular function. Female effects are reviewed in "Cortex Sex" ahead.

Review of the Medical Literature

General tonic... Dong Quai (Angelica sinensis) acts as a blood tonic, and may enhance hematopoiesis [blood formation].[291]

Antioxidant... Dong Quai scavenges superoxide $[O_2^-]$ and hydroxyl $[OH^-]$ free radicals and inhibits lipid peroxidation [lipids: fats and fat related compounds] in mice.[292]

Heart... Dong Quai protects against myocardial [heart muscle] ischaemia-reperfusion [ischaemia: insufficient blood supply; reperfusion: restoration of blood flow, for example, to heart muscles after a heart attack] injury and arrhythmia [abnormal heart beat: too slow, too rapid, too early, irregular] in animals.[293, 294]

Liver... Dong Quai dose-dependently prevents mouse liver toxicity caused by acetaminophen [nonprescription pain medication] and associated with depletion of glutathione [natural internal antioxidant: within cell mitochondria, the main defense against oxidative stress; in the liver, detoxifies toxic oxygen radicals and reduces disulfide groups].[295]

Antiulcer... Dong Quai pretreatment dose-dependently prevents gastric mucous membrane damage in rats from NSAIDs or ethanol. This protective effect can last up to 12 hours.[296]

Immune... Dong Quai is immunostimulating, and shows antitumor activity against Ehrlich ascites tumors [in the animal abdominal cavity, with edema].[297]

Pulmonary fibrosis... Dong Quai reduces alveolitis [inflammation of the small air sacs in the lung] and fibrosis in rat pulmonary fibrosis [chronic lung inflammation and progressive fibrous tissue formation].[298]

Dong Quai/Astragalus… The traditional Chinese 'Dang-Gui Decoction for Enriching the Blood' of Dong Quai and Astragalus stimulates red blood cell production and improves cardiovascular function. Dang-Gui Decoction pretreatment protects against myocardial ischaemia-reperfusion injury in rats.[50] The decoction lowers total cholesterol, triglycerides, low-density lipoproteins [LDL, so-called bad cholesterol] and apolipoprotein [measure of lipoprotein binding, high levels occur in acute angina and heart attack]. This positive regulation of lipid metabolism lessens kidney damage and maintains function in rats with nephrotic syndrome [a type of kidney inflammation characterized by edema, weight gain, high blood pressure, protein in the urine, and anorexia].[299]

Drug interaction… Dong Quai may interact with warfarin [prescription drug, inhibitor of blood clotting].[111]

ASPIRIN

In 1897, Bayer chemist Felix Hoffmann developed aspirin from the American Indian herb, White Willow Bark, whose principal ingredient is salicylic acid. Hoffmann added an acetyl radical and invented acetylsalicylic acid. Interestingly, aspirin gives a better, more predictable therapeutic result than White Willow Bark. Therefore, forget the parent and use the offspring unless you experience aspirin's NSAID side effects, described below.

An aspirin dose of 1300 mg completely relieves a stress or fatigue headache or any other type of adrenal headache, and "gets everything running right" (◊) again within the entire gland. Failure of aspirin to relieve headaches indicates functional exhaustion somewhere in the adrenal gland, probably the cortex, or an unusual cause, as with vasodilation headaches. Two drawbacks to aspirin are: (1) possible soft functioning for up to 30 hours afterward. A soft adrenal gland falls apart easily under stress, leaving you susceptible to more stress and more headaches, and creating a vicious downward spiral. And (2) aspirin can cause gastrointestinal irritation and, in time, ulcers. Taking aspirin with a small meal may ease the irritation. Or instead of aspirin, use safer White Willow Bark, although headache relief is iffy.

Low-dose aspirin therapy helps to prevent blood platelet aggregation, heart attack and cerebrovascular disease. The aspirin medical literature contains over 27,000 articles, a book in itself. Side effects only are summarized below.

Review of the Medical Literature

Aspirin side effects… While an important treatment for pain and inflammation, conventional nonsteroidal anti-inflammatory drugs (NSAIDs) including aspirin are toxic to the gastroduodenal mucous membrane. Factors increasing NSAID toxicity and gastroduodenal risk are high doses, coadministration with anticoagulants or corticosteroids, history of peptic ulcer disease and age.[300] Aspirin causes gastric damage directly by topical irritation and indirectly through microcirculatory damage and inhibition of cyclooxygenase [enzyme found in most tissues; produces prostaglandins and other eicosanoids as part of the normal inflammation process] synthesis. Stomach damage predominates. Gastroduodenal lesions can develop rapidly even with low-dose aspirin, and bleeding is a dose-dependant risk. Upper gastrointestinal complications can include stenosis [narrowing of a passage or vessel] and perforation. Large intestine bleeding, colitis [inflammation of the colon], perforation, and anorectal [anus and rectum] stenosis from aspirin-containing suppositories occur. Esophagitis [inflammation of the esophagus] and esophageal stricture [abnormal narrowing from scar tissue] are also possible. In cirrhosis patients, aspirin may cause varicose vein bleeding. Chronic aspirin consumption can lead to iron deficiency anemia.[301]

Fatigue

Fatigue and its aldosterone hormone can be the first adrenal function to suffer chronic poor functioning and ultimately permanent exhaustion. Besides limiting activities, impaired fatigue function alters breakdown and repair systems, increasing cell oxidation and aging, as explained in Chapter 2. The following symptoms and signs indicate possible fatigue dysfunction or exhaustion: (1) you are chronically cold. This may instead be a thyroid problem, or both aldosterone and thyroid dysfunctions. (2) Edema occurs, usually in the legs and ankles. Other more serious causes of edema are congestive heart failure, kidney disease and cirrhosis.[302] Chronic venous insufficiency can also be causative.[116-119] (3) Hypertension – here high blood pressure results when aldosterone can no longer regulate sodium ⇌ potassium balance. (4) Drinking a lot of water brings on nausea or headache. (5) Severe headaches are frequent; and (6) fatigue develops easily, stamina is non-existent. Life puts great demands on this cortex function, and accordingly you need superior aldosterone nutrition to keep it productive.

Maintaining good aldosterone/fatigue function requires Raw Garlic. Of course, fatigue maintenance also involves nutritional yeasts, Omega 3 fish fatty acids especially salmon, and trace metals. If fatigue becomes palpable during a stressful task, taking sodium salt (table salt) can temporarily boost functioning. However, potassium salt, commonly called "salt substitute," is antithetical to stress and fatigue and actually contributes to aldosterone exhaustion if supplemented during these periods. Potassium must be used only when rest and relaxation lie ahead (aldosterone dormant) to rebalance sodium $\rightleftharpoons$ potassium in the body. See Chapter 11.

RAW GARLIC

Taking Raw Garlic before any fatiguing effort will keep you GOING and GOING... AND GOING! This herb is essential for fatigue ability, and beneficial to healing and immune systems. Raw Garlic also improves stomach digestion and pituitary oversight of adrenal aldosterone. Don't worry about garlic's odor; there is a way around it. The odor and strong therapeutic benefits of Raw Garlic come principally from a compound called allicin. Cooking destroys allicin, leaving only a seasoning herb.

Digestive disturbances and odor. Raw Garlic can cause digestive disturbances with a poorly functioning pancreas. If ingestion becomes indigestion, go to "Plan B" in the next paragraph. Regarding odor, odorless garlic capsules generally do not work as well as the humble garlic clove and they're very pricey. Besides, as little as one-eighth of a clove ingested once to twice a week is sufficient to receive full allicin benefits. With a meal, one-eighth of a well ground up clove is hardly noticeable, adding tang and character to most foods.

Good news, Plan B. You can avoid the digestive disturbances and odor completely by topical application. Yes, strange but effective. The simple truth about skin is that whatever you put on it, whether Raw Garlic, Vitamin E, Vitamin D, gasoline, pesticides, etc., some of that substance will end up inside of you for better or for worse. Garlic's allicin remains unchanged whether ingested or topically applied. Here's an easy how-to. Wet the back of hand or any skin surface. Cut a garlic clove in half and rub the two fresh-cut surfaces on the wet skin in a slow circular motion, each for about 20 seconds. For stronger action, cut and rub in more freshly cut garlic surfaces. Let the garlic oils remain on the skin and continue to be absorbed for five to ten minutes without additional application; twenty minutes or longer is even better. Applying Raw Garlic directly to a pain or inflammation site can be therapeutic. That's it, except for removing the odor from the skin (and stopping all further absorption), which requires a strong soap such as dish detergent. The resulting health benefits are the same as if the Raw Garlic were eaten. Obviously the dosage is much less with topical application, but a little allicin goes a long way!

Review of the Medical Literature

Overview... Garlic (Allium sativum) has been used as a medicinal agent for millennia. Garlic is hypocholesterolemic [lowering blood cholesterol], anti-thrombotic [thrombosis: blood clot formation, as occurs in heart attack and stroke], vasodilatory [opens blood vessels, thereby lowering blood pressure], antiarthritic, antidiabetic, antimicrobial and anticancer.[303-305]

Cardiovascular... The major cardiovascular benefits of garlic are related to its anti-arteriosclerotic [abnormal thickening, loss of elasticity in artery wall] and anti-thrombotic activity. Garlic lowers total and LDL-cholesterol [low-density lipoproteins, so-called bad cholesterol] and triglycerides [completely saturated fat], and raises HDL-cholesterol [high-density lipoproteins, so-called good cholesterol]. Additionally, garlic improves blood viscosity by inhibiting platelet aggregation through decreased fibrinogen [soluble plasma protein, first step in blood coagulation] and increased fibrinolysis [dissolution of fibrin, insoluble protein in blood and the end product of coagulation]. Garlic also decreases arterial blood pressure. In one four-year clinical trial, these garlic therapeutic effects reduced heart attack and stroke risk by more than 50%.[305, 306]

Bacteria and fungi... Louis Pasteur was the first to describe the antibacterial effect of garlic juices. Garlic exhibits broad antibiotic activity including: 1) raw garlic juice is effective against many of common pathogenic intestinal bacteria responsible for diarrhea; 2) garlic shows efficacy even against those bacterial strains that have become resistant to antibiotic drugs; 3) garlic-antibiotic combinations have partial to total synergism; and 4) garlic prevents microorganisms from generating toxins.[307] Helicobacter pylori [H. pylori] is the bacterium responsible for stomach ulcers and cancer. Stomach cancer incidence is lower in populations with a high intake of allium vegetables. Garlic gives good inhibitory activity against H. pylori in vitro [in laboratory vessel], and even some antibiotic-resistant H. pylori strains respond to garlic.[307, 308] Garlic is effective against pneumonia causing bacteria, particularly Streptococcus pneumoniae.[309] Garlic also demonstrates significant antifungal activity.[310]

Cancer... Epidemiological studies indicate that garlic reduces cancer deaths,[305] as do diets rich in fruits, vegetables and fiber, particularly citrus fruits, carrots and leafy green, cruciferous (cabbages, broccoli) and leak (garlic, onions) vegetables. Preventing cancer requires early and long adherence to such nutrition.[311] Garlic stimulates immunity, notably macrophages [relatively long-living, large white blood cells; -phage: anything that devours], NK cells [natural killer lymphocytes: first-line defense against cancer], LAK cells [lymphokine-activated killer cells; lymphokine: hormone-like cell protein factor/signaling molecule], IL-2 [Interleukin 2: hormone-like substance released by T lymphocytes, stimulates more T-cell production and other immune defenses; IL-2 decreases during HIV infection], TNF [tumor necrosis factor; deficiency implicated in cachexia, general ill heath with emaciation], and interferon-gamma [interferon: family of hormone-like glycoproteins that fight virus infection/multiplication]. Garlic's Th1 [Th1 cells: subset of helper/inducer T-lymphocytes] antitumor response is characteristic of all effective cancer therapies.[312] Garlic inhibits proliferation of the human breast cancer cell line (MCF-7) and the human prostate cancer cell line (LNCaP).[313] Garlic even protects against immune suppression during drug chemotherapy and radiation.[312]

Leukemia... Garlic inhibits human promyelocytic leukemia cells (HL-60).[314]

Possible side effects ... The active thiol [sulfur-containing] group present in garlic can cause contact dermatitis, contact urticaria [pale or reddening, irregular patches of skin with itching and hives], pemphigus [blisters and ulcerations], rhinitis [inflammation of the nose or its membrane] and/or allergic asthma.[315]

Drug interaction... Garlic may affect blood clotting, and should not be concomitant with warfarin sodium [prescription drug, inhibitor of blood clotting].[48]

———————

Rebuilding fatigue function. If you cannot put your body through its paces, that is, go from energy to stress and fatigue, and on to stamina and 'second wind' (see Figure 2-C), then fixing fatigue function is Priority One. Priority Two is fixing any energy and stress exhaustions. Energy (adrenaline) and stress (cortisol) often fail after fatigue (aldosterone). These three hormones working together in harmony and at their full capability are the key to feeling young and full of life!

Rebuilding fatigue function requires Raw Garlic, Guarana and Nettle. Guarana and Nettle transform fatigue into stamina and back to energy via the Figure 2-C stamina loop. Ingesting Guarana, Nettle and nutritional yeast together can cure mild fatigue exhaustion or, for more potent therapeutic action, take Raw Garlic and Guarana together. Severe aldosterone exhaustion calls for even more on-target nutrition, complete details in Chapter 12.

Other fatigue herbs. Fatigue function is directly *wired* to stomach digestion, and Ginger and Horseradish along with Raw Garlic can help rebuild this fatigue-stomach link and cure a sour stomach. Cayenne *heats up* aldosterone activity, and vasoconstriction herbs Shepherd's Purse/Woundwort, Heather and 2X Hawthorn Berries boost aldosterone endurance through anti-edema action. Aldosterone regulates sodium ⇌ potassium, and rebalancing these two salts may be needed to improve function.

GUARANA

Guarana wipes out fatigue – TOTAL RELIEF! When you feel a stress/fatigue headache on the way, this amazing herb can reverse that downward spiral into pain. Take 800 mg, as needed. Avoid 2X usage or any product that is not 100% guarana seed. Normally do not take Guarana and Raw Garlic together; this combination creates aldosterone hyperactivity and therefore is appropriate only for curing hypoactivity exhaustion. Raw Garlic several hours before Guarana gives good effect.

800 mg of Guarana supplies approximately 30 mg of caffeine, a jolt to the nervous system, but no problem unless you are already over your caffeine limit from coffee or tea. The caffeine in Guarana triggers adrenaline flow and brings you back to the starting point of all tasks – energy.

Frequent need for Guarana indicates mild to severe fatigue exhaustion. Overuse depletes iron and other related adrenal cortex metals, and may cause sodium-potassium imbalance.

Nature... Guarana (Paullinia cupana) significantly increases the physical capabilities of mice subjected to stressful forced swimming.[316] One hour after oral administration, Guarana raises blood glucose, lowers liver glycogen [short term storage of glucose in the liver], and suppresses exercise-induced hypoglycemia in mice.[317]

Antioxidant, anti-platelet aggregation... Guarana inhibits lipid peroxidation [lipids: fats and fat-related compounds].[318] In rabbits, Guarana reduces blood platelet aggregation.[319]

NETTLE

Nettle, a.k.a. Stinging Nettle, is a secondary fatigue herb. As a nerve herb too, Nettle completes the stamina loop from fatigue back to energy. Nettle evidences strong arthritic and rheumatic pain relief in the medical literature. Occasional use is best, 500 mg in capsule or as a tea, or direct topical application to painful areas. Avoid 2X, and not with Oats.

Review of the Medical Literature

Pain... Applying Stinging Nettle leaf (Urtica dioica) to painful areas reduces osteoarthritic pain,[320] with no side effects except possible transient urticarial rash [see below].[321]

Rheumatoid diseases, anti-inflammatory... Stinging Nettle leaf is registered in Germany as an adjuvant therapy for rheumatoid diseases. Nettle is immunomodulating, mediating T-helper cell derived cytokine [non-antibody protein/signaling molecule] patterns and possibly preventing the inflammatory cascade [series of reactions from one trigger] of autoimmune diseases such as rheumatoid arthritis.[322] Nettle strongly inhibits transcription factor NF-kappaB [common B- and T-cell activator/binder], which is elevated in chronic inflammatory diseases and responsible for pro-inflammatory gene expression.[323]

Possible side effect... Stinging Nettle frequently causes contact urticaria [pale or reddening, irregular patches of skin with itching and hives caused by allergic reaction], accompanied by a stinging sensation often lasting more than 12 hours. Mechanisms are unresolved, but Nettle stings introduce histamine and generate mast cell [resident white blood cells of connective tissue; produce histamine, heparin and serotonin] response.[324]

Nettle Rhizome and Root

Lupus... In animal models, agglutinin lectin [binding protein] present in Nettle rhizomes [horizontal, underground, root-like stems that can send out shoots and roots], unlike classical T-cell lectin mitogens [any substances stimulating cell division], discriminates between CD4+ and CD8+ T-cell [helper T-cells] populations, producing a six-fold increase in V beta 8.3+ T-cells within three days. This agglutinin V beta 8.3+ T-cell response prevents systemic lupus erythematosus [lupus: autoimmune, inflammatory disease of connective tissue with skin eruptions, joint pain, kidney damage] pathology; treated animals do not develop clinical signs of lupus and nephritis [inflammation of the kidney].[325-327]

Prostate... Stinging Nettle root is effective against benign prostatic hyperplasia [BPH: nonmalignant enlargement of the prostate gland] through lignan [dibenzylbutane derivative] binding to human SHBG (sex hormone binding globulin).[328, 329] In addition, Nettle root steroids inhibit membrane $Na+,K(+)$-ATPase [ATPase: enzymes that hydrolyze ATP, the primary energy source within all living cells] prostate activity, which may suppress prostate cell multiplication.[330]

CAYENNE

Cayenne pepper and its active ingredient capsaicin reset adrenal thermoregulation within adrenal cortex fatigue function. If you feel cold for no reason, then aldosterone or thyroid hormones are impaired. The best aldosterone thermal reset is Cayenne. Use at 1X only, as 2X can injury nerves. Supportive nutrients here are nutritional yeast, salmon, Vitamin D, table salt and other aldosterone herbs.

Review of the Medical Literature

Pain... Capsaicin, the principle pungent and active ingredient of hot red and chili peppers (genus Capsicum), is effective in treating the pain of rheumatoid arthritis, osteoarthritis and peripheral neuropathies [injury to the sensation nerves of arms and legs].[331]

Nerves and possible toxicity... Capsaicin depletes stores of substance P [nerve peptide involved in regulating pain threshold] from nociceptive [pain transmission] primary sensory neurons, and can selectively injure dorsal root ganglion (DRG) cells [of the spinal cord], dorsal root nerve fibers, and saphenous [of the legs], chorda tympani [belly] and pulp nerves.[331, 332]

Overactive bladder... Capsaicin neurotoxicity desensitizes neurons that may trigger detrusor [muscle expelling] bladder overactivity. Capsaicin is effective for overactive bladder, with minimal long-term complications.[333]

Antiulcer!... Capsicum evidences clinical efficacy against peptic ulcers.[334]

Cancer... Capsaicin is potently antimutagenic and anticarcinogenic, which may be related to its antioxidant and anti-inflammatory actions.[335, 336]

Leukemia... Adult T-cell leukemia (ATL), associated with human T-cell leukemia virus type 1 (HTLV-1), is resistant to conventional chemotherapy. Capsaicin inhibits the growth of ATL cells, inducing cell cycle arrest and apoptosis [gene-directed, programmed cell death].[337]

Drug interaction... Capsicum may interact with warfarin [prescription drug, inhibitor of blood clotting].[29]

GINGER

Fatigue and stomach digestion are directly linked, and Ginger nourishes this connection. Ginger cures sour stomach and its combination with fatigue, which is a sour stomach headache. Ginger is also effective for motion sickness and morning sickness during pregnancy. Horseradish partners with Ginger in this fatigue-stomach digestion link. Horseradish is therapeutically weaker than Ginger, and a silent partner until you need stronger relief. Frequent need for these herbs indicates stomach-related fatigue exhaustion.

Review of the Medical Literature

Antioxidant... Spices like Ginger (Zingiber officinale) contain antioxidants that protect lipids [fats and fat related compounds] in biological systems.[338] Ginger strongly scavenges superoxide [O_2^-] and hydroxyl [OH^-] free radicals.[339]

Atherosclerosis... Ginger markedly reduces aortic atherosclerosis [depositing plaque on artery walls] lesions, total cholesterol, LDL [low-density lipoproteins, so-called bad cholesterol], VLDL [very LDL] and platelet aggregation in animals.[340, 341]

Arthritis, anti-inflammatory... Ginger shows pronounced antioxidant, anti-inflammatory and antirheumatic activities.[342, 343] Ginger reduces the pain and swelling of rheumatoid arthritis and osteoarthritis with no reported adverse effects. Ginger apparently inhibits synthesis of arachidonic acid-derived prostaglandins [potent eicosanoid mediators of many conduction/transmitter functions regulating cellular activities, especially inflammatory response] and leukotrienes [family of potent hormone-like eicosanoids produced by immune response to antigens; they contribute to defense, inflammation and hypersensitivity]. [344]

Bacteria and fungi... Ginger demonstrates antibacterial activity against respiratory tract pathogens Staphylococcus aureus, Streptococcus pyogenes, Streptococcus pneumoniae and Haemophilus influenzae.[345] Ginger has pronounced activity against a wide variety of fungi.[346]

Cancer and leukemia... Ginger's pungent constituents exhibit antitumor activity,[347] notably against skin tumors.[348, 342] 6-gingerol and 6-paradol constituents inhibit the viability and DNA synthesis of human promyelocytic [bone marrow] leukemia HL-60 cells.[349]

Antiulcer... In animals, Ginger prevents NSAID [nonsteroidal anti-inflammatory drug]-induced gastric ulcers.[350] Zingiberene and 6-gingerol constituents strongly inhibit gastric lesions.[351]

Digestion... Ginger improves gastroduodenal motility [spontaneous movement],[352] with anti-emetic [alleviates nausea and vomiting] effect.[353] Ginger stimulates pancreatic lipase [fat-digesting enzyme], amylase [carbohydrate-digesting enzyme], trypsin [protein-digesting enzyme] and chymotrypsin [specialized protein-digesting] activity. Many spices have a positive effect on pancreatic digestive enzymes. [354]

Motion sickness... Ginger prevents motion sickness nausea, dizziness and vomiting, as well as pregnancy and postoperative vomiting.[355] Motion sickness benefits derive from Ginger's effects on the gastric system.[356] Ginger pretreatment reduces nausea, tachygastria [tachy- 'rapid'], and plasma vasopressin [pituitary anti-diuretic hormone; also constricts blood vessels] induced by spinning motion. And Ginger prolongs the latent period before nausea onset and shortens recovery time.[357] Or oppositely, Ginger possesses no anti-motion sickness activity.[358]

Seasickness, vertigo... Ginger reduces seasickness vomiting and cold sweating significantly better than placebo. Although not statistically significant, seasickness nausea and vertigo [illusion of movement; external world whirling about] symptoms are also fewer.[359] For induced vertigo, Ginger is significantly better than placebo.[360]

Pregnancy and morning sickness... Medical reviewer's conclusions regarding twenty randomized trials: Ginger may be of benefit for nausea and vomiting of early pregnancy, but the evidence is weak.[361]

After surgery... Ginger is an effective anti-emetic [alleviates nausea and vomiting] for surgery, particularly day surgery.[362] Ginger shows statistically significantly fewer incidences of nausea than placebo after gynecological surgery.[363, 364] Or, Ginger is ineffective in reducing postoperative nausea and vomiting.[365, 366]

SHEPHERD'S PURSE and WOUNDWORT

Anti-edema vasoconstriction herbs improve aldosterone fatigue and stamina functioning. Table 7-4 and associated text give full details on the Shepherd's Purse/Woundwort combination. Taking this combination twice, one hour apart, can relieve a vasodilation headache.

HEATHER

Heather complements Shepherd's Purse/Woundwort in satisfying fatigue, stamina and healing-immune vasoconstriction needs and homeostasis. Heather is a proven anti-inflammatory. See Table 7-4 and the text there including review of medical literature.

HAWTHORN BERRIES 2X

Hawthorn at 2X one hour apart benefits fatigue and stamina through vasoconstriction and more stable vasoconstriction $\rightleftharpoons$ vasodilation equilibrium.

Cortex Sex

Nutrition plays an important role in sex. You must nourish both adrenal medulla Energy and cortex Stress functions to achieve your best. And herbs can significantly enhance performance. Medulla sex herbs are described earlier; cortex herbs follow.

SARSAPARILLA

Sarsaparilla is the #1 cortex sex herb for both sexes. Take 500 to 1000 mg once or twice a week, maximum. Combine Sarsaparilla with Oats and separately with

Nettle to revitalize medulla-cortex sexual connections. For males, Sarsaparilla, Saw Palmetto Berries and Pygeum together are a powerful cortex tonic and sexual rejuvenator. For females, Sarsaparilla with Black Cohosh is similarly potent. These herbs combinations can be added to more basic cortex nutrition such as nutritional yeasts and Omega 3 salmon to generate even stronger synergies.

Sarsaparilla medical literature consists of only one informational article… Sarsaparilla (Smilax officinalis) contains three steroidal saponins [see Table 3-3].[367]

AMERICAN GINSENG

American Ginseng is excellent for both sexes; review its profile under "Energy" including the female caveat. This herb "gets things running right"(◐) within both medulla and cortex sexual machinery. Alternating between Sarsaparilla and American Ginseng invigorates and balances sexual performance. Damiana also balances.

NETTLE

Nettle completes the sexual stamina loop back to energy. See its fatigue citation earlier.

♂ Male/ ♀ Female

Male and female herbs nourish the adrenal cortex sexual subfunction as well as testes/ovaries and supporting structures. Males can benefit from small amounts (mild tea) of female herbs, Dong Quai for sure, and vice versa.

MALE – SAW PALMETTO BERRIES, PYGEUM

Not just for the prostate, Saw Palmetto and Pygeum balance male hormones. Take these two herbs as needed, either separately or together, for maintenance and prevention. With benign prostatic hyperplasia (BPH: nonmalignant enlargement of the prostate gland), follow the usage guidelines in the medical literature below. Nettle Root, if you can obtain it, is effective against BPH too. See the Nettle medical literature citation earlier. Recent short-term trials also suggest pumpkin seeds for BPH and lower urinary tract symptoms.[368]

Review of the Medical Literature

Benign Prostatic Hyperplasia... is associated with male pattern baldness.[369] The male sex hormone DHT [dihydrotestosterone] is implicated in the pathogenesis [origin and development] of benign prostatic hyperplasia (BPH), male pattern baldness, acne, and female hirsutism [abnormal hairiness in women]. DHT forms from testosterone through the catalytic action of testosterone 5-alpha-reductase enzyme.[370]

Saw Palmetto Berries

BPH efficacy... In 21 randomized trials involving 3139 men, Saw Palmetto Berries (Serenoa repens) improved BPH-associated urinary tract symptoms and flow measures. Compared to finasteride [drug, active testosterone 5-alpha-reductase inhibitor], Saw Palmetto produced similar symptom and flow improvements, but fewer adverse side effects. Saw Palmetto reduced nocturia [excessive urination during the night] and urinary tract symptom scores, and increased peak urine flow. Saw Palmetto side effects were mild and infrequent; erectile dysfunction was 1.1% for Saw Palmetto vs. 4.9% for finasteride.[371, 372] Saw Palmetto (160 mg twice daily) or finasteride (5 mg once daily) for 6 months evidenced similar efficacy in the only comparative randomized trial of more than 1000 men with moderate BPH. Saw Palmetto at 160 mg twice daily for 1 to 3 months was superior to placebo for dysuria [difficult or painful urination] and other subjective symptoms, as well as objective parameters of nocturia frequency (33 to 74% decrease with Saw Palmetto), urinary frequency during the day (11 to 43% decrease) and peak urinary flow rate (26 to 50% increase). Saw Palmetto is a useful alternative BPH treatment to finasteride and alpha 1-receptor [type 1, described below] antagonists.[373] Saw Palmetto is safe with no recognized side effects.[374]

Europe vs. USA... European doctors treat BPH with Saw Palmetto Berries, while American doctors disregard Saw Palmetto.[375]

Mechanisms... Saw Palmetto Berries contain a complex mixture of pharmacodynamic compounds. Therapeutic action includes inhibiting both type 1 and type 2 isoenzymes [variant enzyme forms] of 5-alpha-reductase and blocking DHT binding to cytosolic [aqueous fluid portion of the cell] androgen receptors in prostate cells,[373, 374] which decreases EGF [epidermal growth factor, especially affects surface tissue lining cells], periurethral region [peri- 'surrounding'; urethra: urine duct from bladder to exterior] enlargement and urinary obstruction.[376] Saw Palmetto produces epithelial contraction, particularly in the transition zone.[377] Inflammatory cells also infiltrate the prostate contributing to BPH development; and Saw

Palmetto exerts anti-inflammatory BPH activity, in part by opposing 5-lipoxygenase [catalyzing enzyme for arachidonic acid conversion to leukotrienes, part of the immune/inflammatory response] metabolism.[378] Saw Palmetto has no effect on serum prostate specific antigen [PSA: simple blood test to detect prostate cancer],[374] and so unlike other 5-alpha-reductase inhibitors, Saw Palmetto does not interfere with PSA screening for prostate cancer.[379]

Cancer… Saw Palmetto shows moderate cytotoxicity against human pancreatic (PACA-2) and renal (A-498) tumor cells, and borderline activity against human prostate (PC-3) tumors.[380]

Side effect… Saw Palmetto may inhibit iron absorption.[48]

Pygeum

BPH mechanisms… Pygeum africanum significantly reduces DHT [dihydrotestosterone] urinary obstructive effects and prostate enlargement in rats. Pygeum decreases prostate weight in the ventral but not the dorsal [back] lobe.[381] Pygeum inhibits rat EGF [epidermal growth factor] and prostatic fibroblast [cell giving rise to connective tissue] proliferation. These therapeutic effects may prevent prostatic overgrowth in man.[382] Pygeum shows anti-inflammatory activity, in part by opposing 5-lipoxygenase [catalyzing enzyme for arachidonic acid conversion to leukotrienes, part of the immune/inflammatory response] metabolism.[383]

Human studies… In a two-month multicenter trial, Pygeum (50 mg twice per day) produced statistically significant improvements in IPSS [International Prostate Symptom Score] (40%), quality of life (31%), nocturnal frequency (32% reduction) and maximum urinary flow, average urinary flow and urine volume. These improvements continued one month past the end of treatment. No adverse side effects occurred, and prostatic volume and quality of sexual life were unchanged throughout treatment.[384] In a placebo-controlled double-blind multicenter study using the same regimen, Pygeum improved quantitative parameters of uroflowmetry, residual urine and daily and nocturnal pollakiuria [urge incontinence]. Micturition [passage of urine] increased a statically significant 66% compared to 31% for placebo. Gastrointestinal side effects occurred in five of 263 patients.[385] In France, Pygeum has been used for over 20 years to treat BPH.[383]

Cancer… Pygeum inhibits cell division of benign prostatic hyperplasia epithelial [surface tissue lining] cells and prostate cancer cells.[386]

Bladder dysfunction… secondary to BPH is a major problem. Partial outlet obstruction causes contractile and metabolic dysfunctions, leading to severe, irreversible changes in bladder function. Pygeum eases the severity of these dysfunctions.[387] Pygeum improves contractility by reversing impaired myosin [contractile protein of muscles] expression.[388] Local ischaemia [insufficient blood supply] may also be a factor in contractile dysfunction, and Pygeum protects against ischemic bladder damage.[389] Pygeum also inhibits bladder hyperreactivity.[383]

FEMALE – BLACK COHOSH

Women are increasingly turning to botanical medicines to treat female conditions. Some traditional herbs for women contain phytoestrogens, which can bind to estrogen receptors with estrogenic and in some cases anti-estrogenic effects.[390] Black Cohosh does not possess hormone or hormone-like activity, yet this herb has proven efficacy for menopausal symptoms and estrogen replacement! And Black Cohosh inhibits breast cancer, unlike conventional hormone replacement therapy.

Review of the Medical Literature

Menopause ... Black Cohosh (Actaea racemosa, formerly Cimicifuga racemosa) shows therapeutic efficacy and a good safety profile for menopausal symptoms including hot flashes, sweating, sleep disturbances and depressive moods. However, Black Cohosh does not possess hormone-like action.[391] In animal models, Black Cohosh does not bind to the estrogen receptor, upregulate estrogen-dependent genes or stimulate the growth of estrogen-dependent tumors.[392] In eight human studies, Black Cohosh is a safe and effective alternative to estrogen replacement therapy for menopausal symptoms.[393] For example, in one randomized trial of 60 women under 40 years of age with hysterectomy, at least one intact ovary and complaining of menopausal symptoms, no significant differences in therapy success occur between Black Cohosh, estriol [produced by the placenta during pregnancy], conjugated estrogens or estrogen-gestagen sequential therapy.[394] Black Cohosh side effects are rare, and there are no known adverse drug interactions.[395]

Breast cancer... Under estrogen-deprived conditions, Black Cohosh significantly inhibits MCF-7 human breast cancer cell proliferation. Furthermore, Black Cohosh inhibits estrogen-induced MCF-7 proliferation and enhances the proliferation-inhibiting effect of tamoxifen [anti-estrogen drug treatment for advanced breast cancer].[396] Black Cohosh, Chaste Berries and Hops inhibit T-47D breast cancer cell growth.[397]

CHASTE BERRIES

A native of the Mediterranean region, berries from the Chaste tree are effective for premenstrual syndrome (PMS) and menopause.

Review of the Medical Literature

PMS… Chaste Berries (Vitex agnus-castus) ease one of the most common premenstrual symptoms, premenstrual mastodynia [breast pain] in double-blind placebo-controlled studies. Chaste Berries reduce premenstrual mastodynia serum prolactin [pituitary hormone for breast development and milk production] levels through dopaminergic action. In addition, in numerous less rigidly controlled studies, Chaste Berries benefit other psychic and physical symptoms of the PMS.[398] Chaste Berries are effective treatment for premenstrual dysphoric disorder (PMDD) [dysphoric: pain, agitation, anguish, malaise], especially its physical symptoms.[399] Well tolerated with few side effects and no serious adverse reactions, Chaste Berries have a very good risk/benefit ratio.[400]

Menopause… Chaste Berries give symptomatic relief from common menopausal symptoms.[401]

Cancer… Chaste Berries cause apoptosis [gene-directed, programmed cell death] and DNA fragmentation of cultured human breast carcinoma (SKOV-3), gastric signet ring carcinoma (KATO-III), colon carcinoma (COLO 201), and small cell lung carcinoma (Lu-134-A-H).[402] Chaste Berries inhibit T-47D breast cancer cell growth.[397]

DONG QUAI

Dong Quai is a traditional uterus tonic and balancer of female hormones. It is also a general stress and blood tonic for both sexes, as reported earlier.

Review of the Medical Literature

Female… Dong Quai (Angelica sinensis) may be of some benefit for PMS [premenstrual syndrome] when employed in traditional Chinese formulations. For relief of menopausal symptoms, Dong Quai has no proven efficacy.[403] Dong Quai does not generate estrogen-like endometrial [membrane lining of the uterus] or vaginal responses.[404] However, phenolic compound ferulic acid in Dong Quai inhibits rat uterine contractions,[405] and Dong Quai stimulates the histamine H1-receptor of the uterus.[406]

Hot flashes... Three-fourths of perimenopausal/menopausal US women experience hot flashes (vasomotor instability), ranging from minor annoyance to an intensely unpleasant, life-disrupting sensations. With decreasing estrogen levels, hot flash results from downward resetting of hypothalamus [gland in the brain, initiator of all things pituitary] thermoregulation, probably by means of norepinephrine [adrenal medulla neurotransmitter/hormone; as a hormone, constricts blood vessels and dilates bronchial tubes] action. The body tries to dissipate unwanted body heat through vasodilation, thereby triggering hot flash. The most successful treatments are hormone replacement with estrogen and progesterone. Alternative therapies of Dong Quai, Vitamin E and evening primrose oil have anecdotal support, but no controlled studies.[407]

Drug interaction... Dong Quai may interact with warfarin [prescription drug, inhibitor of blood clotting].[111]

WILD YAM

Wild Yam topical cream is currently popular for menopausal symptoms.

Review of the Medical Literature

Wild Yam (Dioscorea villosa) is the source of saponin diosgenin, the steroid used in the manufacture of The Pill and other sex hormone preparations. However, over 100,000 tons of Wild Yam must be harvested to provide the 600-700 tons of diosgenin used by the drug industry each year.[408] In a double blind, placebo-controlled study, no statistical difference was found between Wild Yam and placebo for menopausal symptoms of hot flash and nocturnal sweating. Wild Yam produced no changes in weight, blood pressure, blood glucose, FSH [pituitary follicle-stimulating hormone; controls ovary follicle function, egg development], estradiol [potent estrogen of the ovary follicle] or progesterone [female hormone of menstrual cycle].[409]

Gluconeogenesis

Although the adrenal cortex is first and foremost concerned with fat metabolism (fat burning to handle stress), two subfunctions within Primary Stress Function deal with glucose metabolism: (1) gluconeogenesis or the making new glucose to fuel body cells when digested carbohydrates are unavailable, and (2) Glucose Tolerance Factor (GTF), a cortex metabolite of chromium.

The pancreas regulates blood glucose with its insulin and glucagon hormones. Insulin reduces blood glucose, while glucagon raises it through gluconeogenesis. The liver is the first site of glucagon-induced gluconeogenesis, adrenal medulla is second with adrenaline response, and adrenal cortex third, converting glycerol and other substrates into glucose. Failure of gluconeogenesis results in hypoglycemia, which is massive stress. Cortex gluconeogenesis is the last defense before a hypoglycemia headache.

The following herbs can improve cortex gluconeogenesis and prevent hypoglycemia. In practice, relieving hypoglycemia is best accomplished by improving pancreas glucagon functioning and liver glycogen mechanisms, then adrenal medulla adrenaline response, and lastly cortex gluconeogenesis. However, upgrading this cortex subfunction does boost overall stress ability.

YUCCA

Yucca generates strong cortex gluconeogenesis. Yucca is also an immune enhancer (Table 7-6), and rebalances Stress and Immune functions to some extent. Take 500 mg to 1000 mg, as needed.

Combining Yucca with Licorice brings permanent improvement in the cortex gluconeogenesis subfunction. Ingest 500 mg of Yucca, 200 mg of Licorice and 10 mg of Vitamin B6. See Licorice below regarding the need for B6.

> Review of the Medical Literature

Blood antioxidant... Resveratrol and other phenolic compounds from Yucca schidigera inhibit free radical generation in blood platelets.[410]

Immune... Yucca retards Escherichia coli [E. coli, bacteria common in the large intestine] growth.[411] Yucca potently inhibits parasitic skin yeasts and fungi, film-forming yeasts and certain food-deteriorating yeasts.[412] Yucca resveratrol has antimutagenic activity.[413]

LICORICE

Licorice produces palpable cortex gluconeogenesis. To illustrate its effect, the soldiers of both Alexander the Great and Rome chewed Licorice root during battle to boost energy levels. Because of side effects, however, use this herb infrequently and only in low doses. Drawbacks are: (1) Licorice contains Vitamin B2, which can cause pancreatic distress unless balanced with Vitamin B6 (Figure 4-A). Each 500 mg of Licorice needs approximately 25 mg of B6 to protect the pancreas. Furthermore, Licorice in amounts greater than 250 mg: (2) is detrimental to hypoglycemics, (3) induces fatigue exhaustion (complete side effects in the medical literature below) particularly with respect to adrenal thermoregulation, and (4) lessens the effectiveness of aspirin therapies. Normally, ingest only 100 mg of the root for its taste and micronutrient benefits including (5) easing anxiety, as indicated in Table 7-3. Licorice apparently satisfies an endocrine link between cortex gluconeogenesis and anxiety.

> ### Review of the Medical Literature

Nature… Glycyrrhizic acid, the major bioactive triterpene glycoside of Licorice (Glycyrrhiza glabra), possesses antioxidant, antiulcer, anti-inflammatory, anti-allergic, antidote, antiviral and antitumor activity.[414]

Ulcers and side effects… Licorice reduces the symptoms and x-ray evidence of gastric ulcers. However, in experimental animals and then confirmed in patients, approximately 20% of subjects develop facial and leg edema, often with headache, stiffness, pain in the upper abdomen and shortness of breath. Consuming large quantities of Licorice-containing candy, chewing tobacco and other products can also cause this electrolyte and blood pressure homeostatic dysfunction.[415]

Side effects mechanism… Licorice and its active metabolites can induce an acquired form of mineralocorticoid excess (AME) syndrome, which is sodium retention, potassium loss and suppression of the renin-angiotensin-aldosterone system [renin: kidney enzyme released into the blood, catalyst for angiotensin synthesis; angiotensin: vasoconstrictor and stimulator of aldosterone release] with consequences of edema and hypertension [high blood pressure].[416] Another possible symptom is transient visual aberrations/loss.[417] Following Licorice discontinuation, recovery typically takes fourteen days for cortisol [principal stress hormone] metabolism and four months for the renin-angiotensin-aldos-terone system.[418]

Immune... Licorice increases NK lymphocytes [active in spontaneous, non-specific immunity against cancer and viruses, first-line defense against cancer], macrophage [relatively long-living, large white blood cells; -phage: anything that devours] phagocytosis [white blood cell ingestion of bacteria, etc.], macrophage secretion of Interleukin 1[activates/potentiates both B- and T-cells], interferon secretion from spleen cells, and ADCC [antibody-dependent cell-mediated cytotoxicity]. Licorice behaves like a mitogen [any substance stimulating cell division] for B-lymphocytes.[419]

Drug interactions... Licorice can cancel the pharmacological effects of spironolactone [diuretic drug; used to treat low-renin hypertension]. Licorice may interfere with digoxin [digitalis derivative for congestive heart failure with a small margin between therapeutic and toxic dose],[48] and interact with oral and topical corticosteroids.[111]

GLUCOSAMINE

Glucosamine is an amino sugar that relieves hypoglycemia through cortex gluconeogenesis. This therapeutic action revs the Stress side of Immune ⇌ Stress equilibrium, and repeated use can ease Stress exhaustion and its arthritis syndromes. Glucosamine also works on arthritic joints by supplying healing glycosaminoglycans (GAGs) and by stimulating secretion of lubricating and shock-absorbing hyaluronic acid in the synovial fluid around the joint, as explained in the following medical literature review. Glucosamine is not a cure for arthritis, but temporary relief. Adversely, glucosamine forces functioning of the gluconeogenesis mechanism, which can affect blood sugar levels. Still, altered cortex gluconeogenesis is often much gentler with fewer side effects than standard NSAID (nonsteroidal anti-inflammatory drug) arthritis therapy. Of course, curing arthritis and its underlying Stress exhaustion is a better goal and attainable in Chapter 12.

Take 500 mg of glucosamine, up to 1500 mg daily, for temporary relief of arthritic pain and inflammation. Chondroitin, cartilage matrix material, can be added to this regimen to rebuild joint structure, however, healing will remain problematic as long as Stress exhaustion exacts its toll. For anyone suffering from a hypoglycemia syndrome, using glucosamine as little as twice a day forces the adrenal cortex inevitably into a hypoglycemic headache. For those not afflicted by hypoglycemia, gluconeogenesis side effects are unnoticeable. Glucosamine GAGs act as special building block raw materials for a number of systems, not just bones and cartilage. Review Table 7-4 and text there.

Review of the Medical Literature

Background... Approximately 12% of the US population has osteoarthritis [OA]. Current pharmacologic treatments of acetaminophen and other NSAIDs alleviate the pain, but have serious side effects and do not slow or reverse OA degenerative processes.[420, 421] Glucosamine nutritional supplement is a recent alternative treatment option.[421]

Clinical trial evidence... Glucosamine evidences efficacy and safety for OA symptoms in sixteen randomized controlled trials. In thirteen of these trials comparing glucosamine to placebo, glucosamine is superior in all but one. In the four trials comparing glucosamine to NSAIDs, glucosamine is superior in two and equivalent in two.[422] Chondroitin is superior to placebo in four randomized controlled trials. Daily supplementation amounts are typically 1500 mg glucosamine and 1200 mg chondroitin.[423] With abundant in vitro [in laboratory vessel], in vivo [inside the living body] animal and human clinical evidence of their efficacy and safety, glucosamine and chondroitin sulfate deserve a prominent place in the non-surgical treatment of osteoarthritis.[424]

Healing mechanism... Glucosamine is a general, multifunctional precursor of glycosaminoglycans [GAGs: special amino-sugar polysaccharides, an essential element in tissue repair]. Chondroitin incorporates preferentially into cartilaginous tissue.[170]

Synovial mechanism... Glucosamine stimulates synovial [viscous joint fluid] hyaluronic acid (HA) production. High molecular weight HA provides lubricating and shock-absorbing properties to the synovial fluid. HA is analgesic and anti-inflammatory. Many studies show that intra-articular [within the joint] HA injections bring rapid OA pain relief and increased mobility. HA also promotes anabolic [constructive metabolism] healing with chondrocytes [differentiated cells responsible for cartilage formation]. OA decreases synovial HA, and glucosamine reverses that abnormality.[425] Glucosamine gives long-lasting pain reductions and functional improvements through its anti-inflammatory and anabolical mechanisms, and unlike NSAIDs, this therapeutic action is not due to prostaglandin [potent mediators of many conduction/transmitter functions regulating cellular activities, especially inflammatory response] inhibition. Thus, glucosamine treatment is free of adverse side effects. Glucosamine is well tolerated both short-term and long-term by all age groups.[426]

ADRENAL CORTEX IMMUNE

Table 7-6 presents Primary Immune Function herbs under two subheadings: maintain health and rebuild health. The "order of importance" of each herb reflects its basic immune power. These listings are a guide and overview, and not a detailed how-to plan. By necessity, fighting serious immune diseases naturally requires a concentrated research effort for each etiology (cause/origin) and is beyond the scope of this book. However, functional exhaustion or imbalance is a prime factor in many immune failures and Chapter 12 provides effective remedies. General defense is explained below.

TABLE 7-6. ADRENAL CORTEX IMMUNE HERBS.

Subheadings (underlined) specify use. Numbering of herbs indicates potency and "need for" (except #1 = emergencies only). Listed effectiveness in **bold type** is as evidenced in medical literature; listed effectiveness not in bold type is from the herb reference books recommended at the beginning of the chapter. See also Table 3-3 for more immune help.

Herb	Comments
IMMUNE – MAINTAIN HEALTH, i.e. **ESSENTIAL** (in order of importance)	
#1 Goldenseal Root	EMERGENCIES ONLY, usually acute illnesses. See Figure 7-B and text there. Proven efficacy against every invader: **bacteria, viruses, fungi, cancer.**
#2 Blue-Green Algae	Oriental health secret. Also pituitary-immune (Figure 8-B). **Cancer, leukemia, viruses.**
#3 Vitamin C and Bioflavonoids	Synergy when taken together. 500-1000 mg of Vitamin C required daily. 'C' is also an antioxidant (Table 7-4) and liver detoxifier (Table 11-1). **Viruses, cancer, leukemia, bacteria, allergies.** In addition, employ more powerful antioxidants: Pine Bark Extract and Grape Seed Extract against **cancer.**
#4 Echinacea	Also pituitary-immune (Figure 8-B). **Viruses, cancer, fungi, bacteria.**

#5 Astragalus	Also for stress (Table 7-5 and text there). **Viruses, cancer.**
#6 Green Tea	Can replace coffee and common teas. **Cancer, leukemia, viruses, bacteria.**

IMMUNE – REBUILD HEALTH (approximate order of importance).

#7 Lobelia	Helps to restore general well being during any immune/inflammatory distress. Also for '-itis' diseases including pancreatitis (Chapter 10). Occasional use best. Asthma, allergies, pneumonia.
#8 Barley Grass	Cancer, viruses, allergies. Wheat grass and alfalfa are potent immune restorers too.
#9 Raw Garlic	See fatigue (Table 7-5). Also healing (Table 7-4). **Cancer, bacteria, leukemia, fungi.**
#10 Yucca	Also stress (Table 7-5). **Fungi, bacteria,** cancer, allergies.
#11 Aloe vera	Also healing (Table 7-4). **Fungi, cancer, leukemia, bacteria.**
#12 Scullcap	Use Scutellaria baicalensis. Also Adrenal Balance (Table 7-2). **Bacteria, viruses, cancer, fungi.**
#13 Woundwort	Also vasoconstriction (Table 7-4) and fatigue (Table 7-5). **Viruses, cancer.**
#14 Shiitake-Reishi	Good together. Limit Shiitake mushroom intake to 100 mg (neurotoxicity beyond). Cancer, bacteria, allergies, viruses.
#15 Pau D'Arco	Small doses. Fungi, cancer, viruses, allergies.
#16 Saffron	Healing-immune ↑, energy-stress ↓. Take only as tea using 4-8 stigmas maximum. Not before or during any stress. Cancer, bacteria, viruses.
#17 Parsley	Also exocrine liver (Table 11-4). Cancer, viruses, allergies.
#18 Blessed Thistle	Also healing (Table 7-4) and pituitary-healing (Figure 8-B). Bacteria, cancer.
#19 Cayenne	Also fatigue (Table 7-5). **Cancer, leukemia.**
#20 Ginger	Also fatigue (Table 7-5) and stomach and pancreatic digestion. **Cancer, leukemia, bacteria, fungi**.
#21 Heather	Also vasoconstriction (Table 7-4) and fatigue (Table 7-5). **Leukemia.**

Herb	Comments
#22 Yarrow	Also endocrine pancreas glucagon/glucose counterregulation (Table 10-1) and its pituitary control. Viruses, cancer, fungi.
#23 Bee Propolis	Bacteria, viruses, fungi, cancer.
#24 Rosemary	Astringent. Great for seasoning food. Bacteria, viruses, fungi, cancer.
#25 Siberian Ginseng	Also healing (Table 7-4). Cancer, viruses.
#26 Burdock Root	Viruses, bacteria, cancer, allergies.
#27 Chickweed	Allergies, cancer, viruses.
#28 Peppermint and Spearmint	Good together, or separately. Also nerves (Table 7-3). Viruses.
#29 Mullein	Viruses, allergies, bacteria.
#30 Myrrh	Bacteria, fungi, viruses.
#31 Boneset	Viruses, allergies.
#32 Eyebright	Eye problems. Also endocrine pancreas (Table 10-1). Allergies, viruses.
#33 Cranberry juice	Urinary tract infections. Also helpful, eating cranberries (crunch the seeds).

Maintaining Immune Health… Life Insurance

Why are there so many essential immune herbs in Table 7-6, six in all? Immune metabolism depends upon the ingestion of many different plant phyto-compounds to empower defense and achieve protection, as explained in Chapter 3. More phyto-compound variety equals more defense! And what are immune herbs but very powerful, very exotic plant phyto-compounds. The philosophy of Table 7-6 defense and prevention is simple – complexity. The six maintenance herbs here form a solid foundation. Then, add in Table 3-3 phyto-compounds and you have a mighty fortress against disease. Taking a small dose of each of these immune invigorators occasionally generates 24/7 protection. Near the end of his life, Louis Pasteur observed, "The pathogen is nothing, the terrain (immune system) is everything."

GOLDENSEAL ROOT

Save this immune superstar for emergencies, usually acute illnesses. That's how and when Goldenseal Root works best. When the invaders are at the door or already inside and defeating you, Goldenseal Root will shift the Immune $\rightleftharpoons$ Stress equilibrium strongly toward Immune and turn all your defenders into SUPER-lymphocytes! See Figure 7-B and associated text for dosage and medical literature review.

BLUE-GREEN ALGAE

A staple of Oriental diets and one of their secrets to health and long life, Blue-Green Algae is a powerful immune builder and general tonic. These one-celled plankton, rich in green chlorophyll, phycocyanin (blue pigment) and many other vital nutrients, show efficacy against cancer, leukemia and viruses in the medical literature. Popular varieties include Spirulina and Chlorella, which are available in tablet, capsule or bulk powder. Small doses of as little as 50 mg occasionally are sufficient for prevention, but take more, more often with illness or recent exposure to carcinogens and viruses.

> Review of the Medical Literature

Cancer... The antitumor activity of fruits, vegetables and edible marine algae is a reliable cancer prevention strategy.[427] Blue-green algae Spirulina platensis inhibits oral carcinogenesis in animal models. In tobacco chewers of Kerala India, Spirulina at 1 g daily for 12 months reverses oral leukoplakia [pre-cancerous growth, thick white patches on the tongue or other mucous membranes], while showing no toxicity.[428] Spirulina inhibits precancerous colon crypts [small cavities in the wall] in animal studies,[429] and reduces lung metastasis [transfer from one organ/part to another] of B16-BL6 mouse melanoma cells by preventing invasion of the basement membrane [basal lamina: thin membrane underlying epithelium or lining].[430] Through T-cell activation, a glycoprotein extract of Chlorella vulgaris demonstrates antitumor activity against both spontaneous and experimentally-induced mouse metastasis.[431] Algae Lyngbya majuscula and Cladophoropsis vaucheriae inhibit mouse P-388 and L1210 leukemia cells, respectively.[432, 433] Compound 14-keto-stypodiol diacetate from algae Stypopodium flabelliforme arrests DU-145 human prostate tumor cell proliferation.[434] Algae Haslea ostrearia inhibits human solid tumors: lung carcinoma (NSCLC-N6), kidney carcinoma (E39) and melanoma (M96). These carcinoma types are particularly chemoresistant, suggesting the presence of a new potent antitumor agent in Haslea ostrearia.[435]

Viruses... Spirulina platensis inhibits replication of enveloped viruses [envelope: outer layer of some viruses, derived from host cell] including herpes simplex type 1, cytomegalovirus [widespread herpes virus; causes uterus infection, leading to abortion, still-birth or congenital defects], measles, mumps, influenza A and HIV-1. Spirulina selectively prevents virus penetration into host cells.[436] Spirulina maxima inhibits infections of herpes simplex virus type 2 (HSV-2), pseudorabies virus (PRV), human cytomegalovirus (HCMV), and HSV-1.[437] Spirulina platensis possesses antiviral activity against enterovirus 71 infection, which causes significant morbidity and mortality in children worldwide.[438] Allophycocyanin purified from several types of algae Microcystis has remarkable antiviral activity against influenza A virus.[439] Algae sulfated homopolysaccharides and heteropolysaccharides possess anti-HIV activity, as do algae sulfoglycolipids, carrageenans fucoidan, sesquiterpene hydroquinones and others, which receive much less research attention. A sulfate group in the chemical formula is necessary for anti-HIV activity, and potency increases with the degree of sulfation.[440]

Fibromyalgia?... Chlorella reduces average TPI [muscle Tender Point Index] from 32 to 25 after 2 months in a pilot study of 18 patients with moderately severe symptoms of fibromyalgia [common, chronic musculoskeletal disorder of unknown cause/origin]. This 22% decrease in pain intensity is statistically significant.[441]

VITAMIN C and BIOFLAVONOIDS

500 to 1000 mg of Vitamin C daily provides protection against viruses, bacteria, cancer, leukemia, and asthma and allergy flare-ups. Bioflavonoids synergize 'C' in this effort. If invaders get out of control, for instance during a cold or the flu, fight them off with up to 6 grams of Vitamin C daily in 1-2 grams doses. More than 2 grams per day may cause loose stools, but not if this 'C' is used up in the battle. When taking high doses, the gentleness of natural Vitamin C-bioflavonoid supplements such as rose hips and acerola cherries is especially important. With an acid-sensitive stomach, however, use non-acidic Ester-C. Vitamin C's antioxidant activity is reported earlier in this chapter, and Chapter 11 presents its "detox" action and effectiveness against hepatitis viruses.

Review of the Medical Literature

Antioxidant → immune relationship... Strenuous exercise impairs natural immunity, leading to lymphopenia [low white blood cell count], neutrophilia [too many neutrophils], reduced lymphocyte [white blood cell] response to mitogens [promoting cell division], low saliva Immunoglobulin A [IgA: antibody proteins that protect mucous linings from infection], and high pro- and anti-inflammatory cytokines [non-antibody proteins/signaling molecules of the immune system].[442] While conflicting data exist, the preponderance of evidence indicates that exercise increases free-radical generation. Antioxidant supplementation, especially Vitamin C and Vitamin E, reduces lipid peroxidation [lipids: fats and fat-related compounds] following exercise.[443] Vitamin C neutralizes superoxide [O_2^-], hydroxyl [OH^-] and hypochlorous acid [$HOCl$] free radicals in the extracellular fluid and lessens phagocytic [phagocytes: white blood cells that engulf/devour microorganisms and cell fragments] suppression in distance runners.[444] Vitamin C decreases the incidence of upper respiratory tract infection symptoms following competitive distance running events.[445]

The Common Cold... Sixty studies have examined Vitamin C effects on the common cold. No preventative effect was reported in the six largest studies, however, smaller studies found considerable benefit. Common cold incidence dropped an average 50% in three trials involving intense physical activity, and 30% in four other trials. Daily Vitamin C supplementation of one gram or more consistently reduced common cold duration, although results varied widely.[446] Vitamin C produces greater benefit in children than adults. Dose is also important, with greater effect at two grams or more daily compared to one gram daily. In five studies, adults given one gram daily had only a 6% decrease in cold duration, while in two studies, children given two grams daily had a 26% reduction. Three controlled studies reported that Vitamin C lowered pneumonia incidence at least 80%, but preventive effects were apparently limited to individuals with low dietary Vitamin C intake, whereas therapeutic benefits were present across many population subgroups.[446 447]

Asthma... incidence and morbidity have increased in the last decade.[448] Epidemiological studies reveal a link between asthma and the children of smokers, and between oxidant exposure and respiratory infections.[449] Vitamin C protects lung function and airway responsiveness and reduces asthmatic symptoms.[448] Vitamin C improves pulmonary function tests, bronchoprovocation challenges, allergens, histamine levels, white blood cell function and respiratory infections in a number of asthma and allergy studies.[450] However, several studies do not support Vitamin C benefits.

Skin... possesses an elaborate antioxidant defense system to thwart UV-induced oxidative stress. Still, excessive UV/sun exposure can overwhelm cutaneous antioxidant defenses, resulting in oxidative damage, immunosuppression, premature skin aging and skin cancer. One protective strategy is to support the endogenous [arising from within] antioxidant glutathione [within cell mitochondria, the main defense against oxidative stress; also immune modulator].[451] Vitamin C and Vitamin E protect against mitochondrial glutathione oxidation.[204] Vitamin C, Vitamin E and beta-carotene are very effective in photo[sun]protection.[451]

Stomach... Gastric juice and gastric musoca [mucous membrane] maintain high Vitamin C concentrations, suggesting a metabolic role.[452] Helicobacter pylori infection [H. pylori: bacterium implicated in gastric ulcers and cancer] is associated with reduced Vitamin C in gastric juice.[453] Recent studies show that Vitamin C and astaxanthin, a carotenoid, protect against H. pylori.[454] In atrophic gastritis, bacterial overgrowth converts nitrates to carcinogenic nitrites; however, Vitamin C inhibits this conversion.[455]

Cancer... Vitamin C quenches the mutagenic action of free radicals in the stomach.[452] Vitamin C and carotenoids reduce stomach cancer risk,[456, 452] as do fruits and vegetables.[453] Epidemiological studies show that Vitamin C protects against cancer, particularly non hormone-dependent malignancies such as throat tumors.[457] High Vitamin C levels induce apoptosis [gene-directed, programmed cell death] in various tumor cell lines, including salivary gland tumors, oral squamous [scaly, platelike] cell carcinoma,[458] and myelogenous [produced in the bone marrow] leukemia.[459] Vitamin C and Vitamin K [blood clotting vitamin, abundant in dark and green vegetables] act synergistically in apoptosis activity.[458] In one limited terminal cancer study, patients receiving large doses of Vitamin C survived 115 days vs. 48 days for control patients.[460]

Proposed mechanisms... to explain Vitamin C's role in cancer prevention and treatment include: (1) arresting free radical damage, (2) immune system enhancement, (3) neutralizing carcinogenic substances, (4) eliminating oncogenic [mutating a normal gene; can convert a normal cell to tumor cell] viruses, (5) tumor apoptosis, (6) stimulating collagen [fibrous protein of connective tissue] synthesis to 'wall off' tumors, (7) inhibiting hyaluronidase [enzyme that reduces viscosity in tissue spaces], thereby keeping tumors intact and preventing metastasis [transfer from one organ/part to another], and (8) enhancing the activity of certain chemotherapy drugs and reducing toxicity of other chemotherapy agents.[461, 458]

ECHINACEA

When employed early against colds and acute upper respiratory infections, Echinacea is effective in reducing their incidence, severity and duration. This effort must be a short term, 200 to 400 mg at 2X (stimulation dosing) over several days, or if necessary go to 3X to bring the infection under control. An alternative to 3X is taking Echinacea with the other five essential immune herbs in concerted action.

Continuous daily use of Echinacea is counterproductive and slightly toxic. If you have a weak pancreas, even 200 mg can aggravate tissues and lead to pancreatitis. 50 mg of Echinacea occasionally is effective prevention with respect to all invaders: viruses, cancer, fungi and bacteria. Echinacea improves pituitary immune oversight too.

Review of the Medical Literature

Overview... Echinacea purpurea possesses significant immunomodulatory activities, with macrophage [relatively long-living, large white blood cell; -phage: anything that devours] activation demonstrated most convincingly. The following immune responses were reasonably demonstrated: macrophage-derived cytokines [non-antibody protein/signaling molecules of the immune system; include interleukins, lymphokines, interferons and TNF (tumor necrosis factor)], phagocytes [white blood cells that engulf/devour microorganisms and cell fragments], and activation of natural killer cells [NK cells: active in spontaneous, non-specific immunity against cancer and viruses, first-line defense against cancer] and a variety of leukocytes [white blood cells].[462]

Colds, Upper Respiratory Tract Infections... REVIEW #1: From 1961 to 1997, twelve clinical studies concluded that genus Echinacea is effective in treating the common cold, but these results remain ambiguous because of flaws in study design. In three studies of upper respiratory tract infections (URTIs) since 1997, Echinacea reduced the frequency, duration and severity of common cold symptoms, but lacked efficacy in two other studies. Again, uncertainty exists due to methodology with small population groups and use of commercially unavailable, non-standardized dosages.[463] REVIEW #2: In nine URTI Echinacea trials, eight reported generally positive results. In four prevention trials, three reported marginal benefits. Quality of methodology was modest. Echinacea may be beneficial in early treatment of acute URTIs. Little evidence supports prolonged use for prevention.[464]

Viruses... Considerable circumstantial evidence indicates that Echinacea ameliorates virus-mediated illness including the common cold, influenza, AIDS and virus-induced tumors. Echinacea significantly increases natural-killer (NK) cells and monocytes [type of white blood cell, precursor of macrophages] in the bone marrow and spleen of mice as early as one week after treatment. Both NK cells and monocytes kill viruses and mediate nonspecific immunity, suggesting a preventative role for this herb.[465] In vitro [in laboratory vessel] human macrophages cultured in Echinacea produce significantly more IL-1 [Interleukin 1: secreted by various lymphocytes; activates/potentiates both B- and T-cells], IL-6 [stimulates B-cells],

IL-10 [coregulator of mast cell growth; mast cells are involved in histamine release and allergic reaction] and TNF-alpha [tumor necrosis factor-alpha] than controls, consistent with immune-activated antiviral activity.[466] Echinacea angustifolia enhances primary and secondary IgG response [Immunoglobulin G: circulates in the blood giving long-term immunity against previously encountered bacteria, viruses, and other pathogens] in rats.[467]

Cancer... Arabinogalactan, a highly purified Echinacea polysaccharide, activates macrophage tumor cytotoxicity and increased production of IL-1, TNF-alpha and interferon-beta 2 [interferon: family of hormone-like glycoproteins that fight virus infection/multiplication].[468] Or oppositely, Echinacea has no detectable effect on cytokine output in tumor patients.[469] However, natural killer (NK) cells are active in spontaneous, non-specific immunity against tumors and viruses, and Echinacea purpurea increases NK numbers and their anti-tumor lytic [rupture of cell membrane] action in aging mice, reflecting renewed bone marrow production. Echinacea appears to stimulate de novo (quantitatively and functionally rejuvenated) NK cell production in animals of advanced age.[470] Echinacea purpurea and Panax Ginseng significantly enhance NK function in all human population subgroups including healthy patients and those with chronic fatigue syndrome (CFS) [symptoms include weakness, fatigue, muscle pain, lymph node swelling] and AIDS.[44]

Fungi... Echinacea inhibits growth of yeast strains Candida albicans and other Candida, and Saccharomyces cerevisiae.[471] Echinacea purpurea markedly increases in vitro phagocytosis [white blood cell ingestion] of Candida albicans.[472]

Bacteria... Echinacea purpurea stimulates metabolic, phagocytic and bactericidal activities of macrophages in mice.[473]

Toxicity/allergic sensitivity... Echinacea purpurea is non-toxic to rats and mice at many times the human therapeutic dose.[474] In humans, however, 5% of atopic [allergic hypersensitivity] patients have IgE [Immunoglobulin E: associated with hypersensitivity reaction] allergic reactions to Echinacea.[475] If used continuously for more than 8 weeks, Echinacea can cause hepatotoxicity [hepato- prefix meaning 'liver'].[48]

Herb-drug interactions... Echinacea should not be used with other hepatoxic drugs such as steroids, amiodarone [anti-arrhythmic drug], ketoconazole [antifungal] and methotrexate [for leukemia]. However, Echinacea lacks the strongly hepatoxic 1,2 saturated ring of pyrrolizidine alkaloids. Echinacea should not be taken with immunosuppressants such as corticosteroids and cyclosporine [anti-rejection drug after transplant surgery].[48]

ASTRAGALUS

Astragalus uniquely boosts defenses against viruses and cancer while maintaining Immune ⇌ Stress equilibrium and combating stress. As revealed in the following medical literature, Astragalus improves T-lymphocyte, NK (natural killer) lymphocyte, macrophage and TNF (tumor necrosis factor) activity. Its stress benefits are reported earlier.

Review of the Medical Literature

Immune enhancer... Astragalus membranaceus improves cellular immunity and its T-lymphocyte profile in human myocarditis [inflammation of heart muscle from a virus infection].[476] Astragalus enhances antibody response in normal and immunodepressed animals,[477] and phagocyte [white blood cells that engulf/devour microorganisms and cell fragments] function in forced-exercise animals.[478] Astragalus has potent immunorestorative properties.[479]

NK activity/lupus... Astragalus stimulates NK lymphocytes [active in spontaneous, non-specific immunity against cancer and viruses, first-line defense against cancer] in both healthy and SLE [systemic lupus erythematosus] patients. NK activity is significantly lower in SLE patients than healthy controls. The level of NK activity correlates with SLE disease activity.[480]

Cancer... Tumors suppress macrophage [relatively long-living, large white blood cell; -phage: anything that devours] function. In two types of urological tumor, Astragalus reverses this suppression.[481] Astragalus also increases TNF-alpha and TNF-beta [TNF: tumor necrosis factor, deficiency implicated in cachexia, general ill heath with emaciation, which is common in cancer patients].[482]

Recombinant immunotherapy/cancer and AIDS... Recombinant interleukin-2 (rIL-2) [recombinant: resulting from new combinations of genetic material; IL-2: stimulates more T-cell production and other immune defenses] immunotherapy is successful in treating several cancers. rIL-2 generates lymphokine [hormone-like cell protein factor/signaling molecule]-activated killer (LAK) cells to achieve tumor death. However, high doses of rIL-2 cause severe toxicity. rIL-2 plus Astragalus significantly lowers the LAK numbers necessary for tumor death compared to rIL-2 alone. [483] Astragalus potentiates rIL-2-generated LAK activity in both cancer and AIDS patients.[483, 484]

Herpes virus, genital warts... Astragalus is synergic to recombinant interferon [family of hormone-like glycoproteins that fights virus infection/multiplication] for treatment of herpes simplex virus type 2, cytomegalovirus [widespread herpes virus; causes uterus infection, leading to abortion, stillbirth or congenital defects], and chronic inflammation of the cervix from genital warts.[485]

Liver… Astragalus alleviates liver injury from chemical poisoning in mice.[486] Astragalus is effective in delaying chemically-induced hepatocarcinogenesis in rats.[487] Astragalus antioxidant activity protects the mitochondria [cell *organ* responsible for respiration and energy production] membrane.[488]

GREEN TEA

Good tasting and good for you, Green Tea is a daily ritual among Asians, their drink of choice. Green Tea has proven efficacy against cancer, leukemia, viruses and bacteria. Occasional use is sufficient for prevention. Green Tea and Black Tea are both derived from the herb Camellia sinensis. Green Tea is the fresh cut leaf, lightly steamed to deactivate oxidizing enzymes. Black Tea leaves are allowed to oxidize.

Why not replace coffee or ordinary commercial teas with a world tour of refreshing, healthful ones: Green Tea for immune, Peppermint and Spearmint teas for immune and nerves, Chamomile for nerves and sleep, Sage for nerves and healing, and so on. Celestial Seasons® teas give a great tour.

> Review of the Medical Literature

Cancer… Green Tea (Camellia sinensis) contains powerful antioxidants with anticarcinogenic properties. Present in 30-40% of Green Tea extractable solids, polyphenolic catechins [flavonoids, see Table 3-3] epigallocatechin-3-gallate (EGCG), epigallocatechin (EGC), and epicatechin-3-gallate (ECG) profoundly modulate carcinogenic metabolism, intervening in the biochemical and molecular pathways of tumor initiation, promotion and progression. These compounds inhibit cell proliferation, induce apoptosis [gene-directed, programmed cell death], and arrest cell cycle. Many tea polyphenols scavenge reactive oxygen species (ROS) implicated in cancer, neurodegenerative disorders and cardiovascular disease.[489, 490] Camellia sinensis demonstrates anticancer effect in different animal models for different organ sites,[491] specifically esophagus, stomach, duodenum, pancreas, liver, colon, lung, breast and skin cancers induced by chemical carcinogens.[492] However, results vary in epidemiological and human studies. Green Tea has strong efficacy against human esophageal cancer. Six of ten Green Tea stomach cancer studies report inverse association, while three report positive association, although the most comprehensive studies support efficacy. Two of three pancreatic studies suggest inverse association. Three of five colon cancer studies find inverse association, but one positive association. For rectal cancer, only one of four studies gives inverse association, with increased risk in two studies. Two of two studies show inverse association between Green Tea and urinary bladder cancer.[493] Green Tea inhibits human papillomavirus (HPV)-16 associated cervical cancer,[494] and prostate cancer development.[495] Green Tea polyphenols are photoprotective, and can prevent solar UVB-induced skin disorders including skin cancer associated with immune suppression and DNA damage.[496,497]

Leukemia... Green Tea inhibits the growth of human leukemic cell lines,[498] including Jurkat T, HL-60, K562,[499] adult T-cell leukemia (ATL),[500] and eosinophilic leukemia EoL-1.[501]

Viruses... Tea EGCG and theaflavin digallate (TF3) inhibit influenza A and B virus, rotavirus [causes severe, dehydrating diarrhea] and enterovirus [grows in the intestine, includes poliovirus] infections.[502, 503] EGCG and ECG inhibit HIV reverse transcriptase [multiplication], and related DNA and RNA polymerases [catalyzing enzymes for multiplication].[504]

Bacteria... Tea modifies gastrointestinal flora, decreasing undesirable bacteria and increasing beneficial bacteria.[505] Camellia sinensis inhibits a wide range of pathogenic bacteria,[506] including H. pylori [Helicobacter pylori: bacterium implicated in gastric ulcers and cancer] when ingested daily.[507] Green Tea strongly inhibits Escherichia coli [E. coli], Streptococcus salivarius and Streptococcus mutans.[508] Green Tea protects against cariogenic [causing tooth decay] bacteria.[509]

Cardiovascular disease... Green Tea reduces triglycerides, total cholesterol and low and very low-density lipoprotein cholesterols [LDL/VLDL, so-called bad cholesterols], and increases high-density lipoprotein cholesterol [HDL, so-called good cholesterol] in a study of 1371 Japanese men over 40 years of age.[510] Other studies confirm Green Tea preventive effects against high cholesterol, high blood pressure, atherosclerosis and coronary heart disease [CHD].[492] Epidemiological studies of tea in general and tea flavonols are mixed. Three of six studies find clear protection against cardiovascular disease; one study shows protective effect only in the CHD subgroup; and one study of flavonol intake mostly from tea reports increased CHD risk.[511]

304]   Chapter 7: Herbs

Liver… Green Tea protects hepatic cells,[509] including inhibiting chemically-induced damage in animals.[512] This is a modest effect, and not observed with carbon tetrachloride.

Bones and cartilage…Daily tea drinking is protective against osteoporosis.[513] Green Tea EGCG inhibits Interlukin-1beta-induced catabolism [breaking down] of osteoarthritis chondrocytes [differentiated cells responsible for cartilage formation].[514]

Possible side effect… Fluorosis is excessive fluoride intake, and fluoride accumulates in Camellia sinensis leaves.[515] However, fluoride concentrations are very low,[516] ranging from 0.34 to 3.71 ppm for infusions prepared from 44 different teas.[517]

Herb-drug interaction… Green Tea may interact with warfarin [prescription drug, inhibitor of blood clotting].[29]

Rebuilding Immune Health

Rebuilding the immune system and fighting serious disease such as cancer, HIV, shingles and lupus is a daunting, fearful task. Even less threatening afflictions and susceptibilities are very challenging. One contemplative question points out the fundamentals behind immune failure – why now? Why does a person get cancer (disease) now and not one year ago or five years ago? The key factors deciding this question and controlling the outcome of all such primary immune failures are: (a) resistance to, and (b) exposure to the invader.

Limiting exposure to carcinogens is often difficult in today's chemical world. These subtle dangers are highlighted in Table 11-2, "Toxic Load on Liver and Body." Limiting exposure to bacteria, viruses and fungi involves common sense practices by you and public health policies to control and eradicate the most virulent pathogens such as smallpox, polio, Legionnaire's bacteria and the like. Childhood immunization and flu shots build resistance to specific invaders.

For general immunity and a high level of natural internal resistance, you are in charge. Rebuilding a damaged, malfunctioning immune system requires the following superior nutrition:

✓ Chapter 3 fiber and phyto-compound foods using Table 3-3 as your guide.

✓ Chapter 4 'Real Food' B Vitamins with emphasis on nutritional yeasts, green vegetables and no B vitamin supplements, since they lack any immune B factor (Figure 4-A).

✓ Chapter 5 Omega 3 fish fatty acids every day, 2X usage at the start, then 1X. For aggressive intervention, employ Vitamin A in gel capsule, cod liver oil and possibly shark oil. Keep bad fats to a minimum and completely eliminate trans-fatty acids.

✓ Chapter 6 sources of trace metals naturally plus supplementations of zinc (thymus and T-lymphocytes), manganese (primary Immune), nickel (Healing-Immune connector) and selenium (pituitary healing-immune oversight) to be sure defense systems are operating at peak efficiency.

✓ Table 7-6 immune herbs, both maintenance and rebuilding herbs specific to your problem, even to #33 if necessary, and possibly Shepherd's Purse/Woundwort and Heather for vasoconstriction. Adrenal Balance herbs of Table 7-2 help to "get things running right."

After several weeks of this top-quality nutrition, fix any Immune exhaustions and imbalances according to Chapter 12. These immune dysfunctions are vexing because they can involve both hypoactive and hyperactive functioning within the interconnected defense matrix. Only by curing all hypoactive exhaustions and re-supplying abundant nutrients to depleted hyperactive subfunctions can you restore order to your immune system.

Finally, when the crisis is past and your health has thankfully returned to normal, reset Immune ⇌ Stress equilibrium and internal balance perfectly with Goldenseal Root and Devil's Claw of Figure 7-B. All in all, rebuilding the immune system is a difficult, demanding effort... but tomorrow is another day!

OVERVIEW

A paradigm shift is occurring in medicine from the disease-based approach of Western medicine to a prevention- and healing-based approach. Naturopathic medicine is at the forefront of this revolution in health care. Naturopathic medicine uses natural nontoxic methods to build health and prevent disease. The basic principles of naturopathy are:

− Do the patient no harm.

− Nature can heal; the human body has the power to heal within it.

− Treat causes, not effects.

− Prevention is the best cure.

− Treat the whole person. Mind-body-spirit wellness.

Equilibrium Theory adds one more vital principle to this holistic model:

− Internal balance. The body's response to all internal needs and external forces lies within and must adhere to a four-part harmony in Energy, Healing, Stress and Immune functions. This key unlocks the inner world of health.

Life is a balancing act. As we grow older, we learn moderation and limits. These lessons really reflect the necessity for this four-part harmony of tasks. With this new and detailed understanding of the internal mechanisms of homeostasis, we can optimize health using targeted nutrition for each gland and function in the body. Nutrition supplies the raw materials, and physiology turns out the end products of life's amazing chemistry. Good nutrition advances mind-body-spirit wellness, whereas poor nutrition leads to Energy, Healing, Stress and Immune functional weak spots, exhaustions and imbalances, which then cause chronic diseases of autoimmune (hyperactive Immune) and/or degenerative (hypoactive Healing) attack on dependent body systems, acute diseases and premature aging.

Internal balance requires complete nutrition: wholesome, natural macronutrients, B vitamins, fatty acids, trace metals and herbs. Each has a special, singularly important role to play. Variety builds health too. The more different kinds of nutritious and unusual fruits, vegetables, nuts, seeds and botanicals you consume, particularly raw foods, the closer you are to perfect nutrition and internal balance. Perfect nutrition is life giving, restorative and forgiving. Herbs are especially effective in remedying past mistakes. A few are essential, some have the amazing ability "to get things running right" (◖), and the rest provide strong, targeted therapeutic action to correct dysfunctions. Figure out which functions or subfunctions need help, and send in the right herbs and other nutrients to restore health and vitality.

Nutrition does not give instant results. Take time to do it right. Overuse of an herb can turn a fine-tuning vitamin factor into a counterproductive, overdose abuser of health. Caffeine is only the most obvious example. Because of herb potency, small doses are oftentimes optimal. "All things in moderation" applies to macronutrients, B vitamins, fatty acids and trace metals too. Functional hyperactivity from too much nutrition is as bad as the inevitable functional hypoactivity from raw material deprivation. Again, internal balance is your guiding principle – provide for energy, healing, stress and immune needs, but don't overdo it or under do it. Listen to your body for feedback on where functioning is in trouble. Fortunately, Mother Nature's checks and balances allow great latitude once you understand physiology and nutrition. When nutritious foods become habit and then integrated into lifestyle, you can forget all the rules and just live good internal chemistry. Hippocrates' wisdom still holds true, "Let food be your medicine."

The endocrine system as a whole must have internal balance and perfect harmony. Chapters 2-7 describe "how to" for the adrenal gland, as do Chapters 8-11 for pituitary, thyroid, pancreas and liver. This principle of internal balance is identical to that described in traditional Chinese medicine. In fact, Equilibrium Theory fits perfectly into Chinese medicine, the vital force of Qi and the yin and yang duality of life. Equilibrium Theory adds many new yin and yang balances essential for health; first and foremost are the functional balances of Healing ⇌ Energy and Immune ⇌ Stress, followed by corresponding nutrient balances. Life's processes consist of a vast number of homeostatic balances, all working together to create oneness.

The sins of the past may be visiting you today. Years of poor nutrition accumulate a debt of dysfunctions and diseases. Internal balance is lost. The nineteenth-century New England theologian Hosea Ballou got it right when he stated, "disease is the retribution of an outraged nature." Chapter 12 explains how to fix the underlying causes of many dis-eases, instead of the endless folly of treating symptoms. In examining the four-part harmony of Energy, Healing, Stress and Immune functions and what happens if homeostasis is lost, Equilibrium Theory solves the mystery of osteoarthritis, rheumatoid arthritis, multiple sclerosis (MS), lupus, fibromyalgia, chronic fatigue syndrome and many more chronic diseases. Nature's endocrinology can work wonders for you!

***

8. PITUITARY GLAND

The pituitary gland is the master control gland of your endocrine system. While the adrenal gland dictates how your body responds to all internal needs and external forces, the pituitary regulates and unites the entire endocrine system into a single, cohesive unit. Homeostasis is the means, as this gland oversees innumerable feedback mechanisms essential to health. If the pituitary gland suffers from hyperactivity or the opposite, hypoactivity due to exhaustion, suppression or atrophy, then NOTHING inside of you runs right!

Life requires harmony; chaos of any kind is very harmful. The pituitary gland and homeostasis provide this necessary harmony inside the physical body. Nourish your pituitary to keep it young, but to do gently, in line with its purpose.

Common Medical Knowledge

Situated in the deepest part of the brain, at its base, the tiny pituitary gland has two lobes, anterior and posterior pituitary. Above the anterior pituitary and connected directly to it by a stalk of blood vessels is the hypothalamus. Together these three function as a unit, and will be considered as one throughout the rest of the book. Technically called the hypothalamus-pituitary axis, just "pituitary" is sufficient identification beyond the anatomy and physiology of this chapter.

The hypothalamus is an integral part of (directly wired to) the brain and central nervous system, and initiator of all things pituitary. Another important initiator is the pineal gland, located in the forebrain, which regulates biorhythms including sleep with its hormone melatonin. The hypothalamus receives melatonin input along with feedback from glucocorticoids and other hormones, and neurotransmitters such as dopamine and serotonin. Hypothalamus then directs the instinctive functions of body temperature, fluid levels, caloric use, weight regulation and sleep. It also secretes neurohormones (these act as both neurotransmitters and hormones) that control release of the following six anterior pituitary hormones:

- ACTH, adrenocorticotropic hormone, which stimulates the adrenal cortex.
- TSH, thyroid-stimulating hormone, a.k.a. thyrotropin; see Chapter 9.
- GH, growth hormone, for body development from child to adult.
- LH, luteinizing hormone, for sexual maturation and estrogen, progesterone and testosterone release.
- FSH, follicle-stimulating hormone, for ovarian follicle and testicular tubule function, notably egg and sperm development.
- PRL, prolactin, for breast development and milk production.

In addition, the posterior pituitary stores and releases two hypothalamus hormones:

- OXYTOCIN for uterine contractions during childbirth and milk let-down in nursing mothers.
- VASOPRESSIN, or anti-diuretic hormone (ADH), to retain water in the kidneys. Vasopressin also constricts blood vessels.

Hypothalamus-pituitary axis communication with endocrine subordinates is not limited to hormones. Neurotransmitters handle some tasks directly. For example, the adrenal medulla responds to hypothalamus instructions via central nervous system neurotransmitters, and secretes epinephrine (adrenaline) and norepinephrine. Neurotransmitters generate almost instantaneous gland response, while hormones are slower acting, but more long lasting in their effect. The brain, hypothalamus and central nervous system begin all action, and to a significant degree direct the hormonal system.

The activities described above are the basics of pituitary operation. Science knows more, but much more is still unknown.

Nutrition

The complete nutritional program outlined in Table 2-1 sustains not only the adrenal gland and its metabolisms, but also the entire endocrine system. Particulars for the pituitary gland are as follows. Pituitary nutrition adheres to Table 2-1 requirements with one exception; this gland does not use B vitamins in its raw materials → end products chemistry. As for macronutrients and fatty acids, Chapter 3 carbohydrates, proteins, fats and fibers and Chapter 5 good fats satisfy pituitary needs completely. Raw materials special to the pituitary come in just two areas: trace metals and herbs. These are presented ahead in the two main chapter sections: "Pituitary Regulation of Adrenal Gland" and "Pituitary Regulation of Thyroid, Pancreas and Liver."

CAUTION ☛ **Moderation in pituitary nutrition is an ABSOLUTE MUST!** Pituitary exhaustion from nutritional deprivation or pituitary suppression and atrophy from administered steroids such as cortisone are as bad as hyperactivity from overdosing on or overusing these special pituitary raw materials. Both extremes cause severe disruption to endocrine subordinates and their tasks. However, recovery from any pituitary exhaustion, suppression or atrophy can be straightforward with the right trace metal and herb supplementations.

Maintenance and rebuilding are the two ways to utilize this special trace metal and herb pituitary nutrition. For most people, a little maintenance is usually all that's ever needed. Maintenance keeps your pituitary young and fully functional, especially in oversight of the four hard-working adrenal tasks. Rebuilding pituitary function is necessary to overcome long-term raw material deprivation and resulting exhaustion, or to vanquish suppression and atrophy.

PITUITARY REGULATION of ADRENAL GLAND

The adrenal gland operates two action plans: Energy → Stress and Healing → Immune, as explained in Chapter 2. The pituitary gland has two corresponding homeostatic feedback controls for these action plans. In other words, the pituitary is divided into two functional parts (with respect to adrenal control only), and these parts have to be in equilibrium: pituitary healing-immune ⇌ pituitary energy-stress. This pituitary equilibrium is a natural consequence of Figure 2-B adrenal equilibrium in Healing ⇌ Energy and Immune ⇌ Stress. Figure 2-B is the template for many internal balances, not just pituitary adrenal oversight. Pituitary equilibrium moves back and forth as needed responding to internal needs and external forces, and as directed by the biological clock in the pineal gland (see melatonin ahead) and other feedback. Like the adrenal gland, the pituitary gland sustains its internal functions and equilibrium through complete, balanced nutrition.

Trace Metals

Figure 8-A shows pituitary metal chemistry. Follow Chapter 6 guidelines for selenium (Se), germanium (Ge) and titanium (Ti) usage, whether from "trace metals naturally" (for maintenance) or individual supplementation (to rebuild function). Again, for most people, maintenance is all that's ever needed.

Pituitary Gland

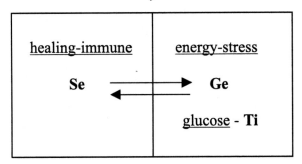

<u>FIGURE 8-A. PITUITARY TRACE METALS.</u>

Dandelion Root, Colloidal Minerals, the organic garden and the other sources of trace metals naturally can maintain pituitary metal health perfectly. Unfortunately, metal concentrations present in these sources cannot restore impaired functioning. That requires a *great leap forward* in functioning, and metal supplementation contributes significantly to rebuilding pituitary activity from long-term nutritional deprivation and exhaustion, or suppression and atrophy. Supplement selenium for healing-immune function and germanium for energy-stress. Selenium and germanium use must be balanced, or pituitary equilibrium goes badly awry. One of the dangers of multi-metal supplements is that most contain selenium, but very few have germanium. A still bigger danger would be a supplement that contains large doses of both. Never take these two metals together; review "One at a Time" in Chapter 6.

Titanium supplementation may or may not be needed to rebuild pituitary health. Titanium metalloenzymes become part of pituitary glucose metabolism and work with vanadium and chromium (Glucose Tolerance Factor, GTF) in regulating blood glucose, as described in Chapter 6. Diabetics should supplement all three of these metals. If titanium is missing, glucose metabolism is shut down at the pituitary *control panel.*

Herbs

Figure 8-B presents nourishing pituitary herbs for oversight regulation of the four primary adrenal functions. While in reality the pituitary gland is divided into only two functional parts as shown in Figure 8-A, the four divisions of Figure 8-B below are also correct! The pituitary at any time can override general action plans, Energy → Stress and Healing → Immune, and write specific instructions for any adrenal function or subfunction, or for any task within the body. That's a lot of switches on the control panel. And each switch, to turn on and off properly, has a satiating herb. For example, ACTH activates adrenal Primary Stress Function and the herb Ginkgo biloba is an ACTH precursor. Unfortunately, most pituitary nutritional factors remain undiscovered. Consequently, the widest variety of foods and exotic plants helps to satisfy the unknown here.

Pituitary Gland

immune	stress
Echinacea **Blue-Green Algae**	**Ginkgo biloba** **Raw Garlic** **Hydrangea**
healing	energy
Aloe vera **Blessed Thistle**	**Wood Betony** **Gotu Kola**

FIGURE 8-B. PITUITARY ADRENAL-OVERSIGHT HERBS.
(in order of importance)

Figure 8-B gives the two or three most powerful herbs for each pituitary adrenal control. All are adrenal herbs too and found in Tables 7-3 to 7-6 except Ginkgo biloba. Raw Garlic nourishes adrenal cortex aldosterone fatigue function and its pituitary regulator. Hydrangea contains nutrients for fat (ester/fatty acid) metabolism and its pituitary control. Gotu Kola, an important balancing herb, feeds pituitary energy and also "gets things running right" (◊) between and within pituitary healing ⇌ pituitary energy and adrenal medulla subordinates. More pituitary food: Suma improves pituitary adrenal cortex oversight.

Moderation in the use of these pituitary adrenal-oversight herbs must always be kept in mind. Once a week to once a month, or even less often, is sufficient to maintain vibrant, youthful functioning. Twice a week, sometimes more often, may be required to rebuild health. Take each herb separately and at 1X dosing ('X' is defined in Chapter 4 "Therapeutic Action"). Daily 1X use of just one pituitary herb, for instance Ginkgo biloba to control stress, over several weeks without balancing with the other Figure 8-B herbs can produce pituitary and adrenal imbalances. The exception for Ginkgo would be with pituitary stress exhaustion or adrenal Stress exhaustion. Then and only then such pituitary stimulation aids in recovery. 2X usage of any pituitary adrenal-oversight herb can be an overdose, causing activation of the dependent adrenal function and related metabolisms. At its worst, 2X produces hyperactivity in the corresponding adrenal function, followed by self-defeating adrenal hypoactivity. This phenomenon happens as follows: normal adrenal functioning → hyperactivity → then hypoactivity, some level of exhaustion from running out of adrenal raw material nutrients and reserves.

GINKGO BILOBA

Ginkgo biloba is first among equals in Figure 8-B. The stress of modern life wears out adrenal cortex Primary Stress Function and its pituitary control. Ginkgo restores vitality to this crucial pituitary function. The herb is 100% pituitary adrenal-stress oversight – A DIRECT HIT – with no *leakage* into other pituitary controls. Still, Ginkgo has proven efficacy elsewhere as evidenced in the medical literature review below. Ginkgo improves memory, concentration and alertness caused by poor blood supply to the brain (cerebral vascular insufficiency), dementia and the early stages of Alzheimer's disease. It also slows aging. Many of these therapeutic actions may be related to its pituitary adrenal-stress role.

Ginkgo biloba supplements are usually sold in standardized extracts: 24% ginkgo flavone, 6% terpene lactones. At 50:1 concentration, 30 mg of Ginkgo is a maintenance dose, 60 mg a rebuilding dose. For stressed adults, maintenance once a week is appropriate. Rebuilding from a long-term deficit requires daily use, as explained in the medical literature.

> ## Review of the Medical Literature

Nature… Ginkgo biloba is one of the oldest living plants. Pharmacologically, Ginkgo has two groups of active compounds: flavonoids, which scavenge free radicals, and terpenes, which inhibit blood platelet activation [progressive changes in platelet shape, adhesiveness and aggregation]. Many studies have examined the effectiveness of Ginkgo biloba EGb 761,[1] a standardized extract of dried Ginkgo leaves containing 24% ginkgo-flavonol glycosides and 6% terpene lactones.[2]

Cerebral/cognitive… EGb 761 shows efficacy for a wide variety of cerebral function disorders including early cognitive decline, mild to moderate senile dementias such as Alzheimer's disease, and multi-infarctual [dead or dying tissue from deprived blood supply] dementias as a result of cerebrovascular insufficiency or stroke.[2] EGb 761 eliminates free radicals, improves blood flow parameters, protects against ischaemia [insufficient blood supply], hypoxia [inadequate oxygen], edema [abnormal accumulation of fluid, swelling] and myelin [insulating fatty acid sheath surrounding nerves] damage, and has positive effects on nerve cell metabolism and various cerebral transmitter and receptor systems.[3] EGb 761 improves memory, attention, alertness, arousal, vigilance and mental fluidity. EGb 761 is also effective in treating auditory and vestibular [front part of the inner ear] disturbances, specifically hypoacusis [decibel hearing impairment], tinnitus [noise in the ears, usually ringing], dizziness, vertigo [illusion of movement; external world whirling about], and other symptoms of vestibulocochlear [cochlea: fluid-filled spiral part of the inner ear] impairment.[2] Treatment with Ginkgo bibola requires a minimum of 4 to 6 weeks to achieve a pronounced effect. Cognitive symptoms and signs improve approximately 25%,[4] however, only 3% in the Alzheimer Disease Assessment Scale subtest.[5] Memory, alertness and concentration correct first, tinnitus and dizziness later. Frequency of side effects is at placebo level.[4] Ginkgo biloba significant improves memory, concentration, fatigue, depressed mood and anxiety in all but one of 40 controlled dementia trials.[6]

Vision… EGb 761 can decrease or prevent retina damage from the sun, diabetic and proliferative retinopathies, and ischaemia-reperfusion injury [reperfusion: restoration of blood flow]. In addition, EGb 761 may improve visual field impairments resulting from diabetes, chronic cerebrovascular insufficiency and AMD [age-related macular degeneration; macula: yellow-pigmented oval area on the central retina, degeneration causes blurring in the center of the visual field and colors to dim].[2] The positive result on AMD is considered equivocal, being one single-blind trial of 20 patients.[7]

Vascular disease… Ginkgo biloba demonstrates effectiveness against intermittent claudication [leg pain brought on by walking, similar in nature to angina] in ten studies of peripheral arterial occlusive disease, most with poor methodology.[2, 8] Preliminary studies indicate that Ginkgo may be useful in preventing and treating cardiovascular disease, especially cardiac ischaemia.[9]

Stress… EGb 761 may help elderly patients cope with the stress of daily life. EGb 761 facilitates adaptive behavior to stress, and may reduce cortisol [principal adrenal cortex stress hormone] release.[2]

Mitochondria and aging… Mitochondria [cell *organ* responsible for respiration and energy production] and particularly mitochondrial DNA (mtDNA) are major targets of free radical attack. Mitochondrial oxidative damage accumulates with aging, with mtDNA damage several times greater than nucleus DNA damage. As a consequence, in the brain and liver, mitochondrial size increases and mitochondrial membrane electrical potential decreases. Ginkgo biloba extract EGb 761, Vitamin E, Vitamin C and sulphur-containing antioxidants protect against this age-related oxidative mtDNA damage, as well as oxidation of mitochondrial glutathione [natural internal antioxidant: the main defense against oxidative stress within cell mitochondria]. Furthermore, EGb 761 extract prevents age-related changes in brain and liver mitochondrial morphology and function. Thus, these antioxidants can prevent mitochondrial aging.[10]

Drug interactions… Self-medication with Ginkgo biloba is not recommended for cardiovascular disease patients who are taking anticoagulants and anti-platelet drugs; consult your physician.[9] Patients taking aspirin, NSAIDs, anticoagulants or other blood platelet inhibitors should use Ginkgo with caution.[11] Ginkgo may affect blood clotting/bleeding time, and should not be taken concomitantly with warfarin sodium [prescription drug: inhibitor of blood clotting].[12]

MELATONIN

Pituitary healing-immune ⇌ energy-stress equilibrium is partly controlled by the pineal hormone melatonin and its rhythmic secretion over the 24-hour period of a day. Located in the posterior forebrain, the pineal gland is your internal clock, regulating sleepiness and wakefulness. Melatonin secretion is stimulated by darkness and suppressed by light to the eyes. Too much darkness produces too much melatonin and Seasonal Affective Disorder (SAD), or the *wintertime blues*. Melatonin pushes pituitary equilibrium toward healing-immune and away from energy-stress, which in excess translates into fewer adrenal medulla Primary Energy Function hormones. Consequently, energy can go AWOL and *the blues* including depression can flood the mind. Providing full-spectrum light indirectly into retinal receptors suppresses pineal melatonin and relieves SAD-ness. Light therapy is the best, most successful therapeutic intervention for SAD.[13]

Too little melatonin from working night shifts or from traveler's jet lag disturbs sleep. Taking melatonin supplement can reset your biological clock, bringing on needed rest, as well as providing antioxidant healing and immune benefits associated with more youthful sleep. Of course, temperance is important when it comes to forced functioning with a hormone supplement. Fortunately, commercial melatonin is an exact copy of nature's hormone and one step removed (before) pituitary-adrenal homeostasis. To yield to the night, take 2 mg of melatonin an hour or two before bedtime, then not again for several weeks. The exception is more frequent dosing with severe sleep disorders, as discussed in the medical literature review below. Melatonin abuse will be SAD and worse. Overall, a good night's sleep lies in the natural transition of the adrenal gland from Energy-Stress to Healing-Immune tasks and in healthy liver functioning (see Chapter 11).

With over 8000 melatonin-related articles in the medical literature, highlights are as follows.

Review of the Medical Literature

Nature… The hormone melatonin (N-acetyl-5-methoxytryptamine) plays a crucial role in providing clock and calendar information for all living organisms including human beings. Synthesized principally in the pineal gland, and to lesser extents in the eye retina and gastrointestinal tract, melatonin output is photosensitive and circadian [regular cycles of about 24 hours] in rhythm with greatest production at night in darkness. Output decreases with age.[14]

Melatonin/circadian rhythm… The circadian system in mammals involves three major components: hypothalamic suprachiasmatic nucleus (SCN) [a densely-packed collection of small cells in the anterior hypothalamus], pineal gland and eye retina.[15] In human physiology, the primary source of rhythmic time is the SCN circadian oscillator.[16] SCN's intrinsic rhythm receives photoperiodic input from the eye retina on ambient lighting conditions and, in a complicated feedback pathway, SCN regulates pineal gland melatonin secretion, which in turn triggers second and third messages that further regulate SCN circadian activity through melatonin receptors within the SCN.[15, 17] Homeostatic activities of body temperature, sleep, blood volume and water balance are all rhythmic, as is the secretion of most hormones. Pineal gland circadian effects and sleep interact to produce the overall rhythmic pattern of the pituitary gland and its hormones. Melatonin, ACTH [adrenocorticotropic hormone; see pituitary hormones at the beginning of the chapter], and cortisol [principal adrenal cortex stress hormone] depend on the pineal circadian clock. TSH [thyroid-stimulating hormone] and PRL [prolactin: for breast development and milk production] are sleep related. GH [growth hormone] is influenced by the first slow wave sleep (SWS) of the night. Delta wave activity, the deepest phase of sleep, generates pulses of GH and PRL, while TSH and ACTH/cortisol pulses occur during more superficial sleep phases.[18] Sleep loss, jet lag, night or shift work, seasonal affective disorder (SAD), aging and various endocrine diseases adversely affect internal timekeeping and sleep-wake homeostasis.[19]

Sleep disorders... Disturbed melatonin rhythm disorders sleep. Low or abnormal melatonin rhythm is present in middle-aged and elderly insomniacs. Melatonin supplementation significantly reduces the time to sleep onset and/or improves sleep efficiency including wake time following onset of sleep. In addition, melatonin replacement often enables discontinuation of benzodiazepine [class of drugs: minor tranquilizers, central nervous system depressants, e.g. Valium].[20] Artificial bright light therapy can also benefit elderly insomniacs.[21] For those suffering from jet lag, early sleep onset, delayed sleep phase syndrome (DSPS) or are blind, melatonin supplementation can synchronize the sleep-wake cycle.[20] In studies of jet lag and shift work, melatonin therapy improves sleep, and in some cases hastens readaptation following shift changes. Melatonin advances the sleep period in DSPS patients, and improves sleep parameters in blind individuals with 24-hour wake disorder.[22]

Antioxidant... Melatonin is a strong free radical scavenger,[23] eliminating hydroxyl radical [OH^-], hydrogen peroxide [H_2O_2], nitric oxide [NO], peroxynitrite [$ONOO^-$], hypochlorous acid [HClO], singlet oxygen [energized but uncharged form of oxygen generated during a metabolic burst of leucocytes], superoxide [O_2^-] and peroxyl radical [OO^{--}], as well as stimulating synthesis of antioxidative enzymes such as superoxide dismutase (SOD) and glutathione peroxidase (GPX).[24, 25] Pinealectomy [-ectomy: excision, removal] decreases endogenous [arising from within the organism] melatonin production and increases free radical damage from oxidative stress.[23]

Neurodegenerative diseases... Oxidative stress is a primary factor in the development of neurodegenerative diseases such as Alzheimer's disease, Parkinson's disease and neurological conditions of stroke, brain damage, neurotrauma and epileptic seizure. Increased oxygen free radical formation coupled with the low antioxidant potential of the central nervous system, especially in aged individuals, account for the oxidative stress seen in neuron cells. Melatonin administration is effective in counteracting neurodegenerative diseases in both experimental models and in patients suffering from such diseases.[25] The brain is highly susceptible to ischaemia [insufficient blood supply, e.g. stroke]. Unless ischaemia is quickly reversed, reperfusion [restoration of blood flow] produces further cerebral damage. Melatonin protects against ischaemia/reperfusion injury.[26]

Immune... Melatonin is the circadian organizer of immune response,[27] and an important hormone in the continuous interaction between nervous and immune systems. Pineal melatonin activation enhances release of Th1 cells [subset of helper/inducer T-lymphocytes] and may counteract stress-induced immunosuppression and other secondary immune deficits. Melatonin shows efficacy in low-dose IL-2 [Interleukin 2 stimulates more T-cell production and other immune defenses] cancer therapy in patients resistant to IL-2 alone.[28] In animal models, pineal gland activation or melatonin administration reduces the incidence and growth of chemically-induced breast cancer, whereas pinealectomy often has the opposite effect.[29]

PITUITARY REGULATION of THYROID, PANCREAS and LIVER

Trace Metals

Metals that the pituitary gland uses in its regulation of the thyroid gland, pancreas and liver remain for the most part unidentified. Fortunately, maintaining metal health here requires only Chapter 6 Dandelion Root, Colloidal Minerals, the organic garden and the other good sources of trace metals naturally. As usual, nature's solution is best.

Rebuilding function is iffy. Pituitary thyroid activity is an integral part of pituitary energy-stress functioning, and so germanium may help overcome the disruption caused by thyroid hormone replacement therapy. Titanium is needed for proper pituitary endocrine-pancreas control. As for exocrine pancreas and liver supervision, these pituitary metals are unknown. Of course, exocrine pancreas digestion requires the metal catalysts tungsten (carbohydrate), molybdenum (protein), niobium/tantalum (fat) and zirconium (fiber), which indirectly affect all internal chemistries, pituitary and otherwise.

Herbs

Pituitary thyroid-oversight herbs are unknown. The widest variety of foods and exotic plants once more helps to satisfy the many unknowns of pituitary nutrition.

Beech Bark and Yarrow from Table 10-1 are a "direct hit" on pituitary endocrine-pancreas functioning. Beech Bark supplies nutrients for glucose/insulin metabolism and its pituitary control, Yarrow for glucagon and its pituitary control. To avoid hyperactivity in the subordinate pancreas, limit Beech Bark and Yarrow use to once every two to three weeks, maximum.

Pituitary exocrine-pancreas herbs are Alfalfa Seeds for carbohydrate digestion, Papaya Seeds for protein digestion, Red Root for fat digestion and Kiwi Seeds for phyto-compound fiber digestion, as detailed in Figure 10-A and associated text. Surprisingly, 2X therapy is required to restore pancreatic enzyme function, and this stimulation does not influence or upset pituitary adrenal oversight.

Regarding pituitary liver herbs, the aromatic seeds of Anise, Caraway, Fennel, Coriander and Dill from Table 11-4 fill this pituitary need and improve bile flow and, to some extent, endocrine liver functions. 2X is appropriate for restoring liver function, once again with no effect on pituitary adrenal oversight.

OVERVIEW

We all need harmony in our lives. This becomes more and more apparent as we grow older and limitations and wisdom overtake youthful immortality. The four-part harmony of Energy, Healing, Stress and Immune systems is a major advance in our understanding of physical self and homeostasis, the internal language of harmony. The pituitary gland oversees homeostasis, uniting the adrenal gland, endocrine system and body into oneness.

Harmony involves more than the "clockwork" human body presented in this book. Utilizing physiology and nutrition to achieve physical harmony is only part of mind-body-spirit wellness. Our glands and organs must have oneness to thrive, and the same is true for our spirit – one with self, one with another and with community, and one with existence, which includes the creator or life force. Oneness is just another word for wholeness. And the search for spiritual nutrition is a large part of life. We are spiritual beings immersed in a human experience.

***

9. THYROID

The thyroid gland manufactures, stores and secretes two hormones, thyroxine (T4) and triiodothyronine (T3). These regulate basal metabolism or your at-rest metabolic rate, and are factors in human growth, particularly early development. Your thyroid and parathyroid glands are located at the base of the neck below the larynx (voice box). Thyroid has two lobes, one on either side of the windpipe; parathyroid has four lobes, two on each side.

The pituitary gland controls thyroid functioning, signaling with TSH (thyroid stimulating hormone) for release of T4 and T3, which then travel throughout the body instructing cells to burn fuel, glucose or esters, at a precise rate. T3 is more potent than T4; therefore the thyroid gland can deliver a broad range of metabolic rates. Stability and equilibrium in this system are achieved through feedback homeostasis. Adrenal cortex fatigue function and the associated stamina loop of Figure 2-C are directly linked to this pituitary-thyroid homeostatic mechanism, and all are part of the endocrine system response to severe stress. No matter the magnitude of stress, your thyroid will increase the metabolic rate to meet it!

The thyroid gland also plays a role in calcium metabolism and bone health. It secretes the hormone calcitonin, which travels to the four surrounding parathyroid lobes. In response, the parathyroid gland and its hormone PTH (parathyroid hormone) adjust and stabilize blood calcium and secondarily blood phosphorus. Vitamin D also regulates PTH. To illustrate calcium homeostasis, low blood calcium reduces thyroid calcitonin, which in turn increases PTH and withdrawal of skeletal calcium. This thyroid role is incidental to its primary function, but shows the complex interweaving of endocrine processes.

NUTRITION and PREVENTION

Thyroid gland end products thyroxine (T4) and triiodothyronine (T3) require only one raw material – IODINE. T4 and T3 are made in the gland's follicles (hollow sacs) by combining iodine with the omnipresent amino acid tyrosine. Of course, many other nutrients aid in thyroid hormone synthesis, activation and metabolism. The trace metal selenium is a good example; its effects are reported in the medical literature citation on "Cretinism" at the end of the chapter.

What can go wrong? Iodine deprivation leads to hyperactive or hypoactive thyroid dysfunction, depending on the degree of undersupply and injury. Both hyperthyroid and hypothyroid syndromes can be mild, insidious and subclinical, or severe and life threatening. Mild symptoms often go undetected for many years – non-specific, they are usually overlooked or assigned to general malaise. Iodine deprivation can also generate nodules in the gland structure, which frequently develop functional autonomy. Eventually, these nodules form into a goiter. Maternal iodine deficiency during pregnancy causes intellectual impairment in the child or, in the extreme, cretinism – irreversible central nervous system damage with resulting stunted growth, spasticity, deaf-mutism and severe mental retardation.

Thyroid disease is epidemic in the United States. Up to 50% of people have microscopic thyroid nodules, 15% develop goiters, 10% have abnormal TSH, 5% of women show overt hyperthyroidism or hypothyroidism, and 3.5% of the population suffer carcinoma. Despite these figures, no major US health agency recommends screening for thyroid disorders.[1] Thyroid dysfunction is widespread in the elderly. Symptoms are often subtle and attributed to normal aging, with subclinical abnormalities more likely than overt disease and atypical presentations common.[2]

Prevention must be your goal. Standard medical treatment (described ahead) is harsh and imperfect, employing antithyroid drugs, radioactive iodine, surgery or synthetic hormone replacement therapy. Medical tests are similarly flawed. The generally accepted total serum thyroxine (T4) by radioimmunoassay is only 80% accurate. Free T4 (metabolically active) by equilibrium dialysis can be near 100%, but this test is expensive, time consuming and not available everywhere. Other tests are also problematic, including finding disease where there is none. Interpretation of the preferred diagnostics – free T4 and pituitary TSH – often requires a specialist. Controversy still exists in this field and family physicians are not trained in the complex clinical presentations.[3, 4]

A much better approach to thyroid health is prevention, with the simplest of ideas: fill up your thyroid gland with iodine, the one and only raw material needed!

Review of the Medical Literature

Recommended daily intake… Iodine is the raw material for synthesis of thyroid hormones thyroxine (T4) and triiodothyronine (T3).[5] The recommended daily iodine intake is 150 mcg [microgram: one one-thousandth of a milligram] or 0.15 mg for adults, 200 mcg during pregnancy, 50 mcg in the first year of life, 90 mcg for ages one to six, and 120 mcg ages seven to twelve. Iodized salt intake should be adjusted to achieve these results.[6]

Possible side effects… The benefits of correcting an iodine deficiency far outweigh the risks from iodine supplementation. However, adverse effects can occur, the worst being iodine-induced hyperthyroidism (IIH), which occurs predominately in older adults with autonomous nodular goiters, particularly after too rapid or too much iodine uptake.[7] Usually mild and self limiting, IIH may become serious and even fatal from cardiovascular complications, specifically thyrotoxicosis [toxic excess of thyroid hormones] can aggravate preexisting cardiac disease and bring on angina [chest pain], thromboembolism [blood vessel blockage], congestive heart failure [ineffective pumping of the heart causes fluid to accumulate in the lungs], atrial fibrillation [chaotic electrical conduction in the atrium heart chambers, loss of pumping], and in rare cases death.[6] IIH arises from mutations in thyroid cells, which develop autonomous functioning. When the mass of these cells becomes sufficient in localized areas or through nodule formation [see goiter, ahead], subsequent iodine supplementation induces thyrotoxicity. IIH can also occur with latent [not expressed because of iodine deficiency] Graves' disease [autoimmune disorder of sustained thyroid hyperactivity, more below].[8] Adequate monitoring of iodine administration can almost entirely prevent IIH and other side effects.[7]

Sources of iodine to feed the thyroid gland? That's the problem. In Japan, where seaweed algae and kelp are dietary staples, thyroid disease is almost nonexistent. All saltwater seafood, both plant and animal, are excellent sources of iodine. In the United States before the introduction of iodized table salt in the 1920s, goiters afflicted half the population of land-locked states. Today, iodine deficiency is more rare, but more insidious, especially as table salt intake falls with blood pressure concerns. Other sources have major disadvantages too. Iodine supplements are limited to 0.15 mg by the Food and Drug Administration (FDA) and of marginal value in rebuilding thyroid health. Elemental iodine, found in the common medicine chest tincture, is poisonous. Dilution to safe level is hard to calculate and even then very harsh in effect. Kelp can also be harsh, and toxic with a poorly functioning liver.

Fortunately, there is a safe, gentle, reliable source of iodine today, although largely unknown. This resource is "Atomidine," a nontoxic iodine trichloride (ICl_3) supplement available at some larger health food stores or by direct order from:

> Heritage Store
> P.O. Box 444
> Virginia Beach, VA 23458
> 800-862-2923

One drop of Atomidine fills the thyroid iodine reservoir for one to three months. One drop taken twice, one week apart, can prevent and cure many hyperactive and hypoactive dysfunctions not yet to goiter, including mild, insidious and subclinical symptoms that medical doctors and medical tests can easily miss. For mild thyroid diseases, Atomidine impregnated with alpha-lipoic acid can be curative. Morning or early afternoon, not close to bedtime, is the best time for one-drop Atomidine dosing. While nontoxic and safe, Atomidine is still iodine and temporarily stimulates thyroid function and basal metabolism.

CAUTION ☞ **Do not take Atomidine more than once in five days.** Too often or too much can produce overstimulation and heat you up like a chimney.

WARNING ☞ **For anyone with autonomous nodules/goiter, Graves' disease or cardiovascular risk (see IIH side effects above), especially older adults, consult your physician before using Atomidine.**

DYSFUNCTIONS and DISEASES

Hyperthyroidism is significantly elevated basal metabolism due to excessive thyroid hormone secretion. All body processes are *running a marathon*, even when you're asleep! Symptoms can include nervousness, irritability, weakness, fatigue, insomnia, hand tremors, rapid pulse, palpations, increased perspiration, heat intolerance, weight loss, malabsorption and loose stools. Atomidine supplementation can correct early hyperthyroidism.

Review of the Medical Literature

Standard USA practice… The most common cause of hyperthyroidism is Graves' disease, an autoimmune disorder of activated immunoglobulins [infection-fighting antibody proteins] that bind to and stimulate TSH receptors, producing sustained thyroid hyperactivity. Toxic nodular goiters [multiple overactive nodules] can also generate hyperthyroidism. Here, autonomous hyperactive functioning develops in localized areas of the gland. The recognized treatments for hyperthyroidism are antithyroid drugs, radioiodine [radioactive isotope, usually I131, which destroys some thyroid follicle cells, thereby relieving hyperactivity], and surgery. All are effective therapies, although no single method is right for all cases. Graves' disease responds to antithyroid drugs, however, drugs are ineffective against toxic nodular goiters. Radioiodine is first-line therapy, and the preferred solution for toxic nodular goiters. It is generally well tolerated and growing in acceptance. The major long-term risk is radioiodine-induced hypothyroidism. Radioiodine can be utilized in all age groups, except children and mothers during pregnancy and lactation. Also, radioiodine may exacerbate Graves' ophthalmopathy,[9] a condition of proptosis [forward displacement of the eyeball], eyelid retraction, ophthalmoplegia [paralysis of eye muscles] and optic neuropathy [nerve disease] present in 2% to 7% of Graves' disease patients.[10] Surgery has limited, specific roles to play in filling gaps in the other modalities, but is rarely utilized in Graves' disease. Partial or near-total thyroidectomy [-ectomy: excision, removal] can achieve euthyroidism [normal thyroid hormone levels].[9]

Hypercalcemia… Hyperthyroidism frequently generates hypercalcemia [excessive calcium in the blood, with bone dissolution] from coincident primary hyperparathyroidism, which normally subsides after successful hyperthyroidism treatment.[11]

In older adults… overt hyperthyroidism can cause cardiovascular angina [chest pain], palpitations, dyspnea [shortness of breath, labored breathing] upon exertion, paroxysmal [recurring spasms or seizures] dyspnea at night, and orthopnea [shortness of breath unless sitting straight or standing erect].[12] Many older adults have abnormal pituitary TSH, while thyroid hormone levels remain normal. This condition is termed subclinical hyperthyroidism (suppressed TSH) or subclinical hypothyroidism (elevated TSH). Affecting less than 2% of elderly adults, subclinical hyperthyroidism causes osteoporosis, cardiovascular symptoms, and eventually progression to overt hyperthyroidism.[13]

Hypothyroidism is slowed metabolism from not enough thyroid hormone secretion. This can cause lethargy, slow speech, loss of appetite, depression, weakness, fatigue, dry scaly skin, menstrual and pregnancy problems, intolerance to cold especially in hands and feet, edema, weight gain and constipation. Synthetic hormone replacement therapy using Synthroid is standard medical practice. Of course, hormone replacement therapy is forced functioning and disruptive to the body compared to nature's perfect pituitary-thyroid homeostatic mechanism, but often necessary when hypothyroidism is discovered late in its presentation.

Review of the Medical Literature

Overview... Hypothyroidism affects 1% to 2% of women and 0.1% to 0.2% of men; however, the incidence of both overt and subclinical hypothyroidism increases dramatically with age, to 5% to 10% of women over 50 and 1.25% of men over 60. Symptoms of slowed metabolic rate can include fatigue, lethargy, changes in memory and mental activity, cold intolerance, weight gain, constipation and goitrous enlargement. Atypical presentations of weight loss, hearing impairment, tinnitus [noise in the ears, usually ringing], and carpal tunnel syndrome occur, especially in elderly adults.[14]

Standard USA practice... Thyroid hormone supplementation is efficacious in patients with documented hypothyroidism.[15] For elderly adults with coronary artery disease, thyroid hormone replacement should be implemented cautiously to avoid hyperthyroid-related angina [chest pain], ventricular arrhythmias [abnormal heart beat: too slow, too rapid, too early, irregular], congestive heart failure [ineffective pumping of the heart causes fluid to accumulate in the lungs], or heart attack.[12]

In older adults... Many older adults have abnormal pituitary TSH, while thyroid hormone levels remain normal. This condition is termed subclinical hyperthyroidism (suppressed TSH) or subclinical hypothyroidism (elevated TSH). Affecting 5% to 10% of the elderly, particularly women, subclinical hypothyroidism causes hyperlipidemia [high fat levels in the blood] and cardiovascular effects, neurological and neuropsychiatric changes, and eventually progression to overt hypothyroidism.[13] Elevated TSH occurs especially in postmenopausal women with about 2.4% having clinical thyroid disease and about 23% subclinical thyroid disease. Among the subclinical group, 74% are hypothyroid and 26% are hyperthyroid. Even mild subclinical hypothyroidism can cause depression, memory loss, cognitive impairment, neuromuscular complaints, increased total cholesterol and low-density lipoproteins [LDL, so-called bad cholesterol] and reduced high-density lipoproteins [HDL, so-called good cholesterol].[16]

Goiter. With characteristic enlargement of the thyroid gland in the neck, goiter is a breakdown, swelling, and inevitable hemorrhaging of follicle cells as a result of iodine deprivation. Scar tissue forms, producing permanent injury and dysfunction. Damaged cells first form into small nodules and later into the visible swelling of goiter. Nodularity leads to functional autonomy. Goiter can occur in both hyper- and hypothyroid states.

Review of the Medical Literature

Epidemiological survey... Nodular goiter risk increases with the age from approximately 1% of schoolchildren to 23% of adults aged 56-75 years.[17] Besides age, goiter is more common in women than men, and following exposure to external radiation.[18] Nodular autonomy and hyperthyroidism develop more often in adults.[17] Four to six percent of US adults have goiters,[17] with estimates of 250,000 new goiters annually.[18]

Nature and development... Iodine deficiency causes goiter and its evolution toward nodularity and functional autonomy.[14] Goiters probably form as a consequence of increased TSH stimulation in reaction to thyroid hormone deficit. A contributing agent may be TSH-related growth factors. Goiters naturally evolve toward nodularity and functional autonomy as more vulnerable thyroid follicle cells, with inherently higher growth rates, are TSH stimulated to hyperactivity.[17] Initial small diffuse goiters develop into multinodular goiters (MNG) of one or more dominant nodules, which may or may not be autonomous. Autonomous functioning thyroid adenomas (AFTA) [benign tumors] usually involve mutation of TSH receptors, which cause rapid growth, hemorrhaging necrosis [tissue death], and nodular fibrosis [forming fibrous tissue].[19] Approximately 5% of all palpable nodules are malignant.[20] The incidence of goiter decreases as iodine intake reaches the estimated adult daily minimum requirement of 150 mcg.[21]

Diagnosis and treatment... Goiter diagnosis and evaluation consists of patient history, physical examination, plasma TSH, free thyroxine [T4] and free triiodothyronine [T3], and imaging studies of goiter anatomy, size and function. Treatment options are L-thyroxine and thionamides [antithyroid drugs], radioiodine I131, surgery and percutaneous [through the skin, as with injection] ethanol injection (PEI). With euthyroidism [normal hormone levels], L-thyroxine can reduce goiter size in some cases, but requires continuous use. Short term, thionamides can control toxic goiter hyperthyroidism. I131 and surgery are most common definitive therapies for toxic and euthyroid MNG, and toxic AFTA. PEI is efficacious in some toxic AFTA.[19] Surgery is the primary treatment for malignancy.[20]

Cretinism is thyroid hormone deprivation during fetal development. This results in stunted growth, spasticity, deaf-mutism and severe mental retardation in the child. Minor hormone deficiency causes less severe consequences of intellectual and neuropsychological impairment. Healthy maternal thyroid function and iodine status are crucial in preventing such irreversible damage.

Review of the Medical Literature

Nature... Material iodine deficiency is the leading cause of infant intellectual impairment in the world.[22] Normal fetal central nervous system development requires adequate exposure to thyroid hormones. With fetal hypothyroid exposure, the resulting neuropathic disorder in the child can vary in degree and features. The full-blown syndrome is called cretinism and includes stunted growth, spasticity, deaf-mutism and severe irreversible mental retardation.[23]

Maternal status and effect... Maternal iodine supplementation during pregnancy significantly reduces infant and early childhood deaths, results in better psychomotor development in four to twenty-five month olds, and decreases the incidence of cretinism at age four years.[22] Maternal iodine deficiency is mild at a daily intake of 50-99 mcg, moderate at 20-49 mcg, and severe with less than 20 mcg.[24] Mild deficiency causes minor neuropsychological damage; severe deficiency results in cretinism.[17]

Cretinism/SIDS/selenium link... Symptoms and signs of cretinism present at age 3-5 months can include delayed development, lethargy, excessive sleepiness, slow feeding, bluish skin discoloration during feeding, flabby musculature, umbilical hernia, enlarged tongue, short stature and delayed union of skull bones. These symptoms and signs have also been reported in low-birth-weight infants and in sudden infant death syndrome (SIDS).[25] Brain neuron aging and degeneration are features of SIDS, and glutathione peroxidase (GSHPx) [H_2O_2-eliminating selenium enzyme]-protected neurons decline in the brain hippocampus [cerebral cortex area involved in long-term memory] and neocortex [six-layered, most highly-developed cortex part] during postnatal development of SIDS infants compared to normal infants. GSHPx protects neurons from free radical attack.[26] In animal studies, selenium deficiency impairs the enzyme activity necessary for brain development and function.[27] In addition, selenium enzyme iodothyronine deiodinase regulates triiodothyronine (T3) synthesis and deactivation.[28] The thyroid gland has the highest selenium content of all organs. Selenium depletion causes thyroid tissue fibrosis [forming fibrous tissue] and necrosis [death] following high iodide loading in animal models. Combined iodide and selenium deficiency may be the cause the myxedematous [swelling around the eyes] form of endemic cretinism in central Zaire.[29]

OVERVIEW

Health care in America is really "disease care." The thyroid gland is the clearest example of the poor application of medical science to the nation's health. Thyroid disease is epidemic in the United States, yet thyroid health requires only one simple raw material ingredient – safe iodine. An adequate solution was developed in the 1920s with iodized table salt, but now its use is falling as blood pressure concerns mount. An effective new solution is Atomidine, nontoxic iodine trichloride (ICl_3).

Prevention is the obvious solution to health when nature's complexity does not blind us; witness the thyroid gland. Prevention gets short shrift from the medical community, yet during the twentieth century, all but 3.7 years of the increase in life expectancy has come as a result of reduced infant mortality.[30] And other preventatives account for most of the remaining increase in life expectancy: vaccinations and flu shots, alcohol and no-smoking programs, cancer and cholesterol screening. The holistic approach to prevention is, of course, nutrition. We must build health, not just fight disease fires!

***

10. PANCREAS

The pancreas regulates glucose (sugar) metabolism with two hormones, insulin and glucagon. Insulin reduces blood glucose levels, while glucagon raises them, i.e. counterregulation. These are critical ENDOCRINE tasks as undisciplined blood glucose, either too high or too low, spells the end of good health. The pancreas also manufactures and secretes digestive enzymes for carbohydrate, protein, fat and phyto-compound breakdown. Production of these enzymes is considered part of the EXOCRINE system (secreting externally) and the specialized field of gastroenterology, because the digestive system is considered external to the body. In a strict technical sense, this is correct. However, pancreatic endocrine and exocrine tissues are closely linked not only anatomically but also functionally. Therefore, this chapter will examine both endocrine and exocrine pancreas – improving one will benefit the other!

Common medical knowledge... The pancreas is long, slender gland sitting almost horizontally in the abdominal cavity, five to six inches in length and centered about one inch below the bellybutton. Digestive enzymes exit through a pancreatic duct at the gland's right end or head into the duodenum, first portion of the small intestine. With distinctive tissue types under the microscope, endocrine pancreas cells are called "islets of Langerhans." Alpha islets make and secrete glucagon; beta islets produce insulin. Homeostatic feedback precisely controls these hormones and blood glucose levels. Exocrine "acinar cells" make and secrete digestive enzymes: amylase for carbohydrates, trypsin for proteins, and lipase for fats, as well as accompanying electrolytes, on average 24 fluid ounces per day. As food passes by the duodenum, hormones from its wall, pacreozymin for enzyme delivery and secretin for electrolyte secretion, enter the bloodstream and signal the exocrine pancreas into action.

NUTRITION

"An ounce of prevention is worth more than a pound of cure." This slightly altered proverb voices absolute truth for the pancreas, which is far more susceptible to injury and scar tissue than the adrenal gland and pituitary gland. There is an unfortunate truth about your body's antioxidant defense system, and that is priorities exist in its protection of glands. The adrenal and pituitary glands come first, and so the lowly pancreas is much more likely to suffer damage from free radical attack and oxidative stress. While inadequate nutrition causes only functional disorders in the adrenal and pituitary glands, the pancreas experiences three bad consequences: function exhaustion, followed closely by injured cells and scar tissue. Functional exhaustion and to some extent injured islet and acinar cells can be fixed, but scar tissue is dead – health forever lost.

Prevention and good nutrition are absolute musts to avoid pancreatic islet and acinar exhaustion, injury and scarring, and their resulting dysfunctions and diseases. Islet impairment causes hypoglycemia and diabetes, and the dependent body system diseases of diabetic neuropathy, diabetic retinopathy, kidney disease, hypertension and increased cardiovascular risk. Acinar impairment causes pancreatic enzyme insufficiency, poor digestion, diarrhea or in some cases constipation, intestinal gas/flatulence, and acute and chronic pancreatitis (inflammation of the pancreas). If your pancreas starts to fail, you're in BIG TROUBLE! Second chances at health abound for the adrenal gland, pituitary, thyroid and liver, but second chances are few and far between for the overworked, indispensable pancreas.

Like the adrenal gland, the pancreas requires nature's complete nutrition: wholesome macronutrients, B vitamins, fatty acids, trace metals and herbs. Table 2.1 introduces these five essential nutrients. Fortunately, meeting basic pancreatic needs is easy, in that adrenal requirements for macronutrients, B vitamins, fatty acids and trace metals satisfy pancreatic requirements too. Chapters 3-6 provide detailed how-to guides. Use specifics for the pancreas are discussed below. As for herbs, special herbs nourish each function and subfunction of the pancreas separately. These are presented later in the chapter under "Endocrine" and "Exocrine" headings. With this complete nutrition, your pancreas will perform flawlessly throughout life.

Macronutrients

Macronutrients play a major positive or a major negative role in pancreatic health – and you get to decide which? Specifically, blood glucose regulation can be easy or hard labor on your pancreas. Simple carbohydrate sugars found in candy, sweets, table sugar, and soft drinks and foods containing high-fructose corn syrup dump too much glucose into the bloodstream too quickly. This overuses and wears out insulin-producing beta islets of Langerhans, bringing on hypoglycemia and eventually diabetes. On the other hand, complex carbohydrates such as whole-grain cereals deliver a slow, steady stream of glucose to the blood over many hours and require little insulin management. There's more ahead in the "Endocrine" section of the chapter on glucose-insulin *wedded bliss*… or what can happen when you let things go terribly wrong.

B Vitamins

B vitamins supply the water-soluble building blocks for insulin and glucagon hormones, digestive enzymes and the other end products of pancreatic chemistry. The adrenal gland B vitamin foods of whole-grain cereals and nutritional yeasts satisfy pancreatic B vitamin needs completely. These foods do not strongly rev or stimulate the pancreas into action; rather they give vitamin nourishment, most importantly Vitamin B6 and biotin in perfect balance.

Vitamin B6 is the primary pancreas B vitamin, sustaining both endocrine and exocrine functions. This is evidenced in the Chapter 4 review of B6 medical literature. Vitamin B6 is richly supplied in nutritional yeasts and to a lesser extent in whole-grain cereals. Supplementation becomes necessary only with pancreatic dysfunctions and diseases. Then, follow Chapter 4 instructions to alleviate the nutritional deficit and resulting functional exhaustion present in endocrine hypoglycemic and diabetic syndromes and/or in impaired exocrine enzyme production and pancreatitis. Of course, functional exhaustion is only one factor in these afflictions; again the other more devastating factors are injured cells and scar tissue.

Biotin aids, connects and facilitates the metabolic pathway between adrenal gland Energy and Stress and the endocrine pancreas. This coenzyme vitamin assists in carbohydrate (glucose) and fat (ester) utilization. There's plenty of biotin in whole grain cereals, so no need for supplementation except with diabetes. Then biotin stimulates insulin-producing beta islets and improves glycemic control. Details are given in the

Chapter 4 biotin presentation and medical literature.

Fatty Acids

Fatty acids supply the fat-soluble building blocks for hormones, enzymes and the other end products of pancreatic chemistry, and for gland maintenance including cell membranes. The pancreas uses both Omega 6 vegetable EFAs (essential fatty acids) and Omega 3 fish fatty acids.[1-3]

Pancreatic dysfunctions and diseases increase fatty acid requirements and the need for discipline in their application. Gamma-linolenic acid (GLA) becomes essential during any endocrine pancreas distress. Chapter 5 medical literature reports the following efficacies: Vitamin E for antioxidant protection and improved diabetic insulin activity and blood platelets, GLA for diabetic neuropathy, beta-carotene to heal diabetic foot ulcers, and Vitamin A for diabetic retinopathy.

Exocrine fatty acid needs are not well understood and may be very complicated. Each of the four exocrine pancreas parts – carbohydrate, protein, fat and phyto-compound digestion – may require the exact same fatty acid as its corresponding adrenal part (compare Figure 3-A and Figure 5-A). For instance, when pancreatitis *jumps all over* this author, Omega 3 salmon brings relief. Coincidentally, the worst or most vulnerable part of my exocrine pancreas dysfunction becomes fat digestion with steatorrhea. And fat digestion is metabolically linked to adrenal cortex Primary Stress Function, which thrives on Omega 3 salmon.

Trace Metals

Black Currants, Dandelion Root, Colloidal Minerals and the other sources of trace metals naturally can maintain pancreatic metal health perfectly, with one exception. Supplementation of cobalt-containing Vitamin B12 becomes necessary as you get older. Review metal sources and the meaning of "occasionally" (best usage) in Chapter 6. The key endocrine and exocrine pancreas metals are as follows.

Glucose Tolerance Factor (GTF), a chromium complex, is a cofactor with insulin in regulating glucose fueling of cells. Unlike insulin, GTF is neither manufactured to meet demand nor later deactivated. Instead, it is always present – or should be! GTF deficiency causes glucose intolerance, giving symptoms of and contributing to diabetes.

Insulin resistance and "brittle diabetes" are frequently GTF related. GTF-impaired insulin utilization also aggravates hypoglycemia, and can produce weight gain. Your brain is most sensitive to glucose disturbance; deficits in short-term memory can be an indication that chromium is running out. Taking "trace metals naturally" corrects this and other maintenance problems. However, with hypoglycemia or diabetes, rebuilding glucose metal mechanisms is essential, and this requires chromium, vanadium and titanium supplementation, as well as Vitamin B12.

Vitamin B12, a cobalt complex, aids, connects and facilitates adrenal medulla Primary Energy Function, adrenal cortex Primary Stress Function and the endocrine pancreas in their common tasks. B12 regulates glucose and ester utilization. Diabetics and sugar lovers need extra B12. Adversely, B12 absorption from food is impaired in most adults, particularly the elderly. The best solution is supplementation by sublingual lozenge, details in Chapter 6.

Metal Catalysts — Exocrine pancreas chemistry especially utilizes the five metal catalysts listed in Table 6-2. Tungsten (W) is catalyst for carbohydrate digestion, molybdenum (Mo) for protein digestion, niobium (Nb) and tantalum (Ta) for fat digestion, and zirconium (Zr) for phyto-compound digestion. Maintaining exocrine pancreas metal health, that is, sufficient amounts of these catalysts for good acinar cell digestive enzyme action, can be accomplished with "trace metals naturally." Rebuilding health requires supplementing the catalysts and possibly the pituitary metals germanium and selenium.

ENDOCRINE PANCREAS

The endocrine pancreas has only one goal, regulating blood glucose. This is called glucose metabolism by the medical profession. The general public often substitutes the word "sugar" for "glucose." In meaning and intent, they are one and the same here.

Before discussing endocrine pancreas herbs, let's look at insulin and glucagon hormone functioning in depth, including the medical literature reviews of their diabetes and hypoglycemia dysfunctions and diseases.

Insulin… Glucose Regulation

Carbohydrate digestion delivers glucose to the bloodstream for cells to burn as fuel, yielding 4 calories of chemical energy per gram of initial carbohydrate in the chemical reaction:

$$\text{glucose} + \text{oxygen} \rightarrow \text{water} + \text{carbon dioxide}$$
$$C_6H_{12}O_6 + 6O_2 \rightarrow 6H_2O + 6CO_2$$

Insulin largely controls this fuel burn. It is necessary to but not part of the chemical reaction. In a sense insulin is a catalyst, although an unusual one, secreted to meet demand and later deactivated by the liver. Actually, insulin and Glucose Tolerance Factor (GTF, discussed above) act together regulating glucose entry into cells. Insulin blood levels mirror glucose levels. As glucose rises, the pancreas adjusts insulin so that both are neither too low nor too high, a very complicated task. Indeed, it is easier to think of the end result; insulin lowers <u>blood</u> glucose by enabling it to enter cells and burn up, creating life-sustaining chemical energy.

The more end product insulin your pancreas produces, the more raw material nutrition you must supply to maintain insulin health. Unfortunately, bad habits such as those enticing simple sugars contain little nutrition, but sharply increase blood glucose levels and necessary insulin response. And here comes big trouble. A lot of insulin gives a quick burst of energy, *a sugar high*, however, both adrenal medulla energy metabolism and pancreas glucose metabolism suffer raw materially.

Raw material deprivation leads to functional exhaustion of beta islets of Langerhans, followed closely by injury and scarring of them. Mild deprivation produces first hyperactive functioning or hyperinsulinism with characteristic delayed insulin response, then overreaction resulting in hypoglycemia. This hyperinsulin hypoglycemia, commonly called reactive hypoglycemia, is precursor to hypoinsulin diabetes, which develops after more severe deprivation and consequent exhaustion, injury and scar tissue.

<u>Diabetes</u> is dangerously elevated blood glucose due to insufficient insulin response. Body cells become starved of their main energy fuel, glucose. As a result,

early symptoms are excessive hunger and thirst, and frequent urination. The thirst and urination come from continuous fat burning, which builds up harmful by-product ketones in the blood. The body calls for water to alleviate ketone poisoning and the kidneys work overtime to flush them out. These early symptoms are rather innocuous compared to what lies ahead.

Diabetes is of two types: Type I, insulin-dependent diabetes mellitus (IDDM), often called juvenile diabetes since it predominately strikes children and adolescents, and Type II, non-insulin-dependent diabetes mellitus (NIDDM), which usually develops after age forty, i.e. adult onset diabetes. Type I is complete destruction of insulin-producing beta islets. The exact cause remains unknown, but evidence suggests an autoimmune antibody attack. Type I requires lifelong insulin injections. Type II is almost always related to obesity and the high sugar, highly refined carbohydrate diet common in the industrialized Western world. Weight loss and improved nutrition can frequently bring Type II under control. This is much safer than insulin injections or drug interventions.

Complications from diabetes are very serious. Acute complications involve either insulin-induced hypoglycemia even to coma (insulin shock) or ketone buildup in the blood, which can also lead to coma and, with severe dehydration, death. Drinking plenty of water to flush ketones is mandatory; the medical profession recommends 8 glasses daily. Chronic complications command constant attention. Kidney disease is the leading cause of death in diabetics, and diabetic retinopathy is the #1 cause of blindness in the United States. High blood glucose increases LDL (bad) cholesterol and blood platelet adhesion and aggregation, contributing to atherosclerosis, cardio-vascular disease, heart attack and stroke. Diabetic neuropathy with characteristic tingling and numbness from loss of nerve function has become epidemic; associated healing problems often manifest as foot ulcers. Many of these complications are related to high blood glucose altering chemical reactions and metabolic processes. Continuous fat burning is constant stress and sooner or later exhausts adrenal Primary Stress Function. Then, the least effort becomes too much stress. Overall, chronic diabetic diseases involve Figure 12-A(2) adrenal dysfunctions of hypoactive Stress and Healing Functions and a hyperactive nervous system.

Review of the Medical Literature

Diabetic emergency/insulin shock… Hypoglycemia resulting from insulin administration and/or efforts at tighter glycemic control is the most common acute side effect in the management of diabetes, and a serious medical emergency with the potential for a fatal outcome.[4] 'Hypoglycemia unawareness,' a common syndrome of severe diabetes, involves reduced perception of the specific symptoms that alert a patient to dangerously low blood glucose and neuroglycopenia [brain glucose deprivation]. Without these warning symptoms, diabetics do not take corrective action of eating food to prevent unconsciousness. 'Hypoglycemia unawareness' results from impaired glucose counterregulation,[5] specifically defective glucagon response becomes nearly universal after five years of severe diabetes, and beyond five to ten years, defective epinephrine [adrenaline] response further compromises counterregulation [see glucagon mechanisms, ahead].[6] Resulting traffic accidents are estimated at 5.2% of the total. Blood glucose awareness training (BGAT) and other intensive education programs can cut traffic accident crash rates from 29.8 to 6.8 per 1,000,000 miles.[7]

Type I juvenile diabetes… is a T cell-mediated autoimmune disease with selective destruction of insulin-producing beta islets of Langerhans. Type I pathology [origin and development] is complex, involving both genetic and environmental factors, many of which remain unidentified. An important hereditary factor is histocompatible [histo- prefix meaning 'tissue'] leukocyte [white blood cell] antigen [any invader eliciting an antibody response] (HLA) alleles [two alleles for each gene trait, one from each parent].[8] Genetic factors are necessary but not sufficient for Type I development. From epidemiological studies, environmental factors include cold climate, infections, high growth rates during adolescence and stressful/traumatic life events. The destructive autoimmunity may begin early in life with exposure to cow's milk, nitrosamines [from sodium nitrite-cured meats], or even fetal events such as blood group incompatibility and viral infections. Type I diabetes is rapidly increasing throughout the Western world.[9]

Type I treatment… Insulin therapy involves an intermediate- or long-acting basal component for nocturnal and between-meal glycemic control and preprandial [before the meal] injections of a short-acting insulin to control meal-stimulated increases in blood glucose.[10] New fasting-acting insulin analogues enable easier and tighter postprandial glucose control, while long half-life analogues improve basal coverage. Eventually, new delivery methods will provide alternatives to the current painful injections.[11, 12]

Type II adult-onset diabetes… is already a worldwide epidemic. By the year 2025, estimates are that 300 million people, mostly in the China, India and the United States, will have Type II diabetes.[13] With early detection, carbohydrate intolerance is manageable, and this holds great promise for preventing Type II onset, progression and complications, but efforts to date have been ineffectual.[14]

Insulin resistance, dual nature of Type II... The majority of Type II patients develop hyperglycemia not only from inadequate beta-islet insulin secretion, but also from insulin resistance, i.e. ineffective insulin action because of its inability to suppress liver glucose production and/or to empower glucose end use in cells. Having both genetic and environmental causes, insulin resistance varies greatly from patient to patient. More insulin secretion can compensate for insulin resistance, while improved insulin activity can mast beta islet defects.[13] The dual endocrine burdens of inadequate insulin secretion and insulin resistance lead to chronic hyperglycemia and full metabolic disarray, with consequent increased morbidity [disease incidence] and premature mortality from cardiovascular disease and microvascular diabetic neuropathy, retinopathy and nephropathy [kidney disease].[15]

Obesity... is the biggest risk factor for Type II diabetes. Preceded by years of impaired glucose tolerance, Type II develops late in obesity as beta islets can no longer sustain high insulin output in the face of high blood glucose levels and insulin resistance.[16] Type II obesity contributes significantly to hypertension [high blood pressure] and high rates of cardiovascular disease.[17]

Type II Treatment... Defective beta islet function, insulin resistance and excessive liver glucose production characterize the Type II derangement. Non-pharmacologic therapy of weight reduction and exercise should be initiated immediately after diagnosis.[12, 17] Regular exercise and a diet of 40% to 50% complex carbohydrates, 10% to 20% protein and polyunsaturated fatty acids are treatment cornerstones. If glycemic goals remain unmet after a three-month diet and exercise regimen, specific pharmacologic agents should be prescribed such as sulfonylurea drugs to stimulate insulin secretion, acarbose to delay carbohydrate absorption from the gut, metformin to inhibit excessive liver glucose production, and troglitazone to reduce insulin resistance. If these agents are insufficient, then insulin therapy becomes necessary.[17] Other important considerations are control of hypertension and cholesterol. Reducing high blood pressure improves cardiovascular and microvascular complications more than glucose control. Cholesterol control utilizing statins [cholesterol-lowering drugs, e.g. Lipitor], aspirin therapy and smoking cessation decreases cardiovascular events.[18]

Cardiovascular disease... is the major cause of morbidity and mortality in diabetic patients. Diabetes increases vascular disease risk 200% to 400%, with disproportionately poor outcomes in women and non-white minorities.[19] Diabetes alters plasma coagulation and fibrinolysis [dissolution of fibrin, the insoluble protein in blood and the end product of coagulation]; of critical importance is greater plasminogen activator inhibitor (PAI-1) [stops the enzyme that breaks down fibrin and dissolves blood clots]. Atherosclerotic plaques formed in the presence of high PAI-1 may be more likely to rupture and result in thrombosis [blood clot]. These modifications in blood platelets, coagulation and fibrinolysis all contribute to the high rate of vascular events seen in diabetic patients.[20] Besides more severe and more diffuse vascular involvement, diabetics have greater frequency of silent ischaemia [insufficient blood supply, as in silent stroke], systolic [left ventricular contraction of the heart] and diastolic [time in between ventricular contractions, when chamber is filling with blood] left ventricular dysfunction, and cardio-neuropathy [heart-nerve disease].[19] Over 11 million Americans suffer diabetes and hypertension together, which contributes significantly to poor cardiovascular outcomes and kidney disease.[21]

Diabetic neuropathy... affects 60% to 70% of diabetic patients, and leads to foot ulcers and in extreme cases to lower limb amputations. Both are preventable.[22] Here, glycation of proteins [sugars reacting with proteins, particularly critical proteins of long-living nerve cells] along with increased free radical activity, decreased neurotrophism [survival of embryonic nerve cells], and vasoactive [opening/narrowing blood vessels] abnormalities cause motor, sensory and autonomic [self-controlling, functionally independent] nerve damage.[23] Correcting underlying metabolic defects is essential, as evidenced with improved peripheral nerve function following pancreas-kidney transplantation. The duration of the diabetic disease, poor glycemic control, hypertension and smoking are all independent risk factors for diabetic neuropathy.[24]

Diabetic retinopathy... Diabetics risk multiple visual complications: glaucoma, cataracts, optic nerve disease, strabismus [deviation of eye orientation including crossed eyes], and especially diabetic retinopathy, which is the leading cause of blindness in the United States. Microvascular damage to the retina from diabetic glucose levels produces microaneurysms [aneurysm: permanent dilation of blood vessel wall at a weak point], hemorrhages and exudate [escaped fluid and cells from blood vessels] deposits such as 'cotton-wool spots' in the visual field. Subsequent neovascularization [new vessel growth] can trigger severe hemorrhage, scarring and permanent visual loss.[25] Good glycemic control is crucial in preventing diabetic retinopathy, or delaying its progression. Other risk factors are hypertension, smoking and proteinuria [-uria: present in the urine].[26] Argon laser photocoagulation is an effective treatment for end stage diabetic retinopathy,[27] reducing development to blindness by over 50%.[28]

Diabetic nephropathy... is the leading cause of end stage kidney disease in the United States, Europe and Japan.[29] Hyperfiltration and albuminuria [albumin protein in the urine] over several years degrade kidney function,[30] with decreasing glomerular filtration rate [glomerulus: filtering kidney capillary] and increasing arterial blood pressure and cardiovascular risk.[29] Genetic predisposition, poor glycemic control, hypertension and smoking are aggravating factors.[31] Diabetic nephropathy is largely preventable, and oftentimes undertreated. Reducing hypertension is key, but not always achievable as the kidneys lose function. Early intervention with ACE-inhibitors [antihypertensive drugs], beta-blockers [class of drugs: blocks adrenaline action, slows heart rate, lowers blood pressure] and diuretics is recommended for all hypertensive diabetic patients to prevent irreversible cardiovascular and nephropathic progression.[32]

Cancer... Epidemiological evidence links Type II diabetes with pancreas, liver, colon, breast and endometrium [membrane lining of the uterus] cancers. Long periods of unregulated hyperglycemia and hyperinsulinemia may be causative, as insulin promotes tumor development in the liver and colon. Hyperinsulinemia could also explain the documented role of a high-fat diet and obesity on cancer risk, as well as the inhibiting effects of high fiber intake and physical exercise.[33]

Endocrine-exocrine link... The endocrine and exocrine pancreas are closely linked both anatomically and functionally.[34] Altered gastrointestinal transit and motility [spontaneous movement] are common in Type I and Type II diabetes. Rapid changes in blood glucose affect motility, while chronic hyperglycemia can induce autonomic [self-controlling, functionally independent] nervous system dysfunction in the gastrointestinal tract. Nausea, vomiting, early satiety, weight loss, diarrhea, constipation and upper gastric pain frequently occur with diabetes.[35] Infection and secondary diseases of the stomach, liver, gallbladder, pancreas, and small and large intestines are also possible.[36] Conversely, exocrine dysfunction such as chronic pancreatitis progressively disrupts islet functioning. In any metabolic partnership, dysfunction in one partner adversely impacts the other.[34]

Glucagon... Glucose Counterregulation

The pancreas manufactures glucagon in the alpha islets of Langerhans. Glucagon secretion raises blood glucose, exactly the opposite of insulin action. This counterregulation first involves insulin suppression by means of the pancreatic hormone somatostatin, after which glucagon stimulates the liver to convert its glucose store of glycogen back into blood glucose as follows:

$$\underline{\text{stored in the liver}} \qquad\qquad \underline{\text{in the blood}}$$
$$\text{glycogen} \; + \; \text{water} \; \rightarrow \; \text{glucose}$$
$$C_6H_{10}O_5 \; + \; H_2O \; \rightarrow \; C_2H_{12}O_6$$

With a healthy liver, glycogen is usually sufficient to prevent hypoglycemia, although approaching hypoglycemia can trigger sympathetic response in adrenal medulla adrenaline to generate energy. If glucagon and adrenaline are insufficient or impaired, then adrenal cortex cortisol becomes involved, producing new glucose from glycerol and other substrates. This triad or three-level approach to counterregulation is called gluconeogenesis. The liver is first-line defense and the key to effective gluconeogenesis.

Hypoglycemia, like diabetes, is of two types: (1) reactive hypoglycemia is a pre-diabetic condition of hyperinsulinism, as injured beta islets over respond. Low blood glucose occurs in reaction to an antecedent event, typically a meal containing carbohydrates. Much more rare is (2) fasting hypoglycemia, a serious often-disabling derangement of the gluconeogenesis triad. During stress such as physical exercise, blood glucose rises with reactive hypoglycemia, but falls with fasting hypoglycemia. Fasting hypoglycemia is also called spontaneous hypoglycemia. Avoiding hypoglycemia is fundamental to clear thinking and long-term cerebral health because glucose is the only fuel the brain normally uses.

Symptoms of hypoglycemia vary from mild to severe, starting with gnawing hunger and weakness, then trembling and nervousness, irritability, cold clammy hands, sweating, blurred vision, dizziness, inability to concentrate, mental confusion and headache as low blood glucose becomes massive stress. Each hypoglycemia syndrome has its own unique pattern and progression of symptoms. Severe symptoms proceed from splitting headache to behavioral changes, stupor, convulsions and coma when blood glucose falls to dangerous and finally lethal levels.

Review of the Medical Literature

Nature and symptoms… Hypoglycemia and its accompanying symptoms develop when blood glucose falls to abnormally low levels, below 0.55 g/l.[37] Hypoglycemia symptoms are neurogenic [of nerve origin] and/or neuroglycopenic [brain glucose deprivation]. Neurogenic symptoms include hunger, trembling, tingling, anxiety, sweating and palpitations from physiological changes in the autonomic [self-controlling, functionally independent] nervous system response to hypoglycemia. Neuroglycopenic symptoms of weakness, fatigue, feeling warm, confusion, cognitive failure, seizures and coma result from brain glucose deprivation. Awareness thresholds shift to lower blood glucose levels following prior episodes of hypoglycemia, causing loss of warning symptoms and 'hypoglycemia unawareness' [see "Diabetic emergency/insulin shock" earlier].[38]

Brain… Glucose is normally the only fuel used by the brain. Hence, a continuous supply is needed for normal cerebral metabolism.[39] During severe and prolonged hypoglycemia, excitatory amino acids damage neurons in the cerebral cortex [outer layers of the brain; where thought processes take place] and hippocampus [cerebral cortex area involved in long-term memory].[40]

Reactive hypoglycemia... Postprandial [after a meal] reactive hypoglycemia can develop in patients with pre-diabetes, gastrointestinal dysfunctions or hormone deficiencies. A large patient group has idiopathic [of unknown cause] reactive hypoglycemia, which is disputed. However, characteristic changes in insulin secretion, either dysinsulinism or hyperinsulinism, accompany each of these conditions. Dietary restriction of refined carbohydrates is the best way to manage meal-related reactive hypoglycemia.[41]

Gluconeogenesis... Averting hypoglycemia involves deactivating insulin and activating the counterregulatory hormones glucagon, epinephrine [adrenaline], cortisol and growth hormone.[6] While all four of these hormones oppose insulin action,[42] a hierarchy exists in counterregulation,[6] with glucagon the primary agent responsible for defense against hypoglycemia.[42] Glucagon strongly stimulates hepatic [liver] glucose output.[43] Absent glucagon, epinephrine becomes essential. Cortisol and growth hormone normally serve during recovery from acute hypoglycemia.[42] The glucose threshold for release of counterregulatory hormones is approximately 0.70 g/l.[6]

Liver... is central to gluconeogenesis and glucose homeostasis. Any disruption in liver metabolism, for example from drug or alcohol toxicity, can affect the glycogenolytic [liver glycogen → blood glucose] pathway and trigger fasting hypoglycemia.[44, 45] Hepatic glycogen storage diseases (GSDs) [rare genetic disorders] disable the enzymes of this pathway and bring on persistent hypoglycemia, hepatomegaly [enlargement of the liver], poor physical growth and abnormal blood and liver function tests. Usually diagnosed in infancy or early childhood, GSDs require a special diet to avoid the glycogenolytic pathway.[45]

Other reasons for hypoglycemia... The most frequent causes of hypoglycemia are diabetic related: over-zealous glycemic control with exogenous [outside the body] insulin and sulphonylurea drugs [hypoglycemic agents for diabetic treatment], or 'hypoglycemic unawareness' from defective gluconeogenesis counterregulation, especially in Type I juvenile diabetes. Hypoglycemia also occurs with alcohol consumption,[46] liver and kidney failure, hormone deficiency diseases, acute cardiac insufficiency,[37] congestive heart failure [ineffective pumping of the heart causing fluid to accumulate in the lungs], sepsis [organisms in the blood, e.g. pathogens and their toxins invading the body], chronic malnutrition and acute calorie deprivation.[47] Insulinoma [beta-islet tumor] produces hyperinsulinemia and persistent hypoglycemia.[37] Ninety percent of insulinomas are benign.[48] Autoimmune hypoglycemia from insulin or insulin-receptor antibodies is rare.[37]

Infants and children... Neonatal [the first four weeks after birth] hypoglycemia is common in both preterm and term infants, and can be symptomatic or asymptomatic.[49] Blood evaluation to identify at-risk newborns is critically important.[50] Serious diseases may be responsible, specifically congenital hyperinsulinism (CHI), which causes hypoglycemia, coma and severe brain damage if left untreated,[51] and persistent hyperinsulinemic hypoglycemia of infancy (PHHI), the most common form of infant hypoglycemia.[52] Diazoxide [drug that is vasodilator, antidiuretic and hypoglycemic agent] is an effective long-term PHHI treatment for many infants, but often ineffective in neonatal forms. Anatomical lesions, either focal or diffuse, are causative.[53] Limited pancreatic resection completely cures focal lesions, whereas diffuse lesions require partial pancreatectomy [surgical removal of the pancreas], which carries diabetic risk.[52] Conservative PHHI management, although difficult for the family and physician, is the best course as long as normal glucose levels can be maintained.[54]

Herbs

Avoiding hypoglycemia and diabetes dysfunctions and diseases is crucial for vigorous health and long life. This requires natural, complete nutrition from complex-carbohydrate macronutrients, B vitamin whole-grain cereals and nutritional yeasts, Omega 6 EFAs and Omega 3 fish fatty acids, trace metals and herbs. Table 10-1 presents effective endocrine pancreas herbs with subheadings indicating specific use.

BILBERRY

Bilberry is the only herb required to maintain pancreatic health. Take 40 mg of standardized 25%-anthocyanin Bilberry extract once a week to once a month, twice a week and possibly more often with diabetes. Bilberry maintains the microvascular structures of the pancreas with its special anthocyanin flavonoids. It also safeguards the retinal capillaries of your eyes as you get older. In fact, this herb is excellent for all microvascular structures of the body. Table 7-4 reports this "Specific Healer" role including medical literature on diabetic retinopathy and other microvascular problems.

Rebuilding endocrine pancreas health is a much more difficult assignment than simple maintenance. Exhausted, injured and dead beta islets of Langerhans give rise to reactive hypoglycemia and diabetes. Herbs #2 through #13 of Table 10-1 can help rebuild islet function.

Two key rebuilding herbs are Beech Bark (#2) for beta islets of Langerhans insulin and its pituitary control, and Yarrow (#3) for alpha islets glucagon and its pituitary control. If necessary, take these powerfully good herbs once every two to three weeks (maximum) to improve insulin and glucagon response.

TABLE 10-1. ENDOCRINE PANCREAS HERBS.

Subheadings (underlined) specify use. Numbering of herbs #1 through #13 indicates "need for."

Herb	Comments
<u>MAINTAIN HEALTH, i.e. **ESSENTIAL**</u>	
#1 Bilberry	For eyes too. Also adrenal medulla nerves (Table 7-3) and healing (Table 7-4).
<u>REBUILD HEALTH – GLUCOSE METABOLISM HORMONES</u>	
#2 Beech Bark	For insulin and its pituitary control (Chapter 8). Improves reactive hypoglycemia and Type II diabetes. Overuse can distress insulin, adrenal medulla-Energy mechanisms and the exocrine pancreas.
#3 Yarrow	For glucagon and its pituitary control (Chapter 8). Improves both reactive and fasting hypoglycemia. Overuse can distress glucagon, liver and adrenal gluconeogenesis mechanisms and the exocrine pancreas. Also for adrenal cortex immune (Table 7-6).
<u>REBUILD HEALTH</u> (approximate order of importance)	
#4 Stevia rebaudiana	Antidiabetic and antihypoglycemic, yet a natural sweetener!
#5 Blueberries	Other blue-pigmented fruits and vegetables helpful, e.g. black seedless grapes, Savoy cabbage.
#6 American Ginseng	Antidiabetic. Also adrenal energy (Table 7-3) and stress (Table 7-5).
#7 Sarsaparilla plus Saw Palmetto Berries for males, Black Cohosh for females.	Sex/endocrine pancreas/glucose link.

Herb	Comments
#8 Buchu	Also nerves (Table 7-3).
#9 Fenugreek	See Diabetes, below.
#10 Strawberry, Raspberry and Blackberry Leaves	Good together or separately. Also nerves (Table 7-3). Eating strawberries, raspberries and blackberries can improve pancreatic functioning too.
#11 Damiana	Antidiabetic and antihypoglycemic. See Adrenal Balance (Table 7-2).
#12 Eyebright	Eye problems. Also immune (Table 7-6).
#13 Uva ursi (Bearberry)	Antidiabetic. A heath family (Ericaceae) leaf like Blueberry Leaf, below.

DIABETES

Gymnema sylvestre	Significantly reduces blood glucose levels. Effective adjunct in Type I and Type II diabetic glucose control.
Fenugreek	Improves blood glucose profiles of both Type I and Type II diabetics. Rebuilds function.

HEALING THE PANCREAS (see Table 7-4 and text there)

Alfalfa Seed Tea	Helps to heal the pancreas, adrenal gland and nervous system. Also for energy (Table 7-3). Seeds for pituitary exocrine pancreas carbohydrate digestion (Figure 10-A ahead).
Bilberry	Helps to heal microvascular structures.

AVOID

Blueberry Leaf	Acts like an insulin injection! Quickly becomes very harsh; depletes Vitamin B12.

Beech Bark and Yarrow are also beneficial in a general maintenance program with Hydrangea (Table 7-5), the micronutrient of fat/fatty acid metabolism and its pituitary control. For any task in life, physiological activity flows naturally from Energy to (→) Stress and finally to gluconeogenesis. Energy comes from glucose metabolism using insulin, Stress from fat burning by cells, and gluconeogenesis is triggered by glucagon. Therefore, on a single day and coinciding with activities and the natural flow of hormones, ingest Beech Bark, later Hydrangea, and lastly Yarrow to develop peak performance in these linked systems. Taking these three herbs out of order frustrates metabolism, while taking them together causes pituitary overstimulation. Of course, healthy Energy → Stress → gluconeogenesis requires many conutrients.

Eyes. For better or worse, eyes are closely tied to pancreatic health. When your pancreas and glucose regulation are in trouble, Bilberry, Vitamins A, C and E and carotenoids lutein and zeaxanthin become essential eye protection. A general carotenoid supplement can fulfill lutein and zeaxanthin requirements. With specific eye disorders such as diabetic retinopathy, check the index at the back of the book for more nutritional help.

Herbs for Diabetes

Getting blood glucose under control is PRIORITY ONE for diabetics, and Gymnema sylvestre has efficacy as an adjunct in diabetic glucose control – without side effects! This herb contains gymnemic acid, an organic acid similar in structure to glucose, and gurmarin, a sweetness-suppressing protein. Gymnemic acid blocks glucose effects in the body, while gurmarin acts on taste cells. You can demonstrate gurmarin's action by applying Gymnema sylvestre to the tongue, then tasting something sweet like table sugar. The expected sweetness of sugar is not there.

Gymnema sylvestre reduces blood glucose levels in both Type I and Type II diabetics. Some Type II diabetics can return to dietary control. Consult your physician before using Gymnema sylvestre. Supplement up to 400 mg daily.

Review of the Medical Literature

Sweetness suppression... Gymnema sylvestre contains gurmarin, a sweetness-suppressing polypeptide.[55] Gurmarin acts on taste cells, possibly binding to sweet-taste receptor proteins.[56]

Intestinal absorption... Gymnema sylvestre also contains gymnemic acid, a group of triterpene glycosides. Gymnemic acid inhibits intestinal absorption of glucose in humans and rats,[57, 58] thereby reducing blood glucose levels.[58] Or differently, gymnemic acid acts in glucose-loaded rats as follows: gymnemoside b and gymnemic acids III, V, and VII show little inhibitory activity on glucose absorption, while principal constituents, gymnemic acid I and gymnemasaponin V, exhibit none.[59] Author's Note: Intestinal glucose absorption effects and blood glucose effects of Gymnema sylvestre are separate actions.

Diabetes... Gymnema sylvestre is used in the treatment of diabetes and in food additives for obesity and tooth decay.[60] In a study of 22 Type II [adult onset] diabetics on conventional oral anti-hyperglycemic drugs, GS4 [a Gymnema sylvestre leaf extract] supplemented at 400 mg daily over 18-20 months significantly decreased blood glucose, glycosylated hemoglobin [important measure of diabetes control] and glycosylated plasma proteins. Conventional drug usage could be cut back in these patients, and five of the 22 discontinued drugs altogether and maintained glycemic control using GS4 alone. GS4 supplementation also increased insulin activity.[61] In another study of 27 Type I [juvenile diabetes] patients on insulin therapy, GS4 at 400 mg daily lowered fasting blood glucose, glycosylated hemoglobin and plasma proteins, and insulin requirements. Blood lipids [fats and fat-related compounds, e.g. cholesterol] improved to near normal levels.[62]

More on cholesterol... In animal studies, Gymnema sylvestre markedly reduces blood cholesterol.[63] High doses of gymnemic acid increase fecal cholesterol excretion.[64]

––––––––––

The herb Fenugreek improves the blood glucose profiles of both Type I and Type II diabetics. As reported in the medical literature, Fenugreek has unique antidiabetic action and works well with the trace metal vanadium in controlling glucose levels. This herb rebuilds beta islet function to some extent, and so benefits both diabetics and hypoglycemics.

Review of the Medical Literature

Insulin/Type II Diabetes... 4-Hydroxyisoleucine, a peculiar amino acid present only in Fenugreek (Trigonella foenum-graecum) seeds and not in human tissue,[65] increases glucose-induced pancreatic insulin release in humans and animals. Ineffective at basal blood glucose levels, 4-hydroxyisoleucine triggers biphasic [both intermediate and fast acting] beta-cell insulin release proportional to glucose, without affecting alpha-cell [secretes glucagon, which raises blood glucose] and delta-cell [secretes somatostatin, which suppresses insulin and inhibits gastric secretion] activity, or other insulin protagonists. 4-Hydroxyisoleucine is a novel drug with potential for treating diabetes.[66, 67]

Type I Diabetes... Fenugreek significantly reduces fasting glucose and 24-hour urinary glucose excretion in Type I [juvenile] diabetics, and improves their Glucose Tolerance Test results. Fenugreek also reduces total blood cholesterol, LDL [low-density lipoproteins, so-called bad cholesterol], VLDL [very LDL] and triglycerides,[68] by inhibiting lipid peroxidation.[69] These results demonstrate Fenugreek usefulness in diabetes management.[68]

Fenugreek/vanadium control... Fenugreek and vanadium [Chapter 6] taken together reverse blood glucose levels and low growth rates in diabetic animals almost to control levels. Fenugreek overcomes vanadium toxicity encountered when the metal is used alone, as their combination requires much lower vanadium dosages. Combined effects restore diabetic parameters better than insulin administration.[70] Fenugreek and vanadium coadministration to diabetic animals also reverses disturbed antioxidant levels and resulting oxidative damage.[71]

Pancreatic digestive enzymes... Fenugreek improves pancreatic lipase [fat digestion] activity,[72] but inhibits three trypsin/chymotrypsin enzymes [protein digestion].[73]

Food intake... Fenugreek contains steroidal saponins.[72] Chronic use increases food intake and the motivation to eat.[74, 72]

Maple Syrup Urine Disease... False positive diagnosis of Maple Syrup Urine Disease [an inherited disorder of branched-chain amino acid metabolism] is possible following Fenugreek ingestion.[75]

Functional Exhaustion

Functional exhaustion of islet of Langerhans cells accounts for part of the dysfunction, disease and symptoms experienced with reactive hypoglycemia and diabetes; injured cells and scar tissue explain the rest. Exhaustion and to some extent injury respond to superior nutrition. Unfortunately, pancreatic dysfunctions and diseases incur more scar tissue than those of adrenal and pituitary glands, and so improvement may be marginal. Results depend significantly upon your body's past and present antioxidant status, as liberal use of antioxidants prevents injury from becoming scar tissue.

Curing functional exhaustion of insulin-producing pancreatic cells is straightforward with the following nutritional regimen. Preliminary nutritional support includes the essential and rebuilding macronutrients, B vitamins, fatty acids and herbs presented earlier in the chapter.

Curing Exhaustion

<u>Biotin-B12 Combination For Hypoglycemia and Diabetes</u>. Combining the B vitamin and trace metal responsible for the same function produces powerful synergy to propel functioning up and over a severe exhaustion "cliff." Good news – the B vitamin biotin and the cobalt metal complex B12 are such a combination for beta islets of Langerhans. Review the facts and medical literature of biotin in Chapter 4 and Vitamin B12 in Chapter 6.

While biotin and B12 taken together can significantly improve beta islet function, exactly how to take them is a little tricky. B12 is effective only in sublingual lozenge, thus producing immediate therapeutic action with no 45-minute delay for digestion and absorption (Figure 4-B). Furthermore, other on-target nutrients beside biotin and B12 contribute to a good outcome here, specifically Bilberry provides microvascular support to beta islets and Oats feed adrenal medulla Energy mechanisms and supply a steady stream of glucose to gentle cycle beta cells in their insulin duties during the *leap forward* in functioning.

HOW-TO: with a small glass of juice or milk, ingest 4000 mcg of biotin supplement, 80 mg of standardized Bilberry extract and one rounded tablespoon of Oats. Allow digestion to take proceed normally and fully by relaxing with your feet up. Then 45 to 50 minutes later, place under the tongue 2000 mcg of Vitamin B12 (sublingual lozenge), and 2000 mcg more after the first lozenge has slowly dissolved away. The synergy of these nutrients immediately impacts beta islets and brings significant improvement in their performance. Higher biotin and B12 dosages generate only slight additional benefit, and use up chromium and other glucose metabolism nutrition at rapid rates. Unfavorably, function exhaustion can reoccur in a weakened pancreas.

<u>Chronic diabetic diseases</u> such as diabetic neuropathy, diabetic retinopathy and

associated kidney disease, hypertension and increased cardiovascular risk involve Figure 12-A(2) adrenal dysfunctions of hypoactive/exhausted Stress and Healing Functions and hyperactive nervous system. Use Chapter 12 therapies to correct this adrenal dis-ease, which contributes strongly to these diabetic complications.

Healing the Pancreas

Apply Chapter 12 "Heal the damage, as much as possible" procedures and regimens to the pancreas using Table 12-5 nutrients. Start with the specified healing for different tissues types, notably protein and fatty acid structures. Then, incorporate specific healers Alfalfa Seed Tea and up to 400 mg of standardized Bilberry extract, and later ingredients such as sunflower seeds, black cherries, "trace metals naturally," zinc, DMAE and alpha-lipoic acid to achieve maximum results. Essential islet nutrition is B vitamin biotin, fatty acids GLA and Omega 3 salmon, possibly Stevia rebaudiana, and later the trace metal Vitamin B12. Vitamin B6 becomes essential if there is significant acinar involvement.

Healing the pancreas is uncertain at best because of its vulnerability to free radical attack and oxidative stress. If you still have a faithful friend in this gland, preventing trouble in the first place must be a prime health objective.

EXOCRINE PANCREAS and DIGESTION

The exocrine pancreas produces digestive enzymes for carbohydrate, protein, fat and phyto-compound (fiber) breakdown. Chapter 3 explains digestion. Pancreatic enzyme production slows down as you get older, and can suffer from the damaging effects of diabetes. Pancreatic enzyme insufficiency causes rapid transit of food and diarrhea, or in some cases constipation, and intestinal gas/flatulence. Over time, enzyme insufficiency can lead to pancreatitis, inflammation of the gland.

Pancreatic digestion improves with the techniques described below. Rapid transit fades first, then diarrhea and constipation, and finally but never completely intestinal gas. Controlling gas is discussed later in the chapter.

Herbs

Herbs are fundamental to rebuilding pancreatic enzyme activity. The macronutrients, B vitamins, fatty acids and trace metals specified earlier compliment and enhance this effort.

fiber	fat
Kiwi Fruit Seeds	**Red Root**
protein	carbohydrate
Papaya Seeds	**Alfalfa Seeds**

FIGURE 10-A. PITUITARY EXOCRINE-PANCREAS HERBS.

Figure 10-A presents the four most important herbs for pancreatic digestion. All are pituitary herbs, restoring normal pituitary function and control over the exocrine pancreas. Only modest control lies in the pancreas itself, therefore stimulating it with digestive enzyme tablets, papaya fruit, bromelain from pineapple, and so forth forces functioning. While this is helpful short term to prime the digestive pump, such technique can be counterproductive long term, further suppressing pituitary oversight and making enzyme supplementation permanently necessary. Only with severe dysfunctions are replacement enzymes an answer too. Provide the necessary nutrition for youthful pituitary oversight and in many cases the exocrine pancreas will leap back to life and good function!

Initial Test of the Pancreas. Once or twice daily over several days, take pancreatic enzyme supplements containing amylase (carbohydrate digestion), trypsin and chymotrypsin or other proteases such as papain and bromelain (protein digestion), lipase (fat digestion), and cellulase (fiber digestion) to see if digestion improves. This will answer the crucial question—is the pancreas part of your digestive problem? If yes, that is, improvement occurs in transit, diarrhea or constipation, intestinal gas or a general sense of well being *down there*, then immediately implement Figure 10-A to consolidate the improvement. If no, consider stomach acid and stomach digestive aids for dyspepsia (ahead) and faulty bile production (Chapter 11).

Figure 10-A herbs are a "direct hit" on pituitary oversight functioning, specifically Alfalfa Seeds for carbohydrate digestion, Papaya Seeds for protein digestion, Red Root for fat digestion, and Kiwi Seeds for phyto-compound digestion. These herbs should be taken together to raise all four digestion "boats" at once, so to speak. 1X dosing is appropriate for minor problems ('X' is defined in Chapter 4 "Therapeutic Action"), but employ at 2X one hour apart for serious dysfunction or complete system failure. Even with regurgitation, some of this medicine will get through. If a particular type of digestion is troublesome, for instance a big carbohydrate meal causes bloating or protein sits down there like a rock, then taking only that particular herb can be corrective.

Alfalfa Seeds rebuild carbohydrate digestion/amylase enzyme production. Ingest 10 to 50 of these small seeds depending on the severity of dysfunction. Use only organic alfalfa seeds for sprouting purposes; any health food store sells them. They can be eaten raw, but be sure to crunch the seeds. An easier way is softening the seeds in hot water; then ingest both seeds and water. The therapeutic action of 10 to 50 seeds is all pituitary control of carbohydrate digestion, whereas the action of thousands of seeds made into tea with no seeds ingested is much broader in effect, and described in Table 7-3, Table 7-4 and texts there.

Papaya Seeds rebuild protein digestion/trypsin and chymotrypsin enzyme production. Papaya fruit can improve protein digestion by supplying plant-based papain enzymes. These enzymes directly stimulate the pancreas and force functioning, which causes pituitary control to become more suppressed, and fruit supplementation more necessary. On the other hand, Papaya Seeds restore pituitary function and oversight control. Ingest the juice from just two or three small black seeds from the center cavity of the fruit. This juice is of unusual taste, although not *ugh* or *yuck*, but perfectly wonderful to your pituitary gland! Crush the seeds in a glass of water, swish vigorously and then strain out the seed material and drink. Or crush the seeds between teeth and suck out the juice. Eating a little of the seed won't hurt.

Red Root rebuilds fat digestion/lipase enzyme production. The first time the author took Red Root; the herb instantly cured not only steatorrhea, but also constant weakness in the lower legs. Both had plagued me for over 15 years. Red Root is available in bulk at herb stores. Chew a very small piece of the hard root or make a mild tea.

Kiwi Seeds rebuild phyto-compound digestion. Kiwi fruit, also known as Chinese gooseberry, is available in every supermarket. Eat the green flesh and the numerous small, black seeds of one fruit. Crunch as many of the seeds as you can since the therapeutic activity lies within them. Kiwi Seeds at 2X dosing have the unexpected side effect of suppressing pituitary carbohydrate digestion. When taking all Figure 10-A herbs at 2X, ingest only 10-15 small Kiwi Seeds in the second dose to eliminate this problem.

Other beneficial herbs—Ginger directly stimulates pancreatic lipase, amylase and trypsin/chymotrypsin production. Fenugreek improves pancreatic lipase activity, but inhibits trypsin/chymotrypsin. Many spices have a positive effect on pancreatic digestion.

Pancreatitis

Pancreatitis is inflammation of the entire gland, although the cause lies with exocrine pancreas functioning or antecedent digestion. Inflammation begins in the pancreatic enzyme duct as it exits into the duodenum. Minor irritation from pancreatic enzyme insufficiency, general digestive insufficiency or obstruction from passing gallstones narrows or completely closes the duct terminus (pancreas head). Juices back up and tissues become irritated and swollen. The inflammation then spreads throughout both exocrine and endocrine parts, producing injury and scar tissue.

Pancreatitis is of two types: acute and chronic. Acute is complete obstruction at the terminus. Enzyme juices begin to digest the pancreas itself, causing excruciating pain. This is life threatening and requires immediate hospitalization. Chronic pancreatitis is a milder smoldering *fire*, oftentimes just a dull pain or awareness at the duct exit.

Chronic pancreatitis responds to these natural modalities:

Digestion. Give your pancreas and digestive system a rest with a water fast, or better yet a plain yogurt fast. Active-culture plain yogurt requires no digestion, yet is soothing and healing to inflamed tissues.

B Vitamins. Functional exhaustion of acinar cells contributes to pancreatitis, and Vitamin B6 supplementation helps to alleviate this exhaustion. Never take B6 alone, except for acute pancreatitis emergency. Use the formula 2 pantothenic acid + 1 B2 + 1 B6 with B2 reduced by one-half to spur pancreatic recovery, as explained in Chapter 4. As for healing, PABA supplementation stimulates repair of injured pancreatic cells.

Fatty Acids act as a healing balm. Vitamin E and beta-carotene promote repair and recovery. If a particular pancreatic enzyme is weak and causative, then its associated fatty acid is needed most. For example, Omega 3 salmon benefits pancreatic lipase insufficiency. Also in this regard, eating salmon fish is superior in its restorative power to supplementing with salmon oil capsules.

Trace Metals. Black Currants, Dandelion Root, Colloidal Minerals and other sources of trace metals naturally support enzyme production and reduce inflammatory symptoms. 2X dosing of "trace metals naturally" is strongly anti-inflammatory. Nickel supplementation can ease pancreatitis and improve healing, particularly if its internal balance partner Vitamin B12 has been taken too often. Supplementing the metal catalysts of Table 6-2 may be needed for a turnaround.

Herbs. Employ Figure 10-A as soon as possible. Ingesting fresh cabbage juice (Green Cabbage, Table 7-4) on an empty stomach can heal and reopen an inflamed pancreatic terminus, and significantly/dramatically relieve pancreatitis. Aloe vera taken internally is also very effective, and these two herbs are excellent together. A fresh aloe poultice on the skin above the pancreas for two hours quenches any smoldering fire in the gland. Again, the gland lies horizontally approximately one inch below the bellybutton and three inches to either side, with the duct exit to the right. Concentrate most of the poultice there. Alfalfa Seed Tea and Bilberry help to heal pancreatitis too. Lobelia helps restore well being during the inflammatory distress of pancreatitis.

Massage. Using the first three fingers (not the thumb) of each hand extended straight out and held together, and with a cotton shirt in-between to reduce friction, gently massage at a 30-degree inclined angle the pancreatic duct exit, which is approximately one inch down and three inches to the right of the bellybutton. First massage to the left with the right-hand fingers, then to the right with left fingers. Find the pain spot, i.e. the "knot" (narrowed terminus), and press down to try to get it to release. Vibrate the fingers on the knot. However, don't overdo it and create more swollen, painful tissues. A little massage every few hours and over several days is the best therapy. When the knot finally releases, pancreatic juices will pour out and leave a tender duodenum behind. Therefore, massaging 45 minutes to one hour after ingestion of fresh cabbage juice or Aloe vera is an effective therapy. Having soothing agents like these in the duodenum when pain knot releases will significantly reduce any resulting tenderness. Pulsating, warm water massage on the skin above the knot is also soothing and corrective.

Digestive Enzymes. Severe chronic pancreatitis and steatorrhea require permanent pancreatic digestive enzyme replacement of amylase, proteases, lipase and possibly cellulase. In the medical literature below, Mayo Clinic reports that large doses of lipase, at least 90,000 USP, are needed to overcome steatorrhea. Pure lipase can be purchased from Internet pharmacies.

> ### Review of the Medical Literature

Acute Pancreatitis (AP)… has many causes, but one basic mechanism: premature activation and retention of proteolytic [splitting of proteins by hydrolysis] enzymes injures acinar [exocrine pancreas] cells. Released cytokines [non-antibody proteins/signaling molecules of the immune system] attract inflammatory agents, particularly neutrophils [specialized white blood cell], and in a cascade more cytokines, inflammation and free radicals including nitric oxide [NO: released during macrophage inflammation] induce pancreatic edema [abnormal accumulation of fluid, swelling] and necrosis [tissue death]. Cytokines also increase acinar cell apoptosis [gene-directed, programmed cell death], further contributing to the necrosis.[76] Metabolic complications can be hypoglycemia, hyperglycemia, diabetic ketoacidosis [ketone buildup with alkaline depletion], hyperlipemia [high blood cholesterol], blood coagulation problems and hypocalcemia [low blood calcium]. Hypocalcemia usually indicates a poor prognosis.[77] Systemic complications can be hypotension [low blood pressure], hypoxia [inadequate oxygen], tachycardia [rapid heartbeat, usually 150-200 beats per minute], capillary leak syndrome and fever.[76] AP can progress to multisystem disease states of respiratory distress, myocardial [heart muscle] depression and shock, and/or acute kidney failure. Recovery from severe AP requires early recognition and management of complications.[77]

Diagnosis and treatment... Alcohol abuse or gallstone obstruction are typical causes of acute pancreatitis. Serum amylase [carbohydrate-digesting enzyme] and serum lipase [fat-digesting enzyme] can confirm the diagnosis, although serum trypsin [protein-digesting enzyme] is the most accurate laboratory test.[78] With severe AP, the primary determinant of outcome is the extent of pancreatic necrosis and subsequent infection.[79] Treatment must include early aggressive fluid resuscitation, intensive support of pancreatic functions, antibiotic prophylaxis [preventative] and surgery in cases of infected pancreatic necrosis or patient deterioration. With gallstone AP, endoscopic [flexible viewing instrument with diagnostic and/or therapeutic roles] removal of the stones is frequently necessary.[80]

Chronic pancreatitis (CP)... involves loss of function from progressive destruction of pancreatic tissues and changes in gland architecture.[81] Pancreatic head enlargement, calcification of functional parts, cysts, stones, fibrosis [forming fibrous tissue] and proliferation of duct cells characterize CP. [82] Diagnosis may be easy or difficult depending on disease severity and its evolution.[81] The most common symptom is pain, at least initially. Recurrent abdominal pain, steatorrhea [visible fat in the stools], fat and protein malabsorption, and diabetes usually emerge in advanced stages of CP, however, atypical presentations are not infrequent.[81, 83] Alcohol abuse is often a factor.[81]

Treatment... Pancreatic duct drainage can normalize duct and tissue pressure and reduce pain in 70% of chronic pancreatitis patients. Drainage by endoscopy may relieve symptoms.[84] About 40% of patients require surgery to preserve functional parts and prevent further decline in enzyme production.[83, 84] Indicators for surgery are intractable pain, duct narrowing, cysts and the presence of an inflammatory mass in the pancreatic head.[85] In 263 CP surgeries at Johns Hopkins over a seventeen year period, the most common symptoms were abdominal pain (88%), weight loss (36%), nausea/vomiting (30%), jaundice (14%), and diarrhea (12%). Overall mortality was 1.9%. Surgery brought improvements in all aspects of quality of life, and is an excellent option for CP patients.[86]

Steatorrhea... In decompensated [inability to maintain functioning] chronic pancreatitis, steatorrhea [visible fat in the stools] and diabetes are dominant symptoms with hypoglycemia and infection possible. Steatorrhea requires pancreatic enzyme replacement therapy, using porcine [from a pig] pancreatin [mixture of pancreatic enzymes and juices] and bacterial and/or acid-resistant fungal lipase enzymes.[87] Recommended lipase dosage for severe insufficiency is at least 90,000 USP units with meals. In most patients, this lipase dose improves fat absorption, and may eliminate steatorrhea.[88]

Exocrine-endocrine link… In the majority of chronic pancreatitis patients, endocrine involvement accompanies the exocrine dysfunction. The incidence of impaired glucose tolerance is 40-70%, and half of these patients develop diabetes. Endocrine onset and severity depend on alcohol consumption and the destruction of functional parts. Severe hypoglycemia also develops in CP diabetic patients from impaired glucagon activity, liver glycogen dysfunction due to alcohol toxicity, and malnutrition. Endocrine insufficiency increases progressively with CP; long-term complications of CP diabetics are similar to those of Type I [juvenile diabetes] patients.[89]

Stomach Acid and Digestion

Too much stomach acid and too little stomach acid are opposite sides of the same coin. Just as hyperinsulin reactive hypoglycemia is precursor to hypoinsulin diabetes, so hyperacidity is precursor to hypoacidity. Hyper function is always the mild state of dysfunction, hypo function the more advanced and serious disorder. Both problems, however, require the same cure.

To normalize stomach acidity, you must restore pituitary control over the stomach acid pump. And the controlling nutrient is found in Citrus Seeds, the white pulp of orange, tangerine, grapefruit, lemon and lime seeds. Each seed type produces a slightly different therapeutic effect, so for best results ingest seed pulp from several different fruits. With hyperacidity, take at 1X dosing only to regain internal control and normalize acid production. With hypoacidity, 2X boosts stomach acid flow. Adding Citrus Seed pulp to the pancreatic therapies of Figure 10-A produces digestive synergy, as does Chapter 11 aromatic seeds of Anise, Caraway, Fennel, Coriander and Dill for strong bile flow.

Antacid preparations for hyperacidity are a major industry – and repeat business! Restoring pituitary control and health with Citrus Seeds and possibly pituitary trace metals are a better answer, or partial answer. "Partial" because dead cells in the stomach acid machinery do not respond to any therapy. Antacids may still be needed, only fewer of them. Calcium oxide and calcium carbonate (which is calcium oxide plus carbon dioxide) are safer antacid choices than magnesium or aluminum-based compounds. Of course, do not use non-chelated calcium oxide or calcium carbonate as a bone supplement, since little of this calcium is absorbed from the digestive tract. Drugs such as acid pump blockers provide more effective acid relief, but with side effects. These drugs are reviewed in the medical literature below.

An acid sensitive stomach may require elimination of all acidic foods and supplements from the diet including Vitamin C and even bone-saving chelated calcium citrate. Substitutes can be non-acidic Ester-C and an amino acid chelated calcium supplement. At the opposite extreme of stomach hypoacidity, consuming oranges, grapefruits and other acid fruits with big meals will sustain protein digestion. These foods are gentler than hydrochloric acid supplements, commonly called bentaine hydrochloride.

Dyspepsia is the medical term for indigestion. Some natural remedies for dyspepsia are:

Alfalfa Seeds or Alfalfa Seed Tea improves both pancreatic and stomach carbohydrate digestion. See exocrine pancreas "Herbs" earlier.

Peppermint and Spearmint. These soothing mints ease carbohydrate indigestion and bloating.

Comfrey stimulates production of the stomach protein-digesting enzyme pepsin.

Ginger settles a sour stomach and improves stomach fat digestion and possibly protein digestion. Ginger can alleviate intestinal cramping. Stomach digestion is directly *wired* to adrenal cortex fatigue function, and Ginger stimulates these functions and the link between them, as does Horseradish.

Horseradish compliments and counterbalances Ginger's therapeutic action. Horseradish promotes gastric secretions.

Raw Garlic. While much more fatigue centered than Ginger and Horseradish, Raw Garlic further compliments the stomach-fatigue-fat link. Sequence Ginger, Horseradish and Garlic to spiral gastric functioning up and back to normal. If these three herbs and/or rebalancing sodium-potassium equilibrium (Na $\rightleftharpoons$ K, presented next) relieve indigestion, then adrenal cortex fatigue exhaustion may be part of the malfunction here. Chapter 12 gives fatigue exhaustion solutions.

Na ⇌ K is another factor in stomach-fatigue interaction. Imbalances in sodium and potassium body salts contribute to stomach hydrochloric acid dysfunction. Chapter 11 explains how to correct this electrolyte problem.

Vasoconstriction ⇌ vasodilation imbalance can cause stomach distress. See Chapter 7 herbs Shepherd's Purse/Woundwort and Heather.

General Tonics. Many spices contain natural digesting enzymes that improve digestion.

Take a Break. Remember Mom's advice, "After you eat, don't go in the pool for 30 minutes!" Basically, activating adrenal hormones adrenaline, cortisol or aldosterone impairs stomach digestion. Keep these hormones quiet during digestion and your stomach will thank you.

When Nothing Will Stay Down. Try plain yogurt. It requires no human digestion, yet gives quality nourishment. However, the taste may be too disagreeable and only add to a difficult circumstance. Chicken soup and eggs are gentle and relatively easy to digest. These may provide enough nutrition to start the turnaround.

Stomach Dysfunctions and Diseases

Review of the Medical Literature

Overview... Gastric acid breaks down the proteins in the food, making them more available to proteolytic enzymes. It also kills ingested pathogens. Gastric acid dysfunction is a major factor in peptic ulcer disease and reflux esophagitis [heartburn].[90] Abnormal secretion of acid and pepsin [protein digestive enzyme of the stomach] alters the mucosal barrier [mucous membrane], thereby contributing to gastric and duodenal ulcer development. Helicobacter pylori [H. pylori] bacterial infection plays a central role in gastric and duodenal ulcers, as well as chronic gastritis [inflammation of the stomach].[91] H. pylori is also associated with gastric cancer, but not with reflux esophagitis and non-ulcer dyspepsia.[92] In the last 30 years, the discoveries of H2-receptors [histamine type2 receptors], the gastric acid pump and its blockers, and H. pylori have revolutionized ulcer treatment. Today, ulcers are more or less solved by antibiotics, whereas reflux disease remains problematic.[93]

Gastritis... H. pylori infection causes nearly all chronic gastritis, as cytotoxic [cyto- prefix meaning 'cell'] and inflammatory agents from the bacterium induce gastric epithelium [surface tissue lining] cell damage. Gastric acid physiology is complex, with gastritis involving interaction of H. pyroli virulence and host and environmental factors. Possible clinical outcomes are asymptomatic gastritis, gastric and duodenal ulcer, gastric carcinoma [malignant tumor that begins in the stomach lining or epithelium] and gastric MALT lymphoma [below]. H. pylori usually increases acid secretion in duodenal ulcer patients, but reduces acid output in gastric cancer patients.[94]

Peptic ulcer disease... Since its 1983 discovery in gastritis mucosa, H. pylori has been found in over 70% of gastric and 90% of duodenal ulcer patients.[95] Stress, aspirin and other NSAIDs [nonsteroidal anti-inflammatory drugs] can also cause peptic ulcers.[96, 97] Antibiotic therapy provides a lifelong cure for most H. pylori-infected ulcer patients.[98] In addition, antibiotics facilitate healing and reduce the risk of bleeding.[95, 97] Acid pump blockers [drug treatment, below] also improve mucosal healing and prevent recurrence when taken long term.[93]

Bleeding ulcers and NSAIDs... Risk factors for upper gastrointestinal tract bleeding and perforation are NSAID use, advanced age, peptic ulcer disease history and being male. NSAID use with advanced age and/or ulcer history carries the greatest risk.[99] NSAIDs damage the gastroduodenal mucosa through topical irritation of the epithelium, impairment of mucosal barrier function and blood flow, and suppression of gastric prostaglandins [potent mediators of many conduction/transmitter functions] and therefore repair.[100] Most harmful of these factors is suppression of cytoprotective prostaglandins PGE2 and PGI2 by inhibiting the COX (cyclo-oxygenase) enzyme.[101] Gastroduodenal ulceration and bleeding are major limitations to NSAID use.[100]

Cancer and H. pylori... H. pylori colonization of the stomach is associated with gastric mucosa-associated lymphoid tissue (MALT) and consequent MALT lymphoma [malignant tumor], gastric adenocarcinoma [tumor involving cells of the wall lining], and even pancreatic adenocarcinoma.[94] The immunological response to H. pylori infection leads to the formation of lymphoid follicles/nodal tissues in the stomach. Early diagnosis of MALT lymphoma is difficult; symptoms are vague and varied. Abdominal pain is a common complaint.[102] H. pylori eradication brings long-term remission of MALT lymphoma in more than 50% of patients.[103] However, reappearance can occur years after treatment, and thus patient follow-up must continue indefinitely.[102]

Acid reflux (heartburn) and treatment... Gastro-esophageal reflux disease (GERD) is among the most common diagnoses in gastroenterology.[104] Here, regurgitation of gastric juices damages the esophagus. Acid neutralization and/or suppression are the cornerstones of GERD treatment. Currently, three classes of drugs eliminate hyperacidity: antacids, histamine2 receptor antagonists (H2RAs), and proton pump inhibitors (PPIs). Antacids neutralize stomach pH, however, their short-term action and limited effectiveness neither prevent nor heal the esophageal injury. Furthermore, many daily doses may be necessary to control symptoms. H2RAs act by inhibiting the histamine-dependent pathway that stimulates gastric acid secretion. Unfortunately, several other pathways promote acid secretion and, as a result, H2RA results are inconsistent. The most effective GERD medication is PPIs, which block acid secretion at its source, the proton pump of the gastric parietal [organ wall] cell. PPIs are more effective than H2RAs in correcting symptoms, preventing esophageal injury and healing esophagitis. PPIs also show efficacy in gastric and duodenal ulcers. The four current PPI drugs in the USA are omeprazole, lansoprazole, rabeprazole and pantoprazole.[105] Pantoprazole is the only PPI that does not interact with other drugs, and therefore is the treatment of choice for patients taking other medications.[106] A possible major GERD complication is Barrett epithelium metaplasia [abnormal surface tissue lining] and its risk of esophageal adenocarcinoma. Affected tissue can be removed by endoscopic thermal ablation, however, this treatment has risks and long-term efficacy studies are lacking.[104]

PPI side effects... PPI long-term side effects can include bacterial overgrowth of the digestive system, intestinal infections, enterochromaffin-like cell [irregular stomach musoca cell that produces histamine] hyperplasia [enlargement due to abnormal cell multiplication], carcinoids [gastrointestinal tumors arising from neuroendocrine cells], gastric adenocarcinoma particularly in H. pylori patients, and malabsorption of vitamins, minerals and fats. Vitamin B12 status should be checked in all PPI patients.[107]

Antacids... Self-prescribed antacid medications contain calcium carbonate and/or magnesium and aluminum compounds. Antacids partially neutralize gastric hydrochloric acid and inhibit pepsin secretion. While antacid usage for GERD and gastric and duodenal ulcers has fallen significantly following H2RA and PPI development, antacids are still of value in treating stress-related gastritis, minor episodes of heartburn (GERD), and non-ulcer dyspepsia [below]. Antacid-drug interactions are a concern and can occur when gastric pH changes affect hydrolysis of drugs and urinary pH changes affect drug elimination, but rescheduling medication times can avoid most interactions. Antacid side effects are generally minor with short-term use; however, large doses over long periods can negatively impact other diseases including chronic kidney failure. Maintaining electrolyte status and avoiding aluminum antacids, which bind to dietary phosphate during chronic kidney failure, minimize any adverse effects.[108]

Non-ulcer dyspepsia (indigestion)... is persistent or recurrent upper abdominal discomfort or pain without structural or biochemical explanation. Exact causes remain unresolved.[109] No strong association exists between H. pylori and non-ulcer dyspepsia,[110] although with H. pylori positive non-ulcer dyspepsia, eradication of the bacterium may correct the dyspepsia.[111] PPIs show effectiveness in twelve dyspepsia trials, but GERD patients may not have been adequately excluded.[112, 113] H2RAs may be superior to placebo, but many of these studies have suboptimal design. Antacids are no more effective than placebo for treatment of non-ulcer dyspepsia.[113]

Intestinal Gas/Flatulence

Intestinal gas is an unfortunate side effect of poor digestion. Undigested organic matter ferments and decays in the presence of putrefactive bacteria, liberating obnoxious gases such as ammonia and methane. These anaerobic bacteria and resulting gases are exactly the same as found in swamp and sewer. Ammonia is particularly damaging; it irritates intestinal membranes and can pass into the blood. Large quantities of gas cause bloating with accompanying discomfort to extreme pain. This contributes to diverticulosis, or small-herniated bulges in the large intestine wall called diverticula.

Stopping the gas. Beyond improving digestion with the therapies for the pancreas, stomach acid and dyspepsia here in Chapter 10 and for bile in Chapter 11, the only solution to intestinal gas is replacing the bad putrefactive bacteria in the gut with good bacteria. Active-culture ("it's alive") yogurt replaces these putrefactive bacteria, shutting down gas formation. Yogurt before or after each meal is especially effective. The more yogurt you eat, the less gas you will have!

Active-culture yogurt contains lactobacillus acidophilus and other friendly probiotic bacteria. These good bacteria *eat* only milk and milk sugar. Yogurt is actually predigested milk, and so requires no further action by the human digestive system. It passes through stomach and intestines as is, and its nutrients are absorbed directly into the bloodstream. Therefore, even adults with lactose intolerance can eat yogurt. Any digestive disturbance from yogurt is due to taste and psychosomatic response. Definitely, it's an acquired taste. Fortunately, yogurt becomes much more palatable when mixed with fruit. Many active-culture fruit combinations are commercially available.

Acidophilus milk and acidophilus capsules are poor, ineffective substitutes for yogurt. While they can contain billions of good bacteria, what's required to control intestinal gas is several orders of magnitude more of these benefactors, from 4 to 8 ounces of yogurt daily and even greater amounts during acute episodes. Acidophilus capsules are slow to achieve such high lactobacillus numbers and overcome bad bacteria, because they must first grow and consume any milk products present; meanwhile the human digestive system is doing the same.

Yogurt provides additional benefits besides gas control. It eliminates most bad breaths, which are in fact caused by the same putrefactive bacteria. The exceptions are bad breaths from diseased gums and tonsils. Yogurt also inhibits the growth of ingested strep, staph, salmonella and other pathogenic bacteria, and helps to alleviate diarrhea. Yogurt has proven efficacy for ulcerative colitis, and generally modulates inflammatory disease processes while strengthening immunity. Yogurt has a soothing, healing effect on gastrointestinal sores, ulcers, diverticula and inflamed tissues. You can feel this soothing and healing by applying yogurt to sunburn – instant relief! Another unusual example is laryngitis. Gargling with plain yogurt will coat the vocal cords, ease the inflammation and kill off the infection.

Review of the Medical Literature

Intestinal health… Microbial balance is an important factor in maintaining intestinal health and homeostasis. In animal models and human studies, yogurt and other fermented milk products ease lactose intolerance, antibiotic-induced diarrhea and bacterial and viral diarrhea, particularly in infants.[114, 115] Or a slightly different assessment, lactobacillus and other probiotics consistently shorten by one day diarrhea resulting from rotavirus [virus of severe, dehydrating diarrhea] infection, but evidence on other bacterial and viral diarrhea is less strong.[116] Or probiotics are effective in preventing and reducing the severity of acute diarrhea in children.[117] Yogurt and other lactic acid bacteria exert positive effects by resisting pathogen multiplication in the digestive tract.[114] Probiotics prevent intestinal overgrowth of pathogenic bacteria.[118]

Gastrointestinal tract and the immune system… Probiotics maintain the delicate balance that exists between the gastrointestinal tract and immune system. When this balance is disrupted, inflammation and disease result. Beneficial intestinal flora inhibits the inflammation and over stimulation of the immune system caused by pathogenic bacteria. Probiobics modulate disease processes and prevent widespread inflammatory disorders.[118] Moreover, these lactic acid bacteria reinforce non-specific immunity and specific immunity such as IgA [Immunoglobulin A: antibody proteins that protect mucous linings from infection] and IgM [Immunoglobulin M: typically the first antibodies in an immune response].[114]

Ulcerative colitis... Convincing evidence from both animal models and human studies implicates pathogenic bacteria in the initiation and continuation of the inflammatory processes of ulcerative colitis.[119] Probiotics are efficacious therapy for ulcerative colitis and pouchitis [acute inflammation of intestinal mucosa].[119, 120] A disturbance in intestinal flora, or in the host response to this flora, plays a definite role in the pathogenesis of inflammatory bowel disease (IBD) [chronic disorder of ulcerative colitis and/or Crohn's disease with abdominal cramping and persistent diarrhea].[121]

Vaginitis, vaginosis... The beneficial effect of yogurt consumption on general health and on the mucosal [mucous membrane] immune system is well established.[122] Lactobacillus recolonization utilizing yogurt or lactobacillus capsules is a promising treatment for both yeast vaginitis [Candida infection] and bacterial vaginosis.[123]

Anticancer... Experimental data indicate probiotic activity against human cancer, but clinical evidence is lacking.[115] In a mouse model, dietary yogurt inhibits the development of a colorectal carcinoma through immunoregulatory mechanisms that reduce the inflammatory response. Yogurt increases IgA, IL-10 [Interlukin-10: its routine function is to limit and ultimately terminate inflammatory responses] and cancer cell apoptosis [gene-directed, programmed cell death].[123]

Food allergies... Allergic food reactions in infants generally manifest in the gastrointestinal tract and cause inflammation of the mucosa. Probiotics such as lactobacillus significantly ameliorate these allergic disorders.[124]

Lactose intolerance... In the gastrointestinal tract, the enzyme lactase coverts lactose [milk sugar] into glucose and galactose, which are then absorbed into the bloodstream. Lactase activity decreases after age 4 to 6 years in most human beings, except for the Caucasian race. Lactose intolerance causes bloating, flatulence, abdominal pain and diarrhea from undigested lactose reaching the large intestine. However, yogurt is well tolerated by lactose intolerant individuals.[125] In these persons, lactose absorption occurs with yogurt and lactase-added milk, but not with acidophilus milk.[115]

OVERVIEW

"We first make our habits, and then our habits make us." –John Dryden. If you have bad habits with regard to consuming simple sugars, you need to break them before they break you with debilitating pancreatic dysfunctions and diseases. Your pancreas is the one indispensable gland that defies nutritional renewal. Second chances at health abound for the adrenal gland, pituitary, thyroid and liver, but second chances are few and far between for the overworked pancreas. Only through sparing use of your insulin and glucagon hormones can you achieve peak energy performance ("in the zone") and preserve pancreatic function throughout life. Nature's perfect whole-grain cereals are the crucial energy food in this effort.

In addition to the metabolic disarray of hypoglycemia and diabetes, simple sugars exhaust Energy/adrenaline functioning, which then compromises the immune system. Simple sugars also increase harmful homocysteine in the blood, alter blood platelets and their aggregation, accelerate atherosclerosis and heart disease, and contribute to eye diseases, nerve degeneration and the beta-amyloid plaques of Alzheimer's disease. Lastly, simple sugars cause glycosylation and glycation of body proteins, which degrade cell functions and bring premature aging. Not a pretty picture, this addiction to sweets.

Don't forget the digestive side of your pancreas. Pancreatic enzyme production slows down as you get older, and can suffer from the damaging effects of diabetes. Correcting problems of pancreatic enzyme insufficiency, pancreatitis, stomach acidity, dyspepsia, lack of liver bile and intestinal gas/flatulence are essential for peace in your intestinal tract and optimal health.

***

11. LIVER

The liver is the largest organ in the body after the skin, and the only one that can regenerate itself. Up to one-quarter can be damaged or removed, and it will soon regrow to original size and shape. With two lobes, the liver occupies the upper right abdomen below the diaphragm, partly under the rib cage. Like the pancreas, the liver performs both endocrine and digestive (exocrine) duties. Many medical books do not consider the liver to be part of the endocrine system because in management terms, it lacks direct *line responsibility*, instead serving a *staff function*. Liver is included in this book for one huge reason – its performance is essential to every other endocrine gland. Your liver is service provider to many metabolisms.

Endocrine liver functions involve: (1) thousands of chemical reactions, making new molecules for use throughout the body and breaking down old worn-out ones such as amino acids, hormones and red blood cells, and flushing them from the body via the kidneys or bile; (2) storage – keeping hundreds of compounds in stock and ready for distribution, for example fatty acids, glycogen for gluconeogenesis, trace metals, sodium and potassium, calcium and magnesium, but not B vitamins; (3) regulation of many endocrine and body processes including blood clotting and parts of glucose, protein and fat metabolism; and (4) filtering impurities from the blood and detoxifying all harmful substances: alcohol, drugs, cigarette smoke, pollution, hydrocarbon vapors, pesticides, food additives and preservatives, and other air, water and food contaminants. The list of tasks the endocrine liver carries out is almost endless.

The exocrine liver, on the other hand, performs only one task, manufacturing and secreting bile, which contributes crucially to fat digestion. Bile flows from the liver through a bile duct into the gallbladder, a storage sac, or directly in the duodenum, first portion of the small intestine. Bile emulsifies fats, keeping them in blood solution and preventing their deposit on artery walls. As with the pancreas, the endocrine and exocrine liver are linked both anatomically and functionally.

NUTRITION

The liver requires few raw material nutrients. While the adrenal gland, pituitary gland and pancreas closely adhere to Table 2-1 nutrition, liver needs are very different. Mostly the liver employs carbohydrates, proteins, fats (here fatty acids), and fibers for the myriad of new molecules it turns out everyday. The liver does not use trace metals or B vitamins, except choline and inositol in bile synthesis. As for herbs, they improve endocrine liver functions only marginally. However, herbs can significantly boost bile flow, and these digestive aids are presented later in the "Exocrine" section of the chapter. Despite not being needy, the liver does have some unusual raw material requirements, which are outlined in Table 11-1 below.

Poisons, chemical and infectious, injure the liver. These bring on JAUNDICE, or yellowing of the skin from the backup of bilirubin, a natural by-product of red blood cell breakdown, into the blood instead of its excretion in bile; and HEPATITIS, which is inflammation of the liver from chemical or viral agent. Toxic hepatitis is due to chemical poisoning through ingestion, inhalation or skin exposure. Viral hepatitis exists in three types. Hepatitis A develops from an infectious virus found in contaminated water or passed on by contact with oral or stool secretions. Symptoms are similar to influenza, but the eyes and skin may become jaundiced. Hepatitis B virus spreads by blood or sexual contact. Much more virulent than type A, Hepatitis B matures into a chronic infection and eventually cirrhosis, or remains in an asymptomatic carrier state. Most destructive is Hepatitis C, a retrovirus that copies its genome into host DNA. Hepatitis C spreads by blood transfusions or exposure to blood products including intravenous drug abuse. Since its discovery in 1989, Hepatitis C has resisted all treatments except interferon and protease inhibitors. Finally, CIRRHOSIS is massive scar tissue, heaps of dead liver cells. Commonly caused by alcohol abuse, cirrhosis can also occur from hepatitis.

Below the *radar screen* of chemically induced jaundice, hepatitis and cirrhosis, the liver must deactivate many subtle environmental poisons such as cigarette smoke, pollution, hydrocarbon vapors, pesticides, and food additives and preservatives, and flush them from the body. Unfortunately, some chemical toxins can only be captured and held for life. These accumulating toxins cause a slow loss of liver function and, most critically, loss of the liver's ability to grow new cells and revitalize old ones, i.e. to regenerate itself. Table 11-1 gives four therapies to protect your liver from this modern chemical gauntlet. The first three maintain health; the last, if needed, rebuilds function. The rebuilding regimen puts a failed liver regeneration mechanism back into action!

TABLE 11-1. REGIMENS FOR GOOD LIVER HEALTH.
Liver's unusual nutritional requirements.

Raw Material	Comments
MAINTAIN HEALTH, **ESSENTIAL**	
#1 Vitamin C, Bioflavonoids	PROTECTS LIVER CELLS by detoxifying harmful substances. Take 500-1000 mg of natural Vitamin C plus bioflavonoids daily. With an acid-sensitive stomach, use non acidic Ester-C
#2 Silymarin	Extra protection during times of liver distress.
#3 Activated Charcoal	For acute chemical poisoning.
REBUILD HEALTH	
#4 Methionine-Activated Charcoal Regimen	REGENERATES LIVER CELLS.

Maintain Health

#1 VITAMIN C and BIOFLAVONOIDS

Human beings are one of the few mammals that cannot manufacture their own Vitamin C internally. This malfunction, ironically in the liver, leaves the organ vulnerable to slow poisoning. The birth of our species included this genetic defect, which apparently was not significant then because the earliest human diet supplied abundant Vitamin C and bioflavonoids. Sadly, modern human diets are woefully deficient in these natural detoxifiers, and at the very time when new and dangerous chemical toxins are every-where – in the air we breathe, in drinking water and in our food. Your liver desperately needs help! At the very least, restore the genetically missing Vitamin C. A daily supple-ment of 500 to 1000 mg of Vitamin C plus bioflavonoids will preserve, protect and defend this vital organ throughout your life.

The liver uses Vitamin C in its primary detoxification process – glutathione detoxi-fication, which is explained in the medical literature review below. In addition, Vitamin C destroys toxic free radicals before they ever reach the liver and do damage, and it kills hepatitis viruses, limiting any infection. Truly "the right stuff" at the right place!

Review of the Medical Literature

Liver detoxification of poisons… Many hepatotoxic [hepato- prefix meaning 'liver'] chem-icals require glutathione [natural internal antioxidant] detoxification.[1] Within cell mitochondria [cell *organ* responsible for respiration and energy production], glutathione is the main defense against oxidative stress and a major target of chemical toxins.[2] Glutathione destroys these toxic oxygen radicals and free radicals in general, and reduces [donates electrons to] disulfide groups [creating more antioxidants]. While present in all cells, glutathione is especially important in organs with intense toxin exposure such as the liver, kidneys, lungs and intestines.[3] Unfortunately, liver mitochondria lack the enzymes necessary for glutathione synthesis, and glu-tathione deficiency causes widespread mitochondrial damage. Vitamin C protects cells against the lethal effects of glutathione deficiency, preserving glutathione and recycling it during defi-ciency. Overall, glutathione and Vitamin C function together in preventing oxidative injury.[4]

What humans CANNOT do… Induced glutathione deficiency in adult mice generates com-pensating internal Vitamin C synthesis in the liver. This rapid and substantial increase in Vitamin C protects tissues from damage. In contrast, newborn rats (like humans) do not synthesize Vitamin C and suffer severe liver and other organ damage under the same study conditions. However, Vitamin C administration prevents this damage in newborn rats.[5]

Chemical poisons in action… In animal studies, glutathione-depleting denatured allyl alco-hol, bromobenzene and diethyl maleate produce liver necrosis [cell and tissue death] including lipid peroxidation [lipids: fats and fat-related compounds].[6] Organochlorine insecticide Dieldrin induces liver tumors through mechanisms not fully understood, but probably related to oxidative stress.[7] PCPs [pentachlorophenols] cause oxidative DNA liver damage, which can be arrested by antioxidants. Vitamin C provides partial PCP protection.[8] Plastics industry di-(2-ethylhexyl) phthalate (DEHP) induces testicular atrophy and liver enlargement. The critical DEHP dose is higher for gonadotoxicity than hepatotoxicity; and Vitamin C and Vitamin E co-administration prevents the testicular injury.[9] High-dose Vitamin C inhibits CC14 [carbon tetrachloride]-induced liver damage, as measured by liver function tests of plasma glucose, bilirubin and proteins.[10] In human studies, Vitamin C reduces the urinary iPs [isoprostanes: free radical catalyzed products of arachidonic acid, an essential fatty acid] characteristic of alcohol-induced chronic liver disease.[11] Indices of free radical-mediated damage such as decreased glutathione and Vitamin C have been documented in patients with alcoholic and viral liver disease. Enhancing the antioxidant ability of hepatocytes [liver cells] counteracts oxidative/nitrosative stress and helps to stop the progression of liver disease. [12]

Acetaminophen [nonprescription pain medication] poisoning... is a significant problem in the United States. The principal clinical feature is hepatotoxicity, which can occur after ingestion of a single large dose or after ingestion of smaller doses in patients with altered liver metabolism as a result of drugs or medical conditions.[13] Acetaminophen depletes mouse liver glutathione and increases liver weight to body weight ratio.[14] Co-administered Vitamin C effectively inhibits acetaminophen-induced hepatotoxicity in mice, completely preventing the 35% mortality observed at 24 hours in control mice.[15] Vitamin C also has antipyretic [reduces or relieves fever] effect.[14]

Hepatitis A... Vitamin C exerts remarkable immunomodulating action against Hepatitis A, and should be an integral part of patient treatment.[16] During the acute phase of Hepatitis A, T-lymphocyte numbers decline significantly, and plasma Vitamin C is low (hypovitaminosis). Vitamin C administration promotes T-lymphocyte recovery.[17]

Hepatitis B... Comparing Vitamin C to placebo, there was no significant difference in post-transfusion Hepatitis B incidence or clinical course in a double-blind controlled trial.[18]

Hepatitis C... Oxidative stress, as measured by a wide range of pro- and antioxidant markers, is a significant factor in Hepatitis C infection. Consequently, antioxidant therapy may be able to slow the progression of the disease to cirrhosis.[19] Author's Note: Hepatitis C is a retrovirus and can copy its genome into host DNA... Free radical-induced mutations are a rich genetic palette for evolutionary forces to select for or against. Millions of years ago when Anthropoidea [primate suborder, includes monkeys, apes and man] lost the ability to produce endogenous [arising from within the organism] Vitamin C, free radicals may have increased the mutation frequency and accelerated primate evolution. Retroviruses and the absence of endogenous Vitamin C may have played a pivotal role in Homo sapien evolution.[20]

Vitamin C's general antioxidation and immune activities are reported in Chapter 7 medical literature. Bioflavonoids are reviewed in Table 3-3.

#2 SILYMARIN

Silymarin, a flavonoid extract from the milk thistle plant, contains potent liver antioxidants. Silymarin can add extra protection against liver injury and scarring during times of severe distress from jaundice, hepatitis, cirrhosis or acute chemical poisoning. Repeated silymarin dosing is very effective in maintaining liver defenses and preserving function. For even more protection, antioxidants Grape Seed Extract and alpha-lipoic acid of Chapter 7 can overcome the free radical lethality of acute intoxication.

Review of the Medical Literature

Overview… Silymarin (from milk thistle plant, Silybum marianum) is a traditional remedy for liver and biliary tract diseases. Silymarin scavenges free radicals, inhibits lipid peroxidation, protects against genome damage, decreases tumorigenesis, stabilizes mast cells [resident white blood cells of connective tissue: produce histamine, heparin and serotonin], increases protein synthesis in the liver, chelates iron and slows calcium metabolism.[21] Silymarin is beneficial in the treatment of toxic hepatitis, viral hepatitis, fatty liver, cirrhosis, radiation toxicity and ischemic [insufficient blood supply] injury.[22] Silymarin has preventive as well as curative activity in animals deliberately intoxicated with mushroom toxins, medicines, toxic organic solvents and heavy metals.[23]

Mechanisms… Silymarin liver protection is well documented. However, little is known of biochemical mechanisms. Proposed silymarin liver actions are: (1) antioxidant, eliminating free radicals and increasing mitochondrial glutathione; (2) preventing cell membrane peroxidation and regulating membrane permeability; and (3) nuclear expression, increasing ribosomal RNA [type of RNA, involved in protein synthesis] synthesis and stimulating DNA polymerase I [enzyme that aids in DNA replication] and DNA transcription.[24, 25]

Alcohol cirrhosis… Approximately 50% of liver cirrhosis in Western societies is due to alcohol abuse. Acetaldehyde, the oxidative metabolite of ethanol, in combination with viral or metabolic liver diseases induces liver fibrogenesis [forming fibrous tissue]. Silymarin, lecithin [see bile later in the chapter], and ursodeoxycholic acid [another constituent of bile] show antifibrotic action and have good safety profiles.[26] Silymarin improves liver functions in alcoholic patients,[27] and gives positive results in diabetics with alcoholic cirrhosis.[28] In alcoholic cirrhosis patients, silymarin corrects impaired superoxide dismutase [SOD: protective enzyme, see Chapter 6] activity and altered immune response,[29] normalizing low T-cell and high CD8+ cell [differentiation antigen; an antigen elicites an antibody response] antibody activity. [30]

Mushroom poisoning... Poisoning from genus Amanita mushrooms is common in North America and Europe. The principal clinical feature is liver damage, with patient death rates reported at 11% to 51%. Supportive therapy for sublethal exposures is hyperbaric oxygen, penicillin and silymarin, with careful management of blood glucose.[31] Penicillin and silymarin are most likely to be effective antidotes for death-cap poisoning [Amanita phalloides].[32]

Cardiovascular... The liver plays a key role in regulating blood lipoproteins [such as cholesterol]. Liver injury often produces secondary hypercholesterolemia and atherogenesis [depositing plaque on artery walls]. Silymarin protects liver functions, and some data suggest that silymarin can directly inhibit liver cholesterol synthesis.[33] Silymarin decreases total cholesterol, LDL [low-density lipoproteins, so-called bad cholesterol] and VLDL [V = very], and increases HDL [high-density lipoproteins, so-called good cholesterol] in hyperlipemic rats.[25]

#3 ACTIVATED CHARCOAL

The liver is not designed for today's environmental poisons. Many of them get stuck there, NOT detoxified, just captured and held for life. This leads to slow loss of function and eventually inability to regenerate new liver cells. Acute poisoning is especially damaging as defense mechanisms are overwhelmed. Common acute episodes include insecticide exposure at home or work and hydrocarbon vapors such as gasoline and kerosene. To combat modern environmental toxins, a modern liver remedy is badly needed.

Activated charcoal is that acute remedy – literally an antidote. It can absorb and instantly detoxify huge amounts of poison in the digestive system and blood. On a personal note, the author's liver was poisoned several times over the years, and is still sensitive to insecticides recently sprayed in stores and to gasoline vapors when fueling the car. If I inhale too much of these, my liver starts to hurt with a dull pain under the right rib cage. Immediately ingesting some activated charcoal gets rid of the pain and poison... before it settles in for *a long stay*.

Acute poisoning right now. For minor episodes of inhaled chemical toxins, take activated charcoal equal in volume to about two or three small green peas. Swallowed poisons require much more charcoal, and professional help is definitely the right call. Many cities have poison control hotlines, or dial 911. Activated charcoal together with large doses of Vitamin C, bioflavonoids, silymarin and other powerful antioxidants can counteract and neutralize severe poisoning.

Entrenched poisons. Activated charcoal sweeps the liver clean of new poisons. Unfortunately, it is much less effective against captured poisons once they are in the liver for more than a few hours. Apparently capture and binding are two separate liver mechanisms. Cleaning out these resistant, long-term chemical toxins and reversing their damage requires the Table 11-1 rebuilding regimen (#4) detailed ahead.

Activated charcoal has few side effects except when ingested in great excess, far beyond need. The liver can tolerate a lot of this antidote. In fact, activated charcoal should be taken as a preventative if you are going into a toxic environment. However, there is a point of too much, and then the liver begins to detoxify charcoal. Not what you want. Therefore, use activated charcoal cautiously, in small single doses and only as needed. It takes about five days for activated charcoal to be eliminated from the liver, so one week between dosing insures against side effects. If necessary, silymarin can relieve symptoms of too much charcoal. *CAUTION* ☛ Large doses and multiple dosing of activated charcoal for the severe poisoning described in the following medical literature require physician care and monitoring.

Review of the Medical Literature

Reversal of hepatic coma… In a study of seventy-six patients with fulminant hepatic failure [a severe and rapid form of hepatitis and liver failure], activated charcoal hemoperfusion resulted in remarkable survival rates: 70% for acetaminophen [nonprescription pain medication] poisoning and 65% overall when signs of stage III hepatic encephalopathy [liver failure causes central nervous system/brain dysfunction; symptoms include confusion to unresponsive coma] were still present. Cerebral edema [abnormal accumulation of fluid, swelling] developed significantly less often in this group than in those starting hemoperfusion when stage IV encephalopathy was evident. Absence of cerebral edema was a major factor in survival. Treatment included activated charcoal hemoperfusion and prostacyclin [an unstable prostaglandin: inhibits platelet aggregation, also vasodilator] for platelet protection. Side effects were minimal; both platelet and white cell counts were unaffected by hemoperfusion.[34] In ten patients with stage IV hepatic encephalopathy, one or more four-hour periods of activated charcoal hemoperfusion resulted in 90% awakening and 40% survival.[35] In one case of seven-day coma from alcohol plus phenobarbital [barbiturate; used as a sedative and anticonvulsant] and diazepam [prescription drug: sedative, antianxiety, muscle relaxant] poisoning, 40 grams of activated charcoal given every 4 hours over 24 hours completely reversed the coma in 12 hours, and serum half life (t1/2) of diazepam was cut from the usual 195 hours to 18 hours.[36] In dogs with fulminant hepatic failure, 8-hour charcoal hemoperfusion significantly delayed the onset of liver encephalopathy and markedly decreased plasma bilirubin and total plasma phenols [e.g. pentachlorophenol or PCP] compared to the controls.[37] Author's Note: Branched-chain amino acids (BCAA: valine, leucine and isoleucine) also aid recovery from hepatic encephalopathy; see Table 3-2.

Chemical poisoning... Activated charcoal is extremely efficient in removing phenols in in-vitro [in laboratory vessel] models.[38] Activated charcoal hemoperfusion is effective in removing paraquat [herbicide] from blood. In one patient, a single hemoperfusion eliminated 99% of circulating paraquat. [39] In six cirrhosis patients with theophylline [prescription drug for bronchial spasms] overdose, activated charcoal decreased serum theophylline t1/2 [half life] from 12 hours to 4 hours.[40] Administered T-2 toxin [potent toxin produced by fungus] caused severe necrosis [cell and tissue death] of the liver, spleen, thymus, stomach, small intestine and adrenal gland in control rats, whereas lesions were minimal or absent in charcoal-treated rats.[41]

Side effects and safety... Possible major side effects of activated charcoal therapy are aspiration [inhaling] of charcoal, gastrointestinal obstruction, and fluid and electrolyte abnormalities.[42] Multiple-dose complications such as pulmonary aspiration, gastrointestinal obstruction, hypernatraemia [high sodium levels in the blood], and hypermagnesemia occur infrequently.[43] Activated charcoal is usually prescribed at 2-10 grams per day, as larger doses can cause nausea, vomiting and constipation.[44] However, large multiple doses are appropriate when the need is great, for example 40 grams of activated charcoal every 4 hours over 24 hours to reverse prolonged coma from alcohol plus phenobarbital and diazepam poisoning.[36] Repeated doses of activated charcoal are relatively more effective in patients with long t1/2 [half life] poisonings.[40] Adverse effects of a 75-gram activated charcoal dose in non-poisoned healthy volunteers were black stool (92%), constipation or abdominal fullness (50%), nausea (21%), headache (17%), vomiting (8%), diarrhea (8%), and anal irritation (8%).[45]

Rebuild Health... Regenerating Liver Tissue

#4 METHIONINE-ACTIVATED CHARCOAL

Methionine, the only sulfur-containing essential amino acid, plays a fundamental role in liver regeneration – and methionine supplementation can put this failed mechanism back to work for you! However, methionine therapy alone will not produce a positive outcome. Activated charcoal is also needed. Why? Methionine brings injured liver cells back to full function. But what injured them in the first place? Poisons. And taking methionine alone expels these poisons back into the bloodstream, only to be captured again by another healthy liver cell. The author learned this zero-sum game the hard way, through trial and error. So, as large amounts of poisons spew out of the liver during methionine healing and regeneration, activated charcoal captures these poisons before they reinjure the liver.

Table 3-2 evidences the essential role of methionine in liver regeneration. SAMe (S-adenosylmethionine) and branched-chain amino acids (BCAA: valine, leucine and isoleucine) also demonstrate liver regenerating activity, and can compliment methionine action.

Symptoms and signs of severe liver damage include sleeplessness, constant nausea (like a hangover), ringing in the ears, persistent pain and tenderness in the right side of chest especially high up under the ribs, and no bile flow as indicated by light yellow stools. With such complaints, immediate rebuilding of the organ is imperative.

Methionine-Activated Charcoal Regimen

If your liver's normal regenerating mechanism has failed and you need to rebuild function, or if you just want to scrub chemical toxins from your liver, ingest 500 mg to 1000 mg L-methionine (more is possible later, as explained below) together with activated charcoal equal in volume to approximately one-third of the methionine. Take methionine and activated charcoal by themselves, with no protein or meal of any substance, although juice is OK. Adding silymarin to the regimen buffers activated charcoal, enabling higher methionine-charcoal doses. Soft functioning (defined in Chapter 4) of the liver can occur for two to three days after treatment, particularly if the organ is in *bad shape*. Eating liver and aromatic seeds such as Anise, Caraway, Fennel, Coriander and Dill (Table 11-4 ahead) can keep functioning up during any temporary adverse soft effects such as glycogen-related hypoglycemia. Wait at least seven days before repeating this methionine-activated charcoal regimen.

Methionine supplementation disturbs amino acid harmony, nature's complex protein equilibriums and interactions. Side effects increase in severity with the degree of liver impairment. Accordingly, begin methionine-activated charcoal therapy with low methionine doses, 500 to 1000 mg, and slowly raise the dosage by 500 mg increments when your body can tolerate more amino acid imbalance without side effects. It may take several months to go from 1000 mg to 1500 mg, and then 2000 mg and beyond. As an adjunct, 200 to 400 mg of SAMe and up to 500 mg of each branched-chain amino acid can augment methionine therapeutic action and regeneration.

Note: Sulfur-containing alpha-lipoic acid of Chapter 7 also heals oxidative liver damage. While not as effective as methionine-activated charcoal treatments, low-dose alpha-lipoic acid in combination with Vitamin C, bioflavinoids, silymarin and protective activated charcoal is therapeutic.

ENDOCRINE LIVER

The endocrine liver is so complex, volumes have been written on it alone. Rather than repeating such lengthy dissertation, discussion here is limited to just two endocrine liver topics and functions: TOXIC LOAD and STORAGE, as these are most germane to well being. Reducing the toxic load your liver faces every day is crucial in keeping this organ young and fully functional. Meanwhile, storage proficiency is a good indicator of overall liver health and whether or not methionine-supplemented regeneration is needed.

Toxic Load

The toxic load experienced by your liver and body involves two factors: defense against poisons and exposure to them. Table 11-1 is defense strategy. Table 11-2 describes exposure with a partial list of environmental poisons and supporting medical evidence. We have just seen how Vitamin C plus bioflavonoids, silymarin and activated charcoal increase defense; now let's reduce offense!

TABLE 11-2. TOXIC LOAD ON LIVER AND BODY.
May involve ingestion, inhalation or skin exposure.
Only a partial listing is possible for many categories.

Agent	Adverse Effects
pollution from elevated nitrogen oxides (NOx), ozone (O3), tobacco smoke, particulatematter and diesel exhaust.	allergies.[46]
tobacco smoke, air pollutants (NO2, O3).	oxidative stress, bronchitis and emphysema.[47]
cigarette smoke	carcinogenegic.[48]
alcohol	chronic liver disease,[11] cirrhosis.[26]

FOOD ADDITIVES

food preservatives	
BHA and BHT	tumor promoters.[49]
gallates	toxic to rat hepatocytes.[50]
nitrites, used in curing meats	hepatotoxic and carcinogenic nitrosamines.[51]
HAA (heterocyclic aromaticamines), found most often in fried foods.	mutagens, animal carcinogens.[52, 53]
MSG (monosodium glutamate), added to many foods.	excitatory neurotoxins.[54]
artificial sweeteners	
saccharin	bladder tumors in rats.[55]
cyclamate	may promote cancer activity in animals.[56]
polyols	rat adrenal medulla lesions.[57]
artificial colors	hyperactive behaviors in children.[58]
food colors erythrosine, allura red, new coccine, brilliant blue, tertrazine and fast green.	toxic to rat hepatocytes, impairs liver gluconeogenesis and urea synthesis.[59]
FD&C Red No. 3 (erythrosine)	sperm abnormalities in mice.[60]
allura red AC	DNA damage in mice.[61]
caramel color III	disturbed immune functions in rodents.[62]
artificial flavors	
acetaldehydes	animal carcinogenic.[63]
furfurals	mutagenic.[64]

potassium bromate, in food products, cosmetics and water disinfection.

rodent carcinogenic, nephro- and neurotoxic in humans.[65]

methyleugenol (MEG), in foods, beverages and cosmetics.

multisite, multispecies carcinogen.[66]

wax, paraffin

increased weight, inflammation and hydrocarbons in rat liver and lymph nodes.[67]

COSMETICS

preservatives
benzoic acid and sodium benzoate
propyl paraben
methyldibromoglutaronitrile (MDGN) in skin care products.

reduced growth in animals.[68]
mild skin irritation.[69]
contact allergy.[70]

sodium dodecyl sulfate, most widely used surfactant in household and industrial cleaners, personal care products and cosmetics.

of cell membrane barrier function, increased permeability to complete cell lysis [antibody destruction].[71]

azo dyes in hair products, lipstick, cosmetics, drug and food products.
CI solvent yellow 7 and 14, CI pigment orange 5, CI pigment red 4 and red 23.
CI pigment red 3
CI pigment red 53:1

mutagenicity.[72]

genotoxic.[73]

carcinogenic.[73]
spleen tumors in male rats.[73]

hair spray: inhaled acrylate copolymer resin.

significantly modified antixenic [against foreign invaders] defense mechanisms of rat respiratory system.[74]

ammonium persulphate, in hair bleaching products.

altered airway responsiveness in rabbits.[75]

potassium bromate and thioglycolate, hair curling solution.

abnormal caloric response in humans; neurotoxic effects on cerebellar-regulated functions of guinea pigs.[76]

zinc pyrithione (Zpt), antidandruff chemical in shampoos.

embryotoxicity in fish.[77]

Agent	Adverse Effects
fragrances musk ketone	concentrates in human fatty tissue and breast milk, may increase susceptibility to carcinogens;[78] increased postimplantation loss and reduced fetal body in rats.[79]
HHCB	skeletal malformations in rats.[79]
AHTN	acute hepatic damage in rats.[80]
HHCB and AHTN in surface waters from fine fragrances, cosmetics, soaps and laundry detergents.	weak estrogenic effects in wildlife and humans at current exposure levels.[81]
antibacterial agents sulphonamides, nalidixic acid, fluoroquinolones, tetracycline.	photo[sun]sensitivity.[82]
sanguinarium, chlorhexidine and tetracycline for periodontal infections.	adversely affect neutrophil viability and functions.[83]
sanguinarine chloride for gingivitis and plaque.	cytotoxic to oral human tissues.[84]
chlorhexidine and sodium hypochlorite in mouthwashs.	cytotoxic to human periodontal ligament cells.[85]
chlorhexidine in mouthwashs, antiseptic wound/skin disinfection.	possible hypersensitivity and anaphylactic shock.[86]
triclosan in deodorants, soaps, mouthrinses and dentifrices.	cytotoxic to human gingival epithelial cells.[87]
topical antifungal, imidazole nitrate	possible contact allergy.[88]
benzophenone-3, common sunscreen chemical.	chromosome aberrations in hamster ovary cells.[89]
titanium dioxide in sunscreens	catalyses human DNA damage.[90]
canthaxanthin, synthetic carotenoid for skin tanning.	possible aplastic anemia [bone marrow defective red blood cells] with fatal outcome.[91]
silicone in cosmetics, toiletries, processed foods, household products, medicalimplantable devices and lubricants in tubing and syringes.	depressed natural killer (NK) cell activity in mice.[92]

nail polish remover, gamma butyrolactone.	irritant and allergic contact dermatitis, skin blisters, tissue inflammation around nail, brittleness, loosening or separating of nail.[93] coma, respiratory depression and bradycardia [abnormally slow heartbeat] possible if inhaled.[94]
fingernail glue remover, acetonitrile	metabolic release of cyanide;[95] animal carcinogen.[96]
ethylene oxide, contaminant in skin-care products.	animal carcinogen[96]
mineral oil	arthritis in rats.[97]
commercial air freshener	exacerbates indoor air pollution via toxic chemicals.[98]

PHARMACEUTICALS

acetaminophen, nonprescription pain medication.	hepatotoxicity,[13] genotoxicity.[99]
NSAIDs (nonsteroidal anti-inflammatory drugs): aspirin, acetaminophen, etc.	upper gastrointestinal (GI) adverse events; also hepatotoxicity, lower GI ulcerations, strictures, colitis, exacerbation of inflammatory bowel disease,[100] and acute renal toxicity.[101]
other OTC (over-the-counter) drugs:	
clonidine, spinal analgesic	fetal abnormalities.[102]
anthraquinone, in laxatives	genotoxicity.[99]
emodin, in laxatives	genotoxicity.[103]
benzoyl peroxide, for common acne	cutaneous tumor promoter.[104]
antibiotics	gastrointestinal disorders, skin reactions, hepatic effects,[105] including:
isoniazid	cytotoxic hepatitis.[105]
sulphonamides	mixed hepatitis.[105]
nitrofurantoin	chronic active hepatitis.[105]
tetracycline	steatosis [fat accumulation within organ].[105]
penicillins, macrolides, clavulanic acid.	intrahepatic cholestasis [arrest of normal bile flow].[105]
chlorpromazine, cyclosporin A	cholestatic injury.[106]
fluoroquinolone antibiotics, chlorpromazine and psoralene.	photomutagens.[107]
tranquilizers, sedatives, anticonvulsants, anesthetics.	liver injury of differing patterns.[108]

Agent	Adverse Effects
anticonvulsants	
felbamate	hepatotoxicity, aplastic anemia.[109]
lamotrigine	hypersensitivity measles-like rashes to multi-organ failure.[109]
topiramate	word-finding difficulties, kidney calculi [abnormal deposits] and bodyweight loss.[109]
vigabatrin	seizure aggravation; rare reports of encephalopathy, language loss, motor disturbances.[109]
valproate, for epilepsy	steatosis.[106]
halothane, anesthetic	immunoallergic liver damage.[106]
chloroform, early anesthetic	hepatoxicant, hepatocellular steatosis and necrosis [death].[110]
anabolic steroids/glucocorticoids	cardiomyopathy, heart failure.[111]
diethylstilbestrol (DES), synthetic estrogen.	vaginal adenocarcinoma.[102]
synthetic retinoids: acitretin and etretinate for psoriasis.	teratogenicity [birth defects]; hair loss, inflamed/cracked lips; less common are hepatotoxicity, pancreatitis and altered blood lipids.[112]
tienilic acid, diuretic	autoimmune hepatitis.[106]
methyldopa, antihypertensive	chronic hepatitis.[106]
amiodarone, anti-arrhythmic drug	alcoholic steatohepatitis-like reactions.[106]
methotrexate, for rheumatoid arthritis and neoplastic [tumor] conditions.	liver fibrosis,[106] possible pulmonary toxicity with inflammation, pneumonia.[113]
chemotherapy	substantial short- and long-term side effects, depending on agents used, dose and duration.[114]
over 1000 drugs	hepatic lesions.[115]
800 different drugs	drug-induced liver injury, 2 to 3% of all hospitalizations.[116]
adverse drug events (ADE) including adverse drug reactions (58%), allergic reactions (19%), medication errors (17%) and drug interactions (6%).	most common causes of death are hepatitis, hepatic failure, cardiopulmonary arrest, overdose and agranulocytosis [poor healing, lesions].[117] estimated 770,000 US hospital patients per year experience ADE.[118] up to 140,000 US inpatient ADE deaths per year.[118]

CHEMICALS

hydrocarbon fuel vapors: gasoline, jet fuel, diesel fuel, kerosene.	neurotoxicity.[119]
unleaded gasoline, vaporized	renal carcinoma in rats; liver tumors in mice.[120]
gasoline exposure	human renal cancer, leukemia.[121]
diesel exhaust, inhaled	pulmonary carcinogen in rats; lung inflammatory and other cellular effects in humans.[122]
MTBE antiknock additive, exhaust inhalation and water contamination.	genotoxic, animal carcinogenic.[123]
MMT gasoline octane enhancer, particulate manganese emitted.	nervous system toxicity, fetal developmental toxicity.[124]
benzene, from active and passive smoking, auto exhaust.	many types of genetic damage, risk of neoplasia [tumor].[125]
benzene derivative, bromobenzene	liver necrosis.[6]
carbon tetrachloride (CC14) and other chlorinated methanes.	hepatoxic, hepatocellular steatosis and necrosis.[110]
acetonitrile, organic solvent	metabolic release of cyanide;[95] animal carcinogen.[96]
denatured allyl alcohol	liver necrosis.[6]
plasticizers	
phthalate esters: DEHP, BBP, DBP and DINP used in cosmetics, medical products, vinyl floors and plastics including food containers and food wraps.	disrupt reproductive development, reproductive tract differentiation of male rat.[126]
DEHP, di-(2-ethylhexyl) phthalate, widely used in plastics industry.	liver enlargement in rats,[9] carcinogenic to rodents.[127]
DINP, diisononyl phthalate, imparts softness and flexibility to polyvinyl chloride (PVC) products.	increase in liver weight and incidence of liver tumors in rodents.[128]
formaldehyde, including urea-formaldehyde foam insulation and pressed wood products.	carcinogenic in animals.[63, 96]
polyurethane	depressed natural killer (NK) cell activity in mice.[92]
ethylene oxide, used as sterilizer, solvent, plasticizer and in antifreeze, polyester resins.	acute toxic alkylating reaction with most organic tissue.[129]
ethylene oxide, vinyl chloride, sulfuric acid, chloromethyl methyl ether, 1,3-butadiene.	animal carcinogens.[96]

Agent	Adverse Effects
dioxins, unwanted impurities from pulp and paper manufacturing and combustion of chlorinated waste.	severe skin lesions, altered liver function and lipid metabolism, immune system depression, general weakness with drastic weight loss, endocrine and nervous system abnormalities.[130]
DEET insect repellents, (N,N-diethyl-m-toluamide).	possible toxic encephalopathy in children.[131]
pesticides	oxidative stress, immunotoxicity and apoptosis [cell death].[132]
polychlorinated biphenyls; also nicotine and alcohol.	impaired neurologic development of children.[133]
PCP (pentachlorophenol), phenols	liver DNA damage in mice.[8]
organochlorine dieldrin	hepatic tumors in mice.[7]
diazinon	high acute toxicity to animals and adverse ecological impacts.[134]
malathion	human chromosome damage.[135]
organophospates, including paraquot	serious toxicity in both acute and chronic exposures; paraquot is the leading cause of death in Taiwan.[136]
organophosphate and carbamate pesticide residues.	wide variability for apples, pears, peaches, nectarines, oranges, bananas and tomatoes.[137]
triazophos residues	wide variability in carrots.[137]
DDT, banned in USA since 1972	human cancers; persists in the environment, bioaccumulates in adipose [human fatty] tissue.[138]
radon gas, ground leakage into residential homes and mines.	lung cancer risk.[139]

TOXIC METALS

lead and mercury	neurotoxic,[140] impaired neurologic development of children.[133]
lead in paint and piping; major sources are dust, paint chips and water.	decrements in children's intelligence, neurodevelopmental deficits;[141] hematological, gastrointestinal and neurological dysfunction; prolonged exposure can cause chronic nephropathy, hypertension and reproductive impairment.[142]

mercury	severe exposure results in erethism [organ irritation/excitement], tremor, and gingivitis; subtle effects involve kidney function and central nervous system cognitive/behavior changes.[143]
methylmercury, bioaccumulates in predatory fish.	neurological brain poisoning of cerebellum (ataxia) and visual cortex (constricted visual fields); prenatal exposure: delayed development and cognitive changes in children.[143]
mercury, in amalgam tooth fillings	releases small quantities of mercury;[144] 3 to 17 mcg/day from dental amalgam is 1.25 to 6.5 times average mercury absorption from dietary sources.[145]
aluminum in cans, cookware, baking powder, antacids, deodorants and cosmetics.	neurotoxicity, Alzheimer's disease development in experimental models; disturbs intracellular signaling, cellular growth and excretory functions; less collagen synthesis and slowing of skeletal mineralization; anemia from low erythropoietin [hormone for red blood cell production], inhibiting of heme-synthesizing enzymes and binding of Al to transferrin (iron carrier in the blood); high Al concentrations found in many neoplastic cells.[146]
iron dietary supplements	most frequent cause of unintentional pediatric fatalities.[147]
organotin, food contaminant	neurotoxic.[140]
nickel contact sensitivity	possible dermatitis.[148]
arsenic, cadmium and lead, common environmental pollutants.	chronic renal disease.[149]
fumes or gaseous forms of many metals	lung diseases.[150]

BIOLOGICAL AGENTS

foodborne diseases	76 million illnesses, 325,000 hospitalizations and 5,000 deaths in the USA each year.[151]
from known pathogens	14 million illnesses, 60,000 hospitalizations and 1,800 deaths.[151]
salmonella, listeria, toxoplasma	1,500 deaths.[151]
salmonella, shigella, campylobacter and other bacteria, parasites and viruses in food.	infectious diarrhea.[152]

Agent	Adverse Effects
salmonella	fatal gastroenteritis or septicemia.[153]
staphylococcus aureus	persistent and relapsing infections.[154]
E. coli (escherichia coli O157:H7)	enterohemorrhagic, fatal hemolytic uremic syndrome.[155]
clostridium botulinum	botulism neurotoxicity.[156]
mold food contaminants (mycotoxins): aflatoxins, ochratoxin A, fumonisins, certain trichothecenes, zearalenone.	allergic responses, immuno-suppression and cancer.[157]
aflatoxin B(1)	hepatocellular carcinoma.[158]
ochratoxin A	nephrotoxicity and carcinogenicity.[159]

Human beings have faced many different toxic threats throughout history. In ancient Rome, wealthy patricians dined on lead tableware – this new wonder metal was the latest status symbol. Lead poisoning is one of the little known contributing factors to the downfall of the Roman Empire. Today, toxic hazards are far greater in variety and subtler in effect, as shown in Table 11-2. You need a proactive strategy of both more defense and less offense. Ingestion, inhalation and skin exposure to a multitude of toxic agents becomes a daily gauntlet for your liver. Insecticides in the home kill the bugs, and a little bit of you too. Meanwhile, many natural safe alternatives such as boric acid for cockroaches can do the job better. Nitrites, used in curing meats and present in all processed meat products, convert to carcinogenic nitrosamines in your body. Cosmetics applied in the morning require liver detoxification throughout the rest of the day. Aluminum and plastics are everywhere now. Table 11-2 reveals that Alzheimer's disease is linked to aluminum, which is found in beverage cans, cookware, baking powder, antacids, deodorants and cosmetics. Plastics are the current wonder material – unfortunately the plasticizers in plastics cause enlarged livers, disrupt reproductive development and are carcinogenic in animals. Plasticizers make plastics soft and formable, but they leach out of plastic food containers and into the food. When the plastic containers become hard and brittle, it's time to throw them out and buy new plasticizer-rich ones! The only truly safe food containers for cooking and storage are glass and stainless steel.

Liver Storage

Table 11-3 presents common liver storage dysfunctions and consequences. Of course, some of problems cited in this table may be due to insufficient nutrient in the first place and not its storage. Standard liver function tests can also help in diagnosing dysfunctions, as can symptomatic clues such as hormonal imbalance, for example, men developing female characteristics and vice versa.

TABLE 11-3. COMMON LIVER STORAGE DYSFUNCTIONS.
A short list of malfunctions that can show up early and obliviously.

Liver storage of...	Storage dysfunction causes...
CARBOHYDRATES	
blood glucose → glycogen (stored in liver) and conversion back (gluconeogenesis) as needed.	fasting hypoglycemia, a debilitating, often disabling condition.
FATTY ACIDS	
Essential Fatty Acids (EFAs) and Omega 3.	dry and scaly skin, cracked lips, poor wound healing.
Beta-carotene	poor healing; no beta-carotene → Vitamin A conversion results in susceptibility to infections.
Vitamin A	susceptibility to infections.
MINERAL BALANCE	
Na (sodium) ⇌ K (potassium).	the liver does not excrete excess sodium; Na ⇌ K equilibrium is lost, and water balance, fatigue function and stamina become impaired.
Ca (calcium) ⇌ Mg (magnesium).	calcium and magnesium unavailable for bones; Ca ⇌ Mg equilibrium is lost, resulting in twitching muscles and leg cramps, i.e. restless leg syndrome.

Gluconeogenesis. Accounting for only a small percentage of all hypoglycemia, fasting hypoglycemia is a serious disorder, requiring immediate medical attention. Severe liver damage impairs liver gluconeogenesis, and this defective storage or conversion of liver glycogen back to blood glucose causes debilitating hypoglycemia following any stressful activity. To ease this hypoglycemic hell, liver function must be rebuilt using the Table 11-1 #4 methionine-activated charcoal regimen. Chapter 10 further explains hypoglycemia and pancreas-mediated gluconeogenesis.

Fatty Acid Problems. The endocrine liver smoothes out the ups and downs of fatty acid availability. For twenty-four hours after any fatty acid intake, normal therapeutic action guarantees availability to all tissues. After that, the liver must supply needs from storage. Dry scaly skin, cracked lips, poor wound healing, scar tissue and premature aging indicate either severe liver damage or severe fatty acid and fatty acid vitamin deprivation to the point that the liver is empty.

Inability to Convert Beta-Carotene into Vitamin A to fight infection is often an early indicator of liver dysfunction. See Chapter 5 "Beta-carotene." An easy test—if large doses of beta-carotene do not defeat an infection, switch to Vitamin A forevermore and implement Table 11-1 defense.

Sodium-Potassium Equilibrium (Na ⇌ K) is controlled by the adrenal cortex hormone aldosterone. However, loss of liver control of sodium and potassium storage and supply to the cortex similarly produces water balance, fatigue and stamina problems. Moreover, if the liver cannot throw off excess dietary sodium through kidney excretion, high blood pressure develops and stroke can occur. Potassium will be ripped from body cells to gain equilibrium by other means. Over 90% of potassium lies within cells, whereas most sodium exists outside of cells in body fluids and blood. Basically, Na ⇌ K equilibrium regulates the flow of fluids through cell membranes and acts as cell electrolyte (*battery fluid*) with changes, for instance, triggering nerve impulses and muscle contractions (see Ca ⇌ Mg below). Hypokalemia or low potassium also degrades kidney function. Sodium-potassium storage and excretion are frequently the first liver function to fail, or partially fail, worn out beyond repair by excessive salt intake over many years. In such cases, you must take over and rebalance sodium and potassium for the rest of your life.

How-To Rebalance Na ⇌ K

With a good liver, Na ⇌ K occurs naturally and automatically through adrenal cortex aldosterone and liver storage mechanisms and homeostasis. Moderate intake of table salt (sodium chloride, NaCl) poses no problem; the liver simply sends any excess to the kidneys for elimination. Only with sweating do your liver and body actually require extra sodium salt. In extreme situations, running out of sodium causes heat exhaustion: pale and damp skin, rapid pulse, dizziness, nausea, and finally collapse. The potassium half of this equilibrium is supplied in sufficient amounts from food unless Na ⇌ K is lost.

Unsure about your liver's Na ⇌ K balance? The following dietary measure is a simple guarantee of equilibrium. No adverse effects, in fact, no effects at all will occur if your liver is OK. If not OK, you should palpably feel a shift back to equilibrium of sodium and potassium between body fluids and cells. On a quiet evening when the stress of the day has past, take a small dose of 50% sodium-50% potassium salt. Potassium salt (potassium chloride, KCl), even if balanced with sodium salt, adversely affects fatigue ability unless your aldosterone hormone is at rest. While few 50% sodium-50% potassium salts exist commercially, you can easily mix your own. Potassium salt is commonly called "salt substitute;" all supermarkets carry it. Use a total salt volume equal to about two green peas, one of salt substitute and one of regular table salt, to rebalance internal Na ⇌ K, then repeat the procedure weekly to maintain this equilibrium if your liver can no longer do the job. Such low dosage works best because high potassium levels, beyond need, can still impact at-rest aldosterone. To illustrate, the rare disorder of hyperactive aldosterone can be corrected back to normal with one teaspoon of 50% sodium-50% potassium salt.

High blood pressure? High blood pressure may be due to Na ← K imbalance. First, take potassium salt alone in the evening until blood pressure comes down. Later, sodium salt may be required because the original hypokalemia overworks and frequently exhausts aldosterone functioning. Chapter 12 gives aldosterone exhaustion cures.

———————

Calcium-Magnesium Equilibrium (Ca ⇌ Mg). Liver and parathyroid glands control calcium metabolism. The liver stores some calcium, but most is held in bones. The liver also controls magnesium metabolism, magnesium storage and Ca ⇌ Mg. Overall, dysfunctions in or caused by the endocrine liver, bile, parathyroid gland, Vitamin D, adrenal cortex (as in arthritis syndromes), and estrogen loss (osteoporosis in postmenopausal women) can upset calcium metabolism. Exact mechanisms remain complex and unresolved.

What is easy to determine is loss of the liver's Ca ⇌ Mg equilibrium. Muscles call up the liver and request an extra supply of calcium to contract, or extra magnesium to relax. As you get older and your liver becomes damaged from chemical toxins in the environment, your muscles still call, but the liver doesn't *answer the phone anymore*, especially in the evening and at night. And so twitching muscles and leg cramps develop. This painful "restless leg syndrome" disrupts sleep endlessly. A secondary cause here can be sodium-potassium imbalance.

Methionine-activated charcoal therapy can eventually restore some muscle peace. In the meantime, imposing Ca ⇌ Mg equilibrium from outside sources is an effective answer to restless leg syndrome. This requires taking a little calcium and a little magnesium together several times in the early evening before bedtime. Calcium source can be an ounce or two of milk or yogurt. A good magnesium source is a chelated supplement such as magnesium citrate or magnesium bound to an amino acid complex. Chelated calcium-magnesium supplements provide an easy all-in-one solution. Most health food stores carry these supplements. Additionally, quinine may relief leg cramps.

<u>Sleep</u>. Ca ⇌ Mg imbalance disturbs sleep. In reality, the entire endocrine liver with its thousands of chemical reactions plays a much bigger role in sleep that can ever be sorted out. Suffice it to say, if you have a liver like a baby, you'll sleep like a baby! Rebuilding liver function with methionine-activated charcoal therapy is a useful tool in rebuilding sleep. Another tool is good circadian rhythm, a gentle natural transition from the energy-stress action plan to the healing-immune action plan as night approaches. This requires healthy adrenal equilibrium and normally functioning pituitary and pineal glands. Temporary adrenal imbalance from caffeine or a disturbing emotional event can upset your circadian rhythm and sleep.

EXOCRINE LIVER

As described at the beginning of the chapter, the liver manufactures bile and secretes it into the gallbladder, a storage sac, or directly into the duodenum, first portion of the small intestine. Bile contributes crucially to fat digestion, and to this end the gallbladder empties its bile when a fat-containing meal passes by the duodenum. Liver and gallbladder bile are carried to the digestive tract through a common bile duct.

It is easy to determine how good your bile flow is – stool color depends almost exclusively on bile. Light yellow in color indicates little or no bile, while dark brown evidences significant flow. The only exceptions are temporary darkening of stools from very dark-colored foods or from bleeding in the digestive tract. Blood usually comes out black and requires immediate medical attention.

Bile is a greenish, sometimes yellowish, alkaline liquid composed of bile salts, cholesterol, lecithin, water, electrolytes, bilirubin and other excreta. Bile salts are the chemical result of liver acids reacting with base compounds, the by-products of the thousands of endocrine liver chemical reactions. In the language of chemistry, an acid + a base = a salt. The digestive action of bile emulsifies fats, reducing them to small globules and making them water-soluble (actually a suspension of one liquid in another). This emulsifying action allows absorbed esters, fatty acids and other lipids to become part of blood, that is, to be in solution.

Inadequate bile or incomplete bile (something's missing?) causes certain fats, namely cholesterol and to a limited extent triglycerides, to become supersaturated (beyond the saturation limit, an unstable condition) in this blood solution. As a result, cholesterol and some triglycerides can precipitate out of solution and deposit on artery walls as plaque. These plaque deposits are known as atherosclerosis, and lead to cardiovascular disease, heart attack and stroke. A heart attack occurs from total blockage of a coronary artery. Triglycerides, or completely saturated fats, are particularly bad with respect to stroke, as *big fat droplets* get stuck in plaque-filled, narrowed blood vessels of the brain, creating blockage and interrupting blood supply. Angina is pain in the heart from restricted blood flow or partial blockage, just as intermittent claudication is pain in the legs from restricted blood flow there.

To prevent atherosclerosis, the medical profession currently recommends a total blood cholesterol of 200 mg/dl or less. Cholesterol can be further classified as high-density lipoproteins (HDL) or so-called good cholesterol, and low-density lipoproteins (LDL) or bad cholesterol. Lp(a) is another bad lipoprotein. Names and numbers aren't as important as the underlying mechanism. Human beings are designed to handle cholesterol. In fact, the liver manufactures it and the body requires it. Cholesterol is a natural constituent of cell membranes, the brain and nervous system, and other tissues. It is essential in many metabolic processes, and for the synthesis of Vitamin D and steroidal and sex hormones. If supply runs short, the liver simply makes more. Thus, the real answer to cholesterol is moderation in intake, and keeping it and other fats in blood solution, which is the fundamental job of bile. And we're back to the recurring theme/nightmare of this chapter, loss of liver function with age and slow chemical poisoning. Not only do endocrine functions suffer and fail from this toxic assault, but so does the one critical exocrine function – bile!

Rebuilding bile output and potency using Table 11-1 #4 methionine-activated charcoal regimen is a long, slow process. The best interim solution is dietary changes and supplementing your current bile to fix the underlying defect of inadequate emulsifying agent. Fixing this bile defect will largely prevent atherosclerosis, cardiovascular disease, heart attack and stroke.

What keeps cholesterol and fat in solution? Three factors:

✓ Obviously less cholesterol and bad fats in the diet. Use Chapter 5 guidelines for fewer bad fats and more good fats.

✓ Bile B vitamins, choline and inositol (ahead), and bile herbs (Table 11-4) produce more and better bile.

✓ Only two substances on earth allow oil and water, or fats and blood, to mix and become one: LECITHIN AND ALCOHOL.

Lecithin is Mother Nature's solution for the human body and bile. The alcohol solution is also known as the French paradox. The French people pleasure in high-cholesterol high-fat fare, yet experience low rates of cardiovascular disease. Wine with the meal provides alcohol to dissolve cholesterol and fat, while flavonoids, particularly in red wine, add antioxidant protection against plaque formation.

You can demonstrate the mixing and fat-dissolving action of lecithin and alcohol by experiment. Just add vegetable oil and water to a sealing, transparent glass jar. Note the clear dividing line, oil on top, water on the bottom. If you like, shake vigorously and within five minutes the oil and water will again separate. Now add lecithin (granular soy lecithin is most effective) or alcohol (high-proof ethanol will work) and shake. Twenty-four hours later, oil and water are still one! For a truer test, use animal fat from the cooking pan, full of cholesterol and triglycerides. The result is the same. Much less shaking is required if the lecithin or alcohol is added before the grease coagulates. Pork grease is the most difficult to keep in solution here, and in your body.

Lecithin

Lecithin, a normal phospholipid constituent of bile, is the human body's answer to mixing oil and water. Inadequate or incomplete bile vis-à-vis atherosclerosis really means inadequate lecithin in the bile. Supplementation can make up for what the liver has lost over the years. Lecithin is well known and perfectly safe, a common ingredient in baking for centuries. The medical literature below evidences the positive action of lecithin supplementation on total cholesterol, LDL, HDL, triglycerides, blood platelets and aggregation, and natural cholesterol elimination by the liver itself, which is called reverse cholesterol transport.

The best lecithin supplement is soy lecithin granules. Do NOT use liquid lecithin; it is not as effective, not as refined as granules, and still contains some bad cholesterol actors. A level tablespoon of granular lecithin is sufficient to completely emulsify a high cholesterol, high fat meal. Lecithin has one potential minor side effect, its high phosphorus content, which can tie up calcium. Phosphorus-calcium equilibrium is complex, however, just a little calcium intake from milk, yogurt or calcium supplement will offset this extra demand on body calcium, even for those with or susceptible to bone and cartilage disorders.

Contrast lecithin, nature's gentle solution, with conventional cholesterol drugs called "statins," which are replete with side effects of liver toxicity and skeletal muscle disorders, as documented in the following medical literature. These drugs inhibit the normal intracellular cholesterol synthesis absolutely necessary to the life of brain and nerve cells and all cell membranes.

Soy lecithin granules are not as powerful as statins in correcting past sins. Nature's solutions never equal the sledgehammer approach of drugs. However, a total effort including lifestyle changes, lecithin supplementation and other natural dietary cholesterol controls, presented ahead, can generate synergies that approach drug action, and with only good consequences for your health.

Lecithin

Soy lecithin in human studies... In hypercholesterolemic patients, soy lecithin at 12 g daily for 3 months reduced blood cholesterol 15% and triglycerides 23%, and increased HDL-cholesterol 16%. In hypertriglyceridemic patients, cholesterol fell 18%, triglycerides 36%, platelet aggregation 27%, while HDL-cholesterol rose 14%. Optimal lipoprotein-lowering effect was achieved at 12 g of soy lecithin per day.[160] In a two-year study, cholesterol decreased 22% and triglycerides 26% using a low-fat, lecithin-supplemented diet. Participants adhered to the dietary protocol willingly and eagerly with no side effects.[161] In hypercholesterolemic patients on a four-week diet replacing animal proteins with textured soy proteins containing 6% lecithin, cholesterol fell 18% with total replacement and 13% with partial replacement.[162] Or oppositely, 20 g per day of soy lecithin over two and four week periods did not significantly alter total cholesterol, triglycerides, HLD, LDL, apolipoprotein A [major protein component of HDL], apolipoprotein B [measure of lipoprotein binding; high levels occur in acute angina and heart attack], lipoprotein (a) levels [another bad lipoprotein like LDL] and fibrinogen [soluble plasma protein, first step in blood coagulation] in hyperlipidemic men.[163]

Extensive animal studies... Cynomolgus monkeys fed the American Heart Association Step I diet (AHA) or a modified AHA Step I diet with 3.4% soy lecithin added (mAHA) over eight weeks had 21% and 18% reductions respectively in total cholesterol and non-HDL for standard AHA compared to 46% and 55% reductions for mAHA.[164] In hypercholesterolemic rats, soy lecithin produced striking reductions in LDL and VLDL [V = very], and an increase in HDL.[165] Soy lecithin fed to rats on a diet containing 0.5% added cholesterol revealed that lecithin reduces dietary cholesterol absorption.[166] In rats with a normal lipid profile, soy lecithin lowered cholesterol by stimulating bile secretion.[167] In guinea pigs fed a six week diet containing 15% lard enriched with 0.5% cholesterol, soy lecithin supplementation at 7.5% of the diet lowered total cholesterol 49% compared to the control group. Dietary lecithin was particularly effective in increasing HDL/total cholesterol ratio.[168] Rabbits fed an atherogenic [depositing plaque on artery walls] diet of 14% hydrogenated coconut oil developed hypercholesterolemia as the lipoprotein distribution shifted from predominately HDL to predominately VLDL. After 18 months of this diet, extensive plaque had formed in main branches of coronary arteries and all parts of the aorta, reducing channel area by almost 50%. Dietary liver damage also occurred with fatty change, cholangitis [inflammation of bile duct] and portal fibrosis [forming fibrous tissue]. Continuing the atherogenic diet but adding 3% soy lecithin for an additional four months resulted in the cholesterol and lipoprotein distribution returning to normal. Also, plaque lesions modified favorably, occupying less space, and there was an absence of foam cells [macrophages take up denatured LDL modified by oxidation or other reactions on the vascular wall] and cholesterol clefts. Dietary lecithin promoted a return to normal lipoprotein distribution and removal of lipids from established atherosclerotic plaque.[169]

Reverse cholesterol transport... is a multi-step process involving the movement of cholesterol from peripheral tissue back to the liver.[170] Apolipoproteins [protein components of lipoproteins, important in lipid transport and metabolism] and two key enzymes, lecithin-cholesterol acyltransferase (LCAT) and cholesteryl ester transfer protein (CETP) mediate these steps. Nascent high-density lipoprotein (HDL) particles gather up free cholesterol in peripheral tissue, which LCAT converts to cholesteryl esters and CETP transfers to apolipoprotein B-containing lipoproteins for liver removal.[171] Soy lecithin increases HDL levels,[160, 165, 168] as well as LCAT.[165] In turn, LCAT increases apolipoprotein B-containing lipoproteins and HDL.[172] HDL cholesterol is anti-atherogenic and an independent predictor of coronary artery disease.[173, 174] having an inverse relationship to coronary events. HLD is not only involved in reverse cholesterol transport, but also has antioxidant properties. HDL prevents endothelial [lining of the heart and blood vessels] dysfunction, and inhibits monocytes [precursor of macrophages, which form LDL-containing foam cells on the vascular wall], apoptosis [gene-directed, programmed cell death], platelet activation [progressive changes in blood platelet shape, adhesiveness and aggregation] and factor X [glycoprotein coagulation factor] activation.[174]

Lipid-Lowering Drugs

Statins, a family of lipid-lowering drugs, inhibit hydroxymethylglutaryl coenzyme A (HMG-CoA) reductase enzyme. This blocks intracellular cholesterol synthesis and stimulates LDL-receptor [binding up LDL] formation and activity.[175] FDA-approved HMG-CoA reductase inhibitors for hypercholesterolemia treatment are fungal metabolites or derivatives: (1) lovastatin [Mevacor], (2) simvastatin [Zocor], and (3) pravastatin [Pravacol]; and synthetic: (4) fluvastatin [Lescol], (5) atorvastatin [Lipitor],[176, 177] and (6) rosuvastatin [Crestor].[178] Many of these drugs reduce LDL by 20-30%. Simvastatin produces LDL reductions greater than 30%,[176] and atorvastatin, a second generation synthetic statin, gives 40-60% reductions depending on dose.[177] In 164 short-term placebo-controlled trials, LDL cholesterol fell 60% with rosuvastatin at 80 mg/day or 40% at 5 mg/day, 55% with atorvastatin at 80 mg/day or 40% at 10 mg/day, and 40% with lovastatin and simvastatin at 40 mg/day. Pravastatin and fluvastatin had smaller reductions.[178] Statins have proven efficacy in reducing the risk of cardiovascular events.[179]

Other uses... Emerging evidence suggests that statins are beneficial in Alzheimer's disease (AD), multiple sclerosis (MS), and ischemic [insufficient blood supply] stroke.[180] High cholesterol is a risk factor for AD in epidemiological studies, and statins can be protective here. Cholesterol is implicated in AD pathogenesis through its physical interaction with amyloid in developing brain plaque deposits; specifically cholesterol levels modulate the processing of amyloid precursor protein (APP), thereby influencing the accumulation of 'A beta' amyloid peptides.[181] For MS, statins are immunomodulatory and reduce the migration of leukocytes into the central nervous system (CNS). Statins also inhibit activation of proinflammatory T-cells, induce Th2 response [Th2: subset of helper/inducer T-lymphocytes; see MS in Chapter 12] and decrease expression of CNS inflammatory mediators such as nitric oxide and tumor necrosis factor alpha (TNF-alpha).[180]

Liver toxicity side effects... HMG-CoA reductase inhibitors are associated with mild, asymptomatic elevation of liver enzymes alanine aminotransferase (ALT) and asparate aminotransferase [these play a key role in protein metabolism]. Case reports show cholestasis [arrest of normal bile flow], jaundice, fatty liver, hepatitis, chronic active hepatitis, cirrhosis and acute liver failure with all lipid-lowering drugs. HMG-CoA reductase inhibitors are also hepatotoxic in some animal studies. Compounding risk factors include alcohol, acetaminophen and pre-existing liver disease. The US Food and Drug Administration (FDA) recommends liver enzyme monitoring for all statins.[182] In one study, 5% of 100 patients on simvastatin and 4.5% of 90 patients on pravastatin develop significant liver toxicity, as evidenced in liver function tests.[183] Lovastatin substantially alters 36 liver proteins in a male rats, with the following study observations: HMG-CoA reductase inhibition (a) provokes a counterregulatory response in the cholesterol synthesis pathway, (b) alters key carbohydrate metabolism enzymes, and (c) modifies cell proteins involved in skeletal musculature, protease [enzyme that splits interior peptide bonds in a protein] inhibition, calcium homeostasis, cell signaling and apoptosis [gene-directed, programmed cell death].[184]

Muscle side effects... Statins are associated with skeletal muscle complaints of myositis [muscle inflammation] and rhabdomyolysis [skeleton muscle cell destruction], mild elevation of blood creatine kinase (CK) [enzyme in muscles catalyzing formation of adenosine triphosphate, the primary energy source within all living cells], myalgia [muscle pain] with and without elevated CK levels, muscle weakness, muscle cramps, and persistent myalgia and CK elevations after statin withdrawal.[185] Pravastatin, lovastatin, and simvastatin are linked to skeletal myopathies [muscle diseases] in humans and rats. Pravastatin is less myotoxic than lovastatin or simvastatin, and this differential toxicity correlates with less pravastatin inhibition of HMG-CoA reductase in nonhepatic tissues.[186]

Cancer... Statins cause cancer in rodents, in some cases at concentrations close to that prescribed to humans. Evidence of human carcinogenicity is inconclusive to date because of inconsistent results and insufficient follow-up duration. Statins should be avoided by all patients except those with high risk of coronary heart disease.[187]

Anticancer... Cholesterol metabolism manipulation opens the possibility of interfering with malignant cell growth. Cholesterol deprivation reduces the development and alters the composition of cell membranes. Malignant cells have a high LDL requirement, which statins address.[188] Lovastatin exerts antitumor activity in experimental models.[189] Lovastatin not only inhibits the hepatic HMG-CoA reductase cholesterol pathway, but also the mevalonate pathway [steroid synthesis; inhibition leads to lack of development] and protein-protein interaction in key regulatory proteins including ras [frequently detected oncogene in animal and human cancers; oncogene: mutated version of a normal gene; can convert a normal cell to tumor cell].[190, 191]

B Vitamins

Liver damage from aging and slow chemical poisoning is only part of the reason for inadequate bile lecithin and damaging cholesterol effects. Ready for a shocker? The liver manufactures its own lecithin by combining two B vitamins, choline and inositol, with fatty acids and phosphoric acid. That's it – that's all we ever needed to prevent cholesterol plaque on artery walls and resulting cardiovascular disease. All the junky white bread, white rice and other denatured cereals we devoured in the past, totally devoid of B vitamin nutrition, was the *slippery slope* to bad cholesterol too!

Choline and inositol are richly supplied in the wholesome B vitamin foods of Chapter 4. Nutritional yeasts are well-endowed and whole-grain cereals are proven cholesterol fighters, not only due to their choline and inositol content, but also through strong antioxidant activity, high soluble fiber especially in oats and barley, and improved gastrointestinal functioning. These quality foods can overcome past deprivation and boost current bile production to some extent, however, lecithin supplement, with its highly concentrated choline and inositol, may always be needed once your liver has been damaged.

<u>Other natural cholesterol controllers</u>. Vitamin C reduces total cholesterol, LDL and triglycerides, as evidenced in its Chapter 7 medical literature review. Here is yet another reason to restore your genetically missing Vitamin C. Vitamin E, Omega 3 and EFAs also have proven efficacy, and so do the herbs American Ginseng, Raw Garlic and others. Supplementing B vitamin niacin decreases triglycerides and LDL, and significantly increases good HDL cholesterol, but with side effects of itching and "flush," a pronounced reddening and warming of the skin.

The medical literature reveals the following about the B vitamins choline and inositol individually.

Review of the Medical Literature

Choline

Membranes and neurons... Phospholipids [phosphate fatty acids] are essential components of cell membranes,[192] and play a critical role in cell membrane signal transduction, which translates external stimulus from hormones, growth factors, etc. into changes in cell transport, metabolism, function, growth or gene expression.[193] Choline is necessary for synthesis of certain phospholipids,[192] including membrane phospholipid lecithin [a phosphatidyl choline, abundant in nerve tissue], sphingomyelin [a phosphoryl choline, found mainly in brain and nervous system], and plasmalogen [glycerol-based, found mainly in brain and spinal cord].[193] Cell membrane breakdown is characteristic of neuron degeneration in acute (stroke) and chronic (senile dementia) neurological disorders. Changes in cell membrane choline phospholipids indicate neuron breakdown,[194] and choline deficit may be responsible for Alzheimer's disease initiatation.[195] Choline is a rate-limiting factor in phospholipid synthesis.[194]

Brain and acetylcholine... Choline is crucial to brain development.[196] Choline is precursor to neurotransmitter acetylcholine [nervous system stimulant, vasodilator, cardiac depressant]. Choline supplementation enhances brain acetylcholine synthesis and release.[192]

Liver... Choline is necessary for normal liver function.[193] Deficiency causes liver cell transformation, proliferation and apoptosis [gene-directed, programmed cell death].[197]

Blood... Choline is involved in lipid transport and platelet activating factor [potent activator of many white blood cell functions and platelet activation: progressive, overlapping changes in blood platelet shape, adhesiveness and aggregation].[193]

Inositol

Membranes... Inositol of cell membrane phospholipid phosphatidylinositol is involved in regulating cell signaling and response to external stimuli and nerve transmission, and in mediating enzyme activity through interaction with various proteins.[198, 199] The cell nucleus is a site for phosphatidylinositol synthesis and hydrolysis [chemical decomposition by reacting with water].[199] Many proteins bind to inositol phosphates.[200]

Nerves... Inositol can be effective in treating central nervous system disorders such as Alzheimer's disease, depression, panic disorder and obsessive-compulsive disorder. Inositol may alleviate some of the negative effects of lithium therapy [antidepressant, suspected of reducing phosphatidylinositol signaling].[198] In human and animal diabetes studies, free inositol and inositol phospholipid deficiency are implicated in nerve conduction deficits.[201] Altered inositol production is documented in patients with diabetes, multiple sclerosis, chronic renal failure and galactosemia [rare genetic disorder; galactose is a glucose isomer converted to glucose by the liver].[198]

Calcium signaling... Inositol trisphosphate (InsP3) is a secondary control for calcium internal release and external entry. InsP3/Ca2+ signaling helps to regulate cell processes including fertilization, development, proliferation and apoptosis [gene-directed, programmed cell death].[202]

Liver and lipids... Inositol deficiency causes intestinal lipodystrophy [-dystrophy: disorder due to defective or faulty nutrition] and liver triglyceride accumulation in animals.[203]

Pregnancy and infants... In preterm RDS [respiratory distress syndrome] infants, inositol supplementation improves neonatal [the first four weeks after birth] outcomes, significantly reducing bronchopulmonary dysplasia [a chronic lung disease, sometimes seen in children who received high-oxygen neonatal respiratory support], retinopathy of prematurity [degenerative eye disease, again related to high-oxygen respiratory support], grade III-IV intraventricular hemorrhage, stage 4 therapy and death rates in two clinical trials.[204] However, inositol use during pregnancy remains controversial, of benefit in preventing neural tube defects [spina bifida] in mice, but with risk of inducing uterine contractions.[198]

Bile Herbs

Table 11-4 lists herbs that improve bile flow. While benefits are most obvious to exocrine functioning, these herbs boost endocrine performance a little too.

TABLE 11-4. EXOCRINE LIVER HERBS.

Herb	Comments
BILE – HELPFUL NUTRIENTS and HERBS (in order of importance)	
eating liver	
Gentian Root	Also found in Swedish Bitters tonic.
Cascara sagrada	Laxative action too, especially at 2X.
Parsley	Also adrenal cortex immune (Table 7-6).
BILE – REBUILDING HEALTH	
The following aromatic seeds:	Rebuild pituitary oversight control.
Anise	
Caraway	
Fennel	
Coriander	
Dill	

Maintaining Bile Health. Eating liver increases bile flow and strengthens endocrine liver functions. In a sense, eating liver is forced functioning of the organ, but a very gentle force. Gentian Root has a powerful effect on bile output – occasional use only, not more than once a week. Cascara sagrada and Parsley are minor players here. Cascara is better known for its laxative action.

Rebuilding Bile Health. The pituitary gland has oversight control of the exocrine liver, just as the pituitary oversees the exocrine pancreas and stomach acid. Aromatic seeds such as *sweet* Anise, Caraway, Fennel, Coriander and Dill supply the pituitary nutrition for this control. These aromatic seeds are used in many food recipes and greatly benefit your liver. When taking the seeds therapeutically, variety is important. The ideal digestive balance is seeds of Anise, Caraway, Fennel and Coriander matched with an equal number of Dill seeds. At 2X dosing, aromatic seeds stimulate bile flow. Combining aromatic seeds with the exocrine pancreas Alfalfa Seeds, Papaya Seeds, Kiwi Seeds and Red Root and stomach acid normalizing Citrus Seeds improves total digestion significantly. Details in Chapter 10.

Gallbladder

Each year surgeons in the United States remove over 300,000 gallbladders because of gallstones. A missing gallbladder impairs fat digestion, since no bile reservoir is available to handle large amounts of ingested fat. Consequently, small low-fat meals are necessary for good digestion and cholesterol control.

Gallstones contain cholesterol, bile salts, calcium bilirubinate, inorganic calcium or other minerals. Guess what they don't contain? Lecithin. Gallstones precipitate out of supersaturated bile in the same way that cholesterol precipitates out of super-saturated blood. Gallstones can cause severe pain, which often starts only years after they first form. Gallbladder inflammation and bile duct obstruction are also possible. Obstruction brings on nausea and jaundice, and requires immediate medical attention. Minor inflammation and partial bile duct obstruction can sometimes be alleviated by massage.

Massage Technique. Use the first three fingers (not the thumb) of the right hand held straight out and together. With cotton shirt in-between to reduce friction, exhale to expose the rib cage and gently push at a 30-degree inclined angle from the ribs to the *valley* below along the right rib cage until you find the "knot" (closure) in the bile duct. Vibrate your fingers on the obstruction, then gently push again, and repeat until the knot releases. However, don't overdo it and aggravate already swollen, inflamed tissues. A little massage every few hours and over several days may be necessary. Pulsating, warm water massage helps too.

Lecithin. Inadequate bile lecithin is the main culprit in gallstones. Higher concentrations of lecithin will relieve supersaturation and prevent stone formation. Rebuild bile lecithin content with the B vitamins and herbs mentioned above, and if necessary with lecithin supplementation as ingested soy lecithin granules will go *full circle* to emulsify bile.

Gallstones... can be asymptomatic or painful with accompanying life-threatening obstruction and infection.[205] Gallstones form when the balance of biliary lipid solubility tips in favor of precipitating out cholesterol, bilirubin [reddish bile pigment, by-product of red blood cell breakdown by the liver], and bacterially degraded biliary lipids. For cholesterol gallstones, changes in liver cholesterol secretion, gallbladder motility [spontaneous movement] and intestinal bacteria degradation of bile salts destabilize cholesterol carriers within bile and nucleate/precipitate cholesterol microcrystals from supersaturated bile.[206, 207] While a necessary condition, bile supersaturation is not sufficient for cholesterol gallstone formation; pronucleating substances such as mucin [albuminoid substance found in mucous secretions] must also be present. Gallbladder stasis [stagnation in fluid flow] is another factor, well-known for its role in pigment stone formation.[208] Black pigment gallstones involve increased bilirubin concentrations in the bile and calcium bilirubinate precipitation. Mechanical obstruction of the biliary tract plays the major role in brown pigment stones, with bacterial degradation and precipitation of biliary lipids.[206] Patients under 40 years of age generate mostly cholesterol stones, whereas pigment stones predominate in patients over 70. Cirrhosis is strongly associated with pigment gallstones. Pigment stones are generally smaller in diameter and fewer in number than cholesterol stones.[209] Gallstones form in 3% to 8% of pregnant women, with 20% to 30% of these stones redissolving postpartum [after childbirth/delivery]. Biliary sludge also disappears following most pregnancies.[210] In epidemiological studies, obesity and alcohol abuse are risk factors for gallstones.[211, 212]

OVERVIEW

Our modern world is a chemical world. Many subtle contaminants in the air we breathe, in drinking water and in our food never threatened previous generations. This daily chemical gauntlet requires a proactive strategy of both more defense and less offense. First line defense is a daily supplement of 500 to 1000 mg of Vitamin C plus bioflavonoids to protect and recycle glutathione, the liver's own internal antioxidant and primary detoxification process. Less offense means limiting your exposure to a wide array of environmental toxins: cigarette smoke, diesel exhaust and particulate matter, gasoline vapors, pesticides, food additives and preservatives, plasticizers, aluminum, and chemicals including many cosmetics. Your overmatched liver cries out for help, "More defense, less offense!"

The liver is the only organ in your body that can regenerate itself. Unfortunately, today's environmental toxins cause a slow loss of liver function and, most critically, loss of liver regeneration. Methionine, the lone sulfur-containing essential amino acid, plays a fundamental role in liver regeneration – and methionine supplementation plus activated charcoal puts the failed mechanism back to work. This revolutionary therapy can bring your liver back to life even in the face of cirrhosis!

Healthy bile is the hidden key to atherosclerosis and cardiovascular disease. Bile emulsifies fats, enabling them to remain in blood solution. Age and slow poisoning of the liver from environmental toxins (again) reduce bile potency and output, causing cholesterol and some triglycerides to precipitate out of blood solution and deposit on artery walls as plaque. Lecithin is the natural emulsifying agent of bile, and supplementation can make up for what your liver has lost over the years. The best lecithin supplement is soy lecithin granules, which improves total cholesterol, LDL, HDL, triglycerides, blood platelets and aggregation, and reverse cholesterol transport, the natural elimination of cholesterol by the liver itself. Lecithin supplementation can also prevent and possibly reverse gallstones.

***

12. CORRECTING DIS-EASE

If it ain't broke, don't fix it! First and foremost build health and stop worrying about disease. Nature put you inside an amazingly resilient self-correcting machine. Generally only years to decades of bad chemistry, with grievous nutritional deprivation, can wreck it. Conversely, good raw material input – macronutrients, B vitamins, fatty acids, trace metals and herbs – produces good end product output: your hormones, neurotransmitters, enzymes, coenzymes, cofactors and the rest of life's chemistry. Chapters 2-7 describe this common sense nutritional approach to health for the adrenal gland, as do Chapters 8-11 for the pituitary, thyroid, pancreas and liver.

Chapter 12 switches emphasis from building the sinews of health to solving endocrine dysfunctions and diseases. Pituitary and adrenal failures involve only functional exhaustions and imbalances because these two glands are protected from injury and scar tissue by the body's strongest antioxidant defenses. As a result, amazing recoveries in function and health are possible. Pituitary exhaustion, suppression or atrophy can easily be corrected by using Chapter 8 trace metal and herb supplementations. Complicated adrenal exhaustions and imbalances cause chronic diseases such as osteoarthritis, rheumatoid arthritis, multiple sclerosis, lupus, fibromyalgia and chronic fatigue syndrome. Starting below, this chapter focuses on solving such debilitating "Adrenal Dis-ease."

With regard to the thyroid gland, pancreas and liver, tissue injury and scarring characterize their dysfunctions and diseases. Reversing such damage is problematic except for the liver, whose regenerating mechanism can be brought back to life even in the face of cirrhosis. Details are given in Chapter 11. Thyroid injury and scar tissue from iodine deprivation lead to hyperthyroidism or hypothyroidism, and goiter. Normal function may be restored with Chapter 9 nutrition, although the standard medical practice of drugs, radioactive iodine, surgery or synthetic hormone replacement therapy eventually proves necessary in many cases. Fortunately, the thyroid gland is a minor endocrine player and loss of homeostasis from these physician solutions is tolerable. Lastly, the pancreas and bad news, second chances at health are few and far between for this crucial endocrine and exocrine performer. Chapter 10 describes a grim reality and some helpful therapies.

ADRENAL DIS-EASE

Inadequate nutrition accumulates a debt of dysfunctions and diseases. Adrenal dysfunctions are permanent errors embedded in the adrenal medulla and cortex, either hypoactive or hyperactive functioning, often requiring extraordinary measures to correct. These breakdowns in primary Energy, Healing, Stress and Immune functions, alone or in combination, or within various subfunctions, cause disease in distant dependent body systems: nerves, muscles and protein structures, bones and cartilage, and connective tissue. To understand the direct relationship between adrenal functions and disease, review Figure 2-B and accompanying "Functions" and "Dependent Body Systems" text in Chapter 2. Sorting out exactly what's wrong with your body is sometimes the most difficult part of any solution to disease. One fact for sure, treating symptoms is not the answer – yes, temporary relief, but long-term counterproductive. Symptoms reveal the problem; cure comes only by finding and correcting its root cause. Discovering underlying mechanisms is a basic tenet of science, and this chapter gives adrenal mechanisms and solutions to many intractable chronic diseases for which Western drugs have no answers.

Adrenal dysfunctions are of only two types: exhaustions and imbalances. Exhaustions are hypoactive functioning in a primary function or subfunction; they can be mild (sub-par functioning, symbolically represented as permanently ↓ or ↓↓) to severe (little or no functioning and output, permanently ↓↓↓ or worse). The key point, exhaustions persist in spite of the fact that all necessary nutrients are now supplied. Basically, raw material input cannot become end product output if gland machinery is nonfunctional. These exhaustions remain unresponsive until targeted, superior nutrition is applied in accordance with this chapter.

Hyperactive-hypoactive imbalances are generally less intractable than exhaustions. They develop between Healing ⇌ Energy, Immune ⇌ Stress or within subfunctions, often energy/nerve or immune response. Their initiating cause is either hyperactivity, mild (permanently ↑ or ↑↑) to severe (permanently ↑↑↑ or worse), or hypoactivity in one of the functions or subfunctions. NOTE: nutrition produces positive therapeutic action, which is symbolically represented as temporarily ↑ or ↑↑.

Hyper and Hypo Ballet. Hyperactivity results when too much of a raw material is supplied, such as caffeine from coffee making nerves hyper. Hyperactivity also occurs if too little nutrition is supplied, as revealed in Chapter 7 "Rebuilding Nerve Function Health." By either account, hyperactive functioning uses up vast quantities of all its raw materials, not just the original causative agent, thereby permanently cementing the dysfunction into adrenal gland physiology. In the primary function where such a permanent error originates, and with continuing deprivation of needed raw materials, hyperactive functioning inevitably decays to hypoactive functioning, i.e. exhaustion develops. Overuse or abuse of a function can also bring on exhaustion; for example Stress exhaustion develops from a lifetime of coping with more stress than the adrenal gland can handle with the nutrition provided. Going full circle, hypoactive exhaustion then produces hyperactive imbalance in the other half of an adrenal equilibrium. Stress exhaustion and consequent hyperactive Immune (autoimmune) activity cause the dependent-body-system disease rheumatoid arthritis. Constant hyperactive or hypoactive functioning is the bane of good health and long life.

All adrenal dysfunctions are some amalgam of exhaustions and imbalances. Needless to say, many complex combinations exist. Adrenal-caused DISEASE, however, goes beyond DYSFUNCTION, and usually involves: (1) long-term nutritional abuse, or (2) some triggering event such as trauma (physiological trauma, not the standard medical definition of physical trauma), which pushes your adrenal gland "over a cliff" and your body into disease. For instance, caffeine can bring on hyper nerves/hypo healing imbalance dysfunction… but hyper nerves/hypo healing disease requires much more to go wrong. When symptoms transfer from adrenal tasks to dependent body systems, then you have welcomed disease into your life. Climbing back up the "disease cliff" demands a quantum leap in corrective measures. Fortunately, good news – it can be done. Superior nutrition using large dose supplementations and combinations of whatever raw materials you ran out of originally "synergize" and can propel you up the steep cliff wall and back to health.

Chronic diseases resulting from adrenal dysfunctions manifest in:

(1) Dependent Body Systems of nerves, muscles and protein structures, bones and cartilage, and connective tissue (from Figure 2-B). Of course, other dependent systems exist and are tied to adrenal functions in more complex ways. Skin depends upon total medulla health, Energy and Healing together. Eyes are linked to adrenal Healing and Immune, and to the endocrine pancreas. Heart and red blood cells rely to some extent on Energy mechanisms, but mostly on Stress ability, while white blood cells require some Healing mechanisms (such as zinc for T-lymphocytes), but mostly Immune function. "Where exactly" chronic disease strikes also depends on specific underlying adrenal causes, including subfunction variations and multiple dysfunctions with a first cause (the setup for disease) and second cause (precipitating event, often trauma). Many more dependent body systems remain hidden in adrenal and endocrine complexity. This necessitates learning all you can about your disease. Answering basic mechanism questions will reveal causes!

(2) Areas of Adrenal Responsibility, that is, NO Energy, NO Healing, NO Stress ability, or NO Immune. A severely exhausted hypoactive function ($\downarrow\downarrow\downarrow$ or worse) can become a disease by itself. One function is particularly critical here. No Immune can unleash a Pandora's box from chronic infections to cancer. In effect, every cell in your body depends on the immune system for its life.

Adrenal diseases dominate medical text pathologies. Western medicine (allopathy), however, is fixated on treating symptoms. Again, such treatment is temporary relief and long-term counterproductive because symptoms are the resulting effect, not the underlying cause. Correct the actor, NOT the receiver of action. Adrenal functions dictate how the body responds to all internal needs and external forces, and this is where the solution lies. Never-ending, incorrect response (chronic dis-ease) has an adrenal root cause and cure. Past deprivation of essential nutrients is the cause, and therefore the means to cure. You must redress nature's long-suffering adrenal chemistry and nutritional needs. By contrast, acute diseases such as heart attack, stroke and other emergency room procedures require a completely different fix – immediate symptomatic countermeasures. Allopathy becomes appropriate and efficacious when chronic disease advances to an acute stage.

Primary Exhaustion-Imbalance Linkages. In their simplest form, severe adrenal exhaustions and imbalances are one hypoactive ($\downarrow \downarrow \downarrow$) and one hyperactive ($\uparrow \uparrow \uparrow$) function in the primary functions, either Healing and Energy or Immune and Stress. However, with continuing nutrient deprivation, primary medulla exhaustion and imbalance or primary cortex exhaustion and imbalance sooner or later engulfs the entire adrenal gland, as shown in Figure 12-A.

IMMUNE	STRESS
$\downarrow \downarrow \downarrow$	$\uparrow \uparrow \uparrow$
HEALING	ENERGY
$\uparrow \uparrow \uparrow$	$\downarrow \downarrow \downarrow$

(1) Energy-Immune Hypolink

IMMUNE	STRESS
$\uparrow \uparrow \uparrow$	$\downarrow \downarrow \downarrow$
HEALING	ENERGY
$\downarrow \downarrow \downarrow$	$\uparrow \uparrow \uparrow$

(2) Stress-Healing Hypolink

FIGURE 12-A.
ADRENAL EXHAUSTION-IMBALANCE LINKAGES.

Figure 12-A reveals that primary hypoactivity and hyperactivity become cross-linked, Energy with Immune and Stress with Healing. This cross-linking is a natural consequence of homeostasis, or stability and equilibrium in a physiological system through feedback. The cross connection can be understood easiest when examining Figure 2-B and how cortex functions act within the pituitary → adrenal medulla → adrenal cortex → pituitary feedback loop for Energy → Stress and Healing → Immune action. For example, hyperactive Immune sends a "too much" message to the pituitary, which shuts down the healing-immune action plan, causing hypoactive Healing. For the energy-stress action plan, hypoactive Stress forces the pituitary into sustained action, thereby generating hyperactive Energy.

The consequences of Figure 12-A are as follows. NO Energy also produces some degree of NO Immune, as depicted in Figure 12-A(1). The resulting poor immune response can range from morning congestion to susceptibility to bacterial infection, colds and flu and even to low-grade leukemia that comes and goes with your energy level. Energy exhaustion is the hidden cause of many immune difficulties, and treating immune symptoms with antibiotics in such cases brings only the briefest respite. Fix your lack of energy and you will fix your immune system too! As an indication of this hypolink, supplementing adrenaline precursor pantothenic acid increases immunoglobulin (antibody proteins that fight infection) and neutrophil (strong against bacteria) phagocyte numbers.[1]

Another linkage outcome is Figure 12-A(2), where NO Stress ability leads to NO Healing too. Of course, Figure 12-A is an idealized end-result. A lifetime of too much stress exhausts Primary Stress Function and induces arthritis; however, Healing starts out normal and only slowly sinks (permanently ↓, then ↓↓) to the severe hypoactivity (↓↓↓) of painful osteoarthritis and joint cartilage degeneration.

Figure 12-A(2) is the *800 pound gorilla* of dysfunction scenarios because both autoimmune assault and degenerative hypoactive healing are possible. Four Figure 12-A(2) AUTOIMMUNE pathologies can develop from first-cause Energy, Healing, Stress and Immune failures:

– Hypoactive Stress exhaustion causes rheumatoid arthritis.

– Hyperactive Immune gives rise to lupus (systemic lupus erythematosus), autoimmune attack on the connective tissue of many organs, especially the kidneys. Here, sustained hyperactivity from an Immune subfunction imbalance uses up vast quantities of immune raw materials, permanently cementing the dysfunction and disease into immune system physiology.

– Hypoactive Healing sooner or later involves autoimmune attack on dependent muscles and body protein structures. This can range from bursitis and forms of rheumatism to fibromyalgia and other muscle diseases.

– Hyperactive Energy can lead to autoimmune attack on the nervous system. Actually, too much energy/adrenaline is a rare commodity, found only in mania. Much more likely are hyperactive nerves, as the nervous system is a near-equal partner with energy in this primary medulla function. Nerve diseases such as multiple sclerosis (MS) and amyotrophic lateral sclerosis (ALS, Lou Gehrig's disease) suffer mild to severe autoimmune attack depending on the degree of cortex involvement and the degree of energy/nerve imbalance (explained later in subfunction "quirks").

Many other more complex autoimmune diseases exist within the Figure 12-A(2) framework; for example autoimmune attack on the skin is due to a total medulla failure, both hypoactive Energy and hypoactive Healing as first cause. The point of attack and the course of autoimmune diseases vary widely, but always occur at the weakest link of targeted dependent systems, usually previously injured tissue. Autoimmune assault seems to be everywhere today and Figure 12-A(2) is the reason.

Figure 12-A(2) can also generate four hypoactive-Healing DEGENERATIVE pathologies from first-cause Energy, Healing, Stress and Immune failures. These severe breakdown and repair failures typically blend with co-conspirator autoimmune to intensify the attack on targeted tissue – a Bonnie and Clyde effect! Hypoactive healing comes immediately to medulla diseases of muscles, nerves and skin, and eventually to cortex diseases of connective tissue, bones and cartilage.

By comparison, Figure 12-A(1) pathologies are relativity benign on dependent body systems. However, primary Immune exhaustion/failure endangers life itself. First-cause hyperactive Stress develops only from administered steroids, including cortisone and prednisone. Hyperactive Healing is also rare, usually the result of trauma such as severe burns, but this can be dealt with by employing vast amounts of healing raw materials before functioning sinks into exhaustion. That leaves only strongly related No Energy = No Immune, and No Immune = No Energy, which because of a more involved metabolic pathway is subtler in its expression.

CURE PRIMER

You are the ultimate overseer of your health. Why not take charge and investigate your chronic disease(s) and any acute manifestations, discovering their mechanisms and tracing them back to adrenal roots. Then take corrective action.

HOW TO PROCEED–the first question is, "where is the disease occurring?" The original negligent adrenal function, the first to go *haywire*, targets its dependent system for attack. Other function failures can pile on further specifying the point of attack. To illustrate, multiple sclerosis (MS) is an attack on the fatty acid myelin sheath of nerves. Understanding a disease mechanism reveals its solution! MS strikes the nervous system; thus the original negligent primary function is Energy/nerves. The modus operandi of attack on a dependent system is almost always Figure 12-A(2) hyperactive Immune (autoimmune) or hypoactive Healing (degenerative) in character, or both. MS demyelination involves some lack of repair, and therefore a hyper nerves/hypo healing imbalance dysfunction… BUT second question, "what turns this relatively harmless dysfunction into debilitating disease?" The MS attack isn't directly on nerves; rather it's slightly altered to the surrounding and insulating fatty acid myelin sheath suggesting a triggering event of Stress trauma, since only Stress function directly affects fatty acid/fat metabolism (Table 3-1). Thus, "where exactly" depends on specific underlying adrenal causes, including multiple mechanisms of first cause, the setup, and second cause or triggering event. A second-cause MS triggering event of Stress trauma (far beyond hyperactive fat burning) quickly depletes cortex nutrients and reserves, bringing on severe Stress exhaustion and consequent severe autoimmune/inflammatory assault, which is the dominate pathology of this disease. More on MS later. The complexity has only just begun.

Severe exhaustion cures combine targeted raw materials – B vitamins, fatty acids, trace metals and herbs – to produce powerful synergies. Taking the B vitamin and trace metal responsible for the same function is particularly effective. For example, ingesting B vitamin pantothenic acid (Figure 4-A) and trace metal copper (Figure 6-A) together will have a powerful effect on Primary Energy Function. It will be a powerful and positive effect IF there is need, i.e. you suffer from severe Energy exhaustion. Energy-related fatty acids and herbs must contribute too, usually by being liberally supplied beforehand. This fills nutrient reserves so complete nutrition is available to participate in the leap back to health. A combined nutritional "direct hit" (↑ ↑ ↑) will then propel a severe adrenal exhaustion up and over the disease cliff (↓ ↓ ↓) of the past and back to precious normalcy, freeing you from the maelstrom forever.

Targeted B vitamin, fatty acid, trace metal and herb combinations achieve potencies equal to Western pharmaceuticals without side effects (again, if there is need). Such amazing positive action, however, brings a *WARNING* ☛ **Take no allopathic**

drugs with these natural cures; interactions occur and can be dangerous. This means NO ℞ drugs for several weeks prior to and for several days after the combination regimens of this chapter. Many over-the-counter drugs are also too strong here, for sure aspirin and other NSAIDs (nonsteroidal anti-inflammatory drugs).

Some ℞ and over-the-counter drugs may be optional in your current health program, while others have natural alternatives. For instance, well-known and proven (insurance companies pay) diet and lifestyle programs exist for cholesterol control and heart disease. If an allopathic drug is necessary and unavoidable, then employ only mild exhaustion cures using Chapter 4 B vitamin supplementations and separately Chapter 6 trace metal supplementations, and correct adrenal imbalances with Chapter 7 herbs. For convenience, these mild "non-combination" exhaustion and imbalance therapies are outlined in concise tables ahead. This route to cure will take longer. Nevertheless, you can slowly work your way back to good health, and in some cases the need for a drug will disappear as you make nutritional improvements.

Another option is commercially available multi-B-vitamin chelated-multi-metal supplements. These are relatively low dose in comparison to Chapter 12 combinations, and can speed recovery from severe exhaustions and imbalances without adversely interacting with ℞ and over-the-counter drugs. Make sure such supplements satisfy Figure 4-A and Figure 6-A nutrition, and then take them only two or three times a week, as side effects occur with continuous use.

Priming the Cure Pump. Powerful combination cures for severe adrenal exhaustion require a foundation of good nutrition beforehand. All maintenance and rebuilding nutrients must be input separately for several weeks before attempting to surmount any disease cliff. This is far beyond nutrition at your pleasure; commitment and discipline are imperatives here. Therefore, add "the right stuff" to your diet, initially at 2X to overcome past deprivation:

✓ Chapter 3 high-quality macronutrients.

✓ Chapter 4 natural, wholesome B vitamin-rich foods of whole-grain cereals, nutritional yeasts and green vegetables.

✓ Chapter 5 good fats of Omega 6 EFA vegetable oils and Omega 3 fish oils including eating fish and seafood – yes, Omega 3 fish every day!

✓ Chapter 6 Colloidal Minerals, Dandelion Root and other sources of trace metals naturally, as well as appropriate metal supplementations.

✓ Chapter 7 herbs to maintain and rebuild key functions.

Incorporate these good foods and nutrients into your diet for at least three weeks before going any further in this chapter. Eating the same old junk food from the supermarket, then taking a pill to fix the past won't work. If that's the shortcut you still desire, consult an MD – they're specialists in pills. Taking any Chapter 12 severe exhaustion cure without a proper nutritional foundation will only further injure your adrenal gland, endocrine system and body, as the cure itself uses up significant raw material reserves. And if all of these nutrients with their own complex interactions are not abundantly present, then the cure isn't going to work.

Learn About Your Disease. Figuring out which adrenal dysfunction(s) and resulting chronic disease(s) you have is often the most difficult and frustrating part of finding a medical solution, whether by conventional methods or this guide. A proper diagnosis is half the battle. Gather as much information from as many sources as you can:

– Symptoms (subjective) and signs (objective, e.g. eczema).

– Established syndromes: arthritis, chronic fatigue syndrome?

– Medical tests: Many endocrine tests evidence dysfunction only during manifest symptoms, not when latent. Endocrine tests are not infallible.

– Past diagnoses.

– Medical books reveal causes and frequently mechanisms.

– Medical literature. The National Institute of Health (NIH) "National Library of Medicine" Internet site, Medline, is very helpful. At this site, you can type in a diagnosis or symptoms and signs and start learning about your disease. Even go to the medical library of a nearby university medical school and study up.

Adrenal Clues. Table 12-1 gives a short list of possible hyperactive and hypoactive symptoms and signs for the four primary adrenal functions and major subfunctions.

TABLE 12-1. COMMON SYMPTOMS AND SIGNS OF ADRENAL DYSFUNCTION AND DISEASE.

IMMUNE	STRESS	
<u>hypoactive</u> — frequent congestion — susceptibility to infections, colds and flu. — yeast infections — serious immune failure, cancer. <u>hyperactive</u> — autoimmune diseases — lupus	<u>stress hypoactive</u> — worn out easily — headaches — arthritis <u>hyperactive</u> — Cushing's syndrome	<u>fatigue hypoactive</u> — quickly exhausted — chronic fatigue — headaches — too cold/too hot (also thyroid?). — edema

HEALING	ENERGY
<u>hypoactive</u> — poor wound healing — premature aging — healing failure in a dependent body system (Figure12-A(2)). — muscle problems, particularly in the hardest working muscle, the heart. — muscle diseases <u>hyperactive</u> — poor wound healing — numbness (and tingling) in arms or legs. — weak flabby muscles; hernias more likely. — heart hurts	<u>hypoactive energy</u> — little or no energy — constant tiredness — dizziness, lightheadedness, feeling of impending fainting. — concussion-like headaches <u>hyperactive nerves</u> — tingling (and numbness) in arms or legs. — hives — nerve diseases

WARNING ☞ **For anyone susceptible to acute disease manifestations such as cardiovascular risk (including angina, heart attack, stroke, fibrillation, arrhythmia, tachycardia and congestive heart failure), especially older adults, consult your physician before using any Chapter 12 cures.**

Order of Battle. Most adrenal disease cures proceed in four stages as shown below. Dysfunctions not yet to the stage of a recognizable disease need only mild exhaustion and/or imbalance remedy. Natural cures usually require that you unwind the disease in reverse order to its original development; the last thing to go wrong is the first to be fixed, and so on. Therefore,

> Step #1—Repair any TRIGGERING EVENTS,
> Step #2—Cure any EXHAUSTIONS,
> Step #3—Correct any IMBALANCES,
> Step #4—HEAL the damage, as much as possible.

Step #1: TRIGGERING EVENTS

Triggering events are often traumas to one or more of the primary adrenal functions or subfunctions. Extreme hyperactivity (far beyond ↑ ↑ ↑) accounts for their pernicious nature. Such frenzied metabolism depletes raw materials quickly, leading to many functional difficulties, chief among them are two priorities: exhaustion (hyper → hypo) and running out of catalysts. Quick-developing exhaustions, those that happen over several weeks to a few months, can be cured exactly the same way as long-term nutritional deprivation exhaustions (Step #2 ahead). Running out of catalysts is the phantom of many diseases. Hyperactivity uses up the catalysts too, whereas normal functioning never depletes the catalysts present in the body.

Causes of Trauma. Stress trauma is the most common shock and ordeal to the endocrine system and body: accident, death in the family, divorce, etc. Basically, upheaval in one's life becomes out-of-control, extreme stress. Energy trauma is intense high-energy use or hyperactive nerves, emotions or mood swings, again personal upheaval, however, this time affecting the nervous system. Healing trauma overwhelms repair systems. Life-threatening burns or tissue damage, or sustained healing without result such as an aneurysm or harsh cosmetics reapplied daily soon exhausts all resources. Immune trauma is usually recurring hyperactivity; a pathogen strikes with ferocity, then hides and cannot be defeated by a weakened immune system. Many subfunction traumas exist particularly within immune lymphocytes, and these can be maddening to solve. A thousand unnatural shocks to mind, body and spirit can wreck adrenal functioning and its four-part harmony. The extreme hyperactivity of trauma requires superior nutrition immediately. If raw material needs are not met throughout the ordeal, you suffer crippling disease consequences.

Multiple sclerosis again provides easy illustration. MS with its original hyper nerves/hypo healing imbalance dysfunction leaps off into disease as a result of Stress trauma with the following over-the-cliff consequences: (1) Stress exhaustion generates autoimmune attack and further aggravates and worsens hypoactive Healing, as indicated in Figure 12-A(2). This leads to progressive healing exhaustion, which is a substantial part of the secondary progressive nature of MS. And (2) missing fatty acid catalysts add the final blow to myelin sheath catabolic and anabolic healing, causing severe impairment of breakdown and repair systems. Stress trauma rapidly depletes niobium and tantalum metal catalysts, now none are available for duties anywhere in the body including stress ability and maintaining the myelin sheath. Rebuilding metal catalytic health requires large-dose supplements as per Chapter 6. Taking trace metals naturally from Colloidal Minerals, Dandelion Root and the like won't do the job of mounting such a steep and high disease cliff.

The herb Hydrangea from Chapter 7 is another fatty acid/fat catalyst that must be replenished following Stress trauma. Table 3-2 amino acid carnitine, which facilitates fat burning by cell mitochondria, can become depleted, although internal manufacture and animal food sources may still be sufficient. The success of the Swank diet[2] in treating MS suggests a catalytic component to the disease. Swank involves ingesting only the good fats of Chapter 5, thus conserving the limited available catalysts for the crucial duty of enabling fatty acids to protect, heal and become part of the myelin sheath. Remaining catalysts are not diluted and wasted on processing bad fats.

Underlying mechanisms and solutions to osteoarthritis, rheumatoid arthritis, multiple sclerosis, lupus, fibromyalgia and chronic fatigue syndrome are presented at the end of this chapter. Because the pathology of most diseases is not as well understood as that of MS, the best Step #1 solution to any chronic disease is to insure no lingering catalytic impairment by supplementing all five metal catalysts – molybdenum (protein), zirconium (fiber), tungsten (carbohydrate) and niobium/tantalum (catabolic and anabolic fat) – according to Chapter 6 guidelines. Energy catalysts Glucose Tolerance Factor (GTF), Beech Bark and Yarrow are also susceptible to depletion.

Not all triggering events are trauma related. Metabolic impairments from nutritional deprivation, age or failure somewhere in endocrine pathways can trigger chronic disease. A triggering event for a number of chronic diseases is immune imbalance. Chronic fatigue syndrome develops from a defect in the metabolic pathway: EFA linoleic acid → phospholipids → arachidonic acid → eicosanoids, which causes T-lymphocyte/B-lymphocyte imbalance and a consequent downward spiral into Immune and Stress exhaustion. While primary function imbalances are usually corrected last (Step #3), immune subfunction imbalances oftentimes must be fixed first to eliminate the cause in "cause and effect." Review of the mild exhaustion cures in Step #2 below reveals many more possible metabolic triggers for chronic disease.

Step #2: EXHAUSTIONS

Adrenal exhaustions are unresponsive nonfunctioning no matter how much good nutrition you now input. Affected adrenal functions or subfunctions have partially shut down (mild exhaustion) or continued on to complete collapse (severe exhaustion). Severe exhaustion is by itself a disease; you went "over a cliff" following years of poor nutrition or the extreme hyperactivity of trauma.

Mild exhaustion symptoms are relatively straightforward. Impaired adrenal hormones cause lack of energy, lack of stress ability, and so on. Severe symptoms develop in both adrenal responsibilities and the dependent body system of the first-cause negligent function in a disease's progression. Table 12-1 gives common hypoactive symptoms and signs for first-cause exhaustions. Second-cause exhaustions are more complicated; resulting syndromes are a blend of characteristics from first cause (the setup) and second cause (triggering event). Multiple sclerosis is a prime example of this blending with its autoimmune and degenerative attack on nervous system myelin sheath.

The most frequent adrenal exhaustions are energy (adrenaline), stress (cortisol) and fatigue (aldosterone) exhaustion, because these three subfunctions and hormones work the hardest every day, and so suffer the most if nutrition is inadequate. Energy exhaustion is as it says, little or no energy for the day's tasks. Symptoms can include constant tiredness, lightheadedness, dizziness, feeling impending fainting and concussion-like headaches. Nerve stimulants such as caffeine, or overuse of simple sugars to generate sugar/energy highs, contribute to adrenaline failure. While these quick energy fixes work short term, in the long run they abuse energy needs and metabolism and hasten its exhaustion. Stress and fatigue exhaustions can occur together, with headaches being the most common symptom. Stress trauma quickly incapacitates the cortisol hormone, however, stress exhaustion most often develops from a lifetime of too much stress for the nutrition provided and, if it's the first function to go *haywire*, spawns arthritis. In all stress-related breakdowns, aldosterone/fatigue function bears the burden too and can become exhausted and unresponsive, making exercise and stamina (Figure 2-C) unpleasant and weight gain and *couch potato-ing* seem normal. Healing exhaustion develops from life-threatening traumas such as severe burns, but also from "endless healing to no avail." For example, harsh cosmetics can wear out repair mechanisms and bring on muscle diseases like fibromyalgia, which is currently epidemic in women. When body proteins (muscles and organ proteins) are broken down only to be used elsewhere rebuilding, then Healing exhaustion is at hand and massive scar tissue and premature aging follow. Immune exhaustion develops as a result of "fighting the same battle endlessly" such as HIV, hepatitis or low-grade infections. Steroids, oral contraceptives and other drugs contribute to poor immune performance. Susceptibility to infections, colds, flu and fungus infestations indicates hypoactivity somewhere in the defense shield. This is serious business because the immune system defends life itself.

All exhaustions must be cured before any imbalances are fixed. And curing exhaustions will go a long way toward correcting imbalances. Unfortunately, plain old good nutrition cannot fix exhaustions. On-target B vitamin and trace metal supplementations are especially needed. However, once health is restored, return to nature's bounty of wholesome B vitamin-rich and metal-rich foods, NOT human-designed pills. Mother Nature is too complicated to interfere with long term.

Mild Exhaustion Cures... summarizing earlier chapters

– Mild exhaustion is chronic low functioning (permanently ↓ or ↓↓), or a glitch in functioning that produces a familiar ebb under similar circumstances.

– Mild exhaustion cures are an attempt to slowly climb back up from an exhaustion "ledge" and restore normal functioning. Slow climbing may not be successful, but should be tried first unless severe exhaustion is certain

– One week, preferably two weeks, of natural wholesome Chapter 3-7 nutrition before attempting any mild exhaustion cure; see "Cure Primer" earlier. And between cure attempts, the same time span and good nutrition.

– ℞ and over-the-counter drugs OK.

Mild exhaustion cures correct an entire primary function with the exception of fatigue, which is handled separately. The text in Chapters 4-7 gives complete details of the following summaries.

Mild Energy Exhaustion Cure

✓ Take Chapter 4 whole-grain cereals especially oats, 2X usage at the start, then 1X. See Table 4-1 and text there.

✓ Chapter 5 good fats every day, 2X at the start and then 1X, with emphasis on Vitamin E, EFAs, GLA and olive oil. See Figure 5-A.

✓ Chapter 6 sources of trace metals naturally, 2X at the start and then 1X. Follow Chapter 6 guidelines.

✓ Input the following Table 7-3 herbs slowly during the period before cure to build Energy health: American Ginseng, Fo-Ti, Alfalfa Seed Tea, Oats, Valerian, Chamomile and Wood Betony. Reread Chapter 7 on how to forge strong adrenal medulla equilibrium as you restore Energy function. Adrenal Balance herbs of Table 7-2 help to "get things running right."

✓ Mild Energy Cure: Supplement B vitamin pantothenic acid and trace metal copper separately, according to guidelines in Chapter 4 and Chapter 6.

✔ Other Concerns…

> Is glucose metabolism OK, specifically pancreas health (Chapter 10) and Vitamin B12, chromium (for GTF), vanadium, titanium, Bilberry, Beech Bark and Yarrow?

> Carbohydrate catalyst: tungsten? Hyperactivity and trauma deplete catalysts.

> Pituitary oversight OK? Review Chapter 8.

Mild Healing Exhaustion Cure

✔ Take Chapter 4 whole-grain cereals especially polysaccharide-rich brown rice and millet, 2X usage at the start, then 1X. See Table 4-1 and text there.

✔ Chapter 5 good fats every day, 2X at the start and then 1X, with emphasis on Vitamin E, EFAs and carotenes. See Figure 5-A.

✔ Chapter 6 sources of trace metals naturally, 2X at the start and then 1X. Follow Chapter 6 guidelines.

✔ Input the following Table 7-4 herbs slowly during the period before cure to build Healing function health: Aloe vera, Blessed Thistle, Passion Flower, Siberian Ginseng, Alfalfa Seed Tea, Hydrangea and possibly Shepherd's Purse/Woundwort and Heather for vasoconstriction. Reread Chapter 7 on how to forge strong adrenal medulla equilibrium as you restore Healing function. Adrenal Balance herbs of Table 7-2 help to "get things running right."

✔ Mild Healing Cure: Supplement B vitamins using the formula 25 pantothenic acid + 1 PABA + 1 B1 (with extra PABA and B1?) according to guidelines in Chapter 4, and separately trace metal zinc according to guidelines in Chapter 6.

✔ Other Concerns…

> Healing-Immune connector/coordinator: nickel?

> Protein catalyst: molybdenum? Hyperactivity and trauma deplete catalysts.

> Pituitary oversight OK? Review Chapter 8.

Mild Stress/Fatigue Exhaustion Cure

✓ Take Chapter 4 nutritional yeasts and green vegetables, 2X usage at the start, then 1X. See Table 4-1 and text regarding balancing with whole-grain cereals.

✓ Chapter 5 good fats every day, 2X at the start and then 1X, with emphasis on Vitamin E, Omega 3, salmon and modest Vitamin D. See Figure 5-A.

✓ Chapter 6 sources of trace metals naturally, 2X at the start and then 1X. Follow Chapter 6 guidelines.

✓ Input the following Table 7-5 herbs slowly during the period before cure to build Stress and fatigue health: American Ginseng, Astragalus (NOT with nutritional yeasts, see severe exhaustion cure ahead), Hawthorn Berries, Hydrangea, Raw Garlic, Sarsaparilla, Yucca and possibly Shepherd's Purse/Woundwort and Heather for vasoconstriction. Adrenal Balance herbs of Table 7-2 help to "get things running right."

✓ Mild Stress Cure: Supplement B vitamins using the formula 2 pantothenic acid + 1 B2 + 1 B6 according to guidelines in Chapter 4, and separately trace metal vanadium according to guidelines in Chapter 6.

✓ Mild Fatigue Cure: Take Guarana, Nettle and nutritional yeast together, or for more potent action, Raw Garlic and Guarana together.

✓ Other Concerns...

Adrenal cortex equilibrium ($\rightleftharpoons$) OK? Adjust with Devil's Claw and Goldenseal Root according to Figure 7-B and text there.

Energy-Stress connector/coordinator: cobalt-containing Vitamin B12?

Fat catalysts: niobium and tantalum? Hyperactivity and trauma deplete catalysts.

GTF metabolism: chromium, vanadium and titanium?

Carnitine OK? See Chapter 3 "Fat Metabolism."

Thyroid OK? Fatigue and stamina problems can be related to thyroid dysfunction; see Chapter 9.

Pituitary oversight OK? Review Chapter 8.

Mild Immune Exhaustion Cure

✓ Take Chapter 3 fiber and phyto-compound foods using Table 3-3 as your guide.

✓ Chapter 4 nutritional yeasts and green vegetables, 2X usage at the start, then 1X. See Table 4-1 and text regarding balancing with whole-grain cereals.

✓ Chapter 5 good fats every day, 2X at the start and then 1X, with emphasis on Vitamin E, Omega 3, Vitamin A, cod liver oil and possibly shark oil. See Figure 5-A.

✓ Chapter 6 sources of trace metals naturally, 2X at the start and then 1X, plus appropriate supplementations. Follow Chapter 6 guidelines.

✓ Input the following Table 7-6 herbs during the period before cure to build Immune health: Blue-Green Algae, Vitamin C/Bioflavonoids, Echinacea, Astragalus (not with nutritional yeasts, see severe exhaustion cure), Green Tea, other problem specific herbs (#7 through #33), and possibly Shepherd's Purse/Woundwort and Heather for vasoconstriction.

✓ Adjust adrenal cortex equilibrium (⇌) with Goldenseal Root and Devil's Claw according to Figure 7-B and text there. Adrenal Balance herbs of Table 7-2 help to "get things running right."

✓ Mild Immune Cure: From Figure 4-A, no Immune B vitamin has been discovered yet. Because of this, combine "B vitamins naturally" nutritional yeasts and green vegetables first with trace metal zinc (for T-lymphocytes) and again an hour later with manganese (primary Immune) using Chapter 4 and Chapter 6 guidelines.

✓ Final adjustment of adrenal cortex equilibrium (⇌) with Goldenseal Root and Devil's Claw, and then Suma.

✓ Other Concerns…

No Energy = No Immune? Figure 12-A(1).

Arachidonic acid metabolism OK? Soy lecithin supplementation may be needed; see Chapter 5.

Thymus atrophy and impaired T-lymphocytes? Zinc supplementation may be needed; see Chapter 6.

Healing-Immune connector/coordinator: nickel?

Fiber catalyst: zirconium? Hyperactivity and trauma deplete catalysts.

Pituitary oversight OK? Review Chapter 8.

Severe Exhaustion Cures

- Severe exhaustion is little or no adrenal functioning (permanently ↓↓↓ or worse), with disease manifesting in a dependent body system.

- Severe exhaustion cures provide the *rocket fuel* (↑↑↑) to propel functioning up the "disease cliff" and back to normal.

- Three weeks of natural wholesome Chapter 3-7 nutrition before attempting any severe exhaustion cure; see "Cure Primer" earlier. And between cure attempts, the same time span and good nutrition.

- No℞ or over-the-counter drugs for several weeks before and several days after cure, dangerous interactions are possible. Low dose commercial multi-B-vitamin chelated-multi-metal supplements are a safe and partially effective alternative to the high dose on-target severe exhaustion cures. Such supplements, if nutritionally complete, are in-between mild and severe exhaustion cures in power and effect.

- For anyone susceptible to acute disease manifestations such as cardiovascular risk, especially older adults, consult your physician before using the following severe exhaustion cures.

Severe exhaustion cures combine B vitamins, trace metals, herbs and fatty acids for the same function or subfunction. Overcoming severe hypoactive functioning involves violating the rules of Table 4-2; specifically harmful overstimulation using 3X is appropriate here! Overstimulation becomes the rocket fuel to propel you back up the disease cliff you fell over in the past. And the bad consequences of overstimulation, mitigated by need, largely disappear. One exception to combining on-target nutrients and producing overstimulation is old age, where the typical exponential increases in free radical activity and oxidative stress leave insufficient function remaining in adrenal gland physiology to handle or benefit from these cures.

Overall, there are hundreds of ways to combine Chapter 4-7 raw materials for the same function and achieve significant benefit in the face of nonfunctioning. The following tables present the few best cures, the ones to try first in your search for renewed health and vigor. However, you may have to invent your own combination cure through trail and error, particularly with regard to the multitude of possible immune lymphocyte exhaustions. The most powerful and successful cures involve ingesting the B vitamin and trace metal responsible for the same function. Unfortunately, the Immune B vitamin remains undiscovered, further complicating any solution to a *haywire* immune system. Sending legions of Table 7-6 herbs and Table 3-3 phyto-compounds may only be the opening immune reconnaissance and battle.

For the two adrenal equilibriums, Healing ⇌ Energy and Immune ⇌ Stress, the powerful therapeutic action (↑ ↑ ↑) of severe exhaustion cures can create new severe imbalances (pantothenic acid + copper generates Healing →→ Energy imbalance), unless both sides of the equilibrium are cured together. Therefore, combined cures for Energy and Healing and for Stress and Immune are the best and most successful therapies, and eliminate much of the complexity of severe exhaustion cures. Basically, you must raise all medulla or all cortex "boats" at the same time. Primary Energy and Healing Functions rise together in Table 12-2, and Primary Stress and Immune in Table 12-3. Of course, individual subfunction cures still have their place, and these do not knock primary equilibriums badly askew. The severe fatigue exhaustion cure of Table 12-4 does not significantly affect the immune system.

CAUTION ☛ **Abuse of the following severe exhaustion cures causes adrenal hyperactivity, which can become as big a problem as hypoactivity exhaustion.** A hyperactive function quickly depletes nutritional reserves and breeds a worse exhaustion. Take time to listen to your body and endocrine system, and then apply just the right amount of the right stuff. The more on-target nutrients you combine, the stronger the cure. A perfect cure will only have to be taken once!

TABLE 12-2. SEVERE ENERGY-HEALING EXHAUSTION CURE.

Necessary nutritional support and "other concerns" are listed earlier in the Mild Energy and Healing Exhaustion Cures.

Item	Protocol/Regimen
1	INGEST EXACTLY 1250 mg pantothenic acid + 50 mg PABA + 50 mg B1 + EXACTLY 2 mg copper + 2 mg zinc at the same time. Rest in bed for the next one hour. Therapeutic action should begin in about 45 minutes (normal digestion) and produce no side effects IF there is need. If any side effects develop from this strong medulla stimulation, STOP, do not continue on to the next item. You can work off the extra medulla hormones/neurotransmitters with energy tasks. Again, R and over-the-counter drug interaction can be dangerous; AVOID THEM.
2	Item 1 must be repeated two more times at one-hour intervals. It takes three doses (3X) to PERMANENTLY eliminate severe Energy and Healing exhaustion and all resultant first-cause dependent body system diseases of nerves, muscles and skin. Never use 4X, which is too much stimulation and goes full circle back to some level of exhaustion.
3	Two days later REBALANCE adrenal medulla and cortex functions with the herbs Angelica and Damiana (Figure 7-A).

Table 12-2. protocol rests on the following raw materials facts between medulla Primary Healing and Energy Functions: 1 PABA + 1 B1 $\rightleftharpoons$ 25 pantothenic acid from Figure 4-C, and Zn $\rightleftharpoons$ Cu from Chapter 6. The interaction of these basic medulla B vitamin and trace metal nutrients is very powerful, and the 3X regimen leaps ($\uparrow \uparrow \uparrow$) almost all medulla "disease cliffs" ($\downarrow \downarrow \downarrow$) in a single bound.

The Table 12-2 protocol will cure NO Energy and NO Healing immediately, and dependent body system diseases of the nervous system, muscles and protein structures in the body, and skin. However, extreme exhaustion (worse than $\downarrow \downarrow \downarrow$) of Energy or Healing may require repeating Table 12-2 three weeks later to achieve complete medulla and dependent body system health. Of course, understand the mechanisms behind your disease completely before attempting any cure. For example, unwinding Step #2 of multiple sclerosis necessitates, first, a severe Stress exhaustion cure, then dealing with the progressive Healing exhaustion resulting from Figure 12-A(2) effects and loss of catalysts. Step #1 has already corrected the catalysts, and the Step #2 severe Stress exhaustion cure eliminates Figure 12-A(2) dynamics, thereby permitting Healing exhaustion to be unwound next. MS targeting of the nervous system developed from an original innocuous Healing → Energy/nerve imbalance (Step #3), which was hardly noticed. Step #3 also must correct any remaining Immune ← Stress imbalance and autoimmune symptoms. Step #4 can then heal the damage, as much as possible. Priming the cure pump for all four of these recovery steps can be carried out simultaneously as you proceed.

Table 12-2 should be the basis for any additional invented medulla exhaustion cure. Some tinkering with nutrients may be needed to get a perfect solution, in particular adding the power of herbs to Items #1 and #2 at 1X and possibly 2X – but never 3X – to achieve a direct hit on the malfunction and past nutritional deprivation. In such cases, preliminary trials of herb-metal combinations are useful and can improve specific medulla subfunctions significantly, sometimes sufficiently. A few examples: copper + Oats for energy and nerve problems, zinc + Aloe vera for poor healing, copper + St. John's Wort for mild depression, copper + Kava for anxiety, and zinc + Shepherd's Purse/Woundwort for defective vasoconstriction. Use herbs cautiously here. To underscore this point, copper + Kudzu (↓) produces instant Energy exhaustion. Lastly, fatty acids are normally input an hour or two before a Table 12-2 cure for some synergy, but adding Omega 6 EFAs, GLA and Vitamin E directly to the cure may be necessary with severe deprivation in the past.

The Table 12-3 protocol for severe cortex exhaustion is not as ideal as the Table 12-2 medulla formulation, and all because there is no known Immune B vitamin. Fortunately, the Table 12-3 alternative raw material combination is very effective. Nutritional yeast contains the missing Immune B vitamin somewhere within its nutritional profile, and supplies strong B nutrition to all Stress and Immune subfunctions. Nutritional yeast *may* aggravate Candida infections, but not here as Table 12-3 combinations correct the underlying cause of Candida, and your immune system should soon kill off the yeast infestation. Review the raw material facts of nutritional yeasts and green vegetables in Chapter 4, and the herb Astragalus in Chapter 7.

TABLE 12-3. SEVERE STRESS-IMMUNE EXHAUSTION CURE.

Necessary nutritional support and "other concerns" are listed earlier in the Mild Stress and Immune Exhaustion Cures. This protocol/regimen does not cure Fatigue Exhaustion; see Table 12-4.

Item	Protocol/Regimen
1	INGEST one heaping tablespoon of nutritional yeast + one small serving of Table 4-1 green vegetables + 500 mg of the herb Astragalus. 1X ONLY for this regimen. Rest in bed for the next one hour. Therapeutic action should begin in about 45 minutes (normal digestion) and produce no side effects IF there is need. If any side effects develop from this strong cortex stimulation, STOP, and ease the distress with abundant antioxidants. Again, R and over-the-counter drug interaction can be dangerous; AVOID THEM. The above regimen at the low end of possible superior cortex nutrition. With the cortex, you must guesstimate how severe your exhaustion is and then apply the right amount of on-target nutrients. So, the right amount may require: ADDING a small 4 oz meal of Omega 3 salmon (for Stress) + 10,000 IU Vitamin A in liquid gel cap (for Immune) to the basic nutritional yeast + green vegetables + Astragalus. And for the worst cases, FURTHER ADDING Chapter 6 full-spectrum sources of trace metals naturally such as Colloidal Minerals (subtle, diffuse effect) or 2 mg vanadium + 2 mg manganese (extremely potent). Remember, too much nutrition for the job at hand generates cortex hyperactivity, followed by hypoactivity exhaustion again. The goal is a measured, balanced Stress-Immune combination of nutrients equal to your particular dysfunction and disease. When in doubt, underestimate and repeat Item #1 three weeks later with a stronger combination.
2	Two days later REBALANCE adrenal medulla and cortex functions with the herbs Angelica and Damiana (Figure 7-A).

Inventing a perfect cortex exhaustion cure for your disease frequently requires adding small doses of on-target herbs and other nutrients to Item #1 to achieve a direct hit on the dysfunction and past nutritional deprivation. This is particularly true for the wide range of possible lymphocyte and immune subsystem exhaustions and consequent imbalances. Researching your disease in the medical literature is crucial, as shown by the examples at the end of the chapter. To illustrate, both chronic fatigue syndrome and lupus evidence low NK (natural killer) lymphocyte activity, but from different causes and, therefore, with different damaging effects. The chronic fatigue syndrome NK triggering event is arachidonic acid impairment, which lies outside of the cortex domain, and so is fixed first and separately. Lupus NK dysfunction lies within the cortex domain and thus produces a connective tissue disease. With lupus, all malfunctioning cortex Immune lymphocytes and subsystems must be fixed at the same time, while maintaining a balanced Immune ⇌ Stress exhaustion cure. Adding extra on-target nutrients to the Table 12-3 regimen can be according to nutrient-specific scientific evidence, or when such detailed understanding is lacking by efficacy against bacteria, viruses, fungi, allergies, cancer and leukemia, as noted in Table 7-6 and Table 3-3. A particular immune dysfunction labyrinth may take weeks to understand. With complicated Stress diseases, the same research effort and targeted nutritional approach is necessary. For example, Vitamin D corrects the autoimmune mechanisms underlying multiple sclerosis and must be part of its Table 12-3 solution.

Table 12-4—Fatigue (aldosterone) exhaustion can manifest in severe and complex ways within a primary Stress malfunction and should be addressed soon after completing the Table 12-3 protocol. In certain situations, Table 12-4 "Severe Fatigue Exhaustion Cure" can be combined with Table 12-3 for an all-in-one, all-at-once cortex solution. A case in point, Astragalus nourishes both cortisol and NK function, and so raises stress and immune "boats" together. Meanwhile, Raw Garlic nourishes aldosterone and NK function, and raises fatigue and immune "boats" together.

Table 12-4 presents the many facets of severe fatigue exhaustion, and how to rebuild aldosterone functioning and its interconnecting links to stomach digestion, pancreas, stamina, vasoconstriction, cortex sex and cortex gluconeogenesis. Review "Fatigue" in Chapter 7 and implement Table 12-4 only after first trying the mild fatigue exhaustion cure.

TABLE 12-4. SEVERE FATIGUE EXHAUSTION CURE.

Necessary nutritional support and "other concerns" are listed earlier in the Mild Stress Exhaustion Cure.

Item	Protocol/Regimen
1	INGEST one heaping tablespoon of nutritional yeast + Raw Garlic + 800 mg of Guarana. 1X ONLY for this regimen. Rest in bed for the next one hour. Therapeutic action should begin in about 45 minutes (normal digestion) and produce no side effects IF there is need. If any side effects develop from this strong aldosterone stimulation, STOP; and ease the overstimulation with a small dose of table salt (sodium) and salt substitute (potassium) in equal amounts. Again, R and over-the-counter drug interactions can be dangerous; AVOID THEM. The above regimen is at the low end of possible superior aldosterone nutrition. You must guesstimate how severe your fatigue exhaustion is and then apply the right amount of on-target nutrients. So, the right amount may require: ADDING a small 4 oz meal of Omega 3 salmon + possibly table salt (dosage volume equal to the size of a green pea). Remember, too much nutrition for the job at hand generates aldosterone hyperactivity and then hypoactivity, i.e. exhaustion again as nutritional reserves become depleted, especially trace metals. The goal is a measured, exact combination of nutrients equal to your particular dysfunction and disease. When in doubt, underestimate and repeat Item #1 and Item #2 three weeks later with a stronger combination.
2	Fatigue function is directly *wired* to many other systems in the body, and a weakness may still exist somewhere in these connections. Therefore, to an appropriate strength of Item #1 nutrients ADD one of the following regimens. STOMACH DIGESTION: Ginger and possibly Horseradish. PANCREAS: Bilberry. STAMINA: Nettle or Cayenne. VASOCONSTRICTION: Shepherd's Purse and Woundwort.

2 Continued	SEX SUBFUNCTION: Sarsaparilla plus male herb Saw Palmetto Berries or female herb Black Cohosh. GLUCONEOGENESIS SUBFUNCTION: Yucca. If necessary, repeat Item #2 three weeks later targeting a different connection, but continue to reduce the power of Item #1 conutrients even to mild cure so that aldosterone raw material reserves are not depleted as a result of functional hyperactivity.

Much is still unknown about natural cures for severe adrenal exhaustion. However, one thing is certain – a synergy of nutrients is fundamental to success. Consider debilitating rheumatoid arthritis, Addison's disease and other extreme forms of Stress exhaustion. These afflictions create extreme Immune ←← Stress imbalance too, and overcoming such metabolic disarray may require a Stress-only Vitamin B2 exhaustion cure. This invented cure would involve the formula: 2 pantothenic acid + 1 B2 +1 B6 from Table 4-3 and Mn ⇌ V from Figure 6-A, probably at 3X dosing in a manner similar to the Table 12-2 protocol. The interaction of Vitamin B2 and vanadium would trigger an extraordinary leap in Stress functioning. Needless to say, more exhaustion cures are needed to solve every adrenal dis-ease.

Step #3: IMBALANCES

Imbalances often develop between primary functions Healing ⇌ Energy or Immune ⇌ Stress, with one function dominating over the other in their equilibrium. Imbalances can also occur within subfunctions, particularly energy/nerve and immune response. Imbalances involve both permanent hyperactive (↑, ↑↑, ↑↑↑ or worse) and hypoactive (↓, ↓↓, ↓↓↓ or worse) functioning. Typically, imbalances are the first step in a disease process, therefore the last step in cure except for healing afterward. Triggering events (Step #1) and severe exhaustions (Step #2) push imbalances over "a cliff of no return" and into dependent body system diseases.

Primary imbalances. The "how to" of restoring healthy medulla Healing ⇌ Energy or cortex Immune ⇌ Stress is explained in Chapter 7. Medulla equilibrium is a very *wishy-washy* mechanism. Every medulla herb, as well as every medulla B vitamin, fatty acid and trace metal, pushes this equilibrium a little one way or the other. Corrective nutrition must nourish and overcome any hyperactivity and hypoactivity in Energy/nerve and Healing, while at the same time forging a strong equilibrium between them. Sometimes medulla imbalances are so far out of whack, either Healing $\rightarrow\rightarrow$ Energy/nerve or Healing $\leftarrow\leftarrow$ Energy/nerve, it is difficult to figure out which way equilibrium lies, because too little or too much healing brings the same result: poor healing, while at the same time hyperactive nerves cause tingling and numbness, or hyperactive healing produces numbness and tingling, only a slight difference. In such cases, you must strongly push Healing $\rightleftharpoons$ Energy/nerve one way or the other to determine where internal balance rests. For instance, ingesting 100,000 IU of healing beta-carotene can reveal what is hyperactive and what is hypoactive. Extreme medulla imbalances require Lavender (Table 7-3) or Saffron (Table 7-4) for correction.

The solution to primary cortex imbalance is very different. Adrenal cortex equilibrium is not a wishy-washy mechanism like that of the medulla. It is rock solid! When "in equilibrium," the cortex stays in equilibrium and is hard to knock off center. When "out of equilibrium" as in arthritis, the cortex is hard to re-center. However, two herbs Devil's Claw and Goldenseal Root can restore Immune $\rightleftharpoons$ Stress equilibrium beautifully, resetting the balance in new *concrete*. See Chapter 7 "Adrenal Balance" and Figure 7-B.

Subfunction imbalances. Subfunction hyperactivity or hypoactivity can remain isolated and not affect the opposite primary function if the subfunction is a minor player. Stress gluconeogenesis is a good example. In contrast, dysfunction in a mainline subfunction such as the stress hormone cortisol always affects immune response and requires primary correction, as described above. Two functions, Energy and Immune, have "quirks" within their makeup that produce unusual subfunction imbalances. Quirkiness is a hyper/hypo split in performance within a primary function.

For Primary Energy Function, energy (adrenaline) and nerve subfunctions diverge from normalcy as follows. Nerves never go hypoactive, and energy never goes hyperactive except in the rare conditions of mania or exogenous adrenaline administration. Still, nerves can be hyperactive while energy remains normal, and energy can be hypoactive while nerves are normal. When both extremes exist together, nerves dictate healing (hyper nerves $\rightarrow$ hypo healing) and energy influences immune (hypo energy → hypo immune), with Figure 12-A(1) and Figure 12-A(2) activities oscillating and deepening the subfunction imbalances over time.

Why does Energy act in this quirky way? Energy and nerves are not the usual primary adrenal function (actor) and dependent body system (receiver of action). Instead, these two are bound together almost as equals. Energy impacts the nervous system and mood, and nerves most certainly affect energy, as demonstrated by caffeine triggering adrenaline flow. Unfortunately, caffeine overuse causes nervous system hyperactivity and inevitably mild to severe energy exhaustion because of inadequate real nutrition. Long term, only good raw material input produces good end product output. An energy/nerve split meets when both are normal and healthy again.

For Primary Immune Function, a hyperactive/hypoactive split can develop between cellular immunity (NK- and T-lymphocyte system) and humoral immunity (B-lymphocyte system), as is the case in chronic fatigue syndrome—see "Disease Examples" ahead. Another possibility is a hyperactive/hypoactive split between Th1 cells (subset of helper/inducer T-lymphocytes) and Th2 cells, as occurs in rheumatoid arthritis, multiple sclerosis and lupus. In all immune dysfunctions and diseases, you must cure the underlying cause of hypoactivity (a Step #2 procedure) and supply a wide variety of immune nutrients to relieve any remaining hyperactivity. The difficulty here cannot be overestimated; proper diagnosis and a thorough medical literature review are essential in order to determine exactly what's wrong. Often cause and cure of hyperactive/hypoactive lymphocyte functioning lie in a distant obscure metabolic pathway. As mentioned earlier, the triggering event for chronic fatigue syndrome is a defect in the fatty acid metabolic pathway: EFA linoleic acid → phospholipids → arachidonic acid → eicosanoids → T-lymphocyte/B-lymphocyte imbalance. Zinc depletion has a similar negative effect on T-lymphocytes.

Step #4: HEAL the damage, as much as possible

Healing is an art. Too much healing is as bad as too little healing; both result in poor healing. The most successful healing of dependent body systems from the assault of past chronic diseases occurs in small incremental steps or leaps forward using combinations of special on-target healers and essential nutrition for the dependent body system in question, preceded by a few days to several weeks of *priming the pump* with general nutrients from Chapters 3-7.

Table 12-5 lists powerful healing nutrients that you can use to heal autoimmune and degenerative damage. Combining just the right Table 12-5 healing nutrients with just the right essential nutrition for the dependent body system often requires an initial best guess followed by some tinkering with ingredients to achieve an effective therapy.

Primary Healing Function must be the only operating function during a "leap forward." Save Energy, Stress and Immune tasks and nutrition for other days. The only exception here is the essential nutrition for the dependent body system necessary to the leap forward. The most needed essential nutrition is that which was the most deprived in the past, usually B vitamins, fatty acids and trace metals.

Tissue types. Healing of each tissue type within a dependent body system is a good starting point. Protein and connective tissue heal on a regimen of complete protein, sulfur supplementation, glucosamine and *gooey* whole-grain polysaccharides, with Aloe vera input a day or two beforehand. For healing cartilage, add the dependent-body-system matrix material, chondroitin. Fatty acid structures and cell membranes heal first and foremost on all good fats and no bad fats, then a regimen of 200-400 IU Vitamin E, 5,000-10,000 IU beta-carotene and on-target Omega 6 EFA and Omega 3 fatty acids. Another effective fatty acid therapy is a 100,000 IU dose of beta-carotene taken alone. Nerve injuries heal on different combinations of complete protein, sulfur supplementation, glucosamine, whole-grain polysaccharides, Alfalfa Seed Tea, Vitamin C, EFAs and Omega 3, sunflower seeds, "trace metals naturally," zinc, DMAE and alpha-lipoic acid. PABA may have to be added to each of these regimens, definitely for nerves, but use it cautiously; PABA is "jet fuel" for healing action. As each tissue type improves, functioning will spiral up and back to life.

Regimens for protein, connective tissue and fatty acid structures can be taken often, every few days. Repeating a regimen containing DMAE or alpha-lipoic acid requires more time, from two to three weeks if both are used together, to refill the countless nutrient reserves used up in the leap forward. Basically, a tincture of time must be part of each healing recipe.

TABLE 12-5. POWERFUL HEALING NUTRIENTS.

See text in Chapters 3-7 for how-to instructions on each nutrient's use.

Type	Special healers to consider using...
Macronutrients	– complete protein. – sulfur supplementation for major repairs.
B Vitamins	– whole-grain cereals except oats. – *gooey* polysaccharides, especially those found in cooked brown rice and millet. – PABA supplementation, "jet fuel" for healing action. Use cautiously, avoid hyperactive healing.
Fatty Acids	– Vitamin E. – beta-carotene including a 100,000 IU "heal-in" taken separately. Carotenoids help too. – EFA fatty acids (Table 5-1). – sunflower seeds and pumpkin seeds provide EFAs plus unknown vital/revitalizing factors. – GLA, Omega 3 and other fatty acids for specific applications (see Figure 5-A). Eating fish and seafood offers hidden synergies not found in Omega 3 capsules alone.
Trace Metals	– "trace metals naturally". – zinc supplementation. – selenium and nickel taken separately. – sufficient metal catalysts for healing: molybdenum, tungsten, niobium/tantalum and zirconium? – other trace metals for specific applications, e.g. copper for nerves (see Figure 6-A).

| Herbs | – Aloe vera.
– Alfalfa Seed Tea helps to heal adrenal gland, pancreas, nervous system and many more systems in unexpected ways.
– Bilberry helps to heal microvascular structures throughout the body.
– Green Cabbage helps to heal gastrointestinal tract including stomach and duodenal ulcers and chronic pancreatitis.
– Horsetail helps to heal bones and connective tissue.
– Vitamin C.
– red seedless grapes: gentle natural antioxidation plus healing.
– black cherries benefits Healing as well as Energy, Stress and Immune in non-quantifiable ways.
– Hydrangea for efficient fatty acid metabolism.
– rebuild Primary Healing Function with Blessed Thistle, Passion Flower, Siberian Ginseng, Sage and other herbs from Table 7-4.
– Scullcap, Angelica, Damiana and Suma taken separately for adrenal balance (Figure 7-A).
– Shepherd's Purse/Woundwort and Heather for vasoconstriction ⇌ vasodilation homeostasis. |
| Special Factors | – glucosamine for major connective tissue matrix repair.
– DMAE for major neuron/nervous system repair and general repair, especially of cell membranes.
– alpha-lipoic acid heals free radical/oxidative stress damage, rejuvenates endocrine machinery. |

After repairing tissue types as much as possible, combine more and more general and targeted healers with essential nutrition to achieve overall repair and maximum results. By reducing dosage amounts, many healing nutrients can work together and still maintain the fine line between not enough healing and too much healing. Too much healing causes harmful overstimulation, nutrient depletion and functional exhaustion. Use DMAE and alpha-lipoic acid sparingly.

With some injuries, large doses of certain healing ingredients can be very effective. Bilberry, Vitamin C and beta-carotene are examples of nutrients that work wonders at high concentrations. Favorably, 400 mg of standardized Bilberry extract and 2000 mg of Vitamin C contribute only modestly to too much healing, while 100,000 IU of beta-carotene, when part of a complete fatty acid regimen, can by offset with GLA fatty acids, an essential nutrient of many tissues. Repair can also proceed in two modest regimens one hour apart with a different emphasis to each regimen, for example start with fatty acid healing, then targeted healers such as Bilberry for microvascular structures. 2X dosing of the gentlest ingredients promotes healing too. Finding the best therapy for a difficult repair problem depends on understanding the underlying causes of the original damage.

Again, healing is art, but nature usually provides an answer for all but dead cells and tissue. Cartilage and fatty acid structures including myelin sheath are relatively easy to heal, nerves and the pancreas among the most difficult. There are no shortcuts to understanding healing. You need to study what the medical literature says about each Table 12-5 healing nutrient and about each type of the essential nutrition for a dependent body system.

NOTE: The above techniques are applicable to any repair effort involving a chronic condition. For acute situations such as severe burns or tissue trauma, the endocrine system already initiates the correct healing response and your job is to supply abundant nutrition to keep up with Primary Healing Function and tissue reconstruction needs.

DISEASE EXAMPLES

Literature reviews, underlying mechanisms and disease solutions are given below for osteoarthritis, rheumatoid arthritis, multiple sclerosis, lupus, fibromyalgia and chronic fatigue syndrome. Many more chronic diseases including amyotrophic lateral sclerosis (ALS, Lou Gehrig's disease), Crohn's disease, scleroderma and Sjogren's syndrome can be cured – instead of endured – by doing a literature review of the disease and applying the techniques of this chapter. While the exact malfunctions leading to a particular dependent body system disease may be obscure, for instance Sjogren's syndrome is immunologic destruction of exocrine glands, the basic mechanisms of Figure 12-A(2) autoimmune and/or degenerative assault apply and must be corrected. Of course, amazing cures are not always possible; ALS requires early intervention because of progressive motor neuron death from free radical cascades.

Primary diseases. Failure in the antioxidant defense shield or in the immune defense shield produces primary, NOT dependent body system, disease. Alzheimer's disease and Parkinson's disease are examples of antioxidant system failure from nutrient deprivation and metal mismanagement. See the index at the back of the book for the mechanisms behind these diseases, and then apply correction. Afterward, Step #4 can be used to heal the damage, as much as possible. Failure in the immune defense shield leads to infections, colds and flu, candidiasis (yeast infection), shingles (herpes zoster), Legionnaire's bacteria, cancers, etc. Two factors control the outcome of all such primary immune failures: (a) resistance to, and (b) exposure to the invader. Use Table 7-6 to rebuild immune resistance and Table 11-2 "Toxic Load on Liver and Body" to reduce your exposure to carcinogens and other immune compromisers. Primary antioxidant and immune failures may require Step #2 exhaustion cures.

Osteoarthritis (OA)

Nature… Osteoarthritis is characterized by slow progressive degeneration of joint cartilage.[3] Structural and functional failure occurs when the dynamic equilibrium between the breakdown and repair of joint tissues is lost.[4] The primary symptom is pain. Ongoing cartilage matrix destruction and joint deformation and misalignment lead to progressive loss of use.[5,6] OA is the most common form of arthritis and affects both men and women, with women more likely to be symptomatic.[3,7] OA incidence in the population correlates directly with age, but OA is not an inevitable consequence of aging.[8] Approximately 12% of the US population suffers from OA.[9]

Mechanisms… OA degradation of the cartilage matrix is caused by increased synthesis and activation of extracellular proteinases [proteolytic enzymes], chiefly metalloproteinases, that breakdown cartilage macromolecules.[3,10] Cartilage consists mainly of a proteoglycan [protein-polysaccharide complex found in structural tissues, important to viscoelastic properties] foundation and a collagen [fibrous protein] network.[6] Cartilage degeneration occurs from loss of matrix tensile strength and stiffness, softening and fraying of the joint surface when chondrocytes [differentiated cells responsible for cartilage formation] cannot maintain and repair tissue, synthesis of smaller less-uniform proteoglycan aggregates and fewer linking collagen proteins, and decreased response to anabolic growth factors.[8] Although OA is considered noninflammatory, a low-grade synovitis [inflammation of viscous fluid membrane surrounding a joint] involving proinflammatory cytokines [non-antibody protein/signaling molecules of the immune system] such as interleukin-1 (IL-1) mediate the disease. In response to IL-1, chondrocytes upregulate production of nitric oxide and prostaglandin E2 [prostaglandins: potent mediators of many conduction/transmitter functions regulating cellular activities, especially inflammatory response], two factors associated with the cellular changes present in OA.[3, 11] Cytokines such as IL-1 and TNF-alpha increase metalloproteinases gene expression and impair chondrocyte compensatory synthesis pathways.[10]

NSAIDs... Despite the fact that a strict definition of osteoarthritis does not include inflammation, epidemiological studies show that synovitis within the joint cavity is a strong predisposing factor for OA cartilage breakdown. Nonsteroidal anti-inflammatory drugs (NSAIDs) demonstrate fast-acting short-term efficacy.[12]

Glucosamine... Current pharmacologic treatments of acetaminophen and other NSAIDs alleviate the pain, but have serious side effects and do not slow or reverse OA degenerative processes.[9, 13] Glucosamine nutritional supplement is a recent alternative treatment option.[9] In 16 randomized controlled trials, glucosamine evidences safety and effectiveness for OA symptoms. In 13 of these trials comparing glucosamine to placebo, glucosamine is superior in all but one. In the four trials comparing glucosamine to NSAIDs, glucosamine is superior in two and equivalent in two.[14] Use of chondroitin [cartilage matrix material] is superior to placebo in four randomized controlled trials. Daily supplementation amounts are typically 1500 mg glucosamine and 1200 mg chondroitin. Although glucosamine is effective alone, combination therapy of glucosamine and chondroitin is reasonable pending further studies.[15]

Glucosamine/chondroitin healing mechanism... Glucosamine is a general, multifunctional precursor of glycosaminoglycans [GAGs: special amino-sugar polysaccharides, an essential element in tissue repair]. Meanwhile, chondroitin incorporates preferentially into cartilaginous tissue.[16]

Glucosamine synovial mechanism... Glucosamine stimulates synovial [viscous joint fluid] hyaluronic acid (HA) production. High molecular weight HA provides lubricating and shock-absorbing properties to the synovial fluid. HA is analgesic and anti-inflammatory. Many studies show that intra-articular [within the joint] HA injections bring rapid OA pain relief and increased mobility. HA also promotes anabolic [constructive metabolism] healing by chondrocytes. OA decreases synovial HA, and glucosamine reverses this abnormality.[17] Glucosamine gives long-lasting pain reductions and functional improvements through its anti-inflammatory and anabolic mechanisms, and unlike NSAIDs, this therapeutic action is not due to prostaglandin inhibition. Thus, glucosamine treatment is free of adverse side effects. Glucosamine is well tolerated both short term and long term by all age groups.[18]

General nutrition… Obesity is associated with OA. A low calorie diet reduces spontaneous development of OA in mice, while a high calorie diet, saturated fats and cholesterol promote the disease. A high-protein diet inhibits OA in mice, but can promote inflammation in humans. Fish oils possess anti-inflammatory and antinociceptive action [nociceptive: pain transmission]. Vitamins E, Vitamin C and B2 inhibit OA in animals. Calcium, zinc and selenium deficits can cause skeletal damage in humans and animals.[19, 20]

Metals… Zinc inhibits TNF production.[21]

Herbs… Capsaicin, the principle pungent and active ingredient of hot red and chili peppers (genus Capsicum), is effective in treating the pain of rheumatoid arthritis, osteoarthritis and peripheral neuropathies [injury to the sensation nerves of arms and legs].[22] Ginger reduces pain and swelling of rheumatoid arthritis and osteoarthritis with no reported adverse effects.[23] See also rheumatoid arthritis nutrition below for more anti-inflammatory help.

Underlying Mechanisms

Where any dependent body system attack comes depends on where the adrenal gland first goes *haywire*. Osteoarthritis (OA) and rheumatoid arthritis (RA) have the same initial dysfunction or first cause of Stress exhaustion, which triggers the attack on joint cartilage. OA and RA, however, have different second causes, and therefore different types and points of attack within the Figure 12-A(2) framework of autoimmune assault and hypoactive healing degeneration. The second cause of OA is a dominant Healing exhaustion, and so a degenerative process occurs within the protein structures (Healing's dependent body system, see Figure 2-B) of cartilage. On the other hand, RA involves a dominant autoimmune attack and that occurs in the connective tissue of cartilage, also as predicted by Figure 2-B.

Disease Solution

Cure usually requires that you unwind the disease in reverse order to its original development; the last thing to go wrong is the first to be fixed, and so on. With OA though, first and second causes can take place almost simultaneously from functional weak spots as a result of inadequate nutrition, and then slowly sink ($\downarrow$, $\downarrow\downarrow$ and $\downarrow\downarrow\downarrow$) into Stress and Healing exhaustions and consequent painful OA. Still another route to OA is Stress trauma. This induces arthritis quickly, followed by progressive Healing exhaustion from Figure 12-A(2) effects and loss of catalysts.

Preliminary nutritional support includes the targeted nutrition specified in the mild Stress and Healing exhaustion cures (Step #2) and the nutrients identified in the literature review above, especially zinc to rebuild Healing function and inhibit TNF production. Glucosamine provides temporary relief from the disease, then permanent healing after all disease mechanisms have been unwound. The following cure steps add detail to the general information on these steps presented earlier in the chapter.

Step #1—Repair any TRIGGERING EVENTS. Stress trauma depletes catabolic and anabolic fat catalysts niobium and tantalum. When OA onset is caused by Stress trauma, supplementing/replenishing all five metal catalysts – molybdenum (protein), zirconium (fiber), tungsten (carbohydrate) and niobium/tantalum (catabolic and anabolic fat) – is necessary to eliminate the disease within the cartilage matrix. Herbal catalyst Hydrangea is needed and possibly amino acid complex carnitine. For a slow developing OA from years of nutritional deprivation, just molybdenum supplementation can be sufficient catalytic help to correct the increased synthesis and activation (hyperactivity) of metalloproteinases. Molybdenum supplements are available at any health food store.

Step #2—Cure any EXHAUSTIONS. Two severe adrenal exhaustions must be overcome, Stress and Healing failure, and these can be accomplished within a week of each other, since one involves the adrenal cortex and the other the medulla. While unwinding disease in reverse order to its development is usually correct, here Stress exhaustion is a major contributing cause to Healing exhaustion through Figure 12-A(2) dynamics, and cause must always be fixed first in a "cause and effect" relationship. Therefore, cure severe Stress exhaustion first by employing Table 12-3 and Table 12-4 protocols. Add the herb Capsaicin (Cayenne) to both regimens, and possibly Ginger later to a Table 12-4 regimen. Then unwind the severe Healing exhaustion using the Table 12-2 protocol.

Step #3—Correct any IMBALANCES. With OA, both Immune ← Stress cortex imbalance and Healing → Energy medulla imbalance need correction. "How to" is as described in Step #3 text earlier.

Step #4—HEAL the damage, as much as possible. Cartilage consists mainly of a proteoglycan (protein-polysaccharide complex) foundation and a collagen (fibrous protein) network. Once the never ending, incorrect metabolic responses of chronic OA disease have ceased, commercially available glucosamine and chondroitin supplements can heal the cartilage matrix quickly. Add complete protein, sulfur supplementation and polysaccharide-rich whole-grain cereal brown rice or millet to glucosamine and chondroitin regimen, with Aloe vera input a day or two beforehand. Aloe vera improves glycosaminoglycan (GAG) and collagen formation, as reported in its medical literature review in Chapter 7.

Rheumatoid Arthritis (RA)

Nature... Rheumatoid arthritis is a chronic inflammatory autoimmune disease of the connective tissue of joints,[24] eventually leading to cartilage and bone destruction.[25] RA ranges from benign remitting to rapidly progressive forms with increased mortality, particularly from infections. Elevated laboratory markers of rheumatoid factor [an immunoglobulin antibody], large numbers of swollen inflamed joints and/or early severe functional impairment suggest an unfavorable disease course.[26]

Mechanisms... Three pathogenic mechanisms characterize RA: (1) chronic inflammation of the synovial [viscous joint fluid] membrane, (2) increased T- and B-cell dependent autoimmune immunoreactions, and (3) hyperplasia [enlargement due to abnormal multiplication of cells] of synovial tissue. Excess CD4+ helper T-cells [Th1 response is promoted by CD4+ Th1 helper T-cells; Th1: subset of helper/inducer T-lymphocytes] and macrophages [long-living, large white blood cells; -phage: anything that devours] play a central role in RA pathogenesis.[24] The degree of cytokine [non-antibody protein/signaling molecule of the immune system; includes interleukins, lymphokines, interferons and TNF (tumor necrosis factor)] imbalance determines RA's erosive nature. TNF-alpha is an important mediator of RA inflammation, while Interleukin-1 (IL-1) has a dominant effect on cartilage destruction occurring later in the disease process.[27] Blocking IL-1 protects joint cartilage and bone from progressive RA destruction.[28] Another pivotal regulator of RA inflammation is transcription factor NF-kappa B [common B- and T-cell activator/binder], which is also involved RA hyperplasia and tissue destruction through promotion of Th1 responses, abnormal apoptosis [programmed cell death], and activation of osteoclast [responsible for bone breakdown] bone resorbing activity. Inhibitors of the NF-kappa B pathway show high therapeutic efficacy against RA.[29] Osteoclasts are key to all forms of RA bone loss. TNF-alpha is a potent osteoclastogenic cytokine. Production of TNF-alpha and other proinflammatory cytokines of RA is largely CD4+ T-cell dependent. TNF-alpha and IL-1, in concert with RANKL (receptor activator of NF-kappaB ligand), powerfully promote osteoclast destructive effects.[30]

Antioxidants... Low antioxidant intake leads to enhanced cytokine production and effects.[31] Antioxidants decrease IL-1 and TNF production.[32]

Omega 3... Omega 3 fatty acids are much less potent in their biological responses than Omega 6, especially in inflammatory response and stimulating cytokines.[33] Omega 3 fatty acids suppress TNF and IL-1 production and actions, while Omega 6 fatty acids exert the opposite effect.[31] In clinical studies, Omega 3 supplementation improves rheumatoid arthritis and inflammatory bowel disease [chronic disorder of ulcerative colitis and/or Crohn's disease with abdominal cramping and persistent diarrhea], reduces cardiovascular disease, arrhythmias [abnormal heart beat: too slow, too rapid, too early, irregular] and hypertension [high blood pressure]; and protects against kidney disease and infection.[33] Dietary Omega 3 supplements consistently reduce morning stiffness and the number of tender joints in RA patients. Benefits do not become apparent until Omega 3 is ingested for 12 weeks or more, with a daily minimum of 3 grams of eicosapentaenoic [EPA] and docosahexaenoic [DHA] acids. In several investigations, RA patients on Omega 3 supplements are able to reduce or discontinue use of NSAIDs [nonsteroidal anti-inflammatory drugs] or antirheumatic drugs.[34, 35]

Vitamin D... Vitamin D hormone [1,25-(OH)2D3] is a natural internal immunoregulator.[36] In animal models, 1,25-(OH)2D3 prevents or markedly suppresses rheumatoid arthritis, lupus [systemic lupus erythematosus: autoimmune, inflammatory disease of connective tissue with skin eruptions, joint pain, kidney damage], experimental autoimmune encephalomyelitis [EAE brain and spinal cord inflammation: a widely accepted mouse model of human multiple sclerosis (MS)], inflammatory bowel disease and Type I diabetes.[37, 25] 1,25-(OH)2D3 complex immunoregulatory mechanisms involve inhibiting cytokines, TNF-alpha [pro-inflammatory protein], IL-1 [Interleukin 1 activates/potentiates both B- and T-cells], IL-6 [stimulates B-cells], and importantly IL-12 [released by macrophages; initiator of cell-mediated immunity T-system]. At the cell level, 1,25-(OH)2D3 decreases Th1 helper cell expression directly or indirectly by inhibiting IL-12 from monocytes [precursor of macrophages, mediator of nonspecific immunity] and increases Th2 helper cells, which generate bone protective cytokines such as IL-4 and IL-10.[36]

Other fatty acids... Vitamin E is beneficial in rheumatic diseases, principally through pain reduction.[38] 300-600 IU daily improves arthritis symptoms.[39] Dietary GLA increases its elongase product dihomo-gamma-linolenic acid (DGLA) in cell membranes without affecting immunostimulatory arachidonic acid. Upon inflammatory stimulation, DGLA is converted to 15-(S)-hydroxy-8,11,13-eicosatrienoic acid and prostaglandin E1, both of which are anti-inflammatory and antiproliferative,[40, 41] thereby giving evening primrose oil and borage oil clinical benefits in rheumatologic disorders.[41]

Herbs... Nettle leaf is registered in Germany as an adjuvant therapy for rheumatoid diseases. Nettle is immunomodulating, mediating T-helper cell derived cytokine patterns and possibly inhibiting the inflammatory cascade [series of reactions from one trigger] of autoimmune diseases such as rheumatoid arthritis.[42] Nettle strongly inhibits transcription factor NF-kappaB, which is often elevated in chronic inflammatory diseases and responsible for pro-inflammatory gene expression.[43] Capsaicin, the principle pungent and active ingredient of hot red and chili peppers (genus Capsicum), is effective in treating the pain of rheumatoid arthritis, osteoarthritis and peripheral neuropathies [injury to the sensation nerves of arms and legs].[22] Ginger shows pronounced antioxidative, anti-inflammatory and antirheumatic activities.[44, 45] Ginger reduces pain and swelling of rheumatoid arthritis and osteoarthritis with no reported adverse effects.[46]

Glucosamine and its anti-inflammatory mechanism... Glucosamine stimulates synovial [viscous joint fluid] hyaluronic acid (HA) production. High molecular weight HA provides lubricating and shock-absorbing properties to the synovial fluid. HA is analgesic and anti-inflammatory.[17] Glucosamine gives long-lasting pain reductions and functional improvements through its anti-inflammatory and anabolic mechanisms, and unlike NSAIDs, this therapeutic action is not due to prostaglandin inhibition. Thus, glucosamine treatment is free of adverse side effects. Glucosamine is well tolerated both short term and long term by all age groups.[18] More on glucosamine under osteoarthritis.

Metals... Selenium and Vitamin E supplementation strongly alleviate joint pain and morning stiffness in RA patients.[47] In clinical trials and private practice, germanium demonstrates efficacy against arthritis, osteoporosis and cancer.[48] Zinc inhibits TNF production.[21]

Vitamin B2... is crucial to erythrocyte [red blood cell] glutathione reductase (EGR) activity. Both basal and stimulated EGR are significantly elevated in rheumatoid arthritis patients. B2 deficiency is associated with increased arthritic activity, suggesting that impaired EGR facilitates continuing inflammation.[49] In fact, B2 can mount significant protection against oxidant-mediated inflammatory injury,[50] whereas deficiency brings on oxidative stress within tissues.[51]

Underlying Mechanisms

Rheumatoid arthritis and osteoarthritis have the same initial dysfunction or first cause of Stress exhaustion, which triggers the attack on joint cartilage. RA and OA, however, have different contributing second causes, and therefore different types and points of attack within the Figure 12-A(2) framework of autoimmune assault and hypoactive healing degeneration. The second cause of RA is Immune subfunction imbalance, specifically Th1 helper cells dominate over Th2 helper cells, thereby generating autoimmune/inflammatory cytokine attack on the connective tissue (Immune's dependent body system) of cartilage. Th1 helper cells become hyperactive, while Th2 helper cells are hypoactive and possibly exhausted.

Disease Solution

The Stress exhaustion and Th1/Th2 Immune subfunction imbalance of RA can develop slowly over many years from functional weak spots due to inadequate nutrition, or quickly from Stress trauma and Th1/Th2 nutritional weakness. Preliminary nutritional support includes the nutrition listed in the mild Stress and Immune exhaustion cures (Step #2) and the nutrients discussed in the literature review above. Vitamin D, Omega 3, Nettle and Capsaicin are especially effective in correcting RA's Th1-Th2 imbalance and autoimmune/inflammatory mechanism.

As usual, cure requires that you unwind the disease in reverse order to its original development. The following cure steps add detail to the general information on these steps given earlier in the chapter.

Step #1—Repair any TRIGGERING EVENTS. Stress trauma depletes catabolic and anabolic fat catalysts niobium and tantalum. To ensure catalytic health and balance, supplementing/replenishing all five metal catalysts – molybdenum, zirconium, tungsten and niobium/tantalum – is necessary. Herbal catalyst Hydrangea is needed and possibly amino acid complex carnitine. Immune subfunction imbalance can be a triggering event for chronic disease, but not here as Th1/Th2 imbalance is not the initiating cause of RA.

Step #2—Cure any EXHAUSTIONS. RA involves only the adrenal cortex. Employ Table 12-3 Severe Stress-Immune Exhaustion Cure utilizing a small 4 oz meal of Omega 3 salmon for Stress + 10,000 IU Vitamin A in liquid gel cap for Immune and add in special nutrients Vitamin D, Nettle and Capsaicin to permanently correct Th1/Th2 imbalance. Then, cure any severe fatigue exhaustion using Table 12-4 and include Nettle, Capsaicin and if necessary Ginger, as explained in that protocol.

Step #3—Correct any IMBALANCES. RA Immune ← Stress cortex imbalance must be fixed to eliminate any remaining autoimmune activity. "How to" is as described in Step #3 text earlier.

Step #4—HEAL the damage, as much as possible. RA healing involves both cartilage and bone repair. Follow the OA guidelines earlier for rebuilding cartilage. Bone rebuilding requires chelated calcium, Vitamin D, boron and other bone nutrients including special "bone builder" formulas available at health food stores. The herb Horsetail helps to heal bone and connective tissue.

Multiple Sclerosis (MS)

Nature... Multiple sclerosis is an autoimmune/inflammatory demyelinating disease [myelin: insulating fatty acid sheath surrounding nerves] of the central nervous system (CNS).[52] This neuropathologic process is continuously active, occurring even during the disease's early subclinical relapsing/remitting phase. In time, 90% of patients develop progressive neurologic disability, termed secondary progressive (SP) MS. SP-MS involves exceeding a threshold in demyelination, after which axon loss [axon: transmits nerve impulses; each nerve cell has one axon that can be over a foot long; large axons are surrounded by myelin sheath] probably contributes to irreversible neurologic decline. Eventually, MS causes moderate to severe disability in the majority of patients.[53-55]

Inflammatory cause... Activated CD4+ helper T-cells [Th1 response is promoted by CD4+ Th1 helper T-cells; Th1: subset of helper/inducer T-lymphocytes] react with myelin, and are the major mediators of this disease.[56] These auto-reactive T-cells migrate into the CNS, disrupt the blood brain barrier (BBB) and produce lesions. Subsequent antigen [any invader eliciting an antibody response] recognition initiates inflammatory responses in which B-cells and their products, along with pro-inflammatory cytokines [non-antibody protein/signaling molecules of the immune system; include interleukins, lymphokines, interferons and TNF (tumor necrosis factor)], cause demyelination and varying degrees of axon loss.[52, 57, 58] The MS cytokine storm is characterized by up-regulation of pro-inflammatory interferon-gamma, TNF-alpha, TNF-beta and IL-12 and down-regulation of TGF-beta and IL-10 cytokines.[59] IL-10 plays a crucial role in regulating immune and inflammatory responses; its routine function is to limit and ultimately terminate inflammatory responses.[60] Th1 cells play a key role in MS and EAE [experimental autoimmune encephalomyelitis (brain and spinal cord inflammation) is a widely accepted mouse model of human MS], while Th2 cells contribute to recovery from the disease.[61] An imbalance between Th1 and Th2 cytokines occurs in several autoimmune diseases. Th1 dominant immune responses cause organ specific autoimmune diseases such as multiple sclerosis (MS) and inflammatory bowel diseases (IBD), while Th2 dominant imbalances cause systemic autoimmune diseases such as systemic lupus erythematosus (SLE) [lupus: autoimmune, inflammatory disease of connective tissue with skin eruptions, joint pain, kidney damage] and Sjogren's syndrome (SS) [immunologic destruction of exocrine glands such as sweat, tear and salivary glands; symptoms include dry eyes, dry mouth, persistent cough].[62]

Repair malfunction... Matrix metalloproteinases (MMPs) are a family of at least fourteen zinc-dependent enzymes, which act as effectors of tissue remodeling and modulators of inflammation.[63, 64] These extracellular matrix remodeling proteases play an important role in normal development, angiogenesis [new capillary blood vessels], wound repair and numerous pathological processes.[65] In neuroinflammatory diseases including MS, MMP dysfunction has been implicated in blood-brain barrier (BBB) and blood-nerve barrier opening, invasion of neural tissue by autoimmune cells, and peripheral and CNS damage.[64] Release of the pro-inflammatory cytokine TNF-alpha is an MMP-dependent process.[63] Excessive proteolytic activity is found in the blood and cerebrospinal fluid of acute MS patients.[65] Down-regulating MMP release may be the basis for the beneficial effect of interferon-beta and corticosteroids [see below] MS treatments.[64]

MRI evidence... Normal-appearing white matter (NAWM) of the brain and spiral cord, as seen in magnetic resonance imaging (MRI), is abnormal in the majority of MS cases.[66] MS lesions on MRI increase by 5% to 10% per year.[53]

Medical treatment... Beta-interferon is effective in treating relapsing-remitting MS, but not as promising for secondary progressive MS. Beta-interferon probably blocks inflammatory neurodegeneration during the relapsing-remitting phase, while other degenerative mechanisms may be at work with secondary progressive disease.[67] Immune system stimulants such as gamma-interferon aggravate MS.[68] Beta-interferon and glatiramer acetate [synthetic polypeptides thought to mimic myelin basic protein] reduce the frequency of attacks. Acute attacks can be treated with corticosteroids.[69]

Vitamin D... Vitamin D hormone [1,25-(OH)2D3] is a natural internal immunoregulator. Its complex immunoregulatory mechanisms involve inhibiting cytokines TNF-alpha [tumor necrosis factor alpha: a pro-inflammatory protein], IL-1 [Interleukin 1 activates/potentiates both B- and T-cells], IL-6 [stimulates B-cells], and importantly IL-12 [released by macrophages; initiator of cell-mediated immunity T-system]. At the cell level, 1,25-(OH)2D3 decreases Th1 helper cell expression directly or indirectly by inhibiting IL-12 from monocytes [precursor of macrophages, mediator of nonspecific immunity] and increases Th2 helper cells, which generate cytokines such as IL-4 and IL-10.[36] Intake of 1,25-(OH)2D3 completely prevents experimental autoimmune encephalomyelitis (EAE), a widely accepted mouse model of human multiple sclerosis. Besides these EAE data, circumstantial evidence is compelling that Vitamin D protects against MS. Vitamin D deficiency and MS have the same striking geographic distribution, nearly zero at the equator and increasing dramatically with latitude in both hemispheres, as well as two geographic anomalies, one in Switzerland with low MS rates at high altitudes and high MS rates at low altitudes, and one in Norway with low MS rates along the coast and high MS rates inland. In Switzerland, ultraviolet (UV) light intensity, greater at high altitudes, results in more Vitamin D synthesis on the skin, thereby accounting for lower MS rates. On the Norwegian coast, fish rich in Vitamin D are consumed at high rates.[70]

Other fatty acids... Fatty acids are essential to central nervous system (CNS) myelinogenesis. Linoleic acid deficit has been found in plasma and erythrocytes [red blood cells] of MS patients, suggesting the need for a diet of increased unsaturated fatty acids and reduced saturated fats.[71] GLA from Borago officinalis [borage oil] strongly inhibits the clinical incidence and histological manifestations [study of tissue at the microscopic level] of acute EAE, as well as clinical relapse of chronic relapsing EAE (CREAE).[72] EFA metabolite depletion contributes to abnormalities in myelin use and replacement, membrane-bound receptors and enzymes, and other axonal structures.[73] In animal and human studies, dietary Omega 3 fatty acids reduce cytokine production,[74] whereas Omega 6 fatty acids increase it.[33] Omega 3 fatty acids suppress TNF and IL-1 production and actions, while Omega 6 fatty acids exert the opposite effect.[31]

Antioxidants… Low antioxidant intake leads to enhanced cytokine production and effects.[31] Antioxidants decrease IL-1 and TNF production.[32]

Metals… Zinc inhibits TNF production.[21] See also MMPs above.

Vitamin B12… MS has been linked to Vitamin B12 deficiency in some studies.[75] Long-term B12 deficiency causes demyelination.[76]

Underlying Mechanisms

Multiple sclerosis is an autoimmune attack on the fatty acid myelin sheath of nerves. MS strikes the nervous system; therefore the original negligent adrenal function is Energy/nerves in accordance with Figure 2-B. And the first cause of MS is hypo Healing → Energy/hyper nerve imbalance. What turned this relatively harmless dysfunction into debilitating disease is a subsequent second-cause triggering event of Stress trauma (far beyond hyper fat burning), which produces severe Stress exhaustion and consequent autoimmune/inflammatory assault through Th1/Th2 imbalance, with Th1 helper cells dominating over Th2 helper cells. Stress trauma modifies the attack from directly in nerves to the surrounding and insulating fatty acid sheath because Stress function directly impacts fatty acid/fat metabolism (Table 3-1). A first-cause Stress disease manifests in bones and cartilage, but a second-cause Stress disease occurs in fatty acid tissue. Stress trauma also depletes all fat-related metal catalysts (now none are available to nourish the myelin sheath) and aggravates and worsens hypoactive Healing through Figure 12-A(2) effects. The disease's matrix metalloproteinase (MMP) repair malfunction evidences the hypoactive Healing. MS is a prime example of combined autoimmune and degenerative attack.

Disease Solution

Preliminary nutritional support includes the nutrition listed in the mild Energy, Healing, Stress and Immune exhaustion cures (Step #2) and the nutrients identified in the literature review above. Zinc supplementation will improve MMP enzyme performance and inhibit TNF production. Vitamin D will help correct the Th1-Th2 imbalance and autoimmune/inflammatory mechanisms. MS suffers from the exact same Th1/Th2 imbalance as rheumatoid arthritis; only the site of the attack is different. Therefore, MS can benefit to some extent from RA's cytokine correcting nutrients of Omega 3, Nettle and Capsaicin. See the RA medical literature for details. Cure requires that you unwind MS in reverse order to its original development; the last thing to go wrong is the first to be fixed, and so on. The following cure steps add detail to the general information on these steps presented earlier in the chapter.

Step #1—Repair any TRIGGERING EVENTS. Stress trauma, the last thing to go wrong, depletes metal catalysts niobium and tantalum. To ensure catalytic health and balance, supplement/replenish all five metal catalysts: molybdenum, zirconium, tungsten, and niobium/tantalum. Herbal catalyst Hydrangea is also needed and possibly amino acid complex carnitine. Immune subfunction imbalance can be a triggering event for chronic disease, but not here as Th1/Th2 imbalance is not an initiating cause of MS.

Step #2—Cure any EXHAUSTIONS. Employ the Table 12-3 protocol to cure severe Stress exhaustion utilizing the small 4 oz meal of Omega 3 salmon for Stress + 10,000 IU Vitamin A in liquid gel cap for Immune and add in special nutrients Vitamin D, Nettle and Capsaicin to permanently correct Th1/Th2 imbalance. Next, cure any severe fatigue exhaustion using Table 12-4 and include Nettle and/or Capsaicin as directed in that protocol. Eventually Ginger may be needed to completely restore fatigue function. Then, deal with progressive Healing exhaustion resulting from Figure 12-A(2) effects and loss of catalysts. Step #1 has already corrected the catalysts and the Step #2 severe Stress exhaustion cure eliminates Figure 12-A(2) dynamics, thereby permitting Healing exhaustion to be unwound using the Table 12-3 protocol.

Step #3—Correct any IMBALANCES. MS Immune ← Stress cortex imbalance must be fixed to eliminate any remaining autoimmune activity. "How to" is as described in Step #3 text earlier. Finally, correct the initial cause or setup for the disease, hypo Healing → Energy/hyper nerve imbalance.

Step #4—HEAL the damage, as much as possible. Demyelination is reversible. Once the negative disease mechanisms are eliminated, a rich 2X fatty acid balm of all good fats and no bad fats can restore myelin integrity. A daily intake of 200-400 IU Vitamin E, 5,000-10,000 IU beta-carotene and balanced Omega 6 EFAs and Omega 3 is excellent for slow-and-easy healing. Occasionally, a 100,000 IU beta-carotene "heal-in" will help too. A low-dose alpha-lipoic acid regimen may be needed late in the myelin repair effort. Any axon loss nerve degeneration associated with secondary progressive MS is more difficult, requiring different combinations of complete protein, sulfur supplementation, glucosamine, whole-grain polysaccharides, PABA, Alfalfa Seed Tea, Vitamin C, EFAs and Omega 3, sunflower seeds, "trace metals naturally," zinc, DMAE and alpha-lipoic acid. If antioxidants have been abundantly supplied throughout the course of secondary progressive MS, most of the affected tissue is injured, not dead, and can be restored to health.

Lupus (systemic lupus erythematosus, SLE)

Nature… Systemic lupus erythematosus is an autoimmune connective tissue disease affecting any organ system, but typically the central and peripheral nervous system, heart, lungs, kidneys, skin and blood. Lupus occurs more often in females.[77, 78]

Natural killer (NK) cells… are a third lymphocyte population, very important in innate immunity and possibly acquired immunity.[79] NK activity is significantly lower in SLE patients than healthy controls. The level of NK activity correlates with SLE disease activity.[80] NK lymphocytes generate large amounts of both active and latent transforming growth factor-beta (TGF-beta), which empower CD8+ helper T-cells to inhibit antibody production. NK-derived TGF-beta is reduced in SLE. In addition to its immunosuppressive effects, TGF-beta may play an important role in generating regulatory T-cells. Defective regulatory T-cell function is characteristic of SLE and other autoimmune diseases.[79]

Types of NK impairment… In autoimmune diseases with localized, organ-specific lesions, increased NK activity occurs at the target organ itself. However, in systemic autoimmune diseases involving various target organs (organ-nonspecific), peripheral blood NK levels are often below normal, which allows expression of autoimmune phenomena such as B-cell hyperactivity and polyclonal antibody production.[81] Decreased NK activity is reported in the peripheral blood and synovial [viscous joint fluid] tissues of patients with autoimmune connective tissue diseases systemic lupus erythematosus (SLE), progressive systemic sclerosis (PSS) or scleroderma [progressive hardening of the connective tissue of skin and other organs, especially lungs, digestive tract, kidneys and heart] and Sjogren's syndrome (SS) [immunologic destruction of exocrine glands such as sweat, tear and salivary glands; symptoms include dry eyes, dry mouth, persistent cough].[78] In such disorders, immunomodulators that increase NK levels should be administered.[81]

Immune imbalance… Imbalance between Th1 and Th2 [T-helper cells] cytokines [non-antibody proteins/signaling molecules of the immune system; include interleukins, lymphokines, interferons and TNF (tumor necrosis factor)] occurs in several autoimmune diseases. Th1 dominant immune responses cause organ specific autoimmune diseases such as multiple sclerosis (MS) and inflammatory bowel diseases (IBD), while Th2 dominant imbalances cause systemic autoimmune diseases such as systemic lupus erythematosus (SLE) and Sjogren's syndrome (SS).[62] While difficult to separate Th1 cells from Th2 cells in humans, some patients with systemic lupus erythematosus (SLE) have higher Interleukin-10 (IL-10) than normal controls.[82] IL-10 plays a crucial role in regulating immune and inflammatory responses; its routine function is to limit and ultimately terminate inflammatory responses.[60] Most likely, increases in IL-10 production cause the disrupted immunity of SLE, with humoral immunity B-lymphocyte hyperactivity and cellular immunity [T-lymphocyte system, NK cells, etc.] hypoactivity producing defective T-lymphocyte production of IL-2 [Interleukin 2 stimulates more T-cell production and other immune defenses] and spontaneous increases in pro-inflammatory cytokines during flare-ups.[83] IL-10 is vigorously overproduced in disseminated lupus erythematosus [advanced form of SLE]. This hyper production has two sources: the immune cells themselves and output from tissues damaged by the inflammatory process.[84]

General nutrition... Excess calories, excess protein, high fat intake, particularly saturated and polyunsaturated Omega-6 fatty acids, zinc [zinc $\rightleftharpoons$ copper required, see below], iron, and L-canavanine (prominent amino acid constituent of alfalfa tablets and alfalfa seed sprouts) aggravate SLE. Beneficial nutrition includes Vitamin E, Vitamin A, Omega 3 fish oils, evening primrose oil, flaxseed, selenium, Chinese herb Tripterygium wilfordii, dehydroepiandrosterone (DHEA), and calcium plus Vitamin D (if using corticosteroids).[85] Omega 3 eicosapetaenoic acid (EPA) and docosahexaenoic acid (DHA) competitively inhibit Omega 6 arachidonic acid inflammatory eicosanoids [prostaglandins and other hormone-like substances] and cytokines.[86]

Herbs... Astragalus stimulates NK lymphocytes in both healthy and SLE patients.[80] Raw Garlic stimulates immunity, notably NK cells and IL-2.[87] Echinacea significantly increases natural-killer (NK) cells.[88] Echinacea appears to stimulate de novo (quantitatively and functionally rejuvenated) NK cell production in animals of advanced age.[89] Echinacea purpurea and Panax Ginseng significantly enhance NK function in all human population subgroups.[90] Aloe vera reduces IL-10.[91] In animal models, agglutinin lectin [binding protein] present in Nettle rhizomes [horizontal, underground, root-like stems that can send out shoots and roots], unlike classical T-cell lectin mitogens [any substances stimulating cell division], discriminates between CD4+ and CD8+ helper T-cell populations, producing a six-fold increase in V beta 8.3+ T-cells within three days. This Nettle agglutinin V beta 8.3+ T-cell response prevents SLE pathology; treated animals do not develop clinical signs of lupus and nephritis [inflammation of the kidney].[92-94]

Fatty acids... Vitamin E significantly improves cellular immunity. [95] Increased intake of Omega 3 fatty acids without adequate antioxidant protection can result in their free radical peroxidation, with accompanying losses in T-cell mediated function and NK cell activity. Cytokines participate in normal immune response and mediate many biological functions through regulated production. Overproduction contributes to acute and chronic inflammatory, autoimmune and neoplastic [uncontrolled growth of abnormal tissue, i.e. tumor] diseases. In animal and human studies, dietary Omega 3 fatty acids reduce cytokine production,[74] whereas Omega 6 fatty acids increase it.[33] Vitamin D hormone [1,25-(OH)2D3] is a natural internal immunoregulator. Through feedback signaling, macrophages [long-living, large white blood cells; -phage: anything that devours] can synthesize D-hormone and reduce immunological overreactions.[36] D-hormone supplementation also exerts this immunosuppressive activity. In animal models, 1,25-(OH)2D3 attenuates SLE.[37] Or contradictorily, at the cell level, 1,25-(OH)2D3 decreases Th1 helper cell expression and increases Th2 helper cells.[36]

Trace metals... Zinc deficiency causes rapid and marked atrophy of the thymus gland [at the base of the neck; synthesizes and releases T-cell lymphocytes],[21] thereby lowering T-cell and overall lymphocyte numbers, as well as IL-2.[96] Copper deficiency reduces IL-2 and probably T-cell proliferation.[97] Selenium increases natural killer (NK) cells.[98] Germanium promotes NK cell and T-suppressor cell [set of T-cells capable of suppressing B-cell antibody formation] activity.[48]

Melatonin... The pineal hormone melatonin enhances release of Th1 cells and may counteract stress-induced immunosuppression and other secondary immune deficits.[99]

Underlying Mechanisms

Where any dependent body system attack comes depends on where the adrenal gland first goes *haywire*. Lupus attacks connective tissue; therefore the first cause of this disease is Immune dysfunction, namely decreased NK cells, Th2/Th1 imbalance with Th2 dominating over Th1 (unlike rheumatoid arthritis and multiple sclerosis where Th1 dominates over Th2), and humoral immunity/cellular immunity imbalance with hyperactive B-cells and polyclonal antibody production, and defective regulatory T-cell function. Lupus likely has a second cause of Energy exhaustion, which would further specify the target as the central and peripheral nervous system, or Healing exhaustion, which would target the protein structures of organ systems including heart, lungs and kidneys, or simultaneous Energy and Healing exhaustion, which would target skin too.

Disease Solution

Preliminary nutritional support includes the nutrition specified in the mild Immune, Stress, Energy and Healing exhaustion cures (Step #2) and the nutrients presented in the literature review above. Increasing NK cell levels is key, and Astragalus, Raw Garlic, Echinacea, agglutinin-containing Nettle rhizomes, Omega 3 fatty acids and Vitamin E are especially effective. Vitamin D medical literature is contradictory on lupus; however, its immunosuppressive activity should prove beneficial, although test Vitamin D alone to be sure this is true for your lupus. As usual, cure requires that you unwind the disease in reverse order to its original development. The following cure steps add detail to the general information on these steps given earlier in the chapter.

Step #1—Repair any TRIGGERING EVENTS. Immune trauma is recurring hyperactivity without resolution. That certainly describes lupus flare-ups. Supplementing/replenishing all five metal catalysts – molybdenum, zirconium, tungsten and niobium/tantalum – may be necessary to ensure catalytic health and balance.

Step #2—Cure any EXHAUSTIONS. Energy and/or Healing exhaustions are probably the last thing to go wrong in lupus. Employ the Table 12-2 protocol (at least Item 1) to guarantee healthy adrenal medulla metabolisms even if this turns out to be an unnecessary step. Then, take the Table 12-3 Severe Stress-Immune Exhaustion Cure utilizing nutritional yeast, green vegetables, Astragalus, a small 4 oz meal of Omega 3 salmon for Stress + 10,000 IU Vitamin A in liquid gel cap and cod liver oil capsule for Immune and small amounts of Raw Garlic, Echinacea and agglutinin-containing Nettle rhizomes to permanently improve the several lupus Immune dysfunctions.

Step #3—Correct any IMBALANCES. Correct any remaining cortex imbalance and autoimmune activity. "How to" is as described in Step #3 text earlier.

Step #4—HEAL the damage, as much as possible. Healing connective tissue and protein structures requires complete protein, sulfur supplementation, glucosamine and *gooey* polysaccharides especially those found in cooked brown rice and millet, with Aloe vera input a day or two beforehand. Any direct nerve damage is a more difficult healing problem, requiring different combinations of complete protein, sulfur supplementation, glucosamine, whole-grain polysaccharides, PABA, Alfalfa Seed Tea, Vitamin C, EFAs and Omega 3, sunflower seeds, "trace metals naturally," zinc, DMAE and alpha-lipoic acid.

Fibromyalgia

Nature… Fibromyalgia is a chronic musculoskeletal disorder characterized by widespread muscle pain particularly at multiple soft-tissue "tender points," muscle weakness, chronic fatigue, and sleep and mood disturbances, notably insomnia and depression.[100-103] Of unknown etiology [causes/origins], fibromyalgia occurs predominately in women, affects approximately 2-4% of persons in industrialized countries, and is associated with high levels of functional disability.[100, 104] Six million Americans suffer from fibromyalgia.[105]

Fibromyalgia muscle abnormalities… can be classified as structural, metabolic and functional. Histological abnormalities in muscle membranes, mitochondria and fiber type have been reported by both light microscopic and ultrastructural methods, and often correlate with biochemical abnormalities and defective energy production, all of which are consistent with neurologic findings and hypothalamic-pituitary-adrenal axis disturbances.[102] Changes in neuroendocrine transmitters such as serotonin [serotonin: central nervous system neurotransmitter/hormone; glucocorticoids rapidly modify serotonergic activity], substance P [nerve peptide involved in regulating pain threshold], growth hormone [GH: pituitary hormone for body development], and cortisol [glucocorticoid, primary adrenal cortex stress hormone] indicate autonomic and neuroendocrine system dysregulation.[103] Adult GH deficiency syndrome has many features similar to fibromyalgia, with low insulin-like growth factor-1 (IGF-1) occurring in about 30% of fibromyalgia patients.[106] With respect to changes in muscle function, pain and psychologic factors often interfere with an accurate assessment by strength and endurance tests, however, decreased muscle efficiency and performance have been verified with P-31 magnetic resonance spectroscopy (MRS) and calculation of the work/energy-cost ratios. During the course of the disease, muscle abnormalities can result from intrinsic changes within the muscle tissue itself and/or extrinsic neurologic and endocrine factors.[102]

Trauma… The strongest evidence supporting a link between fibromyalgia and trauma is a recent Israeli study in which adults with neck injuries suffered a ten-fold increase in fibromyalgia risk within one year of the injury. Several studies on postinjury sleep abnormalities, local injury sites as a source of chronic distant regional pain, and the concept of neuroplasticity hypothesize [proposed, not proven] a link with trauma, but this evidence is not definitive.[107] Women with extracapsular silicone gel have higher risk of fibromyalgia. Silicone-gel breast implant rupture can escape its scar capsule and become extracapsular silicone. [108]

Effective treatments... Supervised aerobic exercise benefits fibromyalgia symptoms and physical capacity with improvements in performance, tender point pain pressure threshold and overall pain. Strength training may also ease some symptoms.[109] Traditional acupuncture demonstrates improvement in myalgic index, number of tender points and quality of life.[110] Low-dose antidepressant therapy can be effective,[103] and serotonergic agents may reduce symptoms.[111]

Blue-Green Algae?... Chlorella reduces average TPI [muscle Tender Point Index] from 32 to 25 after 2 months in a pilot study of 18 patients with moderately severe symptoms of fibromyalgia. This 22% decrease in pain intensity is statistically significant.[112]

Underlying Mechanisms

While little is certain about fibromyalgia, Figure 2-B can reveal cause and cure. Because muscles are targeted, the initial fibromyalgia dysfunction must lie within Primary Healing Function. Healing exhaustion fits with silicone-gel breast implant rupture and the fact that fibromyalgia occurs predominately in women. Women predominately use cosmetics, which reapplied daily can easily become "endless healing to no avail" and cause depletion of healing nutrients and reserves, and functional exhaustion.

If Healing exhaustion alone induces fibromyalgia, the degenerative attack will occur directly in the protein structure of muscles. If fibromyalgia has a second contributing cause of Stress trauma, the resulting autoimmune and degenerative attack will be in the fatty acid parts of muscles. Chronic fatigue symptoms, histological abnormalities in muscle membranes, changes in serotonin and cortisol, and the Israeli study on trauma indicate an adrenal cortex Stress dysfunction, but again little is certain about fibromyalgia. Or fibromyalgia could involve fibrositis, an inflammatory hyperplasia (enlargement due to abnormal multiplication of cells) of white fibrous connective tissue of muscle sheaths. This would develop from a second cause of Immune exhaustion or imbalance and is suggested by the Chlorella pilot study plus some of the Stress indicators above. The best course is to assume both adrenal cortex and adrenal medulla malfunctions and cure both.

Disease Solution

Preliminary nutritional support includes the nutrition listed in the mild Healing, Stress and Immune exhaustion cures (Step #2), and complete adrenal medulla and cortex nutrition in general. As usual, cure requires that you unwind the disease in reverse order to its original development; the last thing to go wrong is the first to be fixed, and so on.

Step #1—Repair any TRIGGERING EVENTS. Possible Stress and Healing trauma require supplementing/replenishing all five metal catalysts – molybdenum, zirconium, tungsten and niobium/tantalum – to ensure catalytic health and balance. Herbal catalyst Hydrangea is also needed and possibly amino acid complex carnitine.

Step #2—Cure any EXHAUSTIONS. First use Tables 12-3 and 12-4 protocols to fix any adrenal cortex exhaustions, adding Chlorella (blue-green algae) to the Table 12-3 regimen. Then take Table 12-2 protocol for the medulla Healing exhaustion.

Step #3—Correct any IMBALANCES. Lingering cortex and medulla imbalances may remain. Correct them as described in Step #3 text earlier.

Step #4—HEAL the damage, as much as possible. Healing protein structures requires complete protein, sulfur supplementation, glucosamine and *gooey* polysaccharides especially those found in cooked brown rice and millet, with Aloe vera input separately. If the connective tissue of muscles is involved, the above ingredients are also effective on the entire protein-connective tissue matrix. If the fatty acid parts of muscles are involved, a rich 2X fatty acid balm of all good fats and no bad fats will start the healing. A daily intake of 200-400 IU Vitamin E, 5,000-10,000 IU beta-carotene and balanced Omega 6 EFAs and Omega 3 is excellent for slow-and-easy healing. A 100,000 IU beta-carotene "heal-in" occasionally will help too. A low-dose alpha-lipoic acid regimen may be needed late in the repair effort.

Chronic Fatigue Syndrome (CFS)

Nature, symptoms and signs... Chronic fatigue syndrome is characterized by severe fatigue, myalgias [muscle pains, -algia: pain], arthritic pains, headaches, recurrent sore throats, lymphadenopathy [swelling of the lymph nodes], chills, fevers and postexertional malaise.[113, 114] The majority of patients describe an infectious onset.[114] Physical and emotional stress exacerbate CFS onset and course.[115]

Immune involvement... CFS shows immune system activation,[114] frequent association with an active viral infection,[116] and low levels of natural killer (NK) cell activity [NK lymphocyte: active in spontaneous, non-specific immunity against cancer and viruses, first-line defense against cancer] in a significant proportion of patients.[117] CFS immunological changes suggest decreased cellular immunity [NK, T-lymphocyte system].[118]

Immune/Essential Fatty Acid (EFA) link... CFS presents hyper- and hypo-responsiveness in immune functions, hypothalamus-pituitary (HP) axes and the sympathetic nervous system [originates in the thoracic and lumbar spinal cord and regulates involuntary actions: breathing rate, heart rate, cardiac output, and blood pressure], all related to impaired EFA metabolism.[119] Normal immune response requires EFA linoleic acid [most essential EFA; see Table 5-1]. EFA metabolite deficiencies impair B- and T-lymphocyte mediated responses.[120] Three clinical observations about viral infections are well known but poorly understood: (1) susceptibility of people with atopic eczema [inflammatory skin condition; redness, itching and oozing lesions] to viral infections, (2) viral infections precipitating an atopic syndrome, and (3) the development of CFS following viral infections. A unifying hypothesis is interaction between viral infections and EFA metabolism.[121] Growing evidence suggests that the PGE group of prostaglandins are a negative feedback modulator of immune response, while eicosanoids [general term for prostaglandins and other hormone-like substances] derived from arachidonic acid are immunostimulatory.[122] EFA dietary changes can adjust the ratios of both cell membrane EFAs and EFA metabolites [arachidonic acid → immunostimulatory eicosanoids] and thereby correct CFS hypo-responsive immune functioning.[119]

Stress involvement... Baseline cortisol [glucocorticoid, primary adrenal cortex stress hormone] is significantly low in approximately one-third of CFS patients. A more consistent finding is reduced HPA [hypothalamus-pituitary-adrenal] function and enhanced 5-HT function [5-hydroxytryptamine: neurotransmitter/hormone related to serotonin] in challenge tests.[123] CFS involves impaired HPA activation with recent work suggesting disturbed serotonergic neurotransmission [serotonin: central nervous system neurotransmitter/hormone; glucocorticoids rapidly modify serotonergic activity] and altered AVP [arginine vasopressin antidiuretic hormone: part of the AVP-renin-angiotensin-aldosterone system; aldosterone is an adrenal cortex hormone that relieves fatigue]. Both AVP and CRH [corticotropin-releasing hormone: hypothalamus neuropeptide; CRH-ACTH-cortisol system fights stress] influence HPA axis function.[115]

Herbs... Astragalus stimulates NK lymphocytes.[80] Raw Garlic stimulates immunity, notably NK cells.[87] Echinacea significantly increases natural-killer (NK) cells.[88] Echinacea appears to stimulate de novo (quantitatively and functionally rejuvenated) NK cell production in animals of advanced age.[89] Echinacea purpurea and Panax Ginseng significantly enhance NK function in all human population subgroups.[90]

Fatty acids... Vitamin E significantly improves cellular immunity.[95] Increased intake of Omega 3 fatty acids without adequate antioxidant protection can result in their free radical per-oxidation, with accompanying losses in T-cell mediated function and NK cell activity.[74] Vitamin A is necessary for resistance to and recovery from infection.[124]

Trace metals... Selenium increases natural killer (NK) cells.[98] Germanium promotes NK cell and T-suppressor cell [set of T-cells capable of suppressing B-cell antibody formation] activity.[48]

Underlying Mechanisms

The triggering event or first cause (the setup) of CFS is impairment in the meta-bolic pathway: EFA linoleic acid → phospholipids → arachidonic acid → eicosanoids → effective cellular immunity (NK- and T-lymphocyte system). This causes decreased NK-lymphocytes and cellular immunity, with consequent cellular immu-nity/humoral immunity (B-lymphocyte system) imbalance. Sooner or later a viral infection occurs, which triggers a downward spiral in Stress and Immune function-ing, as follows. Insufficient NK cellular immunity forces Immune function into hyperactivity to fight even the most harmless or undetected viral infection. Immune hyperactivity demands more and more adrenal cortex resources, leaving fewer and fewer cortex resources to handle the daily stress of life. In turn, Stress function must become hyperactive just to meet everyday needs. Unfortunately, such back and forth hyperactivity uses up vast quantities of nutrition and reserves, quickly bringing on exhaustions in both cortex functions, which then grow worse with each new immune and stress episode. Continuing on with the stressful tasks of life produces first mild and eventually severe stress (cortisol) and fatigue (aldosterone) exhaustion.

Disease Solution

Cure usually requires that you unwind the disease in reverse order to its original development. However, impaired EFA metabolism is the triggering event for CFS and must be fixed first to eliminate the cause in "cause and effect." Preliminary nutritional support includes the nutrition specified in the mild Stress and Immune exhaustion cures (Step #2) and the nutrients identified in the literature review above. The following cure steps add detail to the general information on these steps given earlier in the chapter.

Step #1—Repair any TRIGGERING EVENTS. The defect in the metabolic pathway of EFA linoleic acid → phospholipids → arachidonic acid → eicosanoids → effective NK/cellular immunity occurs in phospholipid production. A healthy liver normally produces phospholipid precursors of arachidonic acid from linoleic acid and omnipresent phosphorus. However, this liver function can falter or fail with age and liver damage from years of slow environmental poisoning by chemical toxins in the air, water and food. Supplementing phospholipid-rich lecithin restores normalcy to the arachidonic acid-eicosanoid system. As revealed in Chapter 11, soy lecithin granules are your best lecithin supplement choice to satisfy phospholipid nutrition. Another consideration, hyperactivity in Immune and Stress functions depletes catalysts, and these may have to be replenished.

Step #2—Cure any EXHAUSTIONS. CFS involves only adrenal cortex exhaustions. These develop in NK/cellular immunity of Primary Immune Function and cortisol and aldosterone hormones of Primary Stress Function. Because Astragalus raises NK immune and cortisol stress functions together, and Raw Garlic raises NK and aldosterone fatigue functions together, the Table 12-3 Severe Stress-Immune Exhaustion Cure and Table 12-4 Severe Fatigue Exhaustion Cure can be combined into all-in-one, all-at-once cortex leap back to health. Follow Table 12-3 and Table 12-4 protocols ingesting Astragalus, Raw Garlic and Guarana with nutritional yeast, green vegetables and a small 4 oz meal of Omega 3 salmon for Stress + 10,000 IU Vitamin A in liquid gel cap for Immune. If necessary, cure any lingering fatigue exhaustion using Table 12-4 with Nettle, Capsaicin and eventually Ginger, as directed in that protocol.

Step #3—Correct any IMBALANCES. Use Step #3 procedures to fix any remaining cortex imbalance.

Step #4—HEAL the damage, as much as possible. Table 12-3 and Table 12-4 regimens heal all cortex damage. Maintaining and rebuilding liver function is worthwhile using Table 11-1 "Regimens for Good Liver Health." Any damage to fatty acid metabolic pathways will respond to a rich 2X fatty acid balm of all good fats and no bad fats and a daily intake of 200-400 IU Vitamin E, 5,000-10,000 IU beta-carotene and balanced Omega 6 EFAs and Omega 3 fish oils.

OVERVIEW

The great philosophers throughout history teach harmony - in your life, in your mind and in your relations with others. Your body with its network of glands and organs needs harmony too; chaos of any kind is very harmful. This physical harmony is achieved by means of "HOMEOSTASIS: (medical definition) stability and equilibrium in a physiological system through feedback." Homeostasis is the internal dialogue of harmony going on inside all of us all the time. Homeostasis is also the basis of natural therapeutics including nutrition and acupuncture, and therefore an important key in finding natural solutions to health and disease. By achieving physical harmony, that is, working with and not against your own internal homeostasis, you nurture and build mind-body-spirit wellness.

Equilibrium Theory provides the following new understanding of the inner workings of homeostasis. Within the endocrine system and adrenal gland physiology, four interconnected functions - ENERGY, HEALING, STRESS and IMMUNE - work in healthy equilibrium, or internal balance. The body's response to all internal needs and external forces lies within and must adhere to this four-part harmony. Moreover, these tasks are the template for all nutrition. For example, each food type nourishes one of the four functions: carbohydrates for energy, proteins for healing, fats for stress, and fibers for immune. The same direct relationship and necessary equilibrium apply to all other nutrients and their nutritional categories: B vitamins, fatty acids, trace metals and herbs.

Also significant, in examining the four-part harmony of Energy, Healing, Stress and Immune functions and what happens if homeostasis is lost, Equilibrium Theory solves the mystery of chronic diseases, revealing the mechanisms behind and solutions to osteoarthritis, rheumatoid arthritis, multiple sclerosis (MS), lupus, fibromyalgia, chronic fatigue syndrome and many more!

Universal in its application, Equilibrium Theory agrees with the wisdom of traditional medicine and the science of Western medicine. In particular, Equilibrium Theory fits perfectly into Chinese medicine, the principles of Qi and the yin and yang duality of life. The theory reveals new yin and yang balances essential for health; first and foremost are the functional balances of Healing ⇌ Energy and Immune ⇌ Stress. Equilibrium Theory also conforms to modern Western medical science, and then goes beyond that science to resolve baffling physiological evidence.

Like all theories, Equilibrium Theory involves subjective insight and discovery, and will require objective testing and confirmation. However, two objective findings give immediate credence and weight to Equilibrium Theory: (1) the theory correctly predicts the pathologies of chronic diseases, for example it reveals why arthritis divides into two types, and then describes the nature of both osteoarthritis and rheumatoid arthritis precisely, i.e. osteoarthritis is a degenerative (hypoactive Healing) disease in the protein structures of cartilage, while rheumatoid arthritis is an autoimmune (hyperactive Immune) disease in the connective tissue of cartilage. And (2) the central concept of a four-part harmony in Energy, Healing, Stress and Immune functions explains all observed human physiology including zinc-copper antagonism and beta-carotene cancer and cardiovascular studies.

Equilibrium Theory is a revolutionary solution to human health and chronic disease, a new key to the inner world of health and harmony. Its simple, common sense nutrition can build health and eliminate dysfunctions and disease from the human body. It can help everyone live healthier lives, and especially help those with debilitating chronic diseases get a second chance at life. Equilibrium Theory goes a long way toward achieving Hippocrates' ideal, "Let food be your medicine." And not surprisingly, the mystery of health seems to move in never-ending circles - balance, equanimity, harmony - the spiritual teachings of the great philosophers may be rooted in our physical nature, the internal physiology of homeostasis and a four-part harmony in crucial energy, healing, stress and immune systems.

***

REFERENCES

Chapter 1 – Health and Harmony

1   Dateline NBC, July 11 1995
2   CBS 48 Hours, September 15 1995
3   Adverse Drug Events in Hospitalized Patients. Classen DC et al; JAMA, 1997 Jan 22-29, 277(4):301-06
4   Interactions of Retinoid Binding Proteins and Enzymes in Retinoid Metabolism. Napoli JL; Biochim Biophys Acta, 1999 Sep 22, 1440(2-3):139-62 Review
5   Free Radicals, Antioxidant Enzymes, and Carcinogenesis. Sun Y; Free Radic Biol Med, 1990;8(6):583-99 Review
6   Anthocyanosides in the Treatment of Retinopathies. Scharrer A et al; Klin Monatsbl Augenheilkd, 1981 May, 178(5):386-89

Chapter 2 – Adrenal Gland Prescribes Health

1   Williams Textbook of Endocrinology. 8th Edition, edited by Wilson JD and Foster DW; W.B. Saunders Company, 1992, Catecholamines and the Adrenal Medulla:621-22
2   The Trigeminovascular System in Humans: Pathophysiologic Implications for Primary Headache Syndrome of the Neural Influences on the Cerebral Circulation. May A et al; J Cereb Blood Flow Metab, 1999 Feb, 19(2):115-27 Review
3   Symptomatology and Pathogenesis of Migraine. Spierings EL; J Pediatr Gastroenterol Nutr, 1995, 21, Supp 1:S37-41 Review
4   Treatment of Edematous Disorders with Diuretics. Rasool A et al; Am J Med Sci, 2000 Jan, 319(1):25-37 Review
5   Intimate Partners. Scarf M; Random House, New York, 1987:253-59
6   Natural Killer Cells Wear Different Hats: Effector Cells of Innate Resistance and Regulatory Cells of Adaptive Immunity and of Hematopoiesis. Trinchieri G; Semin Immunol, 1995 Apr, 7(2):83-88 Review
7   Natural Killer Cells. Role in Resistance to Cancer and Infection. Djeu JY; J Fla Med Assoc, 1991 Nov, 78(11):763-65 Review
8   Effect of Age on Human Neutrophil Function. Wenisch C et al; J Leukoc Biol, 2000 Jan, 67(1):40-45
9   Mast Cells Mediate Acute Inflammatory Responses to Implanted Biomaterials. Tang L et al; Proc Natl Acad Sci USA, 1998 Jul 21, 95(15):8841-46
10   Williams Textbook of Endocrinology. 8th Edition, edited by Wilson JD and Foster DW; W.B. Saunders Company, 1992, The Adrenal Cortex:574
11   Effects of Coenzyme Q10 in Early Parkinson Disease: Evidence of Slowing of the Functional Decline. Shults CW et al; Arch Neurol, 2002 Oct, 59(10):1541-50
12   Obesity Drugs and the Heart. Connolly HM et al; Curr Probl Cardiol, 1999 Dec, 24(12):745-92 Review
13   Synergistic Interactions between Fenfluramine and Phentermine. Wellman PJ et al; Int J Obes Relat Metab Disord, 1999 Jul, 23(7):723-32 Review
14   Current Status of Fenfluramine/Dexfenfluramine-Induced Cardiac Valvulopathy. Pallasch TJ; J Calif Dent

---

Assoc, 1999 May, 27(5):400-404 Review

15 Ma Huang, from Dietary Supplement to Abuse. Arditti J et al; Acta Clin Belg Suppl, 2002, (1):34-36 Review

16 Antioxidants, Oxidative Damage and Oxygen Deprivation Stress. Blokhina O et al; Ann Bot (Lond), 2003 Jan, 91 Spec No:179-94 Review

17 Protein Turnover by the Proteasome in Aging and Disease. Shringarpure R et al; Free Radic Biol Med, 2002 Jun 1, 32(11):1084-89 Review

18 Free Radicals and Grape Seed Proanthocyanidin Extract: Importance in Human Health and Disease Prevention. Bagchi D et al; Toxicology, 2000 Aug 7, 148(2-3):187-197 Review

Chapter 3 – Macronutrients

1 Newer Concepts of the Indispensable Amino Acids. Laidlaw SA et al; Am J Clin Nutr, 1987 Oct, 46(4):593-605 Review

2 Preventing Coronary Artery Disease by Lowering Cholesterol Levels. Steinberg D et al; JAMA, 1999 Dec 1, 282(21):2043-50 Review

3 Physical and Metabolic Factors in Gallstone Pathogenesis. Donovan JM; Gastroenterol Clin North Am, 1999 March, 28(1):75-93 Review

4 A Prospective Study of Dietary Fiber Type and Symptomatic Diverticular Disease in Men. Aldoori WH et al; J Nutr, 1998 Apr, 128(4):714-19

5 Vegetarianism, Dietary Fibre and Gastro-Intestinal Disease. Nair P et al; Dig Dis, 1994 May-Jun, 12(3):177-85 Review

6 Long-Term Blood Cholesterol-Lowering Effects of a Dietary Fiber Supplement. Knopp RH et al; Am J Prev Med, 1999 Jul, 17(1):18-23

7 Dietary Fiber in Management of Diabetes. Vinik AI et al; Diabetes Care, 1988 Feb, 11(2):160-73 Review

8 Dietary Fiber and the Chemopreventative Modelation of Colon Carcinogenesis. Alabaster O et al; Mutat Res, 1996 Feb 19, 350(1):185-97

9 Chemo- and Dietary Prevention of Colorectal Cancer. Schatzkin A et al; Eur J Cancer, 1995 Jul-Aug, 31A(7-8):1198-1204 Review

10 Glycemic Index, Cardiovascular Disease and Obesity. Morris KL et al; Nutr Rev, 1999 Sept, 57(9 Pt 1):273-76 Review

11 Diabetes and Diet. We are Still Learning. Quinn S; Med Clin North Am, 1993 Jul, 77(4):773-82 Review

12 DNA-Dependent Protein Kinase: A Major Protein Involved in the Cellular Response to Ionizing Radiation. Muller C et al; Bull Cancer, 1999 Dec, 86(12):977-83 Review

13 TGF-beta Receptors: Structure and Function. Lin HY et al; Cell Mol Biol, 1994 May, 40(3):337-49 Review

14 The I Kappa B Kinase (IKK) and NF-kappa B: Key Elements of Proinflammatory Signalling. Karin M et al; Semin Immunol, 2000 Feb, 12(1):85-98 Review

15 Editing of Errors in Selection of Amino Acids for Protein Synthesis. Jakubowski H et al; Microbiol Rev, 1992 Sep, 56(3):412-29 Review

16 Polymorphisms of N-acetyltransferases, Glutathione S-transferases, Microsomal Epoxide Hydrolase and Sulfotransferases: Influence on Cancer Susceptibility. Hengstler JG et al; Recent Results Cancer Res, 1998, 154:47-85 Review

17 Mutation Analysis of Amyloid Precursor Protein in Early-Onset Familial Alzheimer's Disease. Naruse S et al; Nippon Rinsho, 1993 Sep, 51(9):2445-51 Review

18 Alzheimer's Disease Families with Amyloid Precursor Protein Mutations. Rossor MN et al; Ann N Y Acad Sci, 1993 Sep 24, 695:198-202 Review

19 Liver Transplantation for Hereditary Transthyretin Amyloidosis. Suhr OB et al; Liver Transpl, 2000 May, 6(3):263-76 Review

20 Transthyretin Amyloidosis: A New Mutation Associated with Dementia. Petersen RB et al; Ann Neurol, 1997 Mar, 41(3):307-13 Review

21 Intracerebral Distribution of the Abnormal Isoform of the Prion Protein in Sporadic Creutzfeldt-Jakob Disease and Fatal Insomnia. Parchi P et al; Microsc Res Tech, 2000 Jul 1, 50(1):16-25 Review

22 Leucine Supplementation and Intensive Training. Mero A; Sports Med, 1999 Jun, 27(6):347-58 Review

23 Mechanisms of Myocardial Protection by Amino Acids. Pisarenko OI; Clin Exp Pharmacol Physiol, 1996 Aug, 23(8):627-33 Review

24 Brain Metabolism of Branched-Chain Amino Acids. Yudkoff M; Glia, 1997 Sep, 21(1):92-98 Review

25 Clinical Use of Branched-Chain Amino Acids in Liver Disease, Sepsis, Trauma, and Burns. Sax HC et al; Arch Surg, 1986 Mar, 121(3):358-66 Review

26 Nutritional Modulation of Liver Regeneration by Carbohydrates, Lipids, and Amino Acids: A Review. Holecek M; Nutrition, 1999 Oct, 15(10):784-88 Review

27 Use of Branched Chain Amino Acids for Treating Hepatic Encephalopathy: Clinical Experiences. Rossi Fanelli F et al; Gut, 1986 Nov, 27 Suppl 1:111-15 Review

28 Upper Gastrointestinal Bleeding: An Ammoniagenic and Catabolic Event due to the Total Absence of Isoleucine in the Haemoglobin Molecule. Olde Damink SW et al; Med Hypotheses, 1999 Jun, 52(6):515-19 Review

29 Homocysteine. Finkelstein JD et al; Int J Biochem Cell Biol, 2000 Apr, 32(4):385-89 Review

30 Homocysteine and Risk of Cardiovascular Disease. Andreotti F et al; J Thromb Thrombolysis, 2000 Jan, 9(1):13-21 Review

31 Hyperhomocysteinemia: Atherothrombosis and Neurotoxicity. Fridman O; Acta Physiol Pharmacol Ther Latinoam, 1999, 49(1):21-30 Review

32 Hyperhomocysteinemia and Pregnancy: A Dangerous Association. Aubard Y et al; J Gynecol Obstet Biol Reprod (Paris), 2000 Jun, 29(4):363-72 Review

33 Cephalosporin C Production by Cephalosporium acremonium: The Methionine Story. Demain AL et al; Crit Rev Biotechnol, 1998, 18(4):283-94 Review

34 Alcoholic Liver Disease: New Insights in Pathogenesis Lead to New Treatments. Lieber CS; J Hepatol, 2000, 32(1 Suppl):113-28 Review

35 Brain Function in the Elderly: Role of Vitamin B12 and Folate. Weir DG et al; Br Med Bull, 1999, 55(3):669-82 Review

36 Methioninase: A Therapeutic for Diseases Related to Altered Methionine Metabolism and Transmethylation: Cancer, Heart Disease, Obesity, Aging, and Parkinson's Disease. Hoffman RM; Hum Cell, 1997 Mar, 10(1):69-80 Review

37 S-adenosylmethionine. Lu SC; Int J Biochem Cell Biol, 2000 Apr, 32(4):391-95 Review

38 Regulation of Hepatic Glutathione Synthesis. Lu SC; Semin Liver Dis, 1998, 18(4):331-43 Review

39 Mitochondrial Glutathione: Importance and Transport. Fernandez-Checa JC et al; Semin Liver Dis, 1998, 18(4):389-401 Review

40 S-adenosyl-L-methionine–A New Therapeutic Agent in Liver Disease? Osman E et al; Aliment Pharmacol Ther, 1993 Feb, 7(1):21-28 Review

41 S-adenosyl-L-methionine Synthetase and Methionine Metabolism Deficiencies in Cirrhosis. Mato JM et al; Adv Exp Med Biol, 1994, 368:113-17 Review

42 Changes of tRNA Population during Compensatory Cell Proliferation: Differential Expression of Methionine-tRNA Species. Kanduc D; Arch Biochem Biophys, 1997 Jun 1, 342(1):1-5

43 Carnitine: Vitamin or Doping? Krahenbuhl S; Ther Umsch, 1995 Oct, 52(10):687-92 Review

44 Carnitine: An Overview of its Role in Preventive Medicine. Kendler BS; Prev Med, 1986 Jul, 15(4):373-90 Review

45 Effects of Creatine Supplementation on Exercise Performance. Demant TW et al; Sports Med, 1999 Jul, 28(1):49-60 Review

46 Immunomodulating Effects of Methionine Enkephalin. Li XY; Chung Kuo Yao Li Hsueh Pao, 1998 Jan, 19(1):3-6 Review

47 Transcription Factors C/EBP alpha, C/EBP beta, and CHOP (Gadd153) Expressed during the Differentiation

Program of Keratinocytes in Vitro and in Vivo. Maytin EV et al; J Invest Dermatol, 1998 Mar, 110(3):238-46 Review

48 Cyclic AMP Signalling and Cellular Proliferation: Regulation of CREB and CREM. Della Fazia MA et al; FEBS Lett, 1997 Jun 23, 410(1):22-24 Review

49 Nucleocytoplasmic Protein Transport and Recycling of Ran. Yoneda Y et al; Cell Struct Funct, 1999 Dec, 24(6):425-33 Review

50 Protein Metabolism and Liver Disease. Charlton MR; Baillieres Clin Endocrinol Metab, 1996 Oct, 10(4):617-35 Review

51 Leucine-Rich Repeat Glycoproteins of the Extracellular Matrix. Hocking AM et al; Matrix Biol, 1998 Apr, 17(1):1-19 Review

52 Toll Receptors: An Expanding Role in our Understanding of Human Disease. Schuster JM et al; J Leukoc Biol, 2000 Jun, 67(6):767-73 Review

53 Biochemical and Molecular Basis of Bernard-Soulier Syndrome. de la Salle C et al; Nouv Rev Fr Hematol, 1995, 37(4):215-22 Review

54 Advances in the Molecular Understanding of Gonadotropins-Receptors Interactions. el Tayar N; Mol Cell Endocrinol, 1996 Dec 20, 125(1-2):65-70 Review

55 Innervation and Effects of Dilatory Neuropeptides on Cerebral Vessels. New Aspects. Edvinsson L; Blood Vessels, 1991, 28(1-3):35-45 Review

56 Peptidergic Cells in the Mammalian Pineal Gland. Morphological Indications for a Paracrine Regulation of the Pinealocyte. Moller M; Biol Cell, 1997 Dec, 89(9):561-67 Review

57 Neuro-Immuno-Cutaneous System. Misery L; Pathol Biol (Paris), 1996 Dec, 44(10):867-74 Review

58 Effect of Matrigel and Laminin Peptide YIGSR on Tumor Growth and Metastasis. Yamamura K et al; Semin Cancer Biol, 1993 Aug, 4(4):259-65 Review

59 Transcriptional Analysis of Purified Histone Acetyltransferase Complexes. Steger DJ et al; Methods 1999 Nov;19(3):410-16 Review

60 ATP Sensitive Potassium Channel and Myocardial Preconditioning. Day YJ et al; Acta Anaesthesiol Sin, 1999 Sep, 37(3):121-31 Review

61 Cholesterolemic Effects of the Lysine/Arginine Ratio in Rabbits after Initial Early Growth. Sanchez A et al; Arch Latinoam Nutr, 1988 Jun, 38(2):229-38 Review

62 Peptides as Weapons against Microorganisms in the Chemical Defense System of Vertebrates. Nicolas P et al; Annu Rev Microbiol, 1995, 49:277-304 Review

63 Lysyl Oxidase: Mechanism, Regulation and Relationship to Liver Fibrosis. Kagan HM; Pathol Res Pract,1994 Oct, 190(9-10):910-19 Review

64 Hormonal Control of Collagen Metabolism. Kucharz EJ; Endocrinologie 1988 Oct-Dec, 26(4):229-37 Review

65 Potential Use of Biaromatic L-Phenylalanyl Derivatives as Therapeutic Agents in the Treatment of Sickle Cell Disease. Votano JR et al; Proc Natl Acad Sci U S A, 1984 May, 81(10):3190-94

66 Tetrahydrobiopterin Biosynthesis, Regeneration and Functions. Thony B et al; Biochem J, 2000 Apr 1, 347 Pt 1:1-16 Review

67 Enzymology of the Phenylalanine-Hydroxylating System. Kaufman S; Enzyme, 1987, 38(1-4):286-95 Review

68 Phenylketonuria Revisited. Gerrard JW; Clin Invest Med, 1994 Oct, 17(5):510-13

69 Iatrogenic and Transient Hyperglycinemia in Patients with Phenylketonuria. Nagata N et al; Eur J Pediatr, 1979 Sep, 132(1):17-20

70 5-Hydroxytryptophan: A Clinically-Effective Serotonin Precursor. Birdsall TC; Altern Med Rev, 1998 Aug, 3(4):271-80 Review

71 Serotonin Activity in Anorexia and Bulimia Nervosa: Relationship to the Modulation of Feeding and Mood. Kaye WH et al; J Clin Psychiatry, 1991 Dec, 52 Suppl:41-48 Review

72 Importance of L-tryptophan Metabolism in Trypanosomiasis. Vincendeau P et al; Adv Exp Med Biol, 1999, 467:525-31 Review

73 Serotonin and Amino Acids: Partners in Delirium Pathophysiology? van der Mast RC et al; Semin Clin

Neuropsychiatry, 2000 Apr, 5(2):125-31 Review

74   New Approaches in the Management of Hyperkinetic Movement Disorders. Fahn S; Adv Exp Med Biol, 1977, 90:157-73 Review

75   L-tryptophan: A Rational Anti-Depressant and a Natural Hypnotic? Boman B; Aust N Z J Psychiatry, 1988 Mar, 22(1):83-97 Review

76   Utilization of Superoxide Anion by Indoleamine Oxygenase-Catalyzed Tryptophan and Indoleamine Oxidation. Hayaishi O; Adv Exp Med Biol, 1996, 398:285-89 Review

77   Physiological Importance of Quinoenzymes and the O-quinone Family of Cofactors. Stites TE et al; J Nutr, 2000 Apr, 130(4):719-27 Review

78   The Metabolic Roles, Pharmacology, and Toxicology of Lysine. Flodin NW; J Am Coll Nutr, 1997 Feb, 16(1):7-21 Review

79   Success of L-lysine Therapy in Frequently Recurrent Herpes Simplex Infection. Treatment and Prophylaxis. Griffith RS et al, Dermatologica, 1987, 175(4):183-90

80   Subjective Response to Lysine in the Therapy of Herpes simplex. Walsh DE et al; J Antimicrob Chemother,1983 Nov, 12(5):489-96

81   Topical Treatment of Recurrent Mucocutaneous Herpes with Ascorbic Acid-Containing Solution. Hovi T et al; Antiviral Res, 1995 Jun, 27(3):263-70

82   Use of Water-Soluble Bioflavonoid-Ascorbic Acid Complex in the Treatment of Recurrent Herpes labialis. Terezhalmy GT et al; Oral Surg Oral Med Oral Pathol, 1978 Jan, 45(1):56-62

83   Tryptophan Produced by Showa Denko and Epidemic Eosinophilia-Myalgia Syndrome. Kilbourne EM et al; J Rheumatol Suppl, 1996 Oct, 46:81-88 Review

84   Management of Diabetic Ketoacidosis. Kitabchi AE et al; Am Fam Physician, 1999 Aug, 60(2):455-64 Review

85   Alcoholic Ketoacidosis at Autopsy. Pounder DJ et al; J Forensic Sci, 1998 Jul, 43(4):812-16

86   Carnitine: An Overview of its Role in Preventive Medicine. Kendler BS; Prev Med, 1986 Jul, 15(4):373-90 Review

87   Therapeutic Strategies in Multiple Sclerosis. II. Long-Term Repair. Scolding N; Philos Trans R Soc Lond B Biol Sci, 1999 Oct 29, 354(1390):1711-20 Review

88   Mechanisms of Damage and Repair in Multiple Sclerosis. Zajicek J et al; Mult Scler, 1995 Jun, 1(2):61-72 Review

89   Stable Isotope Techniques for the Study of Gluconeogenesis in Man. Landau BR; Horm Metab Res, 1997 July, 29(7):334-36

90   Vegetables, Fruit, and Cancer Prevention. Steinmetz KA et al; J Am Diet Assoc, 1996 Oct, 96(10):1027-39 Review

91   Increases in Human Plasma Antioxidant Capacity after Consumption of Controlled Diets High in Fruit and Vegetables. Cao G et al; Am J Clin Nutr, 1998 Nov, 68(5):1081-87

92   Mechanisms of Action of Antioxidants as Exemplified in Vegetables, Tomatoes and Tea. Weisburger JH; Food Chem Toxicol, 1999 Sep-Oct, 37(9-10):943-48 Review

93   Fruit and Vegetable Intake and Incidence of Bladder Cancer in a Male Prospective Cohort. Michaud DS et al; J Natl Cancer Inst, 1999 Apr 7,91(7):605-13

94   Antioxidant Properties of the Major Polyphenolic Compounds in Broccoli. Plumb GW et al; Free Radic Res, 1997 Oct, 27(4):429-35

95   Dietary Flavonoid Intake and Risk of Cardiovascular Disease in Postmenopausal Women. Yochum L et al; Am J Epidemiol, 1999 May 15, 149(10):943-49

96   Broccoli Sprouts: An Exceptionally Rich Source of Inducers of Enzymes that Protect against Chemical Carcinogens. Fahey JW et al; Proc Natl Acad Sci U S A, 1997 Sep 16, 94(19):10367-372

97   Polymethoxylated Flavones Derived from Citrus Suppress Tumor Necrosis Factor-Alpha Expression by Human Monocytes. Manthey JA et al; J Nat Prod, 1999 Mar, 62(3):441-44

98   Antiproliferative Activity of Flavonoids on Several Cancer Cell Lines. Kawaii S et al; Biosci Biotechnol

Biochem,1999 May, 63(5):896-99

99 Effect of Citrus Flavonoids on HL-60 Cell Differentiation. Kawaii S et al; Anticancer Res, 1999 Mar-Apr, 19(2A):1261-69

100 Inhibition of Mammary Cancer by Citrus Flavonoids. Guthrie N et al; Adv Exp Med Biol, 1998, 439:227-36 Review

101 Biological Effects of Hesperidin, a Citrus Flavonoid: Antiinflammatory and Analgesic Activity. Galati EM et al; Farmaco, 1994 Nov, 40(11):709-12

102 Inhibition of Bacterial Mutagenesis by Citrus Flavonoids. Calomme M et al; Planta Med, 1996 Jun, 62(3):222-26

103 Antiproliferative Effects of Citrus Flavonoids on a Human Squamous Cell Carcinoma in Vitro. Kandaswami C et al; Cancer Lett, 1991 Feb, 56(2):147-52

104 Citrus Flavone Tangeretin Inhibits Leukaemic HL-60 Cell Growth Partially Through Induction of Apoptosis with Less Cytotoxicity on Normal Lymphocytes. Hirano T et al; Br J Cancer,1995 Dec, 72(6):1380-88

105 Intake of Flavonoids and Lung Cancer. Le Marchand L et al; J Natl Cancer Inst, 2000 Jan 19, 92(2):154-60

106 Effect of Concentrated Red Grape Juice Consumption on Serum Antioxidant Capacity and Low-Density Lipoprotein Oxidation. Day AP et al; Ann Nutr Metab, 1997, 41(6):353-57

107 Grape Juice, but Not Orange Juice or Grapefruit Juice, Inhibits Human Platelet Aggregation. Keevil JG et al; J Nutr, 2000 Jan, 130(1):53-56

108 Comparison of Antioxidant Potentials of Red Wine, White Wine, Grape Juice and Alcohol. Durak I et al; Curr Med Res Opin, 1999, 15(4):316-20

109 Red Wine Inhibits the Cell-Mediated Oxidation of LDL and HDL. Rifici VA et al; J Am Coll Nutr, 1999 Apr, 18(2):137-43

110 The Effect of Red Wine on Blood Antioxidant Potential. Durak I et al; Curr Med Res Opin, 1999, 15(3):208-13

111 Cardioprotection of Red Wine: Role of Polyphenolic Antioxidants. Das DK et al; Drugs Exp Clin Res, 1999, 25(2-3):115-20 Review

112 Red-Wine Polyphenols and Inhibition of Platelet Aggregation: Possible Mechanisms, and Potential Use in Health Promotion and Disease Prevention. Halpern MJ et al; J Int Med Res, 1998 Aug-Sep, 26(4):171-80

113 Biological Effects of Resveratrol. Fremont L; Life Sci, 2000 Jan 14, 66(8):663-73 Review

114 Resveratrol, an Antioxidant Present in Red Wine, Induces Apoptosis in Human Promyelocytic Leukemia (HL-60) Cells. Surh YJ et al; Cancer Lett, 1999 Jun 1, 140(1-2):1-10

115 The Effect of Red Wine and its Components on Growth and Proliferation of Human Oral Squamous Carcinoma Cells. Elattar TM et al; Anticancer Res, 1999 Nov-Dec, 19(6B):5407-4146

116 Alcohol, Ischemic Heart Disease, and the French Paradox. Constant J; Coron Artery Dis, 1997 Oct, 8(10):645-49 Review

117 Intake of Flavonols and Flavones and Risk of Coronary Heart Disease in Male Smokers. Hirvonen T et al; Epidemiology, 2001 Jan, 12(1):62-67

118 Inhibitory Effect of Tea Flavonoids on the Ability of Cells to Oxidize Low Density Lipoprotein. Yoshida H et al; Biochem Pharmacol, 1999 Dec 1, 58(11):1695-703

119 Tea Flavonoids may Protect against Atherosclerosis: The Rotterdam Study. Geleijnse JM et al; Arch Intern Med,1999 Oct 11,159(18):2170-74

120 Mechanistic Studies of Catechins as Antioxidants Against Radical Oxidation. Kondo K et al; Arch Biochem Biophys, 1999 Feb 1, 362(1):79-86

121 Effects of Catechins on Human Blood Platelet Aggregation and Lipid Peroxidation. Neiva TJ et al; Phytother Res, 1999 Nov, 13(7):597-600

122 Scavenging of Hydrogen Peroxide and Inhibition of Ultraviolet Light-Induced Oxidative DNA Damage by Aqueous Extracts from Green and Black Teas. Wei H et al; Free Radic Biol Med, 1999 Jun, 26(11-12):1427-35

123 Induction of Apoptosis in Human Stomach Cancer Cells by Green Tea Catechins. Hibasami H et al; Oncol

Rep, 1998 Mar-Apr, 5(2):527-29

124 Green Tea (Camellia sinensis) Extract and its Possible Role in the Prevention of Cancer. Brown MD; Altern Med Rev, 1999 Oct, 4(5):360-70 Review

125 Mechanistic Findings of Green Tea as Cancer Preventive for Humans. Fujiki H et al; Proc Soc Exp Biol Med, 1999 Apr, 220(4):225-28 Review

126 Green Tea Regulates Cell Cycle Progression in Oral Leukoplakia. Khafif A et al; Head Neck, 1998 Sep, 20(6):528-34

127 Growth Inhibition of Leukemic Cells by (-)-Epigallocatechin Gallate, the Main Constituent of Green Tea. Otsuka T et al; Life Sci, 1998, 63(16):1397-403

128 Molecular Targets for Green Tea in Prostate Cancer Prevention. Adhami VM et al; J Nutr, 2003 Jul,133(7 Suppl):2417S-2424S

129 Green Tea Polyphenols: DNA Photodamage and Photoimmunology. Katiyar SK et al; J Photochem Photobiol B, 2001 Dec 31, 65(2-3):109-14 Review

130 RELIEF Study: First Consolidated European Data. Reflux Assessment and Quality of Life Improvement with Micronized Flavonoids. Jantet G; Angiology, 2000 Jan, 51(1):31-37

131 Clinical Efficacy of Micronized Purified Flavonoid Fraction. Struckmann JR; J Vasc Res, 1999, 36 Suppl 1:37-41 Review

132 Daflon 500 mg in the Treatment of Hemorrhoidal Disease: A Demonstrated Efficacy in Comparison with Placebo. Godeberge P; Angiology, 1994 Jun, 45(6 Pt 2):574-78

133 Effects of Flavonoids and Vitamin C on Oxidative DNA Damage to Human Lymphocytes. Noroozi M et al; Am J Clin Nutr, 1998 Jun, 67(6):1210-18

134 Antibacterial Activity of Pure Flavonoids Isolated from Mosses. Basile A et al; Phytochemistry, 1999 Dec, 52(8):1479-82

135 Chemopreventive Drug Development: Perspectives and Progress. Kelloff GJ et al; Cancer Epidemiol Biomarkers Prev, 1994 Jan-Feb, 3(1):85-98 Review

136 Oxidant-Induced Apoptosis of Glomerular Cells: Intracellular Signaling and its Intervention by Bioflavinoid. Kitamura M et al; Kidney Int, 1999 Oct, 56(4):1223-29 Review

137 IkappaB Kinases Alpha and Beta Show a Random Sequential Kinetic Mechanism and are Inhibited by Staurosporine and Quercetin. Peet GW et al; J Biol Chem, 1999 Nov 12, 274(46):32655-661

138 Quercetin in Men with Category III Chronic Prostatitis. Shoskes DA et al; Urology, 1999 Dec, 54(6):960-63

139 Quercetin Inhibits p21-RAS Expression in Human Colon Cancer Cell Lines and in Primary Colorectal Tumors. Ranelletti FO et al; Int J Cancer, 2000 Feb 1, 85(3):438-45

140 Quercetin-Induced Apoptosis in Colorectal Tumor Cells: Possible Role of EGF Receptor Signaling. Richter M et al; Nutr Cancer, 1999, 34(1):88-99

141 Effects of Luteolin and Quercetin, Inhibits of Tyrosine Kinase, on Cell Growth and Metastasis-Associated Properties in A431 Cells Overexpressing Epidermal Growth Factor Receptor. Huang YT et al; Br J Parmacol, 1999 Nov, 128(5):999-1010

142 Antioxidant Properties of Flavonol Glycosides from Green Beans. Plumb GW et al; Redox Rep, 1999, 4(3):123-27

143 The Potential of Soybean Foods as a Chemoprevention Approach for Human Urinary Tract Cancer. Su SJ et al; Clin Cancer Res, 2000 Jan, 6(1):230-36

144 Genistein-Induced G2-M Arrest, p21WAF1 Upregulation, and Apoptosis in a Non-Small-Cell Lung Cancer Cell Line. Lian F et al; Nutr Cancer, 1998, 31(3):184-91

145 Determining Efficacy of Cancer Chemopreventive Agents using a Cell-Free System Concomitant with DNA Adduction. Smith WA et al; Mutat Res, 1999 Mar 10, 425(1):143-52

146 Soy, Disease Prevention, and Prostate Cancer. Moyad MA et al; Semin Urol Oncol, 1999 May, 17(2):97-102 Review

147 Growth Inhibition of Human Breast Cancer Cells by Herbs and Phytoestrogens. Dixon-Shanies D et al; Oncol Rep, 1999 Nov-Dec, 6(6):1383-87

148 Symptomatic Efficacy of Avocado/Soybean Unsaponifiables in the Treatment of Osteoarthritis of the Knee and Hip. Maheu E et al; Arthritis Rheum, 1998 Jan, 41(1):81-91

149 Phytoestrogen Intake and Prostate Cancer. Strom SS et al; Nutr Cancer, 1999, 33(1):20-25

150 Clinical Effects of Phytoestrogens. Knight DC et al; Obstet Gynecol, 1996 May, 87(5 Pt 2):897-904 Review

151 Antioxidant Efficacy of Phytoestrogens in Chemical and Biological Model Systems. Mitchell JH et al; Arch Biochem Biophys,1998 Dec 1, 360(1):142-48

152 Synergistic Effect of Flavones and Flavonols against Herpes Simplex Virus Type 1 in Cell Culture. Comparison with the Antiviral Activity of Propolis. Amoros M et al; J Nat Prod, 1992 Dec, 55(12):1732-40

153 Antibacterial, Antifungal and Antiviral Activity of Propolis of Different Geographic Origin. Kujumgiev A et al; J Ethnopharmacol, 1999 Mar, 64(3):235-40

154 Protection by the Flavoniods Myricetin, Quercetin, and Rutin against Hydrogen Peroxide-Induced DNA Damage in Caco-2 and Hep G2 Cells. Aherne SA et al; Nutr Cancer, 1999, 34(2):160-66

155 Investigation of the Efficacy of Oxerutins Compared to Placebo in Patients with Chronic Venous Insufficiency Treated with Compression Stockings. Unkauf M et al; Arzneimittelforschung,1996 May, 46(5):478-82

156 Hydroxyethylrutosides in Elderly Patients with Chronic Venous Insufficiency: Its Efficacy and Tolerability. MacLennan WJ et al; Gerontology, 1994, 40(1):45-52

157 Growth Inhibitory Effects of Flavonoids in Human Thyroid Cancer Cell Lines. Yin F et al; Thyroid, 1999 Apr, 9(4):369-76

158 Luteolin-Rich Artichoke Extract Protects Low Density Lipoprotein from Oxidation in Vitro. Brown JE et al; Free Radic Res, 1998 Sep, 29(3):247-55

159 Pharmacological Properties and Therapeutic Profile of Artichoke. Wegener T et al; Wien Med Wochenschr, 1999, 149(8-10):241-7 Review

160 Milk Thistle (Silybum marianum) for the Therapy of Liver Disease. Flora K et al; Am J Gastroenterol, 1998 Feb, 93(2):139-43 Review

161 Antioxidant Functions of Vitamins. Vitamins E and C, Beta-Carotene, and Other Carotenoids. Sies H et al; Ann N Y Acad Sci, 1992 Sep 30, 669:7-20 Review

162 Protective Dietary Factors and Lung Cancer. Fontham ET; Int J Epidemiol, 1990, 19 Suppl 1:S32-42

163 Lutein and Zeaxanthin as Protectors of Lipid Membranes against Oxidative Damage: The Structural Aspects. Sujak A et al; Arch Biochem Biophys, 1999 Nov 15, 371(2):301-07

164 Carotenoids and Colon Cancer. Slattery ML et al; Am J Clin Nutr, 2000 Feb, 71(2):575-82

165 Consumption of Vegetables Reduces Genetic Damage in Humans: First Results of a Human Intervention Trial with Carotenoid-Rich Foods. Pool-Zobel BL et al; Carcinogenesis, 1997 Sep, 18(9):1847-50

166 Tomato Consumption Modulates Oxidative DNA Damage in Humans. Rehman A et al; Biochem Biophys Res Commun, 1999 Sep 7, 262(3):828-31

167 Does Tomato Consumption Effectively Increase the Resistance of Lymphocyte DNA to Oxidative Damage? Riso P et al; Am J Clin Nutr, 1999 Apr, 69(4):712-18

168 Modulation of Human T-Lymphocyte Functions by the Consumption of Carotenoid-Rich Vegetables. Watzl B et al; Br J Nutr, 1999 Nov, 82(5):383-89

169 The Anti-Carcinogenic Role of Lycopene, Abundantly Present in Tomato. Sengupta A et al; Eur J Cancer Prev,1999 Aug, 8(4):325-30 Review

170 An Ecologic Study of Dietary Links to Prostate Cancer. Grant WB; Altern Med Rev, 1999 Jun, 4(3):162-69

171 Tomatoes, Tomato-Based Products, Lycopene, and Cancer: Review of the Epidemiologic Literature. Giovannucci E; J Natl Cancer Inst, 1999 Feb 17, 91(4):317-31 Review

172 Antioxidant Effects of Isoflavonoids and Lignans, and Protection against DNA Oxidation. Harper A et al; Free Radic Res,1999 Aug, 31(2):149-60

173 Mammalian Lignans Inhibit the Growth of Estrogen-Independent Human Colon Tumor Cells. Sung MK et al; Anticancer Res, 1998 May-Jun, 18(3A):1405-08

174 Antiproliferative Activity of Mammalian Lignan Derivatives against the Human Breast Carcinoma Cell Line, ZR-75-1. Hirano T et al; Cancer Invest, 1990, 8(6):595-602

175   Experimental Studies on Lignans and Cancer. Thompson LU; Baillieres Clin Endocrinol Metab, 1998 Dec, 12(4):691-705 Review

176   Immunomodulatory Effect of Arctigenin, a Lignan Compound, on Tumour Necrosis Factor-Alpha and Nitric Oxide Production, and Lymphocyte Proliferation. Cho JY et al; J Pharm Pharmacol, 1999 Nov, 51(11):1267-73

177   Priming Effect of 2,3-Dibenzylbutane-1,4-diol (Mammalian Lignan) on Superoxide Production in Human Neutrophils. Morikawa M et al; Biochem Biophys Res Commun, 1990 Apr 16, 168(1):194-99

178   Phytosterol Compounds having Antiviral Efficacy. Eugster C et al; Panminerva Med, 1997 Mar, 39(1):12-20

179   Dietary Phytosterols as Cholesterol-Lowering Agents in Humans. Jones PJ et al; Can J Physiol Pharmacol, 1997 Mar, 75(3):217-27 Review

180   Effects of Dietary Phytosterols on Cholesterol Metabolism and Atherosclerosis: Clinical and Experimental Evidence. Moghadasian MH et al; Am J Med, 1999 Dec, 107(6):588-94 Review

181   Functional Foods: Cholesterol-Lowering Benefits of Plant Sterols. Thurnham DI; Br J Nutr, 1999 Oct, 82(4):255-56

182   Cholesterol-Lowering Efficacy of a Sitostanol-Containing Phytosterol Mixture with a Prudent Diet in Hyperlipidemic Men. Jones PJ et al; Am J Clin Nutr, 1999 Jun, 69(6):1144-50

183   Plant Sterols and Sterolins: A Review of their Immune-Modulating Properties. Bouic PJ et al; Altern Med Rev, 1999 Jun, 4(3):170-77 Review

184   Efficacy of Beta-Sitosterol and its Glucoside as Adjuvants in the Treatment of Pulmonary Tuberculosis. Donald PR et al; Int J Tuberc Lung Dis,1997 Dec, 1(6):518-22

185   Beta-Sitosterol (Phytosterol) for the Treatment of Benign Prostatic Hyperplasia. Klippel KF et al; Br J Urol, 1997 Sep, 80(3):427-32

186   Anti-Elastase and Anti-Hyaluronidase Activities of Saponins and Sapogenins from Hedera Helix, Aesculus Hippocastanum, and Ruscus Aculeatus: Factors Contributing to their Efficacy in the Treatment of Venous Insufficiency. Facino RM et al; Arch Pharm (Weinheim), 1995 Oct, 328(10):720-24

187   Medical Edema Protection–Clinical Benefit in Patients with Chronic Deep Vein Incompetence. Diehm C et al; Vasa, 1992, 21(2):188-92

188   Anti-Inflammatory Activity of Aqueous Extracts and Steroidal Sapogenins of Agave Americana. Peana AT et al; Planta Med, 1997 Jun, 63(3):199-202

189   Effect of a Novel Saponin Adjuvant Derived from Quillaja Saponaria on the Immune Response to Recombinant Hepatitis B Surface Antigen. So HS et al; Mol Cells, 1997 Apr 30, 7(2):178-86

190   Cytotoxicity of Triterpenoid Saponins: Activities against Tumor Cells in Vitro and Hemolytical Index. Bader G et al; Pharmazie, 1996 Jun, 51(6):414-17

191   Pharmacological and Biochemical Actions of Simple Coumarins: Natural Products with Therapeutic Potential. Hoult JR et al; Gen Pharmacol, 1996 Jun, 27(4):713-22 Review

192   Facilitation of Retinal Function Recovery by Coumarin Derivatives. Liu SX et al; J Ocul Pharmacol Ther, 1997 Feb, 13(1):69-79

193   Protective Actions of 5'-n-alkylated Curcumins on Living Cells Suffering from Oxidative Stress. Oyama Y et al; Eur J Pharmacol, 1998 Oct 30, 360(1):65-71

194   The Effect of Chelidonium- and Turmeric Root Extract on Upper Abdominal Pain due to Functional Disorders of the Biliary System. Niederau C et al; Med Klin, 1999 Aug 15, 94(8):425-30

195   Sulphydryl-Containing Agents: A New Approach to the Problem of Refractory Peptic Ulceration. Salim AS; Pharmacology, 1992, 45(6):301-06

196   Sulfhydryl-Containing Agents in the Treatment of Gastric Bleeding Induced by Nonsteroidal Anti-Inflammatory Drugs. Salim AS; Can J Surg, 1993 Feb, 36(1):53-58

197   Role of Sulphydryl-Containing Agents in the Management of Recurrent Attacks of Ulcerative Colitis. Salim AS; Pharmacology, 1992, 45(6):307-18

198   Therapeutic Values of Onion (Allium cepa L.) and Garlic (Allium sativum L.). Augusti KT; Indian J Exp Biol, 1996 Jul, 34(7):634-40 Review

199 Differential Induction of NAD(P)H:Quinone Oxidoreductase by Anti-Carcinogenic Organosulfides from Garlic. Singh SV et al; Biochem Biophys Res Commun, 1998 Mar 27, 244(3):917-20

200 Carbohydrate Ingestion and Muscle Glycogen Depletion during Marathon and Ultramarathon Racing. Noakes TD et al; Eur J Appl Physiol, 1988, 57(4):482-9

201 The Marathon: Dietary Manipulation to Optimize Performance. Sherman WM et al; Am J Sports Med, 1984 Jan-Feb, 12(1):44-51 Review

202 Calorie Restriction, Aging, and Cancer Prevention: Mechanisms of Action and Applicability to Humans. Hursting SD et al; Annu Rev Med, 2003;54:131-52 Review

203 Calorie Restriction in Nonhuman Primates: Mechanisms of Reduced Morbidity and Mortality. Hansen BC et al; Toxicol Sci, 1999 Dec, 52(2 Suppl):56-60 Review

204 Calorie Restriction and Aging. Heilbronn LK et al; Am J Clin Nutr, 2003 Sep,78(3):361-69 Review

205 The Inflammation Hypothesis of Aging: Molecular Modulation by Calorie Restriction. Chung HY et al; Ann N Y Acad Sci, 2001 Apr, 928:327-35 Review

206 Caloric Restriction and Aging in Primates: Relevance to Humans and Possible CR Mimetics. Lane MA et al; Microsc Res Tech, 2002 Nov 15, 59(4):335-38 Review

207 Implications of Protein Degradation in Aging. Goto S et al; Ann N Y Acad Sci, 2001 Apr, 928:54-64 Review

208 Calorie Restriction Enhances the Expression of Key Metabolic Enzymes Associated with Protein Renewal during Aging. Spindler SR; Ann N Y Acad Sci, 2001 Apr, 928:296-304 Review

209 Amyloidosis: Prognosis and Treatment. Gertz MA et al; Semin Arthritis Rheum, 1994 Oct, 24(2):124-38 Review

210 Amyloidoses that Infiltrate the Heart. McCarthy RE 3rd et al; Clin Cardiol, 1998 Aug, 21(8):547-52 Review

Chapter 4 – B Vitamins

1 Carbohydrates, Dietary Fiber, and Incident Type 2 Diabetes in Older Women. Meyer KA et al; Am J Clin Nutr, 2000 Apr, 71(4):921-930

2 Wholemeal versus Wholegrain Breads: Proportion of Whole or Cracked Grain and the Glycaemic Response. Jenkins DJ et al; BMJ, 1988 Oct 15, 297(6654):958-60

3 Encyclopedia Britannica: Human Nutrition, Classes of Food, Cereals; britannica.com ©1999-2000

4 Rice Bran Proteins: Properties and Food Uses. Prakash J; Crit Rev Food Sci Nutr, 1996 Jul, 36(6):537-52 Review

5 Glycemic Index, Cardiovascular Disease and Obesity. Morris KL et al; Nutr Rev, 1999 Sept, 57(9 Pt 1):273-76 Review

6 Cereal Grains and Coronary Heart Disease. Truswell AS; Eur J Clin Nutr, 2002 Jan, 56(1):1-14 Review

7 Whole Grain Consumption and Weight Gain: A Review of the Epidemiological Evidence, Potential Mechanisms and Opportunities for Future Research. Koh-Banerjee P et al; Proc Nutr Soc, 2003 Feb, 62(1):25-29 Review

8 Refined-Cereal Intake and Risk of Selected Cancers in Italy. Chatenoud L et al; Am J Clin Nutr, 1999 Dec, 70(6):1107-10

9 Whole-Grain Consumption and Chronic Disease: Protective Mechanisms. Slavin J et al; Nutr Cancer, 1997, 27(1):14-21 Review

10 Antioxidant Activity and Total Phenolics in Selected Cereal Grains and their Different Morphological Fractions. Zielinski H et al; J Agric Food Chem, 2000 Jun, 48(6):2008-16

11 Plasma Lipid Lowering Effects of Wheat Germ in Hypercholesterolemic Subjects. Cara L et al; Plant Foods Hum Nutr, 1991 Apr, 41(2):135-50

12 Use of an Expanded-Whole-Wheat Product in the Reduction of Body Weight and Serum Lipids in Obese Females. Fordyce-Baum MK et al; Am J Clin Nutr, 1989 Jul, 50(1):30-36

13 Protection Against Cancer by Wheat Bran: Role of Dietary Fibre and Phytochemicals. Ferguson LR et al; Eur J Cancer Prev, 1999 Feb, 8(1):17-25 Review

14 A Possible Role of the Dietary Fibre Product, Wheat Bran, as a Nitrite Scavenger. Moller ME et al; Food Chem Toxicol, 1988 Oct, 26(10):841-45

15 Potential of Wheat-Based Breakfast Cereals as a Source of Dietary Antioxidants. Baublis AJ et al; J Am Coll Nutr, 2000 Jun, 19(3 Suppl):308S-311S Review

16 Wholewheat Flour Ensures Higher Mineral Absorption and Bioavailability than White Wheat Flour in Rats. Levrat-Verny MA et al; Br J Nutr, 1999 Jul, 82(1):17-21

17 Isolation and Identification of Novel Tocotrienols from Rice Bran with Hypocholesterolemic, Antioxidant, and Antitumor Properties. Qureshi AA et al; J Agric Food Chem, 2000 Aug, 48(8):3130-40

18 Petrovic G; Med Pregl, 2000 Mar-Apr, 53(3-4):207-14

19 Rye Bread Decreases Serum Total and LDL Cholesterol in Men with Moderately Elevated Serum Cholesterol. Leinonen KS et al; J Nutr, 2000 Feb, 130(2):164-70

20 Rye Bread Improves Bowel Function and Decreases the Concentrations of Some Compounds that are Putative Colon Cancer Risk Markers in Middle-Aged Women and Men. Grasten SM et al; J Nutr, 2000 Sep,130(9):2215-21

21 Whole-Grain Rye and Wheat Foods and Markers of Bowel Health in Overweight Middle-Aged Men. McIntosh GH et al; Am J Clin Nutr, 2003 Apr, 77(4):967-74 Review

22 Glycaemic Response to Maize, Bajra and Barley. Shukla K et al; Indian J Physiol Pharmacol, 1991 Oct, 35(4):249-54

23 Can Dietary Oats Promote Health? Welch RW; Br J Biomed Sci, 1994 Sep, 51(3):260-70 Review

24 The Role of Viscous Soluble Fiber in the Metabolic Control of Diabetes. A Review with Special Emphasis on Cereals Rich in Beta-Glucan. Wursch P et al; Diabetes Care, 1997 Nov, 20(11):1774-80 Review

25 The Role of Fiber in the Treatment of Hypercholesterolemia in Children and Adolescents. Kwiterovich PO Jr; Pediatrics, 1995 Nov, 96(5 Pt 2):1005-09 Review

26 Oats can be Included in Gluten-Free Diet. Hallert C et al; Lakartidningen, 1999 Jul 28, 96(30-31):3339-40

27 Do Oats Belong in a Gluten-Free Diet? Thompson T; J Am Diet Assoc, 1997 Dec, 97(12):1413-16 Review

28 Candida Albicans Pathogenicity: A Proteomic Perspective. Niimi M et al; Electrophoresis 1999 Aug, 20(11):2299-308 Review

29 Candida Albicans, the Opportunist. A Cellular and Molecular Perspective. Dupont PF; J Am Podiatr Med Assoc, 1995 Feb, 85(2):104-15 Review

30 Effect of Beta-Glucan from Oats and Yeast on Serum Lipids. Bell S et al; Crit Rev Food Sci Nutr, 1999 Mar, 39(2):189-202 Review

31 Effect of Addition of Brewer's Yeast to Soy Protein and Casein on Plasma Cholesterol Levels of Rabbits. De Abreu J et al; Arch Latinoam Nutr, 1994 Mar, 44(1):18-22

32 Effect of Preoperative Oral Immune-Enhancing Nutritional Supplement on Patients at High Risk of Infection After Cardiac Surgery. Tepaske R et al; Lancet 2001, Sep 1, 358(9283):696-701

33 Nutritional Role of Chromium. Anderson RA; Sci Total Environ, 1981 Jan, 17(1):13-29 Review

34 Vitamin Supplementation and Athletic Performance. Williams MH; Int J Vitam Nutr Res Suppl, 1989, 30:163-91 Review

35 Pantothenic Acid Metabolic Disorder and its Relation to the Change in Energy Processes in Patients with Ischemic Heart Disease and Hypertension. Borets VM et al; Vopr Pitan, 1983, (1):45-49

36 Pantothenic Acid in Health and Disease. Tahiliani AG et al; Vitam Horm, 1991, 46:165-228 Review

37 Panthenol and Glucocorticoids. Fidanaza A et al; Boll Soc Ital Biol Sper, 1981 Sep 30, 57(18):1869-72

38 The Quebec Cooperative Study of Friedreich's Ataxia: 1974-1984–10 Years of Research. Barbeau A; Can J Neurol Sci, 1984 Nov, 11(4 Suppl):646-60

39 Role of the B Vitamins in the Immune Response. Axelrod AE; Adv Exp Med Biol, 1981, 135:93-106 Review

40 Nutrition and the Immune Response. Dreizen S; Int J Vitam Nutr Res, 1979, 49(2):220-28 Review

41 The Use of Pantothenic Acid Preparations in Treating Patients with Viral Hepatitis A. Komar VI; Ter Arkh, 1991, 63(11):58-60

42   Studies on Wound Healing: Effects of Calcium D-Pantothenate on the Migration, Proliferation and Protein Synthesis of Human Dermal Fibroblasts in Culture. Weimann BI et al; Int J Vitam Nutr Res,1999 Mar, 69(2):113-19

43   Role of Pantothenic and Ascorbic Acid in Wound Healing Processes: In-Vitro Study on Fibroblasts. Lacroix B et al; Int J Vitam Nutr Res, 1988, 58(4):407-13

44   Topical Use of Dexpanthenol in Skin Disorders. Ebner F et al; Am J Clin Dermatol, 2002, 3(6):427-33 Review

45   Pantothenic Acid Deficiency as the Pathogenesis of Acne Vulgaris. Leung LH; Med Hypotheses,1995 Jun, 44(6):490-92

46   Study of Pantothenic Acid Derivatives as Cardiac Protectors in a Model of Experimental Ischemia and Reperfusion of the Isolated Heart. Kumerova AO et al; Biull Eksp Biol Med, 1992 Apr, 113(4):373-75

47   Pantothenic Acid as a Weight-Reducing Agent: Fasting Without Hunger, Weakness and Ketosis. Leung LH; Med Hypotheses, 1995 May, 44(5):403-05

48   Antioxidative Vitamins in Prematurely and Maturely Born Infants. Bohles H; Int J Vitam Nutr Res, 1997, 67(5):321-28 Review

49   Effect of Antioxidative Vitamins on Immune Function with Clinical Applications. Grimble RF; Int J Vitam Nutr Res, 1997, 67(5):312-20 Review

50   Glutathione Reductase Activity, Riboflavin Status, and Disease Activity in Rheumatoid Arthritis. Mulherin DM et al; Ann Rheum Dis, 1996 Nov, 55(11):837-40

51   Protection by Vitamin B2 against Oxidant-Mediated Acute Lung Injury. Seekamp A et al; Inflammation, 1999 Oct, 23(5):449-60

52   Acute Ethanol Exposure Alters Hepatic Glutathione Metabolism in Riboflavin Deficiency. Dutta P et al; Alcohol, 1995 Jan-Feb, 12(1):43-47

53   Effects of Exercise on Riboflavin Requirements of Young Women. Belko AZ et al; Am J Clin Nutr, 1983 Apr, 37(4):509-17

54   Riboflavin and Vitamin B-6 Intakes and Status and Biochemical Response to Riboflavin Supplementation in Free-Living Elderly People. Madigan SM et al; Am J Clin Nutr, 1998 Aug, 68(2):389-95

55   Effectiveness of High-Dose Riboflavin in Migraine Prophylaxis. Schoenen J et al; Neurology, 1998 Feb, 50(2):466-70

56   Vitamins, Iron, and Physical Work. Bates CJ et al; Lancet, 1989 Aug 5, 2(8658):313-14

57   The Role of Vitamins in the Prevention and Control of Anaemia. Fishman SM et al; Public Health Nutr, 2000 Jun, 3(2):125-50

58   Riboflavin Deficiency: Mucocutaneous Signs of Acute and Chronic Deficiency. Roe DA; Semin Dermatol, 1991 Dec, 10(4):293-95 Review

59   Riboflavin. Rivlin RS; Adv Exp Med Biol, 1986, 206:349-55

60   Vitamin B6 Requirements and Recommendations. Bender DA; Eur J Clin Nutr, 1989 May, 43(5):289-309 Review

61   Diabetes and Vitamin Levels. Tamai H; Nippon Rinsho, 1999 Oct, 57(10):2362-65 Review

62   Failure of Pyridoxine to Improve Glucose Tolerance in Diabetics. Rao RH et al; J Clin Endocrinol Metab, 1980 Jan, 50(1):198-200

63   Glucose Tolerance in Subclinical Pyridoxine Deficiency in Man. Rao RH; Am J Clin Nutr, 1983 Sep, 38(3):440-44

64   Improvement of Oral Glucose Tolerance in Gestational Diabetes by Pyridoxine. Bennink HJ et al; Br Med J,1975 Jul 5, 3(5974):13-15

65   Effect of Oral Contraceptives and Vitamin B6 Deficiency on Carbohydrate Metabolism. Rose DP et al; Am J Clin Nutr, 1975 Aug, 28(8):872-78

66   A Deficiency of Vitamin B6 is a Plausible Molecular Basis of the Retinopathy of Patients with Diabetes Mellitus. Ellis JM et al; Biochem Biophys Res Commun, 1991 Aug 30, 179(1):615-19

67   The AGE Inhibitor Pyridoxamine Inhibits Development of Retinopathy in Experimental Diabetes. Stitt A et al; Diabetes, 2002 Sep, 51(9):2826-32

68 Pharmacotherapy of Hyperhomocysteinaemia in Patients with Thrombophilia. O'Donnell J et al; Expert Opin Pharmacother, 2002 Nov, 3(11):1591-98 Review

69 B Vitamins and Homocysteine in Cardiovascular Disease and Aging. Wilcken DE et al; Ann N Y Acad Sci, 1998 Nov 20, 854:361-70 Review

70 The Effect of a Subnormal Vitamin B-6 Status on Homocysteine Metabolism. Ubbink JB et al; J Clin Invest, 1996 Jul 1, 98(1):177-84

71 Low Circulating Folate and Vitamin B6 Concentrations: Risk Factors for Stroke, Peripheral Vascular Disease, and Coronary Artery Disease. European COMAC Group. Robinson K et al; Circulation, 1998 Feb 10, 97(5):437-43

72 Prevention of Myocardial Infarction by Vitamin B6. Ellis JM et al; Res Commun Mol Pathol Pharmacol, 1995 Aug, 89(2):208-20

73 Deregulation of Homocysteine Metabolism and Consequences for the Vascular System. Nicolas JP et al; Bull Acad Natl Med, 1997 Feb, 181(2):313-29

74 Homocysteine and Coronary Heart Disease in the Caerphilly Cohort: A 10 Year Follow Up. Fallon UB et al; Heart, 2001 Feb, 85(2):153-158

75 The Controversy over Homocysteine and Cardiovascular Risk. Ueland PM et al; Am J Clin Nutr, 2000 Aug, 72(2):324-32 Review

76 Homocysteine, Vitamins, and Coronary Artery Disease. Comprehensive Review of the Literature. Taylor BV et al; Can Fam Physician, 2000 Nov, 46:2236-45 Review

77 Pyridoxine Improves Endothelial Function in Cardiac Transplant Recipients. Miner SE et al; J Heart Lung Transplant, 2001 Sep, 20(9):964-69

78 Folate, Vitamin B12, and Neuropsychiatric Disorders. Bottiglieri T; Nutr Rev, 1996 Dec, 54(12):382-90 Review

79 Neuropsychiatric Manifestations of Folate, Cobalamin and Pyridoxine Deficiency Mediated through Imbalances in Excitatory Sulfur Amino Acids? Santhosh-Kumar CR et al; Med Hypotheses, 1994 Oct, 43(4):239-44

80 Relation between Cytokines (TNF-alpha, IL-1 and 6) and Homocysteine in Android Obesity and the Phenomenon of Insulin Resistance Syndromes. Hrnciar J et al; Vnitr Lek, 1999 Jan, 45(1):11-16

81 Interventions for Nausea and Vomiting in Early Pregnancy. Jewell D et al; Cochrane Database Syst Rev, 2000;(2):CD000145 Review

82 Prenatal High-Dose Pyridoxine may Prevent Hypertension and Syndrome X in-utero by Protecting the Fetus from Excess Glucocorticoid Activity. McCarty MF; Med Hypotheses, 2000 May, 54(5):808-13

83 The Importance of Vitamin B6 for Development of the Infant. Human Medical and Animal Experiment Studies. Gerster H; Z Ernahrungswiss, 1996 Dec, 35(4):309-17 Review

84 Vitamin B6 and Cognitive Development: Recent Research Findings from Human and Animal Studies. Guilarte TR; Nutr Rev, 1993 Jul, 51(7):193-98 Review

85 Disturbance of GABA Metabolism in Pyridoxine-Dependent Seizures. Kurlemann G et al; Neuropediatrics, 1992 Oct, 23(5):257-59

86 Pyridoxine-Dependent Epilepsy in an Infant. van Waarde WM et al; Ned Tijdschr Geneeskd, 1995 Aug 19, 139(33):1694-97

87 Pyridoxine-Dependent Seizures: A Clinical and Biochemical Conundrum. Baxter P; Biochim Biophys Acta, 2003 Apr 11, 1647(1-2):36-41 Review

88 Experimental Model of Pyridoxine (B6) Deficiency-Induced Neuropathy. Dellon AL et al; Ann Plast Surg, 2001 Aug, 47(2):153-60

89 Nutrition and Immunity with Emphasis on Infection and Autoimmune Disease. Harbige LS; Nutr Health, 1996, 10(4):285-312 Review

90 Pyridoxine Deficiency: New Approaches in Immunosuppression and Chemotherapy. Trakatellis A et al; Postgrad Med J, 1997 Oct, 73(864):617-22 Review

91 Antitumor Effect of Vitamin B6 and its Mechanisms. Komatsu S et al; Biochim Biophys Acta, 2003 Apr 11,

1647(1-2):127-30 Review

92 Vitamin B6 (Pyridoxine) Therapy for Carpal Tunnel Syndrome. Jacobson MD et al; Hand Clin, 1996 May, 12(2):253-57 Review

93 Vitamin B6, Vitamin C, and Carpal Tunnel Syndrome. Keniston RC et al; J Occup Environ Med, 1997 Oct, 39(10):949-59

94 High-Dose Pyridoxine as an Anti-Stress Strategy. McCarty MF; Med Hypotheses, 2000 May, 54(5):803-07

95 Metabolism of Vitamin B6 and its Requirement in Chronic Renal Failure. Mydlik M et al; Kidney Int Suppl, 1997 Nov, 62:S56-59

96 The Pathogenesis of Decreased Aspartate Aminotransferase and Alanine Aminotransferase Activity in the Plasma of Hemodialysis Patients: The Role of Vitamin B6 Deficiency. Ono K et al; Clin Nephrol, 1995 Jun, 43(6):405-08

97 Effect of Vitamin B6 Supplementation on Plasma Oxalate and Oxalate Removal Rate in Hemodialysis Patients. Costello JF et al; J Am Soc Nephrol, 1992 Oct, 3(4):1018-24

98 Vitamin B6 Status in Uremia. Laso Guzman FJ et al; Klin Wochenschr, 1990 Feb 1, 68(3):183-86

99 Vitamin B6 Requirements of Patients on Chronic Peritoneal Dialysis. Ross EA et al; Kidney Int, 1989 Oct, 36(4):702-06

100 Para-Aminobenzoic Acid Inhibits the Manifestation of Inducible SOS Functions in Escherichia Coli K-12. Vasil'eva SV et al; Genetika, 1983 Nov, 19(11):1778-85

101 Para-Aminobenzoic Acid Inhibits a Set of SOS Functions in Escherichia Coli K12. Vasilieva S; Mutat Res, 2001 Sep 20, 496(1-2):89-95

102 Para-Aminobenzoic Acid Intensification of DNA Repair Processes in Escherichia Coli K-12. Vasil'eva SV et al; Genetika, 1982 Mar, 18(3):381-91

103 Repair Effect of P-Aminobenzoic Acid and Aminobenzhydrazide. Ivanov SD et al; Biull Eksp Biol Med, 1982 Apr, 93(4):37-39

104 Concepts and Models for DNA Repair: from Escherichia Coli to Mammalian Cells. Hanawalt PC; Environ Mol Mutagen, 1989, 14 Suppl 16:90-98

105 The Effect of Para-Aminomethylbenzoic Acid (Amben) on Peripheral Nerve Regeneration. Chaikovskii IuB et al; Patol Fiziol Eksp Ter, 1989 Sep-Oct, (5):60-62

106 Comparative Assessment of Antioxidant Activity of Para-Aminobenzoic Acid and Emoxipin in Retina. Akberova SI et al; Vestn Oftalmol, 1998 Nov-Dec, 114(6):39-44

107 The Antithrombotic Activity of Para-Aminobenzoic Acid in Experimental Thrombosis. Stroeva OG et al; Izv Akad Nauk Ser Biol, 1999 May-Jun, (3):329-36

108 Para-Aminobenzoic Acid Suppression of Cis-Diamminedichloroplatinum(II) Nephrotoxicity. Esposito M et al; Carcinogenesis, 1993 Dec, 14(12):2595-99

109 UVA-Potentiated Damage to Calf Thymus DNA by Fenton Reaction System and Protection by Para-Aminobenzoic Acid. Shih MK et al; Photochem Photobiol, 1996 Mar, 63(3):286-91

110 The Photochemistry of P-Aminobenzoic Acid. Shaw AA et al; Photochem Photobiol, 1992 May, 55(5):647-56

111 The Inhibiting Effect of PABA on Photocarcinogenesis. Flindt-Hansen H et al; Arch Dermatol Res, 1990, 282(1):38-41

112 Photocarcinogenesis is Retarded by a Partly Photodegraded Solution of Para-Aminobenzoic Acid. Flindt-Hansen H et al; Photodermatol, 1989 Dec, 6(6):263-67

113 The Effect of a Sunscreen Containing Para-Aminobenzoic Acid on the Systemic Immunologic Alterations Induced in Mice by Exposure to UVB Radiation. Morison WL; J Invest Dermatol, 1984 Dec, 83(6):405-08

114 Ability of PABA to Protect Mammalian Skin from Ultraviolet Light-Induced Skin Tumors and Actinic Damage. Synder DS et al; J Invest Dermatol, 1975 Dec, 65(6):543-46

115 New Biological Properties of P-Aminobenzoic Acid. Akberova SI; Izv Akad Nauk Ser Biol, 2002 Jul-Aug, (4):477-81 Review

116 Study of Interferon-Inducing Activity of Para-Aminobenzoic Acid Injected Subconjunctivally in Rabbits.

Akberova SI et al; Vestn Oftalmol, 1999 Jan-Feb, 115(1):24-26

117   Neuropathology of Thiamine Deficiency Disorders. Kril JJ; Metab Brain Dis, 1996 Mar, 11(1):9-17 Review

118   Thiamine Treatment Today. Tallaksen CM et al; Tidsskr Nor Laegeforen, 1998 Oct 20, 118(25):3946-49 Review

119   Wernicke-Korsakow Syndrome: Clinical Aspects, Pathophysiology and Therapeutic Approaches. Preuss UW et al; Fortschr Neurol Psychiatr, 1997 Sep, 65(9):413-20 Review

120   Wernicke's Encephalopathy. Andersson JE; Ugeskr Laeger, 1996 Feb 12, 158(7):898-901 Review

121   The Korsakoff Syndrome. Kopelman MD; Br J Psychiatry, 1995 Feb, 166(2):154-73 Review

122   Metabolic Impairment Elicits Brain Cell Type-Selective Changes in Oxidative Stress and Cell Death in Culture. Park LC et al; J Neurochem, 2000 Jan, 74(1):114-24

123   Mechanisms of Selective nNeuronal Cell Death due to Thiamine Deficiency. Todd K et al; Ann N Y Acad Sci, 1999, 893:404-11

124   Mechanisms of Neuronal Cell Death in Wernicke's Encephalopathy. Hazell AS et al; Metab Brain Dis, 1998 Jun 13(2):97-122 Review

125   Chronic Ethanol Consumption: from Neuroadaptation to Neurodegeneration. Fadda F et al; Prog Neurobiol, 1998 Nov, 56(4):385-431

126   B Vitamin Deficiency and Neuropsychiatric Syndromes in Alcohol Misuse. Cook CC et al; Alcohol Alcohol, 1998 Jul-Aug, 33(4):317-36 Review

127   Clinical and Neuropathological Aspects of Wernicke-Korsakoff Syndrome. Zubaran C et al; Rev Saude Publica, 1996 Dec, 30(6):602-08

128   Wernicke's Encephalopathy Associated with Hemodialysis. Ihara M et al; Clin Neurol Neurosurg, 1999 Jun, 101(2):118-21 Review

129   Plasma Thiamine Deficiency Associated with Alzheimer's Disease but not Parkinson's Disease. Gold M et al; Metab Brain Dis, 1998 Mar, 13(1):43-53

130   The History of Healing; Beriberi: 'Kind of Paralysis'. de Knecht-van Eekelen A; Ned Tijdschr Geneeskd, 1997 Jun 14, 141(24):1199-203

131   Shoshin Beriberi. A Rapidly Curable Hemodynamic Disaster. Meurin P; Presse Med, 1996 Jul 6-13, 25(24):1115-18 Review

132   Failure in Self Care and Heart Failure, Thiamine Deficiency in Geriatric Patients. te Water W et al; Tijdschr Gerontol Geriatr, 1996 Jun, 27(3):97-101

133   Thiamin Status, Diuretic Medications, and the Management of Congestive Heart Failure. Brady JA et al; J Am Diet Assoc, 1995 May, 95(5):541-44

134   Metabolic Acidosis and Thiamine Deficiency. Romanski SA et al; Mayo Clin Proc, 1999 Mar, 74(3):259-63

135   Optimum Nutrition: Thiamin, Biotin and Pantothenate. Bender DA; Proc Nutr Soc,1999 May, 58(2):427-33 Review

136   Thiamine-Deficient Lactic Acidosis with Brain Tumor Treatment. Kuba H et al; J Neurosurg, 1998 Dec, 89(6):1025-28

137   The Effects of Nutrients on Mood. Benton D et al; Public Health Nutr, 1999 Sep, 2(3A):403-09 Review

138   Anaphylaxis to Parenteral Thiamine (Vitamin B1). Morinville V et al; Schweiz Med Wochenschr, 1998 Oct 31, 128(44):1743-44

139   Parenteral Thiamine and Wernicke's Encephalopathy: the Balance of Risks and Perception of Concern. Thomson AD et al; Alcohol Alcohol, 1997 May-Jun, 32(3):207-09

140   Folate Deficiency beyond Megaloblastic Anemia: Hyperhomocysteinemia and Other Manifestations of Dysfunctional Folate Status. Green R et al; Semin Hematol, 1999 Jan, 36(1):47-64 Review

141   Folate and Vitamin B12. Scott JM; Proc Nutr Soc, 1999 May, 58(2):441-48 Review

142   Megaloblastic Anemia in Children. de Lumley L et al; Arch Pediatr, 1994 Mar, 1(3):281-88 Review

143   Anemia in Pregnancy. Lops VR et al; Am Fam Physician, 1995 Apr, 51(5):1189-97 Review

144   Megaloblastic Anemia in Pregnancy. Campbell BA; Clin Obstet Gynecol, 1995 Sep, 38(3):455-62 Review

145   Folic Acid: Influence on the Outcome of Pregnancy. Scholl TO et al; Am J Clin Nutr, 2000 May, 71(5 Suppl):1295S-303S Review

146   Folate Status and Neural Tube Defects. Molloy AM et al; Biofactors, 1999, 10(2-3):291-94

147   Spina Bifida, Sarwark JF; Pediatr Clin North Am, 1996 Oct, 43(5):1151-58 Review

148   Neural Tube Defects, Vitamins and Homocysteine, Eskes TK; Eur J Pediatr, 1998 Apr, 157 Suppl 2:S139-41 Review

149   Cobalamin and Folate Deficiency: Acquired and Hereditary Disorders in Children. Rosenblatt DS et al; Semin Hematol, 1999 Jan, 36(1):19-34 Review

150   Folic Acid Antagonists during Pregnancy and the Risk of Birth Defects. Hernandez-Diaz S et al; N Engl J Med, 2000 Nov 30, 343(22):1608-1614

151   Folate Deficiencies and Cardiovascular Pathologies. Durand P et al; Clin Chem Lab Med, 1998 Jun, 36(7):419-29 Review

152   Folate Supplementation and the Risk of Masking Vitamin B12 Deficiency. Brantigan CO; JAMA, 1997 Mar 19, 277(11):884-85

153   How Safe are Folic Acid Supplements? Campbell NR; Arch Intern Med, 1996 Aug 12-26, 156(15):1638-44 Review

154   Further Evidence on the Effects of Vitamin B12 and Folate levels on Episodic Memory Functioning: Population-Based Study of Healthy Very Old Adults. Hassing L et al; Biol Psychiatry, 1999 Jun 1, 45(11):1472-80

155   Folate, Vitamin B12, and Homocysteine in Major Depressive Disorder. Fava M et al; Am J Psychiatry, 1997 Mar, 154(3):426-28

156   Reduced Red-Cell Folate in Mania. Hasanah CI et al; J Affect Disord, 1997 Nov, 46(2):95-99

157   Folate and Cobalamin in Psychiatric Illness. Hutto BR; Compr Psychiatry, 1997 Nov-Dec, 38(6):305-14 Review

158   Folate, Vitamin B12, and Neuropsychiatric Disorders. Bottiglieri T; Nutr Rev, 1996 Dec, 54(12):382-90 Review

159   Homocysteine, Folate Deprivation and Alzheimer Neuropathology. Shea TB et al; J Alzheimers Dis, 2002 Aug, 4(4):261-67 Review

160   Hyperhomocysteinemia and Thrombosis. Makris M; Clin Lab Haematol, 2000 Jun, 22(3):133-43 Review

161   Homocysteine, Vitamins, and Coronary Artery Disease. Taylor BV et al; Can Fam Physician, 2000 Nov, 46:2236-45 Review

162   Erythropoietin, Folic Acid Deficiency and Hyperhomocysteinemia: Is There a Possible Relationship in Chronically Hemodialyzed Patients? Korzets A et al; Clin Nephrol, 2000 Jan, 53(1):48-54

163   Folate: Effects on Carcinogenesis and the Potential for Cancer Chemoprevention. Mason JB et al; Oncology (Huntingt), 1996 Nov, 10(11):1727-36, 1742-43 Review

164   Folic Acid as a Cancer-Preventing Agent. Jennings E; Med Hypotheses, 1995 Sep, 45(3):297-303 Review

165   Folate and Carcinogenesis: An Integrated Scheme. Choi SW et al; J Nutr, 2000 Feb, 130(2):129-32 Review

166   Folate Deficiency Causes Uracil Misincorporation into Human DNA and Chromosome Breakage: Implications for Cancer and Neuronal Damage. Blount BC et al; Proc Natl Acad Sci U S A, 1997 Apr 1, 94(7):3290-95

167   Folate-Responsive Optic Neuropathy. Golnik KC et al; J Neuroophthalmol, 1994 Sep, 14(3):163-69

168   Age-Related Hearing Loss. Vitamin B-12, and Folate in Elderly Women, Houston DK et al; Am J Clin Nutr, 1999 Mar, 69(3):564-71

169   High-Dose Biotin, an Inducer of Glucokinase Expression, may Synergize with Chromium Picolinate to Enable a Definitive Nutritional Therapy for Type II Diabetes, McCarty MF; Med Hypotheses, 1999 May, 52(5):401-06 Review

170   Evidence for a Pathogenic Role of Omega 6 Polyunsaturated Fatty Acid in the Cutaneous Manifestations of Biotin Deficiency. Mock DM; J Pediatr Gastroenterol Nutr, 1990 Feb, 10(2):222-29

171   Abnormal Fatty Acid Composition of Biotin-Responsive Multiple Carboxylase Deficiency Fibroblasts.

Packman S et al; J Inherit Metab Dis, 1989, 12(1):47-57

172 Effects of Biotin Deficiency on Serum Fatty Acid Composition: Evidence for Abnormalities in Humans. Mock DM et al; J Nutr, 1988 Mar, 118(3):342-48

173 Biotin in Metabolism and its Relationship to Human Disease. Pacheco-Alvarez D et al; Arch Med Res, 2002 Sep-Oct, 33(5):439-47 Review

174 Biotin Deficiency in an Infant Fed with Amino Acid Formula and Hypoallergenic Rice. Higuchi R et al; Acta Paediatr, 1996 Jul, 85(7):872-74 Review

175 Biotin Deficiency Complicating Parenteral Alimentation: Aiagnosis, Metabolic Repercussions, and Treatment. Mock DM et al; J Pediatr, 1985 May, 106(5):762-69

176 Cell-Mediated Immunity in Nutritional Deficiency. McMurray DN; Prog Food Nutr Sci, 1984, 8(3-4):193-228

177 Biotin Status: Which are Valid Indicators and How Do We Know? Mock DM; J Nutr 1999 Feb, 129(2S Suppl):498S-503S Review

178 Marginal Biotin Deficiency is Teratogenic. Zempleni J et al; Proc Soc Exp Biol Med, 2000 Jan, 223(1):14-21 Review

179 Increased Urinary Excretion of 3-Hydroxyisovaleric Acid and Decreased Urinary Excretion of Biotin are Sensitive Early Indicators of Decreased Biotin Status in Experimental Biotin Deficiency. Mock NI et al; Am J Clin Nutr, 1997 Apr, 65(4):951-58

180 Pellagra: Diagnosis Still Valid. Llancapi P et al; Rev Med Chil, 1998 Apr, 126(4):435-38

181 Pellagra and Pellagralike Dermatoses: Etiology, Differential Diagnosis. Dermatopathology, and Treatment, Hendricks WM; Semin Dermatol, 1991 Dec, 10(4):282-92 Review

182 Pellagra may be a Rare Secondary Complication of Anorexia Nervosa. Prousky JE; Altern Med Rev, 2003 May, 8(2):180-185 Review

183 Special Reference to Niacin Deficiency Encephalopathy. Meador KJ et al; South Med J, 1988 Aug, 81(8):1042-46

184 Crohn's Disease Associated with Pellagra and Increased Excretion of 5-Hydroxyindolacetic Acid. Abu-Qurshin R et al; Am J Med Sci, 1997 Feb, 313(2):111-13

185 Pellagra as the Presenting Manifestation of Crohn's Disease. Pollack S et al; Gastroenterology, 1982 May, 82(5 Pt 1):948-52

186 Pathological Effects of Pellagra on the Esophagus. Segal I et al; Nutr Cancer, 1990, 14(3-4):233-38

187 Pellagra Encephalopathy among Tuberculous Patients: its Relation to Isoniazid Therapy. Ishii N et al; J Neurol Neurosurg Psychiatry, 1985 Jul, 48(7):628-34

188 Tryptophan Metabolism in Alcoholic Pellagra Patients: Measurements of Urinary Metabolites and Histochemical Studies of Related Muscle Enzymes. Vannucchi H et al; Am J Clin Nutr, 1982 Jun, 35(6):1368-74

189 Nutritional Factors that Regulate on the Conversion of L-Tryptophan to Niacin. Shibata K; Adv Exp Med Biol, 1999, 467:711-16

190 The Effects of Administration of Drugs Influencing Haemostasis during Treatment of Patients with Burns. Iashvili BP et al; Burns Incl Therm Inj, 1986 Feb, 12(3):184-87

191 Evaluating the Role of Niacin in Human Carcinogenesis. Jacobson EL et al; Biochimie, 1995, 77(5):394-98 Review

192 Niacin as a Potential AIDS Preventive Factor. Murray MF; Med Hypotheses, 1999 Nov, 53(5):375-79

193 Schizophrenia: a Biochemical Disorder? Horrobin DF; Biomedicine, 1980 May, 32(2):54-55

194 Essential Fatty Acids, Lipid Membrane Abnormalities, and the Diagnosis and Treatment of Schizophrenia. Fenton WS et al; Biol Psychiatry, 2000 Jan 1, 47(1):8-21 Review

195 Nicotinic Acid and Pyridoxine Modulate Arachidonic acid Metabolism in Vitro and ex Vivo in Man. Saareks V et al; Pharmacol Toxicol, 1999 Jun, 84(6):274-80

196 New Extended-Release Niacin (Niaspan): Efficacy, Tolerability, and Safety in Hypercholesterolemic Patients. Morgan JM et al; Am J Cardiol, 1998 Dec 17, 82(12A):29U-34U; discussion 39U-41U

197 Effects of Nonstatin Lipid Drug Therapy on High-Density Lipoprotein Metabolism. Rader DJ; Am J Cardiol,

2003 Apr 3, 91(7A):18E-23E Review

198   Atherosclerosis: The Importance of HDL Cholesterol and Prostacyclin: A Role for Niacin Therapy. Luria MH; Med Hypotheses, 1990 May, 32(1):21-28 Review

199   Effect of Orotic Acid, Calcium Pangamate, and Lipamide on Ultrastructural Changes in Lipocytes in Hepatic Dystrophy. Posokhova EA; Biull Eksp Biol Med, 1981;91(1):76-78

200   Effect of Vitamin B15 on Cholesterol Levels in the Intestinal Wall of Rabbits. Nagorna-Stasiak B et al; Pol Arch Weter, 1983, 23(4):63-71

201   Studies on the Chemical Identity and Biological Functions of Pangamic Acid. Schneider D et al; Arzneimittelforschung, 1999 Apr, 49(4):335-43

202   Examination of Toxicity of Diisopropylammonium Dichloracetate (DADA), Remedies for Cardiac Diseases, Toward Isolated Rat Hepatocytes. Hatano M et al; Meikai Daigaku Shigaku Zasshi, 1990, 19(1):137-44

203   The Effect of Pangamic Acid on Maximal Treadmill Performance. Gray ME et al; Med Sci Sports Exerc, 1982, 14(6):424-27

204   Unproven Methods of Cancer Management. Laetrile. CA Cancer J Clin, 1991 May-Jun, 41(3):187-92 Review

205   A Clinical Trial of Amygdalin (Laetrile) in the Treatment of Human Cancer. Moertel CG et al; N Engl J Med, 1982 Jan 28, 306(4):201-06

206   Accidental Choke-Cherry Poisoning: Early Symptoms and Neurological Sequelae of an Unusual Case of Cyanide Intoxication. Pentore R et al; Ital J Neurol Sci, 1996 Jun, 17(3):233-35

207   Neuromyopathy of Cyanide Intoxication due to "Laetrile" (Amygdalin). A Clinicopathologic Study. Kalyanaraman UP et al; Cancer, 1983 Jun 1, 51(11):2126-33

208   A Pharmacologic and Toxicological Study of Amygdalin. Moertel CG et al; JAMA, 1981 Feb 13, 245(6):591-94

209   Laetrile Intoxication and Hepatic Necrosis: A Possible Association. Leor R et al; South Med J, 1986 Feb, 79(2):259-60

210   Amygdalin (Laetrile): Effect on Clonogenic Cells from Human Myeloid Leukemia Cell Lines and Normal Human Marrow. Koeffler HP et al; Cancer Treat Rep, 1980 Jan, 64(1):105-09

211   Effects of Cyanate, Thiocyanate, and Amygdalin on Metabolite Uptake in Normal and Neoplastic Tissues of the Rat. Lea MA et al; J Natl Cancer Inst, 1979 Nov, 63(5):1279-83

Chapter 5 – Fatty Acids

1   Cyclic AMP and Arachidonic Acid: a Tale of Two Pathways. Wang X et al; Mol Cell Endocrinol, 1999 Dec 20, 158(1-2):7-12 Review

2   Essential Unsaturated Fatty Acids. Yamamoto S; Nippon Rinsho, 1999 Oct, 57(10):2242-46 Review

3   Biochemical Functions of a Pool of Arachidonic Acid Associated with Triglycerides in Human Inflammatory Cells. Triggiani M et al; Int Arch Allergy Immunol, 1995 May-Jun, 107(1-3):261-63 Review

4   Cellular Regulation of Arachidonate Mobilization and Metabolism. Rosenthal MD et al; Prostaglandins Leukot Essent Fatty Acids, 1995 Feb-Mar, 52(2-3):93-98 Review

5   Atherosclerosis. Yamada N; Nippon Rinsho, 1999 Oct, 57(10):2345-48 Review

6   Preventing Coronary Artery Disease by Lowering Cholesterol Levels: Fifty Years from Bench to Bedside. Steinberg D et al; JAMA, 1999 Dec 1, 282(21):2043-50 Review

7   Cholesterol Management in the Era of Managed Care. Grundy SM; Am J Cardiol, 2000 Feb 10, 85(3A):3A-9A Review

8   Antiatherogenic Role of High-Density Lipoprotein Cholesterol. Kwiterovich PO; Am J Cardiol, 1998 Nov 5, 82(9A):13Q-21Q Review

9   Hypertriglyceridemia: Danger for the Arteries. Chanu B; Presse Med, 1999 Nov 20, 28(36):2011-17 Review

10   Pathophysiology of Triglyceride-Rich Lipoproteins in Atherothrombosis: Cellular Aspects. Gianturco SH et al; Clin Cardiol, 1999 Jun, 22(6 Suppl):II7-14 Review

11   Pathophysiology of Acute Coronary Syndromes Leading to Acute Myocardial Infarction. Doering LV; J

Cardiovasc Nurs, 1999 Apr,13(3):1-20 Review

12   Dietary Fat and Prostate Cancer Progression and Survival. Fradet Y et al; Eur Urol, 1999, 35(5-6):388-91 Review

13   Dietary Fat and Prostate Cancer Survival. Meyer F et al; Cancer Causes Control, 1999 Aug, 10(4):245-51

14   Dietary Fat and Advanced Prostate Cancer. Bairati I et al; J Urol, 1998 Apr, 159(4):1271-75

15   Monounsaturated and Other Types of Fat, and the Risk of Breast Cancer. La Vecchia C et al; Eur J Cancer Prev, 1998 Dec, 7(6):461-64

16   Intake of Conjugated Linoleic Acid, Fat, and Other Fatty Acids in Relation to Postmenopausal Breast Cancer: The Netherlands Cohort Study on Diet and Cancer. Voorrips LE et al; Am J Clin Nutr, 2002 Oct, 76(4):873-82

17   A Prospective Study of Association of Monounsaturated Fat and Other Types of Fat with Risk of Breast Cancer. Wolk A et al; Arch Intern Med, 1998 Jan 12, 158(1):41-45

18   Specific Fatty Acids and Risks of Breast and Prostate Cancer: Dietary Intake. Willett WC; Am J Clin Nutr, 1997 Dec, 66(6 Suppl):1557S-1563S Review

19   Nutrition and Cancer. Willett WC; Salud Publica Mex, 1997 Jul-Aug, 39(4):298-309 Review

20   Fried, Well-Done Red Meat and Risk of Lung Cancer in Women (United States). Sinha R et al; Cancer Causes Control, 1998 Dec, 9(6):621-30

21   Dietary Fat and Chronic Diseases: Epidemiologic Overview. Kuller LH; J Am Diet Assoc, 1997 Jul, 97(7 Suppl):S9-15 Review

22   Hypercholesterolemia. Dietary Advice for Patients Regarding Meat. Keenan JM et al; Postgrad Med, 1995 Oct, 98(4):113-14, 117-18, 120-21

23   Best Food: Tender Is The Loin. Tallmadge K; article 8430, http://www.ediets.com

24   Previous Milk Consumption is Associated with Greater Bone Density in Young Women. Teegarden D et al; Am J Clin Nutr, 1999 May, 69(5):1014-17

25   Calcium and Bone Health in Children. Stallings VA; Am J Ther, 1997 Jul-Aug, 4(7-8):259-73 Review

26   Dairy Calcium, Bone Metabolism, and Prevention of Osteoporosis. Renner E; J Dairy Sci, 1994 Dec, 77(12):3498-505

27   Calcium Needs of Adolescents. Key JD et al; Curr Opin Pediatr, 1994 Aug, 6(4):379-82

28   Osteoporosis and Bone Metabolic Parameters in Dependence upon Calcium Intake Through Milk and Milk Products. Stracke H et al; Eur J Clin Nutr, 1993 Sep, 47(9):617-22

29   Dietary Cholesterol–the Role of Eggs in the Prudent Diet. Vorster HH et al; S Afr Med J, 1995 Apr, 85(4):253-56

30   Effects of Two Eggs per Day in Moderately Hypercholesterolemic and Combined Hyperlipidemic Subjects Taught the NCEP Step I Diet. Knopp RH et al; J Am Coll Nutr, 1997 Dec, 16(6):551-61

31   Consumption of Eggs with Meals Increases the Susceptibility of Human Plasma and Low-Density Lipoprotein to Lipid Peroxidation. Levy Y et al; Ann Nutr Metab, 1996, 40(5):243-51

32   A Prospective Study of Egg Consumption and Risk of Cardiovascular Disease in Men and Women. Hu FB et al; JAMA, 1999 Apr 21, 281(15):1387-94

33   Serum Lipids and Eggs. Flynn MA et al; J Am Diet Assoc, 1986 Nov, 86(11):1541-48

34   Food Processing and Lipid Oxidation. German JB; Adv Exp Med Biol, 1999, 459:23-50 Review

35   Routes of Formation and Toxic Consequences of Lipid Oxidation Products in Foods. Kubow S; Free Radic Biol Med, 1992, 12(1):63-81 Review

36   Occurrence of Lipid Oxidation Products in Foods. Addis PB; Food Chem Toxicol, 1986 Oct-Nov, 24(10-11):1021-30 Review

37   Trans-Fatty Acids and Health. Pedersen JI et al; Tidsskr Nor Laegeforen, 1998 Sep 20, 118(22):3474-80 Review

38   Dietary Fat Consumption and Health. Lichtenstein AH et al; Nutr Rev, 1998 May, 56(5 Pt 2):S3-19 Review

39   Trans Fatty Acids, Lipoproteins, and Coronary Risk. Zock PL et al; Can J Physiol Pharmacol, 1997 Mar,

75(3):211-16 Review

40 Trans Fatty Acids and Coronary Heart Disease Risk. Am J Clin Nutr, 1995 Sep, 62(3):655S-708S Review

41 Adipose Fatty Acids and Cancers of the Breast, Prostate and Colon: EURAMIC Study Group. Bakker N et al; Int J Cancer, 1997 Aug 7, 72(4):587-91

42 Association of Dietary Intake of Fat and Fatty Acids with Risk of Breast Cancer. Holmes MD et al; JAMA, 1999 Mar 10, 281(10):914-20

43 Fatty Acid Composition of the Subcutaneous Adipose Tissue and Risk of Proliferative Benign Breast Disease and Breast Cancer. London SJ et al; J Natl Cancer Inst, 1993 May 19, 85(10):785-93

44 Food Heating and the Formation of Heterocyclic Aromatic Amine and Polycyclic Aromatic Hydrocarbon Mutagens/Carcinogens. Knize MG et al; Adv Exp Med Biol, 1999, 459:179-93 Review

45 Carcinogenic Heterocyclic Amines in Model Systems and Cooked Foods: Formation, Occurrence and Intake. Skog KI et al; Food Chem Toxicol, 1998 Sep-Oct, 36(9-10):879-96 Review

46 Isomeric Trans Fatty Acids in the U.S. Diet. Enig MG et al; J Am Coll Nutr, 1990 Oct, 9(5):471-86

47 Similar Distribution of Trans Fatty Acid Isomers in Partially Hydrogenated Vegetable Oils and Adipose Tissue of Canadians. Chen ZY et al; Can J Physiol Pharmacol, 1995 Jun, 73(6):718-23

48 Trans Fatty Acid Isomers in Canadian Human Milk. Chen ZY et al; Lipids, 1995 Jan, 30(1):15-21

49 Olestra and its Gastrointestinal Safety. Thomson AB et al; Aliment Pharmacol Ther, 1998 Dec, 12(12):1185-200 Review

50 Olestra, a Nonabsorbed, Noncaloric Replacement for Dietary Fat. Lawson KD et al; Drug Metab Rev, 1997 Aug, 29(3):651-703 Review

51 Utilization of Vitamin E. Traber MG; Biofactors, 1999, 10(2-3):115-20 Review

52 Synthetic as Compared with Natural Vitamin E is Preferentially Excreted as Alpha-CEHC in Human Urine: Studies using Deuterated Alpha-Tocopheryl Acetates. Traber MG et al; FEBS Lett, 1998 Oct 16, 437(1-2):145-48

53 Human Plasma and Tissue Alpha-Tocopherol Concentrations in Response to Supplementation with Deuterated Natural and Synthetic Vitamin E. Burton GW et al; Am J Clin Nutr, 1998 Apr, 67(4):669-84

54 Toxicology of the Synthetic Antioxidants BHA and BHT in Comparison with the Natural Antioxidant Vitamin E. Kahl R et al; Z Lebensm Unters Forsch, 1993 Apr, 196(4):329-38 Review

55 Carcinogenicity and Modification of the Carcinogenic Response by BHA, BHT, and Other Antioxidants. Ito N et al; Crit Rev Toxicol, 1985, 15(2):109-50 Review

56 Control of Polyunsaturated Acids in Tissue Lipids. Holman RT; J Am Coll Nutr, 1986, 5(2):183-211 Review

57 Essential Fatty Acids as Determinants of Lipid Requirements in Infants, Children and Adults. Uauy R et al; Eur J Clin Nutr, 1999 Apr, 53 Suppl 1:S66-77 Review

58 Eicosanoids: A Historical Overview. Baker RR; Clin Biochem, 1990 Oct, 23(5):455-58 Review

59 Essential Fatty Acids in Pregnancy and Early Human Development. Hornstra G et al; Eur J Obstet Gynecol Reprod Biol, 1995 Jul, 61(1):57-62 Review

60 Essential Fatty Acid Consideration at Birth in the Premature Neonate and the Specific Requirement for Preformed Prostaglandin Precursors in the Infant. Friedman Z; Prog Lipid Res, 1986, 25(1-4):355-64 Review

61 Exogenous Lipids in Myelination. Di Biase A et al; Kao Hsiung I Hsueh Ko Hsueh Tsa Chih, 1997 Jan, 13(1):19-29 Review

62 Essential Fatty Acids, Prostaglandins, and Alcoholism. Horrobin DF; Alcohol Clin Exp Res, 1987 Feb, 11(1):2-9 Review

63 Behavioral Methods used in the Study of Long-Chain Polyunsaturated Fatty Acid Nutrition in Primate Infants. Carlson SE; Am J Clin Nutr, 2000 Jan, 71(1 Suppl):268S-74S Review

64 Long-Chain Polyunsaturated Fatty Acids in Children with Attention-Deficit Hyperactivity Disorder. Burgess JR et al; Am J Clin Nutr, 2000 Jan, 71(1 Suppl):327S-30S Review

65 Relationship between Schizophrenia and Essential Fatty Acid and Eicosanoid Metabolism. Horrobin DF; Prostaglandins Leukot Essent Fatty Acids, 1992 May, 46(1):71-77 Review

66   Could Diet be One of the Causal Factors of Alzheimer's Disease? Newman PE; Med Hypotheses, 1992 Oct, 39(2):123-26 Review

67   Estrogen, Statins and Polyunsaturated Fatty Acids: Similarities in Their Actions and Benefits - Is There a Common Link? Das UN; Nutrition, 2002 Feb, 18(2):178-88 Review

68   Diet and Coronary Heart Disease. Oliver MF; Hum Nutr Clin Nutr, 1982, 36(6):413-27 Review

69   Food Use and Health Effects of Soybean and Sunflower Oils. Meydani SN et al; J Am Coll Nutr, 1991 Oct, 10(5):406-28 Review

70   Polyunsaturated Fatty Acid Deficiency in Liver Diseases: Pathophysiological and Clinical Significance. Cabre E et al; Nutrition, 1996 Jul-Aug, 12(7-8):542-48 Review

71   Metabolism and Function of Skin Lipids. Ziboh VA et al; Prog Lipid Res, 1988, 27(2):81-105 Review

72   Post-Viral Fatigue Syndrome, Viral Infections in Atopic Eczema, and Essential Fatty Acids. Horrobin DF; Med Hypotheses, 1990 Jul, 32(3):211-7 Review

73   Essential Fatty Acids and Immune Response. Hwang D; FASEB J, 1989 Jul, 3(9):2052-61 Review

74   Essential Fatty acids, Lipid Peroxidation and Apoptosis. Das UN; Prostaglandins Leukot Essent Fatty Acids, 1999 Sep, 61(3):157-63 Review

75   Eicosanoids and Essential Fatty Acid Modulation in Chronic Disease and the Chronic Fatigue Syndrome. Gray JB et al; Med Hypotheses, 1994 Jul, 43(1):31-42 Review

76   Altered Glucocorticoid Regulation of the Immune Response in the Chronic Fatigue Syndrome. Visser JT et al; Ann N Y Acad Sci, 2000, 917:868-75 Review

77   The Estrogen Connection: Etiological Relationship between Diabetes, Cancer, Rheumatoid Arthritis and Psychiatric Disorders. Holden RJ; Med Hypotheses, 1995 Aug, 45(2):169-89 Review

78   Premenstrual Syndrome and Premenstrual Breast Pain (Cyclical Mastalgia): Disorders of Essential Fatty Acid (EFA) Metabolism. Horrobin DF et al; Prostaglandins Leukot Essent Fatty Acids, 1989 Sep, 37(4):255-61

79   Calcium Metabolism, Osteoporosis and Essential Fatty Acids. Kruger MC et al; Prog Lipid Res, 1997 Sep, 36(2-3):131-51 Review

80   Fatty Acid Metabolism in Health and Disease: the Role of Delta-6-Desaturase. Horrobin DF; Am J Clin Nutr, 1993 May, 57(5 Suppl):732S-736S Review

81   Essential Fatty Acid Metabolism and its Modification in Atopic Eczema. Horrobin DF; Am J Clin Nutr, 2000 Jan, 71(1 Suppl):367S-72S Review

82   Treatment of Atopic Eczema with Evening Primrose Oil: Rationale and Clinical Results. Kerscher MJ et al; Clin Investig, 1992 Feb, 70(2):167-71 Review

83   A Chance for the Prevention of Atopic Diseases. Melnik BC; Monatsschr Kinderheilkd, 1990 Mar, 138(3):162-66 Review

84   Nutrition Supplements and the Eye. Brown NA et al; Eye, 1998, 12 (Pt 1):127-33 Review

85   Essential Fatty Acid and Prostaglandin Metabolism in Sjogren's Syndrome, Systemic Sclerosis and Rheumatoid Arthritis. Horrobin DF; Scand J Rheumatol Suppl, 1986, 61:242-45 Review

86   Importance of Dietary Gamma-Linolenic Acid in Human Health and Nutrition. Fan YY et al; J Nutr, 1998 Sep, 128(9):1411-14 Review

87   Evening Primrose Oil and Borage Oil in Rheumatologic Conditions. Belch JJ et al; Am J Clin Nutr, 2000 Jan, 71(1 Suppl):352S-56S Review

88   Diet and Asthma: Has the Role of Dietary Lipids been Overlooked in the Management of Asthma? Spector SL et al; Ann Allergy Asthma Immunol, 2003 Apr, 90(4):371-77 Review

89   Use of Gamma Linolenic Acid in the Prevention and Treatment of Diabetic Neuropathy. Jamal GA; Diabet Med, 1994 Mar, 11(2):145-49 Review

90   Essential Fatty Acids in the Management of Impaired Nerve Function in Diabetes. Horrobin DF; Diabetes, 1997 Sep, 46 Suppl 2:S90-93 Review

91   Treatment of Diabetic Neuropathy. Frati-Munari AC et al; Gac Med Mex, 1998 Jan-Feb, 134(1):85-92 Review

92   Nitric Oxide Deficiency, Leukocyte Activation, and Resultant Ischemia are Crucial to the Pathogenesis of Diabetic Retinopathy/Neuropathy–Preventive Potential of Antioxidants, Essential Fatty Acids, Chromium,

Ginkgolides, and Pentoxifylline. McCarty MF; Med Hypotheses, 1998 May, 50(5):435-49 Review

93   Effects of Antioxidants on Nerve and Vascular Dysfunction in Experimental Diabetes. Cameron NE et al; Diabetes Res Clin Pract, 1999 Sep, 45(2-3):137-46 Review

94   Protective Effects of Omega-6 Fatty Acids in Experimental Autoimmune Encephalomyelitis (EAE) in Relation to Transforming Growth Factor-Beta 1 (TGF-Beta1) Up-Regulation and Increased Prostaglandin E2 (PGE2) Production. Harbige LS et al; Clin Exp Immunol, 2000 Dec, 122(3):445-52

95   Gamma-Linolenic Acid, Arachidonic Acid, and Eicosapentaenoic Acid as Potential Anticancer Drugs. Das UN; Nutrition, 1990 Nov-Dec, 6(6):429-34 Review

96   Effects of Gamma-Linolenic Acid on Breast Pain and Diabetic Neuropathy: Possible Non-Eicosanoid Mechanisms. Horrobin DF; Prostaglandins Leukot Essent Fatty Acids, 1993 Jan, 48(1):101-04 Review

97   Hypothesis: Cis-Unsaturated Fatty Acids as Potential Anti-Peptic Ulcer Drugs. Das UN; Prostaglandins Leukot Essent Fatty Acids, 1998 May, 58(5):377-80 Review

98   Herbal Medicinals: Selected Clinical Considerations Focusing on Known or Potential Drug-Herb Interactions. Miller LG; Arch Intern Med, 1998 Nov 9, 158(20):2200-11 Review

99   Vitamin E: Beyond Antioxidant Function. Traber MG et al; Am J Clin Nutr, 1995 Dec, 62(6 Suppl):1501S-1509S Review

100   Vitamin E as a Universal Antioxidant and Stabilizer of Biological Membranes. Evstigneeva RP et al; Membr Cell Biol, 1998, 12(2):151-72 Review

101   Vitamin E: Function and Metabolism. Brigelius-Flohe R et al; FASEB J, 1999 Jul, 13(10):1145-55 Review

102   Gamma-Tocopherol: An Efficient Protector of Lipids against Nitric Oxide-Initiated Peroxidative Damage. Wolf G; Nutr Rev, 1997 Oct, 55(10):376-78 Review

103   Vitamin E and Human Health: Rationale for Determining Recommended Intake Levels. Weber P et al; Nutrition, 1997 May, 13(5):450-60 Review

104   Relationship between Vitamin E Requirement and Polyunsaturated Fatty Acid Intake in Man. Valk EE et al; Int J Vitam Nutr Res, 2000 Mar, 70(2):31-42 Review

105   Mitochondria, Oxidative Stress and Aging. Sastre J et al; Free Radic Res, 2000 Mar, 32(3):189-98 Review

106   The Role of Vitamin E in the Prevention of Heart Disease. Emmert DH, et al; Arch Fam Med, 1999 Nov-Dec, 8(6):537-42 Review

107   Regulation of Cell Signalling by Vitamin E. Rimbach G et al; Proc Nutr Soc, 2002 Nov, 61(4):415-25 Review

108   Prevention of Platelet Dysfunction by Vitamin E in Diabetic Atherosclerosis. Gerster H; Z Ernahrungswiss, 1993 Dec, 32(4):243-61 Review

109   Antioxidant Vitamins and the Prevention of Coronary Heart Disease. Adams AK et al; Am Fam Physician, 1999 Sep 1, 60(3):895-904 Review

110   Vitamins E plus C and Interacting Conutrients Required for Optimal Health. A Critical and Constructive Review of Epidemiology and Supplementation Data Regarding Cardiovascular Disease and Cancer. Gey KF; Biofactors, 1998, 7(1-2):113-74 Review

111   Vitamin E and Heart Disease: Basic Science to Clinical Intervention Trials. Pryor WA; Free Radic Biol Med, 2000 Jan 1, 28(1):141-64 Review

112   Use and Safety of Elevated Dosages of Vitamin E in Adults. Machlin LJ; Int J Vitam Nutr Res Suppl, 1989, 30:56-68 Review

113   Diabetes, Coagulation and Vascular Events. Nenci GG et al; Recenti Prog Med, 2000 Feb, 91(2):86-90 Review

114   Pathophysiology of Vascular Complications in Diabetes. Yasunari K et al; Nippon Rinsho, 1999 Jul, 57(7):1642-47 Review

115   Oxidative Stress and Glycemic Regulation. Ceriello A; Metabolism, 2000 Feb, 49(2 Suppl 1):27-29 Review

116   Can Protein Kinase C Inhibition and Vitamin E Prevent the Development of Diabetic Vascular Complications? Bursell SE et al; Diabetes Res Clin Pract, 1999 Sep, 45(2-3):169-82 Review

117   Antioxidant Modulation of Cytokines and their Biologic Function in the Aged. Meydani SN et al; Z Ernahrungswiss, 1998, 37 Suppl 1:35-42 Review

118   Role of Vitamin E in T-cell Differentiation and the Decrease of Cellular Immunity with Aging. Moriguchi S;

Biofactors, 1998, 7(1-2):77-86 Review

119   Vitamin E and Immunity. Moriguchi S et al; Vitam Horm, 2000, 59:305-36 Review

120   Nutrients and HIV: Part Two–Vitamins A and E, Zinc, B-Vitamins, and Magnesium. Patrick L; Altern Med Rev, 2000 Feb, 5(1):39-51 Review

121   The Keys of Oxidative Stress in Acquired Immune Deficiency Syndrome Apoptosis. Romero-Alvira D et al; Med Hypotheses, 1998 Aug, 51(2):169-73 Review

122   High Doses of Multiple Antioxidant Vitamins: Essential Ingredients in Improving the Efficacy of Standard Cancer Therapy. Prasad KN et al; J Am Coll Nutr, 1999 Feb, 18(1):13-25 Review

123   Diet, Androgens, Oxidative Stress and Prostate Cancer Susceptibility. Fleshner NE et al; Cancer Metastasis Rev, 1998-99, 17(4):325-30 Review

124   Chemoprevention of Urological Cancer. Kamat AM et al; J Urol, 1999 Jun, 161(6):1748-60 Review

125   Lung Cancer Chemoprevention. Khuri FR et al; Semin Surg Oncol, 2000 Mar, 18(2):100-05 Review

126   Experimental Basis for Cancer Prevention by Vitamin E. Shklar G et al; Cancer Invest, 2000, 18(3):214-22 Review

127   Tocopherols and the Etiology of Colon Cancer. Stone WL et al; J Natl Cancer Inst, 1997 Jul 16, 89(14):1006-14 Review

128   Effect of Antioxidative Vitamins on Immune Function with Clinical Applications. Grimble RF; Int J Vitam Nutr Res, 1997, 67(5):312-20 Review

129   Rheumatoid Arthritis and Metal Compounds–Perspectives on the Role of Oxygen Radical Detoxification. Aaseth J et al; Analyst, 1998 Jan, 123(1):3-6 Review

130   Vitamin E in Therapy of Rheumatic Diseases. Sangha O et al; Z Rheumatol, 1998 Aug, 57(4):207-14 Review

131   Relationship of Carotenoid and Vitamins A and E with the Acute Inflammatory Response in Acute Pancreatitis. Curran FJ et al; Br J Surg, 2000 Mar, 87(3):301-05

132   Nutritional Antioxidants as Therapeutic and Preventive Modalities in Exercise-Induced Muscle Damage. Goldfarb AH; Can J Appl Physiol, 1999 Jun, 24(3):249-66 Review

133   Free radicals, Exercise and Antioxidant Supplementation. Kanter M; Proc Nutr Soc, 1998 Feb, 57(1):9-13 Review

134   Vitamin E Supplementation and Endurance Exercise. Takanami Y et al; Sports Med, 2000 Feb, 29(2):73-83 Review

135   Vitamin E in the Treatment of Tardive Dyskinesia. Boomershine KH et al; Ann Pharmacother, 1999 Nov, 33(11):1195-202 Review

136   High Doses of Vitamin E in the Treatment of Disorders of the Central Nervous System in the Aged. Vatassery GT et al; Am J Clin Nutr, 1999 Nov, 70(5):793-801 Review

137   Antioxidant Defense of the Brain: A Role for Astrocytes. Wilson JX; Can J Physiol Pharmacol, 1997 Oct-Nov, 75(10-11):1149-63 Review

138   Biochemical and Therapeutic Effects of Antioxidants in the Treatment of Alzheimer's Disease, Parkinson's Disease, and Amyotrophic Lateral Sclerosis. Di Matteo V et al; Curr Drug Target CNS Neurol Disord, 2003 Apr, 2(2):95-107 Review

139   Vitamin E and Alzheimer Disease. Grundman M; Am J Clin Nutr, 2000 Feb, 71(2):630S-636S Review

140   Oxidative Stress and Alzheimer Disease. Christen Y; Am J Clin Nutr, 2000 Feb, 71(2):621S-629S Review

141   Vitamin E as an Antioxidant/Free Radical Scavenger against Amyloid Beta-Peptide-Induced Oxidative Stress in Neocortical Synaptosomal Membranes and Hippocampal Neurons in Culture: Insights into Alzheimer's Disease. Butterfield DA et al; Rev Neurosci, 1999, 10(2):141-49 Review

142   Neuroprotective Approaches in Experimental Models of Beta-Amyloid Neurotoxicity: Relevance to Alzheimer's Disease. Harkany T et al; Prog Neuropsychopharmacol Biol Psychiatry, 1999 Aug, 23(6):963-1008 Review

143   Vitamins in Pregnancy. Yoshioka T; Nippon Rinsho, 1999 Oct, 57(10):2381-84 Review

144   Oxidative Damage in Chemical Teratogenesis. Wells PG et al; Mutat Res, 1997 Dec 12, 396(1-2):65-78 Review

145 Antioxidative Vitamins in Prematurely and Maturely Born Infants. Bohles H; Int J Vitam Nutr Res, 1997, 67(5):321-28 Review

146 Natural Therapies for Ocular Disorders: Diseases of the Retina. Head KA; Altern Med Rev, 1999 Oct, 4(5):342-59 Review

147 Potential Preventive Effects of Vitamins for Cataract and Age-Related Macular Degeneration. Jacques PF; Int J Vitam Nutr Res, 1999 May, 69(3):198-205 Review

148 Use of Antioxidants in Healing. Martin A; Dermatol Surg, 1996 Feb;22(2):156-60 Review

149 Depletion of Reduced Glutathione, Ascorbic Acid, Vitamin E and Antioxidant Defence Enzymes in a Healing Cutaneous Wound. Shukla A et al; Free Radic Res, 1997 Feb, 26(2):93-101

150 Specific Nutritional Factors in Wound Healing. Thomas DR; Adv Wound Care, 1997 Jul-Aug, 10(4):40-43 Review

151 Use of Endogenous Antioxidants to Improve Photoprotection. Steenvoorden DP et al; J Photochem Photobiol B, 1997 Nov, 41(1-2):1-10 Review

152 Antioxidant Vitamins and Prevention of Lung Disease. Menzel DB; Ann N Y Acad Sci, 1992 Sep 30, 669:141-55 Review

153 Male Infertility: Nutritional and Environmental Considerations. Sinclair S; Altern Med Rev, 2000 Feb, 5(1):28-38 Review

154 Potential for Dietary Supplements to Reduce Premenstrual Syndrome (PMS) Symptoms. Bendich A; J Am Coll Nutr, 2000 Feb, 19(1):3-12 Review

155 Pathophysiology and Treatment of Hot Flashes. Shanafelt TD et al; Mayo Clin Proc, 2002 Nov, 77(11):1207-18 Review

156 Safety of Oral Intake of Vitamin E. Bendich A et al; Am J Clin Nutr, 1988 Sep, 48(3):612-19 Review

157 Tolerance and Safety of Vitamin E: A Toxicological Position Report. Kappus H et al; Free Radic Biol Med, 1992, 13(1):55-74 Review

158 Hypervitaminosis E, Murphy BF; JAMA, 1974 Mar 25, 227(12):1381

159 Necrotizing Myopathy with Paracrystalline Inclusion Bodies in Hypervitaminosis E. Bardosi A; Acta Neuropathol (Berl), 1987, 75(2):166-72

160 Carotenoids: Metabolism and Physiology. Faure H et al; Ann Biol Clin (Paris), 1999 Mar-Apr, 57(2):169-83 Review

161 Current Controversies in Carotene Nutrition. Sivakumar B; Indian J Med Res, 1998 Nov, 108:157-66 Review

162 Beta-Carotene and Other Carotenoids as Antioxidants. Paiva SA et al; J Am Coll Nutr, 1999 Oct, 18(5):426-33 Review

163 Beta Carotene: From Biochemistry to Clinical Trials. Pryor WA et al; Nutr Rev, 2000 Feb, 58(2 Pt 1):39-53 Review

164 Procarcinogenic and Anticarcinogenic Effects of Beta-Carotene. Wang XD et al; Nutr Rev, 1999 Sep, 57(9 Pt 1):263-72 Review

165 Beta-Carotene and Lung Cancer. Albanes D; Am J Clin Nutr, 1999 Jun, 69(6):1345S-1350S Review

166 Beta-Carotene, Carotenoids and the Prevention of Coronary Heart Disease. Kritchevsky SB; J Nutr, 1999 Jan, 129(1):5-8 Review

167 Beta-Carotene and Risk of Coronary Heart Disease. Tavani A et al; Biomed Pharmacother, 1999 Oct, 53(9):409-16 Review

168 Safety Evaluation of Synthetic Beta-Carotene. Woutersen RA et al; Crit Rev Toxicol, 1999 Nov, 29(6):515-42 Review

169 Effect of Dietary Retinyl Acetate, Beta-Carotene and Retinoic Acid on Wound Healing in Rats. Gerber LE et al; J Nutr, 1982 Aug, 112(8):1555-64

170 High Glucose-Induced Growth Factor Resistance in Human Fibroblasts can be Reversed by Antioxidants and Protein Kinase C-Inhibitors. Hehenberger K et al; Cell Biochem Funct, 1997 Sep, 15(3):197-201

171 Use of Water-Soluble Beta-Carotene in the Combined Treatment of Patients with Duodenal Peptic Ulcer and Chronic Proctosigmoiditis at Krainka General Health Resort. Neliubin VV et al; Vopr Kurortol Fizioter Lech

Fiz Kult, 1994 Jul-Aug, (4):20-22

172 Gastric Alpha-Tocopherol and Beta-Carotene Concentrations in Association with Helicobacter pylori Infection. Zhang ZW et al; Eur J Gastroenterol Hepatol, 2000 May, 12(5):497-503

173 Chemoprevention of Oral Cancer: Beta-Carotene and Vitamin E in Leukoplakia. Garewal H; Eur J Cancer Prev, 1994 Mar, 3(2):101-07 Review

174 Diet Potentiates the UV-Carcinogenic Response to Beta-Carotene. Black HS et al; Nutr Cancer, 2000, 37(2):173-78

175 Effects of Beta-Carotene Supplementation for Six Months on Clinical and Laboratory Parameters in Patients with Cystic Fibrosis. Renner S et al; Thorax, 2001 Jan, 56(1):48-52

176 Improved Antioxidant and Fatty Acid Status of Patients with Cystic Fibrosis after Antioxidant Supplementation is Linked to Improved Lung Function. Wood LG et al; Am J Clin Nutr, 2003 Jan, 77(1):150-59

177 Nutrients, Age and Cognitive Function. Riedel WJ et al; Curr Opin Clin Nutr Metab Care, 1998 Nov, 1(6):579-85 Review

178 Safety of Antioxidant Vitamins. Meyers DG et al; Arch Intern Med, 1996 May 13, 156(9):925-35 Review

179 Importance of N-3 Fatty Acids in Health and Disease. Connor WE; Am J Clin Nutr, 2000 Jan, 71(1 Suppl):171S-75S Review

180 Immunonutrition: The Role of Omega-3 Fatty Acids. Alexander JW; Nutrition, 1998 Jul-Aug, 14(7-8):627-33 Review

181 Fatty Acid Modulation of Endothelial Activation. De Caterina R et al; Am J Clin Nutr, 2000 Jan, 71(1 Suppl):213S-23S Review

182 Unsaturated Fatty Acids Omega-3: Structure, Sources, Determination, Metabolism in the Organism. Bartnikowska E et al; Rocz Panstw Zakl Hig, 1997;48(4):381-97 Review

183 Essential Fatty Acids in Health and Chronic Disease. Simopoulos AP; Am J Clin Nutr, 1999 Sep, 70(3 Suppl):560S-569S Review

184 Essential Fatty Acids and the Brain. Haag M; Can J Psychiatry, 2003 Apr, 48(3):195-203 Review

185 Health Benefits of Docosahexaenoic Acid. Horrocks LA; Pharmacol Res, 1999 Sep, 40(3):211-25 Review

186 N-3 Fatty Acids and Serum Lipoproteins: Human Studies. Harris WS; Am J Clin Nutr, 1997 May, 65(5 Suppl):1645S-1654S Review

187 Effect of N-3 Polyunsaturated Fatty Acids on Cytokine Production and their Biologic Function. Meydani SN; Nutrition, 1996 Jan, 12(1 Suppl):S8-14 Review

188 Omega-3 Fatty Acids as Cancer Chemopreventive Agents. Rose DP et al; Pharmacol Ther, 1999 Sep, 83(3):217-44 Review

189 Dietary Polyunsaturated Fatty Acids and Cancers of the Breast and Colorectum: Emerging Evidence for their Role as Risk Modifiers. Bartsch H et al; Carcinogenesis, 1999 Dec, 20(12):2209-18 Review

190 Weight Loss in Cancer and Alzheimer's Disease is Mediated by a Similar Pathway. Knittweis J; Med Hypotheses, 1999 Aug, 53(2):172-74 Review

191 Some Biological Actions of Alkylglycerols from Shark Liver Oil. Pugliese PT et al; J Altern Complement Med, 1998 Spring, 4(1):87-99 Review

192 Dietary Fatty Acids and Allergy. Kankaanpaa P et al; Ann Med, 1999 Aug, 31(4):282-87 Review

193 Prevention of Asthma. Peat JK; Eur Respir J, 1996 Jul, 9(7):1545-55 Review

194 N-3 Fatty Acid Supplements in Rheumatoid Arthritis. Kremer JM; Am J Clin Nutr, 2000 Jan, 71(1 Suppl):349S-51S Review

195 Effects of Dietary N-3 Polyunsaturated Fatty Acids on Neutrophils. Sperling RI; Proc Nutr Soc, 1998 Nov, 57(4):527-34 Review

196 Polyunsaturated Fatty Acids and Inflammatory Bowel Disease. Belluzzi A et al; Am J Clin Nutr, 2000 Jan, 71(1 Suppl):339S-42S Review

197 N-3 Fatty Acids and the Prevention of Coronary Atherosclerosis. von Schacky C; Am J Clin Nutr, 2000 Jan, 71(1 Suppl):224S-27S Review

198 Fish Consumption and Coronary Heart Disease Mortality. Marckmann P et al; Eur J Clin Nutr, 1999 Aug, 53(8):585-90 Review

199 Long-chain N-3 Polyunsaturated Fatty Acids and Triacylglycerol Metabolism in the Postprandial State. Roche HM et al; Lipids, 1999, 34 Suppl:S259-65 Review

200 Fish, Fish Oils, Arrhythmias and Sudden Death. Landmark K; Tidsskr Nor Laegeforen, 1998 Jun 10, 118(15):2328-31 Review

201 Antiarrhythmic and Anticonvulsant Effects of Dietary N-3 Fatty Acids. Leaf A et al; J Membr Biol, 1999 Nov 1, 172(1):1-11 Review

202 Health Benefits of Docosahexaenoic Acid. Horrocks LA; Pharmacol Res, 1999 Sep, 40(3):211-25 Review

203 Role of Essential Fatty Acids in the Function of the Developing Nervous System. Uauy R et al; Lipids, 1996 Mar, 31 Suppl:S167-76 Review

204 Essential Fatty Acid Deficiency in Erythrocyte Membranes from Chronic Schizophrenic Patients, and the Clinical Effects of Dietary Supplementation. Peet M et al; Prostaglandins Leukot Essent Fatty Acids, 1996 Aug, 55(1-2):71-75 Review

205 Essential Fatty Acids, Lipid Membrane Abnormalities, and the Diagnosis and Treatment of Schizophrenia. Fenton WS et al; Biol Psychiatry, 2000 Jan 1, 47(1):8-21 Review

206 Omega-3 Fatty Acids and Bipolar Disorder. Stoll AL et al; Prostaglandins Leukot Essent Fatty Acids, 1999 May-Jun, 60(5-6):329-37 Review

207 Vitamin A, Infectious Disease, and Childhood Mortality. Sommer A; J Infect Dis, 1993 May,167(5):1003-07 Review

208 Interactions of Retinoid Binding Proteins and Enzymes in Retinoid Metabolism. Napoli JL; Biochim Biophys Acta, 1999 Sep 22, 1440(2-3):139-62 Review

209 Optimal Nutrition: Vitamin A and the Carotenoids. Thurnham DI et al; Proc Nutr Soc, 1999 May, 58(2):449-57 Review

210 Vitamin A as an Immunomodulating Agent. Rumore MM; Clin Pharm, 1993 Jul, 12(7):506-14 Review

211 Measles Severity and Serum Retinol (Vitamin A) Concentration among Children in the United States. Butler JC et al; Pediatrics, 1993 Jun, 91(6):1176-81

212 Vitamin A Deficiency Disorders. McLaren DS; J Indian Med Assoc, 1999 Aug, 97(8):320-23 Review

213 Xerophthalmia and Vitamin A Status. Sommer A; Prog Retin Eye Res, 1998 Jan, 17(1):9-31 Review

214 Retinitis Pigmentosa: Defined from a Molecular Point of View. van Soest S et al; Surv Ophthalmol, 1999 Jan-Feb, 43(4):321-34 Review

215 Management of Hereditary Retinal Degenerations. Sharma RK et al; Surv Ophthalmol, 1999 Mar-Apr, 43(5):427-44 Review

216 Nutrition and Retinal Degenerations. Berson EL; Int Ophthalmol Clin, 2000 Fall, 40(4):93-111

217 Lutein Improves Visual Function in Some Patients with Retinal Degeneration. Dagnelie G et al; Optometry, 2000 Mar, 71(3):147-64

218 Vitamin A Homeostasis and Diabetes Mellitus. Basu TK et al; Nutrition, 1997 Sep, 13(9):804-06 Review

219 Vitamin A and Retinoids in Antiviral Responses. Ross AC et al; FASEB J, 1996 Jul, 10(9):979-85 Review

220 Retinoic acid–A Player that Rules the Game of Life and Death in Neutrophils. Mehta K; Indian J Exp Biol, 2002 Aug, 40(8):874-81 Review

221 Vitamin A, Immunity, and Infection. Semba RD; Clin Infect Dis, 1994 Sep, 19(3):489-99 Review

222 Vitamin A and Immunity to Viral, Bacterial and Protozoan Infections. Semba RD; Proc Nutr Soc, 1999 Aug, 58(3):719-27 Review

223 Neutrophil Maturation and the Role of Retinoic Acid. Lawson ND et al; Exp Hematol, 1999 Sep, 27(9):1355-67 Review

224 Retinoic Acids Regulate Apoptosis of T Lymphocytes Through an Interplay between RAR and RXR Receptors. Szondy Z et al; Cell Death Differ, 1998 Jan, 5(1):4-10 Review

225 Nutrition and Immunity with Emphasis on Infection and Autoimmune Disease. Harbige LS; Nutr Health,

1996, 10(4):285-312 Review

226 Retinoids and Mammalian Development. Morriss-Kay GM et al; Int Rev Cytol, 1999, 188:73-131 Review

227 Role of Vitamin A in the Formation of Congenital Heart Defects. Sinning AR; Anat Rec, 1998 Oct, 253(5):147-53 Review

228 Retinoids and their Receptors in Skeletal Development. Underhill TM et al; Microsc Res Tech, 1998 Oct 15, 43(2):137-55 Review

229 Retinoid-Regulated Gene Expression in Neural Development. Clagett-Dame M et al; Crit Rev Eukaryot Gene Expr, 1997, 7(4):299-342 Review

230 Antioxidative Vitamins in Prematurely and Maturely Born Infants. Bohles H; Int J Vitam Nutr Res, 1997, 67(5):321-28 Review

231 Role of Retinoids in Renal Development: Pathophysiological Implication. Merlet-Benichou C et al; Curr Opin Nephrol Hypertens, 1999 Jan, 8(1):39-43 Review

232 Safety of Vitamin A: Recent Results. Wiegand UW et al; Int J Vitam Nutr Res, 1998, 68(6):411-6 Review

233 Periconceptional Vitamin A Use: How Much is Teratogenic? Miller RK et al; Reprod Toxicol, 1998 Jan-Feb, 12(1):75-88 Review

234 Vitamin A and its Congeners. Monga M; Semin Perinatol, 1997 Apr, 21(2):135-42 Review

235 Current Use and Future Potential Role of Retinoids in Dermatology. Orfanos CE et al; Drugs, 1997 Mar, 53(3):358-88 Review

236 The Interaction of Ethanol and Vitamin A as a Potential Mechanism for the Pathogenesis of Fetal Alcohol Syndrome. Zachman RD et al; Alcohol Clin Exp Res, 1998 Oct, 22(7):1544-56 Review

237 Overview of the Potential Role of Vitamin A in Mother-to-Child Transmission of HIV-1. Semba RD; Acta Paediatr Suppl, 1997 Jun;421:107-12 Review

238 Breastfeeding and Vertical Transmission of HIV-1. Kreiss J; Acta Paediatr Suppl, 1997 Jun, 421:113-17 Review

239 Significance of Vitamin A and Carotenoid Status in Persons Infected by the Human Immunodeficiency Virus. Nimmagadda A et al; Clin Infect Dis, 1998 Mar, 26(3):711-18 Review

240 Maternal Vitamin A Nutriture and the Vitamin A Content of Human Milk. Haskell MJ et al; J Mammary Gland Biol Neoplasia, 1999 Jul, 4(3):243-57 Review

241 Vitamin A Supplementation for Preventing Morbidity and Mortality in Very Low Birthweight Infants. Darlow BA et al; Cochrane Database Syst Rev, 2000, 2:CD000501 Review

242 Modulation of B-cell Immunoglobulin Synthesis by Retinoic Acid. Ballow M et al; Clin Immunol Immunopathol, 1996 Sep, 80(3 Pt 2):S73-81 Review

243 Chronic Diarrhea in Infancy and Childhood. Mehta DI et al; J La State Med Soc, 1998 Sep, 150(9):419-29 Review

244 Three Independent Lines of Evidence Suggest Retinoids as Causal to Schizophrenia. Goodman AB; Proc Natl Acad Sci U S A, 1998 Jun 23, 95(13):7240-44 Review

245 Vitamin A Functions in the Regulation of the Dopaminergic System in the Brain and Pituitary Gland. Wolf G; Nutr Rev, 1998 Dec, 56(12):354-55 Review

246 Use of Retinoids in the Pediatric Patient. Ruiz-Maldonado R et al; Dermatol Clin, 1998 Jul, 16(3):553-69 Review

247 What are Natural Retinoids? Vahlquist A; Dermatology, 1999, 199 Suppl 1:3-11 Review

248 Retinoids and Psoriasis: Novel Issues in Retinoid Pharmacology and Implications for Psoriasis Treatment. Saurat JH; J Am Acad Dermatol, 1999 Sep, 41(3 Pt 2):S2-6 Review

249 Retinoids. Photodamaged Skin and the Prevention of Nonmelanotic Skin Cancer. Taranu T et al; Rev Med Chir Soc Med Nat Iasi, 1998 Jul-Dec, 102(3-4):56-59 Review

250 Retinoids: Renaissance and Reformation. Griffiths CE; Clin Exp Dermatol, 1999 Jul, 24(4):329-35 Review

251 Intervention Studies on Cancer. Young KJ et al; Eur J Cancer Prev, 1999 Apr, 8(2):91-103 Review

252 Roles of Retinoids and their Nuclear Receptors in the Development and Prevention of Upper Aerodigestive

Tract Cancers. Lotan R; Environ Health Perspect, 1997 Jun, 105 Suppl 4:985-88 Review

253 Retinoids and the Control of Growth/Death Decisions in Human Neuroblastoma Cell Lines. Melino G et al; J Neurooncol, 1997 Jan, 31(1-2):65-83 Review

254 Retinoid Chemoprevention of Second Primary Tumors. Benner SE et al; Semin Hematol 1994 Oct;31(4 Suppl 5):26-30 Review

255 Chemoprevention of Head and Neck Cancer. Armstrong WB et al; Otolaryngol Head Neck Surg, 2000 May, 122(5):728-735

256 Nutritional Pharmacotherapy of Chronic Liver Disease: From Support of Liver Failure to Prevention of Liver Cancer. Moriwaki H et al; J Gastroenterol, 2000, 35 Suppl 12:13-17

257 Retinoids in the Treatment of Acute Promyelocytic Leukemia. Graf N et al; Klin Padiatr, 1995 Mar-Apr, 207(2):43-47 Review

258 All Trans Retinoic Acid in Acute Promyelocytic Leukemia. Degos L et al; Oncogene, 2001 Oct 29, 20(49):7140-45 Review

259 Mechanism-based Therapy for Leukemia: A Lesson from ATRA Therapy. Naoe T; Nagoya J Med Sci, 2001 Nov, 64(3-4):103-08 Review

260 Retinoids: Pleiotropic Agents of Therapy for Vascular Diseases? Streb JW et al; Curr Drug Targets Cardiovasc Haematol Disord, 2003 Mar, 3(1):31-57

261 Dietary Iron Absorption. Role of Vitamin A. Garcia-Casal MN et al; Arch Latinoam Nutr, 1998 Sep, 48(3):191-96 Review

262 Importance of Adequate Vitamin A Status during Iron Supplementation. Nutr Rev, 1997 Aug, 55(8):306-07 Review

263 Vitamin D and Retinoids in Parathyroid Glands. Hellman P et al; Int J Mol Med, 1999 Apr, 3(4):355-61 Review

264 Subclinical Hypervitaminosis A Causes Fragile Bones in Rats. Johansson S et al; Bone, 2002 Dec, 31(6):685-89

265 Vitamin A Hepatotoxicity: A Cautionary Note Regarding 25,000 IU Supplements. Kowalski TE et al; Am J Med, 1994 Dec, 97(6):523-28 Review

266 Rheumatologic Complications of Vitamin A and Retinoids. Nesher G et al; Semin Arthritis Rheum, 1995 Feb, 24(4):291-96 Review

267 The Vitamin D Story: A Collaborative Effort of Basic Science and Clinical Medicine. DeLuca HF; FASEB J, 1988 Mar 1, 2(3):224-36 Review

268 New Analogs of Vitamin D3. Slatopolsky E et al; Kidney Int Suppl, 1999 Dec, 73:S46-51 Review

269 Perspective on Assessment of Vitamin D Nutrition. Rao DS; J Clin Densitom, 1999 Winter, 2(4):457-64 Review

270 Vitamin D Therapy of Osteoporosis: Plain Vitamin D Therapy versus Active Vitamin D Analog (D-hormone) Therapy. Lau KH et al; Calcif Tissue Int, 1999 Oct, 65(4):295-306 Review

271 Vitamins in Pregnancy. Yoshioka T; Nippon Rinsho, 1999 Oct, 57(10):2381-84 Review

272 Vitamin D Supplementation in Pregnancy: A Necessity. Arch Pediatr, 1995 Apr, 2(4):373-76 Review

273 Metabolic Bone Disease of Prematurity. Backstrom MC et al; Ann Med, 1996 Aug, 28(4):275-82 Review

274 Is Low Prenatal Vitamin D a Risk-Modifying Factor for Schizophrenia? McGrath J; Schizophr Res, 1999 Dec 21, 40(3):173-77 Review

275 Nutritional and Metabolic Rickets. Teotia M et al; Indian J Pediatr, 1997 Mar-Apr, 64(2):153-57 Review

276 Nutritional Rickets. Feldman KW et al; Am Fam Physician, 1990 Nov, 42(5):1311-18 Review

277 Nutritional Aspects of Calcium and Vitamin D from Infancy to Adolescence. Saggese G et al; Ann Ist Super Sanita, 1995, 31(4):461-79 Review

278 Calcium, Phosphorus and Vitamin D Administration in Infancy: Unsolved Questions. Haschke F et al; Monatsschr Kinderheilkd, 1992 Sep, 140(9 Suppl 1):S13-16 Review

279 Vitamin D and the Skin. Kira M et al; J Dermatol, 2003 Jun, 30(6):429-37 Review

280 Future of Vitamin D in Dermatology. Kragballe K; J Am Acad Dermatol, 1997 Sep, 37(3 Pt 2):S72-76 Review

281 Vitamin D Analogues. Brown AJ; Am J Kidney Dis, 1998 Oct, 32(2 Suppl 2):S25-39 Review

282 An Update on Vitamin D3 Analogues in the Treatment of Psoriasis. van de Kerkhof PC; Skin Pharmacol Appl Skin Physiol, 1998 Jan-Feb, 11(1):2-10 Review

283 Update on Synovitis. Szekanecz Z et al; Curr Rheumatol Rep, 2001 Feb, 3(1):53-63 Review

284 Osteoporosis in Rheumatoid Arthritis–Significance of Alfacalcidol in Prevention and Therapy. Schacht E; Z Rheumatol, 2000, 59 Suppl 1:10-20 Review

285 1,25-Dihydroxyvitamin D3–A Hormone with Immunomodulatory Properties. Lemire J; Z Rheumatol, 2000, 59 Suppl 1:24-27 Review

286 Vitamin D and Prostate Cancer: Biologic Interactions and Clinical Potentials. Miller GJ; Cancer Metastasis Rev, 1998-99, 17(4):353-60 Review

287 Calcium and Vitamin D. Their Potential Roles in Colon and Breast Cancer Prevention. Garland CF et al; Ann N Y Acad Sci, 1999, 889:107-19 Review

288 Vitamin D and Multiple Sclerosis. Hayes CE et al; Proc Soc Exp Biol Med, 1997 Oct, 216(1):21-27 Review

289 Pathogenesis of Secondary Hyperparathyroidism. Slatopolsky E et al; Kidney Int Suppl, 1999 Dec, 73:S14-19 Review

290 Vitamin D Analogs: Perspectives for Treatment. Brown AJ et al; Miner Electrolyte Metab, 1999 Jul-Dec, 25(4-6):337-41 Review

291 Parathyroid Hormone, Vitamin D, and Cardiovascular Disease in Chronic Renal Failure. Rostand SG et al; Kidney Int, 1999 Aug, 56(2):383-92 Review

292 Mechanism of Atherosclerotic Calcification. Shioi A et al; Z Kardiol, 2000, 89 Suppl 2:75-79 Review

293 Osteoporosis. Lane JM et al; Clin Orthop, 2000 Mar, (372):139-50 Review

294 Secondary Osteoporosis and its Treatment–Diabetes Mellitus. Kumeda Y et al; Nippon Rinsho, 1998 Jun, 56(6):1579-86 Review

295 Effective Strategies for the Prevention of Osteoporosis across the Life Span. Dombrowski HT; J Am Osteopath Assoc, 2000 Jan, 100(1 Suppl):S8-15 Review

296 Osteoporosis Management. Rozenberg S et al; Int J Fertil Womens Med, 1999 Sep-Oct, 44(5):241-49 Review

297 Therapy of Osteoporosis: Strategies for Individualized Treatment. Weber K et al; Wien Med Wochenschr, 1999, 149(16-17):489-92 Review

298 Use of Fluoride in the Treatment of Osteoporosis. Bohatyrewicz A; Chir Narzadow Ruchu Ortop Pol, 1998, 63(3):267-71 Review

299 Osteoporosis: Treatment Options Today. Meiner SE; Adv Nurse Pract, 1999 Jul, 7(7):26-31, 80 Review

300 Corticosteroid Osteoporosis. Sambrook PN; Z Rheumatol, 2000, 59 Suppl 1:45-47 Review

301 Bone Demineralization in Crohn's Disease, its Diagnosis, Therapy and Prevention. Kocian J et al; Cas Lek Cesk, 1999 Aug 30, 138(17):522-24 Review

302 Hypervitaminosis D. Morita R et al; Nippon Rinsho, 1993 Apr, 51(4):984-88 Review

303 The Vitamin D Allowance of Premature Infants and their Phosphorus-Calcium Metabolic Status with Different Types of Feeding and Rickets Prevention. Shakirova EM et al; Vopr Pitan, 1990 Mar-Apr, (2):37-41 Review

304 Williams Syndrome: An Historical Perspective of its Evolution, Natural History, and Etiology, Jones KL; Am J Med Genet Suppl, 1990, 6:89-96 Review

Chapter 6 – Trace Metals

1 http://www.suga-lik.com/molasses/composition.html

2 Nation-Wide Survey of the Chemical Composition of Drinking Water in Norway. Flaten TP; Sci Total Environ, 1991 Feb, 102:35-73

3 Survey for Cadmium, Cobalt, Chromium, Copper, Nickel, Lead, Zinc, Calcium, and Magnesium in Canadian Drinking Water Supplies. Meranger JC et al; J Assoc Off Anal Chem, 1981 Jan, 64(1):44-53

4 Lithium: Occurrence, Dietary Intakes, Nutritional Essentiality. Schrauzer GN; J Am Coll Nutr, 2002 Feb,

21(1):14-21 Review

5   Justification for Providing Dietary Guidance for the Nutritional Intake of Boron. Nielsen FH; Biol Trace Elem Res, 1998 Winter, 66(1-3):319-30 Review

6   In Vivo and In Vitro Effects of Boron and Boronated Compounds. Benderdour M et al; J Trace Elem Med Biol, 1998 Mar, 12(1):2-7 Review

7   Delay of Natural Bone Loss by Higher Intakes of Specific Minerals and Vitamins. Schaafsma A et al; Crit Rev Food Sci Nutr, 2001 May, 41(4):225-49 Review

8   Scientific American. April 2001, 284(4):85

9   Dietary Titanium and Infant Growth. Schwietert CW et al; Biol Trace Elem Res, 2001 Nov, 83(2):149-67

10   Vanadium and Diabetes. Thompson KH; Biofactors, 1999, 10(1):43-51 Review

11   Nutritional Factors that Can Favorably Influence the Glucose/Insulin System: Vanadium. Verma S et al; J Am Coll Nutr, 1998 Feb, 17(1):11-18 Review

12   Vanadium and Diabetes. Poucheret P et al; Mol Cell Biochem, 1998 Nov, 188(1-2):73-80 Review

13   Long-term Antidiabetic Activity of Vanadyl after Treatment Withdrawal: Restoration of Insulin Secretion? Cros GH et al; Mol Cell Biochem, 1995 Dec 6-20, 153(1-2):191-95 Review

14   Multifunctional Actions of Vanadium Compounds on Insulin Signaling Pathways. Fantus IG et al; Mol Cell Biochem, 1998 May, 182(1-2):109-19 Review

15   Vanadium. Barceloux DG; J Toxicol Clin Toxicol, 1999, 37(2):265-78 Review

16   Dietary Supplements and the Promotion of Muscle Growth with Resistance Exercise. Kreider RB; Sports Med, 1999 Feb, 27(2):97-110 Review

17   Nutritional Supplements to Increase Muscle Mass. Clarkson PM et al; Crit Rev Food Sci Nutr, 1999 Jul, 39(4):317-28 Review

18   Vanadium: Review of its Potential Role in the Fight against Diabetes. Badmaev V et al; J Altern Complement Med, 1999 Jun, 5(3):273-91 Review

19   Haematological Effects of Vanadium on Living Organisms. Zaporowska H et al; Comp Biochem Physiol C, 1992 Jun, 102(2):223-31 Review

20   Role of Chromium in Nutrition and Therapeutics and as a Potential Toxin. Jeejeebhoy KN; Nutr Rev,1999 Nov, 57(11):329-35 Review

21   Chromium and Parenteral Nutrition. Anderson RA; Nutrition, 1995 Jan-Feb, 11(1 Suppl):83-86 Review

22   Effects of Chromium on the Immune System. Shrivastava R et al; FEMS Immunol Med Microbiol, 2002 Sep 6, 34(1):1-7

23   Chromium Metabolism. Ducros V; Biol Trace Elem Res, 1992 Jan-Mar, 32:65-77 Review

24   Chromium in Human Nutrition. Mertz W; J Nutr, 1993 Apr, 123(4):626-33 Review

25   Therapeutic Potential of Glucose Tolerance Factor. McCarty MF; Med Hypotheses, 1980 Nov, 6(11):1177-89

26   Chromium Update. Preuss HG et al; Curr Opin Clin Nutr Metab Care, 1998 Nov, 1(6):509-12 Review

27   Chromium Content of Foods and Diets. Kumpulainen JT; Biol Trace Elem Res, 1992 Jan-Mar, 32:9-18 Review

28   Chromium in the Prevention and Control of Diabetes. Anderson RA; Diabetes Metab, 2000 Feb, 26(1):22-27 Review

29   Nutritional Factors Influencing the Glucose/Insulin System: Chromium. Anderson RA; J Am Coll Nutr, 1997 Oct, 16(5):404-10 Review

30   Safety and Efficacy of High-Dose Chromium. Lamson DS et al; Altern Med Rev, 2002 Jun, 7(3):218-35 Review

31   Effects of Chromium on Body Composition and Weight Loss. Anderson RA; Nutr Rev, 1998 Sep, 56(9):266-70 Review

32   Effects of Exercise on Chromium Levels. Clarkson PM; Sports Med, 1997 Jun, 23(6):341-49 Review

33   Anabolic Effects of Insulin on Bone Suggest a Role for Chromium Picolinate in Preservation of Bone Density. McCarty MF; Med Hypotheses, 1995 Sep, 45(3):241-46 Review

34 Effects of Glucose/Insulin Perturbations on Aging and Chronic Disorders of Aging. Preuss HG; J Am Coll Nutr, 1997 Oct, 16(5):397-403 Review

35 Chromium in the Elderly. Offenbacher EG; Biol Trace Elem Res, 1992 Jan-Mar, 32:123-31 Review

36 Chromium Content of Foods and Diets. Kumpulainen JT; Biol Trace Elem Res, 1992 Jan-Mar, 32:9-18 Review

37 Recent Advances in the Clinical and Biochemical Effects of Chromium Deficiency. Anderson RA; Prog Clin Biol Res, 1993, 380:221-34 Review

38 Manganese, Barceloux DG; J Toxicol Clin Toxicol, 1999, 37(2):293-307 Review

39 Nutritional Aspects of Manganese from Experimental Studies. Keen CL et al; Neurotoxicology, 1999 Apr-Jun, 20(2-3):213-23 Review

40 Biosynthesis and Regulation of Superoxide Dismutases. Hassan HM; Free Radic Biol Med, 1988, 5(5-6):377-85 Review

41 Superoxide Dismutase and Pulmonary Oxygen Toxicity. Tsan MF; Proc Soc Exp Biol Med, 1993 Jul, 203(3):286-90 Review

42 The Role of Manganese Superoxide Dismutase in Health and Disease. Robinson BH; J Inherit Metab Dis, 1998 Aug, 21(5):598-603 Review

43 Free Radicals, Antioxidant Enzymes, and Carcinogenesis. Sun Y; Free Radic Biol Med, 1990;8(6):583-99 Review

44 Trace Elements in Spinocerebellar Degeneration. Nakashima K; Nippon Rinsho, 1996 Jan, 54(1):129-33 Review

45 Superoxide and Iron: Partners in Crime. Liochev SI et al; IUBMB Life, 1999 Aug, 48(2):157-61 Review

46 Manganese Superoxide Dismutase Protects nNOS Neurons from NMDA and Nitric Oxide-Mediated Neurotoxicity. Gonzalez-Zulueta M et al; J Neurosci, 1998 Mar 15, 18(6):2040-55 Review

47 Existing and Emerging Mechanisms for Transport of Iron and Manganese to the Brain. Malecki EA et al; J Neurosci Res, 1999 Apr 15, 56(2):113-22 Review

48 Free Radicals: Important Cause of Pathologies Refer to Ageing. Venarucci D et al; Panminerva Med, 1999 Dec, 41(4):335-39 Review

49 Manganese Neurotoxicity in Industrial Exposures: Proof of Effects, Critical Exposure Level, and Sensitive Tests. Iregren A; Neurotoxicology, 1999 Apr-Jun, 20(2-3):315-23 Review

50 Brief History of the Neurobehavioral Toxicity of Manganese. McMillan DE; Neurotoxicology, 1999 Apr-Jun, 20(2-3):499-507 Review

51 Atherogenic and Anti-Atherogenic Factors in the Human Diet. Addis PB et al; Biochem Soc Symp, 1995, 61:259-71 Review

52 Analysis of Cellular Responses to Free Radicals: Focus on Exercise and Skeletal Muscle. Powers SK et al; Proc Nutr Soc, 1999 Nov, 58(4):1025-33 Review

53 Nutrition versus Toxicology of Manganese in Humans: Evaluation of Potential Biomarkers. Greger JL; Neurotoxicology, 1999 Apr-Jun, 20(2-3):205-12 Review

54 Dietary Standards for Manganese: Overlap between Nutritional and Toxicological Studies. Greger JL; J Nutr, 1998 Feb, 128(2 Suppl):368S-371S Review

55 Erythrocyte Free Radical and Energy Metabolism. Siems WG et al; Clin Nephrol, 2000 Feb, 53(1 Suppl):S9-17 Review

56 Physiology of Oxygen Transport. Habler OP et al; Transfus Sci, 1997 Sep, 18(3):425-35 Review

57 Role of Free Radical Reactions with Haemoglobin and Thalassaemia. Anastassopoulou J et al; J Inorg Biochem, 2000 Apr, 79(1-4):327-29 Review

58 Anaemia and Iron Deficiency Disease in Children. Olivares M et al; Br Med Bull, 1999, 55(3):534-43 Review

59 Current Data on Iron Metabolism. Loreal O et al; Ann Endocrinol (Paris), 1999 Sep, 60(3):197-203 Review

60 Iron-Regulatory Proteins, Iron-Responsive Elements and Ferritin mRNA Translation. Thomson AM et al; Int J Biochem Cell Biol, 1999 Oct, 31(10):1139-52 Review

61   Defining Optimal Body Iron. Cook JD; Proc Nutr Soc, 1999 May, 58(2):489-95 Review

62   Nutritional Assessment of Iron Status. Cook J; Arch Latinoam Nutr, 1999 Sep, 49(3 Suppl 2):11S-14S Review

63   Anemia in Pregnancy. Sifakis S et al; Ann N Y Acad Sci, 2000, 900:125-36 Review

64   Potential Impact of Iron Supplementation during Adolescence on Iron Status in Pregnancy. Lynch SR; J Nutr, 2000 Feb, 130(2S Suppl):448S-451S Review

65   Anemia and Iron Deficiency: Effects on Pregnancy Outcome. Allen LH; Am J Clin Nutr, 2000 May, 71(5 Suppl):1280S-84S Review

66   Iron Status and Iron Balance during Pregnancy. Milman N et al; Acta Obstet Gynecol Scand, 1999 Oct, 78(9):749-57 Review

67   Iron Deficiency: The Global Perspective. Cook JD et al; Adv Exp Med Biol, 1994, 356:219-28 Review

68   Effect of Iron Deficiency on Cognitive Development in Children. Grantham-McGregor S et al; J Nutr, 2001 Feb, 131(2S-2):649S-666S Review

69   Iron Deficiency and the Intellect. Gordon N; Brain Dev, 2003 Jan, 25(1):3-8 Review

70   Iron Requirements in Adolescent Females. Beard JL; J Nutr, 2000 Feb, 130(2S Suppl):440S-442S Review

71   Anemia and Coagulation Disorders in Adolescents. Hord JD; Adolesc Med, 1999 Oct, 10(3):359-67, ix Review

72   Effects of Nutrients on Mood. Benton D et al; Public Health Nutr, 1999 Sep, 2(3A):403-09 Review

73   Anaemia and Iron Deficiency in Athletes. Chatard JC et al; Sports Med, 1999 Apr, 27(4):229-40 Review

74   Iron Deficiency in Europe. Hercberg S et al; Public Health Nutr, 2001 Apr, 4(2B):537-45 Review

75   Iron-Deficiency Anaemia. Cook JD; Baillieres Clin Haematol,1994 Dec, 7(4):787-804 Review

76   Stomach and Iron Deficiency Anaemia. Annibale B et al; Dig Liver Dis, 2003 Apr, 35(4):288-95

77   'Common' Uncommon Anemias. Abramson SD et al; Am Fam Physician, 1999 Feb 15, 59(4):851-58 Review

78   New Perspectives on Iron. Boldt DH; Am J Med Sci, 1999 Oct, 318(4):207-12 Review

79   Cellular Iron Metabolism. Ponka P; Kidney Int Suppl, 1999 Mar, 69:S2-11 Review

80   Iron Absorption and Transport. Conrad ME et al, Am J Med Sci, 1999 Oct, 318(4):213-29 Review

81   Role of Iron in Neurodegeneration: Prospects for Pharmacotherapy of Parkinson's Disease. Jellinger KA; Drugs Aging, 1999 Feb, 14(2):115-40 Review

82   Alzheimer's Disease. Beta-Amyloid Protein and Zinc, Huang X et al; J Nutr, 2000 May, 130(5S Suppl):1488S-92S Review

83   Oxidative Stress and Alzheimer Disease. Christen Y; Am J Clin Nutr, 2000 Feb, 71(2):621S-629S Review

84   Friedreich Ataxia. Delatycki MB et al; J Med Genet, 2000 Jan, 37(1):1-8 Review

85   Benefits and Dangers of Iron during Infection. Brock JH; Curr Opin Clin Nutr Metab Care, 1999 Nov, 2(6):507-10 Review

86   Iron and Infection. Patruta SI et al; Kidney Int Suppl, 1999 Mar, 69:S125-30 Review

87   Importance of Adequate Vitamin A Status during Iron Supplementation. Nutr Rev, 1997 Aug, 55(8):306-07 Review

88   Iron Metabolism and HIV Infection. Savarino A et al; Cell Biochem Funct, 1999 Dec, 17(4):279-87 Review

89   Iron Therapy and Cancer. Weinberg ED; Kidney Int Suppl, 1999 Mar, 69:S131-34 Review

90   Interactions of Retinoid Binding Proteins and Enzymes in Retinoid Metabolism. Napoli JL; Biochim Biophys Acta, 1999 Sep 22, 1440(2-3):139-62 Review

91   Dietary Iron Absorption. Role of Vitamin A. Garcia-Casal MN et al; Arch Latinoam Nutr, 1998 Sep, 48(3):191-96 Review

92   Meat from the Nutritional Medicine Viewpoint. Weigand K; Z Gesamte Inn Med, 1993 Jan, 48(1):29-34 Review

93   Nutritional Adequacy of Plant-Based Diets. Sanders TA; Proc Nutr Soc, 1999 May, 58(2):265-69 Review

94   Iron Status of Vegetarians. Craig WJ; Am J Clin Nutr, 1994 May, 59(5 Suppl):1233S-1237S Review

95   Animal- and Plant-food-based Diets and Iron Status. Hambraeus L; Proc Nutr Soc, 1999 May, 58(2):235-42

Review

96 Effectiveness and Strategies of Iron Supplementation during Pregnancy. Beard JL; Am J Clin Nutr, 2000 May, 71(5 Suppl):1288S-94S Review

97 Ferrous Sulfate Toxicity: A Review of Autopsy Findings. Pestaner JP et al; Biol Trace Elem Res, 1999 Sep, 69(3):191-98 Review

98 Pediatric Iron Poisonings in the United States. Morris CC; South Med J, 2000 Apr, 93(4):352-58 Review

99 Vitamin B12. Watanabe F et al; Nippon Rinsho, 1999 Oct, 57(10):2205-10 Review

100 Vitamin B12 Metabolism and Deficiency States. Swain R; J Fam Pract, 1995 Dec, 41(6):595-600 Review

101 Staging Vitamin B-12 (Cobalamin) Status in Vegetarians. Herbert V; Am J Clin Nutr, 1994 May, 59(5 Suppl):1213S-1222S Review

102 Cobalamin. Markle HV; Crit Rev Clin Lab Sci, 1996, 33(4):247-356 Review

103 Vitamin Supplementation and Athletic Performance. Williams MH; Int J Vitam Nutr Res Suppl, 1989, 30:163-91 Review

104 Folate/Vitamin B12 Inter-Relationships. Scott J et al; Essays Biochem, 1994, 28:63-72 Review

105 Folate, Vitamin B12, and Neuropsychiatric Disorders. Bottiglieri T; Nutr Rev, 1996 Dec, 54(12):382-90 Review

106 Folate and Cobalamin in Psychiatric Illness. Hutto BR; Compr Psychiatry, 1997 Nov-Dec, 38(6):305-14 Review

107 How to Diagnose Cobalamin Deficiency. Nexo E et al; Scand J Clin Lab Invest Suppl, 1994, 219:61-76 Review

108 Neurological Disorders of Vitamin B12 Deficiency. Tomczykiewicz K et al; Neurol Neurochir Pol, 1998 Nov-Dec, 32(6):1473-84 Review

109 Biochemical Basis of the Neuropathy in Cobalamin Deficiency. Weir DG et al; Baillieres Clin Haematol, 1995 Sep, 8(3):479-97 Review

110 Subtle Vitamin-B12 Deficiency and Psychiatry: A Largely Unnoticed but Devastating Relationship? Dommisse J; Med Hypotheses, 1991 Feb, 34(2):131-40 Review

111 Type 1 Diabetes and Latent Pernicious Anaemia. Davis RE et al; Med J Aust, 1992 Feb 3, 156(3):160-62

112 Vitamin B12 Deficiency in the Elderly. Baik HW et al; Annu Rev Nutr, 1999, 19:357-77 Review

113 Diet Peculiarities. Vegetarianism, Veganism, Crudivorism, Macrobiotism. Debry G; Rev Prat, 1991 Apr 11, 41(11):967-72 Review

114 Blood Folic Acid and Vitamin B12 in Relation to Neural Tube Defects. Wald NJ et al; Br J Obstet Gynaecol, 1996 Apr, 103(4):319-24 Review

115 Vitamin B12 Insufficiency and the Risk of Fetal Neural Tube Defects. Ray JG et al; QJM, 2003 Apr, 96(4):289-95 Review

116 Cobalamin and Folate Deficiency: Acquired and Hereditary Disorders in Children. Rosenblatt DS et al; Semin Hematol, 1999 Jan, 36(1):19-34 Review

117 Vitamins and Brain Development. Ramakrishna T; Physiol Res, 1999, 48(3):175-87 Review

118 Effects of Methylcobalamin on Diabetic Neuropathy. Yaqub BA et al; Clin Neurol Neurosurg, 1992, 94(2):105-11

119 Clinical Usefulness of Intrathecal Injection of Methylcobalamin in Patients with Diabetic Neuropathy. Ide H et al; Clin Ther, 1987, 9(2):183-92

120 Multiple Sclerosis and Vitamin B12 Metabolism. Reynolds EH; J Neuroimmunol, 1992 Oct, 40(2-3):225-30 Review

121 Selected Vitamins in HIV Infection. Tang AM et al; AIDS Patient Care STDS, 1998 Apr, 12(4):263-73 Review

122 DNA Damage from Micronutrient Deficiencies is Likely to be a Major Cause of Cancer. Ames BN; Mutat Res, 2001 Apr 18, 475(1-2):7-20 Review

123 Vitamin B12 Deficiency: A New Risk Factor for Breast Cancer? Choi SW; Nutr Rev, 1999 Aug, 57(8):250-53 Review

124 Hyperhomocysteinemia: Atherothrombosis and Neurotoxicity. Fridman O; Acta Physiol Pharmacol Ther Latinoam, 1999;49(1):21-30 Review

125 Homocysteine and Atherosclerotic Disease: The Epidemiologic Evidence. Saw SM; Ann Acad Med Singapore, 1999 Jul, 28(4):565-68 Review

126 Homocysteine Metabolism and Risk of Cardiovascular Diseases: Importance of the Nutritional Status on Folic Acid, Vitamins B6 and B12. Aleman G et al; Rev Invest Clin, 2001 Mar-Apr, 53(2):141-51 Review

127 Pharmacotherapy of Hyperhomocysteinaemia in Patients with Thrombophilia. O'Donnell J et al; Expert Opin Pharmacother, 2002 Nov, 3(11):1591-98 Review

128 Vitamin B 12 Deficiency in the Aged. Pautas E et al; Presse Med, 1999 Oct 23, 28(32):1767-70 Review

129 Hyperhomocysteinemia: A New Risk Factor for Degenerative Diseases. Herrmann W et al; Clin Lab, 2002, 48(9-10):471-81 Review

130 Vitamin B12 Deficiency. Recognizing Subtle Symptoms in Older Adults. Dharmarajan TS et al; Geriatrics, 2003 Mar, 58(3):30-4, 37-38 Review

131 Danger of B12 Deficiency in the Elderly. Wynn M et al; Nutr Health, 1998, 12(4):215-26 Review

132 Vitamin B12 Deficiency in Geriatrics. Bopp-Kistler I et al; Schweiz Rundsch Med Prax, 1999 Nov 4, 88(45):1867-75 Review

133 Plasma Homocysteine as a Risk Factor for Dementia and Alzheimer's Disease. Seshadri S et al; N Engl J Med, 2002 Feb 14, 346(7):476-83

134 Vitamin B12 Transporters. Russell-Jones GJ et al; Pharm Biotechnol, 1999, 12:493-520 Review

135 Absorption, Distribution and Excretion of Vitamin B12. Nicolas JP et al; Ann Gastroenterol Hepatol (Paris), 1994 Nov-Dec, 30(6):270-76 Review

136 Selective Cobalamin Malabsorption and the Cobalamin-Intrinsic Factor Receptor. Grasbeck R; Acta Biochim Pol, 1997, 44(4):725-33 Review

137 Analogues, Ageing and Aberrant Assimilation of Vitamin B12 in Alzheimer's Disease. McCaddon A et al; Dement Geriatr Cogn Disord, 2001 Mar-Apr, 12(2):133-37

138 Vitamin B12 Deficiency in Untreated Celiac Disease. Dahele A et al; Am J Gastroenterol, 2001 Mar, 96(3):745-50

139 Folate Supplementation and the Risk of Masking Vitamin B12 Deficiency. Brantigan CO; JAMA, 1997 Mar 19, 277(11):884-85

140 How Safe are Folic Acid Supplements? Campbell NR; Arch Intern Med, 1996 Aug 12-26, 156(15):1638-44 Review

141 Pernicious Anemia Revisited. Pruthi RK et al; Mayo Clin Proc, 1994 Feb, 69(2):144-50 Review

142 Diagnosis of Vitamin B12 Deficiency. Bachli E et al; Schweiz Med Wochenschr, 1999 Jun 12, 129(23):861-72 Review

143 Sublingual Therapy for Cobalamin Deficiency as an Alternative to Oral and Parenteral Cobalamin Supplementation. Delpre G et al; Lancet 1999, Aug 28, 354(9180):740-41

144 Nickel. Barceloux DG; J Toxicol Clin Toxicol, 1999, 37(2):239-58 Review

145 Nickel–An Essential Element. Anke M et al; IARC Sci Publ, 1984, (53):339-65 Review

146 Nickel, An Essential Trace Element. Metabolic, Clinical and Therapeutic Considerations. Mancinella A; Clin Ter, 1991 Aug 15-31, 138(3-4):159-65 Review

147 Possible Roles of Nitric Oxide and Redox Cell Signaling in Metal-Induced Toxicity and Carcinogenesis. Buzard GS et al; J Environ Pathol Toxicol Oncol, 2000, 19(3):179-99 Review

148 Intracellular Copper Routing: The Role of Copper Chaperones. Harrison MD et al; Trends Biochem Sci, 2000 Jan, 25(1):29-32 Review

149 Copper Chaperones: Function, Structure and Copper-Binding Properties. Harrison MD et al; J Biol Inorg Chem, 1999 Apr, 4(2):145-53 Review

150 Role of Copper in Neurodegenerative Disease. Waggoner DJ et al; Neurobiol Dis, 1999 Aug, 6(4):221-30 Review

151 Mutation Spectrum of ATP7A, the Gene Defective in Menkes Disease. Turner Z et al; Adv Exp Med Biol, 1999, 448:83-95 Review

152 Clinical Manifestations and Treatment of Menkes Disease and its Variants. Kodama H et al; Pediatr Int, 1999 Aug, 41(4):423-29 Review

153 Molecular Mechanisms of Copper Metabolism and the Role of the Menkes Disease Protein. Harrison MD et al; J Biochem Mol Toxicol, 1999, 13(2):93-106 Review

154 Recognition, Diagnosis, and Management of Wilson's Disease. Brewer GJ; Proc Soc Exp Biol Med, 2000 Jan, 223(1):39-46 Review

155 Wilson's Disease. Update of a Systemic Disorder with Protean Manifestations. Cuthbert JA; Gastroenterol Clin North Am, 1998 Sep, 27(3):655-81 Review

156 Treatment and Management of Wilson's Disease. Shimizu N et al; Pediatr Int, 1999 Aug, 41(4):419-22 Review

157 Novel Copper Superoxide Dismutase Mimics and Damage Mediated by O2-. Athar M et al; Nutrition, 1995 Sep-Oct, 11(5 Suppl):559-63 Review

158 Mutant CuZn Superoxide Dismutase in Motor Neuron Disease. Gurney ME et al; J Inherit Metab Dis, 1998 Aug, 21(5):587-97 Review

159 Role of Copper, Zinc, Selenium and Tellurium in the Cellular Defense against Oxidative and Nitrosative Stress. Klotz LO et al; J Nutr, 2003 May, 133(5 Suppl 1):1448S-51S Review

160 Amyotrophic Lateral Sclerosis: Copper/Zinc Superoxide Dismutase (SOD1) Gene Mutations. Orrell RW; Neuromuscul Disord, 2000 Jan, 10(1):63-68 Review

161 Amyloid Precursor Protein, Copper and Alzheimer's Disease. Multhaup G; Biomed Pharmacother, 1997, 51(3):105-11 Review

162 Neuropathology of Amyotrophic Lateral Sclerosis. Chou SM; J Formos Med Assoc, 1997 Jul, 96(7):488-98 Review

163 Requirements and Toxicity of Essential Trace Elements, Illustrated by Zinc and Copper. Sandstead HH; Am J Clin Nutr, 1995 Mar, 61(3 Suppl):621S-624S Review

164 Metal Ion Metabolism. The Copper-Iron Connection, Chang A et al; Curr Biol, 1994 Jun 1, 4(6):532-33 Review

165 Copper. Barceloux DG; J Toxicol Clin Toxicol, 1999, 37(2):217-30 Review

166 Metals and Neuroscience. Bush AI; Curr Opin Chem Biol, 2000 Apr, 4(2):184-91 Review

167 Oxidative Stress and Motor Neuron Disease. Cookson MR et al; Brain Pathol, 1999 Jan, 9(1):165-86 Review

168 Molecular Pathogenesis of Prion Diseases. Kretzschmar HA; Eur Arch Psychiatry Clin Neurosci, 1999, 249 Suppl 3:56-63 Review

169 Sudden Infant Death Syndrome: Oxidative Stress. Reid GM et al; Med Hypotheses, 1999 Jun, 52(6):577-80 Review

170 Copper and Immunity. Percival SS; Am J Clin Nutr, 1998 May, 67(5 Suppl):1064S-1068S Review

171 Cysteine, Glutathione (GSH) and Zinc and Copper Ions together are Effective, Natural, Intracellular Inhibitors of (AIDS) Viruses. Sprietsma JE; Med Hypotheses, 1999 Jun, 52(6):529-38 Review

172 Rheumatoid Arthritis and Metal Compounds–Perspectives on the Role of Oxygen Radical Detoxification. Aaseth J et al; Analyst, 1998 Jan, 123(1):3-6 Review

173 Cardiovascular Effects of Dietary Copper Deficiency. Saari JT et al; Biofactors, 1999, 10(4):359-75 Review

174 Lack of a Recommended Dietary Allowance for Copper may be Hazardous to your Health. Klevay LM; J Am Coll Nutr, 1998 Aug, 17(4):322-26 Review

175 Copper Intake and Assessment of Copper Status. Milne DB; Am J Clin Nutr, 1998 May, 67(5 Suppl):1041S-1045S Review

176 Copper Absorption and Bioavailability. Wapnir RA; Am J Clin Nutr, 1998 May, 67(5 Suppl):1054S-1060S Review

177 Gastrointestinal Tract and Acute Effects of Copper in Drinking Water and Beverages. Pizarro F et al; Rev Environ Health, 1999 Oct-Dec, 14(4):231-38 Review

178   Neutropenia Caused by Copper Deficiency: Possible Mechanisms of Action. Percival SS; Nutr Rev, 1995 Mar, 53(3):59-66 Review

179   Zinc and the Gene. Dreosti IE; Mutat Res, 2001 Apr 18, 475(1-2):161-67 Review

180   Antioxidant Properties of Zinc. Powell SR; J Nutr, 2000 May, 130(5S Suppl):1447S-54S Review

181   Extracellular and Immunological Actions of Zinc. Rink L et al; Biometals, 2001 Sep-Dec, 14(3-4):367-83 Review

182   Zinc, Exercise, and Thyroid Hormone Function. Ganapathy S et al; Crit Rev Food Sci Nutr, 1999 Jul, 39(4):369-90 Review

183   Zinc Protoporphyrin: A Metabolite with a Mission. Labbe RF et al; Clin Chem, 1999 Dec, 45(12):2060-72 Review

184   Antioxidant Role of Metallothioneins. Viarengo A et al; Cell Mol Biol, 2000 Mar, 46(2):407-17 Review

185   Nuclear Trafficking of Metallothionein. Ogra Y et al; Cell Mol Biol, 2000 Mar, 46(2):357-65 Review

186   Function of Zinc Metallothionein: A Link between Cellular Zinc and Redox State. Maret W; J Nutr, 2000 May, 130(5S Suppl):1455S-58S Review

187   Antioxidant Function of Metallothionein in the Heart. Kang YJ; Proc Soc Exp Biol Med, 1999 Dec, 222(3):263-73 Review

188   Antiatherogenic Properties of Zinc: Implications in Endothelial Cell Metabolism. Hennig B et al; Nutrition, 1996 Oct, 12(10):711-17 Review

189   Zinc Status in Human Immunodeficiency Virus Infection. Baum MK et al; J Nutr, 2000 May, 130(5S Suppl):1421S-23S Review

190   Zinc: An Overview. Prasad AS; Nutrition 1995, Jan-Feb, 11(1 Suppl):93-99 Review

191   Evidence Supporting Zinc as an Important Antioxidant for Skin. Rostan EF et al; Int J Dermatol, 2002 Sep, 41(9):606-11 Review

192   Dynamic Link between the Integrity of the Immune System and Zinc Status. Fraker PJ et al; J Nutr, 2000 May, 130(5S Suppl):1399S-406S Review

193   Interactions between Zinc and Vitamin A. Christian P et al; Am J Clin Nutr, 1998 Aug, 68(2 Suppl):435S-441S Review

194   Zinc Gluconate and the Common Cold. Review of Randomized Controlled Trials. Marshall S; Can Fam Physician, 1998 May,44:1037-42 Review

195   Zinc Lozenges Reduce the Duration of Common Cold Symptoms. Nutr Rev, 1997 Mar, 55(3):82-85 Review

196   Role of Zinc in Wound Healing. Andrews M et al; Adv Wound Care, 1999 Apr, 12(3):137-38 Review

197   Matrix Metalloproteinases, Tumor Necrosis Factor and Multiple Sclerosis. Chandler S et al; J Neuroimmunol, 1997 Feb, 72(2):155-61 Review

198   Matrix Metalloproteinases: Multifunctional Effectors of Inflammation in Multiple Sclerosis and Bacterial Meningitis. Leppert D et al; Brain Res Brain Res Rev, 2001 Oct, 36(2-3):249-57 Review

199   Matrix Metalloproteinases and Neuroinflammation in Multiple Sclerosis. Rosenberg GA; Neuroscientist, 2002 Dec, 8(6):586-95 Review

200   Metabolic Responses and Nutritional Therapy in Patients with Severe Head Injuries. Wilson RF et al; J Head Trauma Rehabil, 1998 Feb, 13(1):11-27 Review

201   Zinc–A New Therapeutic Principle in Dermatology? Leyh F; Z Hautkr, 1987 Jul 15, 62(14):1064, 1069-72, 1075 Review

202   Zinc Finger Proteins: Watchdogs in Muscle Development. Krempler A et al; Mol Gen Genet, 1999 Mar, 261(2):209-15 Review

203   Importance of Zinc in the Central Nervous System: The Zinc-Containing Neuron. Frederickson CJ et al; J Nutr, 2000 May, 130(5S Suppl):1471S-83S Review

204   Regulation of Zinc Metabolism and Genomic Outcomes. Cousins RJ et al; J Nutr, 2003 May, 133(5 Suppl 1):1521S-6S Review

205   Molecular Basis for the Role of Zinc in Developmental Biology. Falchuk KH; Mol Cell Biochem, 1998 Nov,

496]   References

188(1-2):41-48 Review

206   Chimeric Restriction Enzymes. Chandrasegaran S et al; Biol Chem, 1999 Jul-Aug, 380(7-8):841-48 Review

207   Zinc Nutrition and Apoptosis of Vascular Endothelial Cells: Implications in Atherosclerosis. Hennig B et al; Nutrition, 1999 Oct, 15(10):744-48 Review

208   Cellular Zinc Fluxes and the Regulation of Apoptosis/Gene-Directed Cell Death. Truong-Tran AQ et al; J Nutr, 2000 May, 130(5S Suppl):1459S-66S Review

209   Regulation of Caspase Activation and Apoptosis by Cellular Zinc Fluxes and Zinc Deprivation. Chai F et al; Immunol Cell Biol, 1999 Jun, 77(3):272-78 Review

210   Zinc Deficiency in Liver Cirrhosis. Marchetti P et al; Ann Ital Med Int, 1998 Jul-Sep, 13(3):157-62 Review

211   Zinc and Brain Injury. Choi DW et al; Annu Rev Neurosci, 1998, 21:347-75 Review

212   Zinc Deficiency in Women, Infants and Children. Prasad AS; J Am Coll Nutr, 1996 Apr, 15(2):113-20 Review

213   Zinc Supplementation and Growth of the Fetus and Low Birth Weight Infant. Castillo-Duran C et al; J Nutr, 2003 May,133(5 Suppl 1):1494S-7S Review

214   Zinc Transfer to the Breastfed Infant. Krebs NF; J Mammary Gland Biol Neoplasia, 1999 Jul, 4(3):259-68 Review

215   Dietary Zinc and Iron Sources, Physical Growth and Cognitive Development of Breastfed Infants. Krebs NF; J Nutr, 2000 Feb, 130(2S Suppl):358S-360S Review

216   Zinc and Diarrhea in Infants. Folwaczny C; J Trace Elem Med Biol, 1997 Jun, 11(2):116-22 Review

217   Zinc and Micronutrient Supplements for Children. Allen LH; Am J Clin Nutr, 1998 Aug, 68(2 Suppl):495S-498S Review

218   Zinc, Copper and Selenium in Reproduction. Bedwal RS et al; Experientia, 1994 Jul 15, 50(7):626-40 Review

219   Diet, Micronutrients, and the Prostate Gland. Thomas JA; Nutr Rev, 1999 Apr, 57(4):95-103 Review

220   Zinc: Pathophysiological Effects, Eeficiency Status and Effects of Supplementation in Elderly Persons. Abbasi A et al; Z Gerontol Geriatr, 1999 Jul, 32 Suppl 1:I75-79 Review

221   Zinc, T-cell Pathways, Aging: Role of Metallothioneins. Mocchegiani E et al; Mech Ageing Dev, 1998 Dec 1, 106(1-2):183-204 Review

222   Nutrition Supplements and the Eye. Brown NA et al; Eye, 1998, 12 (Pt 1):127-33 Review

223   Zinc and the Elderly. Ripa S et al; Minerva Med, 1995 Jun;86(6):275-78 Review

224   Zinc Status in Athletes: Relation to Diet and Exercise. Micheletti A et al; Sports Med, 2001, 31(8):577-82 Review

225   Assessment of Marginal Zinc Status in Humans. Wood RJ; J Nutr, 2000 May,130(5S Suppl):1350S-54S Review

226   Zinc. Barceloux DG; J Toxicol Clin Toxicol, 1999, 37(2):279-92 Review

227   Antioxidant Status in Vegetarians versus Omnivores. Rauma AL et al; Nutrition, 2000 Feb, 16(2):111-19 Review

228   Consideration in Estimates of Requirements and Critical Intake of Zinc. Adaption, Availability and Interactions. Sandstrom B; Analyst, 1995 Mar, 120(3):913-15 Review

229   Dietary Factors Influencing Zinc Absorption. Lonnerdal B; J Nutr, 2000 May, 130(5S Suppl):1378S-83S Review

230   Zinc Toxicity. Fosmire GJ; Am J Clin Nutr, 1990 Feb, 51(2):225-27 Review

231   Herbal Medicinals: Selected Clinical Considerations Focusing on Known or Potential Drug-Herb Interactions. Miller LG; Arch Intern Med, 1998 Nov 9, 158(20):2200-11 Review

232   Therapeutic Effects of Organic Germanium. Goodman S; Med Hypotheses, 1988 Jul, 26(3):207-15 Review

233   Hazard Assessment of Germanium Supplements. Tao SH et al; Regul Toxicol Pharmacol, 1997 Jun, 25(3):211-19 Review

234   Complexes of Metals Other than Platinum as Antitumour Agents. Kopf-Maier P; Eur J Clin Pharmacol, 1994, 47(1):1-16 Review

235   Carcinogenesis as the Result of the Deficiency of Some Essential Trace Elements. Marczynski B; Med

Hypotheses, 1988 Aug, 26(4):239-49 Review

236 Selenium in Health and Disease. Foster LH et al; Crit Rev Food Sci Nutr, 1997 Apr, 37(3):211-28 Review

237 Developments in Selenium Metabolism and Chemical Speciation. Patching SG et al; J Trace Elem Med Biol, 1999 Dec, 13(4):193-214 Review

238 Selenium in Uremia. Bonomini M et al; Artif Organs, 1995 May, 19(5):443-48 Review

239 Essentiality of Selenium in the Human Body: Relationship with Different Diseases. Navarro-Alarcon M et al; Sci Total Environ, 2000 Apr 17, 249(1-3):347-71 Review

240 RNA and Protein Requirements for Eukaryotic Selenoprotein Synthesis. Berry MJ et al; Biomed Environ Sci, 1997 Sep, 10(2-3):182-89 Review

241 The Diverse Role of Selenium within Selenoproteins. Holben DH et al; J Am Diet Assoc, 1999 Jul, 99(7):836-43 Review

242 Thioredoxin Reductase. Mustacich D et al; Biochem J, 2000 Feb 15, 346 Pt 1:1-8 Review

243 Selenoprotein Metabolism and Function: Evidence for More than One Function for Selenoprotein P. Burk RF et al; J Nutr, 2003 May,133(5 Suppl 1):1517S-20S Review

244 Nutrition and Development: Other Micronutrients' Effect on Growth and Cognition. Wasantwisut E; Southeast Asian J Trop Med Public Health, 1997, 28 Suppl 2:78-82 Review

245 Selenium Intake, Mood and Other Aspects of Psychological Functioning. Benton D; Nutr Neurosci, 2002 Dec, 5(6):363-74 Review

246 Role of Selenium Depletion in the Etiopathogenesis of Depression in Patient with Alcoholism. Sher L; Med Hypotheses, 2002 Sep, 59(3):330-33 Review

247 Effects of Dietary Antioxidants on the Immune Function of Middle-Aged Adults. Hughes DA; Proc Nutr Soc, 1999 Feb, 58(1):79-84 Review

248 Expression of Selenoproteins in Monocytes and Macrophages–Implications for the Immune System. Ebert-Dumig R et al; Med Klin, 1999 Oct 15, 94 Suppl 3:29-34 Review

249 Selenium and Immune Function. Kiremidjian-Schumacher L et al; Z Ernahrungswiss, 1998, 37 Suppl 1:50-56 Review

250 Chemopreventive Mechanisms of Selenium. Combs GF Jr; Med Klin, 1999 Oct 15, 94 Suppl 3:18-24 Review

251 Recent Advances in Cancer Chemoprevention, with Emphasis on Breast and Colorectal Cancer. Decensi A et al; Eur J Cancer, 2000 Apr, 36(6):694-709 Review

252 What Causes Prostate Cancer? A Brief Summary of the Epidemiology. Chan JM et al; Semin Cancer Biol, 1998 Aug, 8(4):263-73 Review

253 Cancer of the Prostate: A Nutritional Disease? Fair WR et al; Urology, 1997 Dec, 50(6):840-48 Review

254 Diet and the Prevention and Treatment of Breast Cancer. Nicholson A; Altern Ther Health Med, 1996 Nov, 2(6):32-38 Review

255 Hypothesis: Iodine, Selenium and the Development of Breast Cancer. Cann SA et al; Cancer Causes Control, 2000 Feb, 11(2):121-27 Review

256 Thyroid Function. Arthur JR et al; Br Med Bull, 1999, 55(3):658-68 Review

257 Trace Element Selenium and the Thyroid Gland. Kohrle J; Biochimie, 1999 May,81(5):527-33 Review

258 Male Infertility: Nutritional and Environmental Considerations. Sinclair S; Altern Med Rev, 2000 Feb, 5(1):28-38 Review

259 Selenium and Cardiovascular Diseases. Huttunen JK; Biomed Environ Sci, 1997 Sep, 10(2-3):220-26 Review

260 Interacting Nutritional and Infectious Etiologies of Keshan Disease. Levander OA et al; Biol Trace Elem Res, 1997 Jan, 56(1):5-21 Review

261 Synergistic Effects of Vitamin E and Selenium in Iron-Overloaded Mouse Hearts. Bartfay WJ et al; Can J Cardiol, 1998 Jul, 14(7):937-41 Review

262 Function of Zinc Metallothionein: A Link between Cellular Zinc and Redox State. Maret W; J Nutr, 2000 May, 130(5S Suppl):1455S-58S Review

263 Selenium in the Treatment of Heavy Metal Poisoning and Chemical Carcinogenesis. Whanger PD; J Trace

Elem Electrolytes Health Dis, 1992 Dec, 6(4):209-21 Review

264 Selenium Requirements as Discussed in the 1996 Joint FAO/IAEA/WHO Expert Consultation on Trace Elements in Human Nutrition. Levander OA; Biomed Environ Sci, 1997 Sep, 10(2-3):214-19 Review

265 Selenium: A Quest for Better Understanding. Badmaev V et al; Altern Ther Health Med, 1996 Jul, 2(4):59-62, 65-67 Review

266 Selenium. Barceloux DG; J Toxicol Clin Toxicol, 1999, 37(2):145-72 Review

267 Nutritional Importance of Selenium. Ortuno J et al; Arch Latinoam Nutr, 1997 Mar, 47(1):6-13 Review

268 Recent Developments in Selenium Metabolism and Chemical Speciation. Patching SG et al; J Trace Elem Med Biol, 1999 Dec, 13(4):193-214 Review

269 Environmental Implications of Excessive Selenium. Lemly AD; Biomed Environ Sci, 1997 Dec, 10(4):415-35 Review

270 Free Radical Generation by Selenium Compounds and their Prooxidant Toxicity. Spallholz JE; Biomed Environ Sci, 1997 Sep, 10(2-3):260-70 Review

271 On the Nature of Selenium Toxicity and Carcinostatic Activity. Spallholz JE; Free Radic Biol Med, 1994 Jul, 17(1):45-64 Review

272 Zirconium. An Abnormal Trace Element in Biology. Ghosh S et al; Biol Trace Elem Res, 1992 Dec, 35(3):247-71 Review

273 Role of Lysosomes in the Selective Concentration of Mineral Elements. Berry JP; Cell Mol Biol, 1996 May, 42(3):395-411 Review

274 Tungsten in Biological Systems. Kletzin A et al; FEMS Microbiol Rev, 1996 Mar, 18(1):5-63 Review

275 Molybdenum-Cofactor-Containing Enzymes. Kisker C et al; Annu Rev Biochem, 1997, 66:233-67 Review

276 Distribution and Pathophysiologic Role of Molybdenum-Containing Enzymes. Moriwaki Y et al; Histol Histopathol, 1997 Apr, 12(2):513-24 Review

277 Free Radicals Generated by Xanthine Oxidase Mediate Pancreatitis-Associated Organ Failure. Folch E et al; Dig Dis Sci, 1998 Nov, 43(11):2405-10

278 Xanthine Oxidase Deficiency (Hereditary Xanthinuria), Molybdenum Cofactor Deficiency. Sumi S et al; Nippon Rinsho, 1996 Dec, 54(12):3333-36 Review

279 Hereditary Xanthinuria, Rare Cause of Hypo-Uric Acidemia. Mayaudon H et al; Presse Med, 1998 Apr 11, 27(14):661-63

280 Genetics of Molybdenum Cofactor Deficiency. Reiss J et al; Hum Genet, 2000 Feb, 106(2):157-63

281 Active Sites of Molybdenum- and Tungsten-Containing Enzymes. McMaster J et al; Curr Opin Chem Biol, 1998 Apr, 2(2):201-07 Review

282 Xanthine Oxidase-Derived Oxygen Radicals Play Significant Roles in the Development of Chronic Pancreatitis in WBN/Kob Rats. Zeki S et al; J Gastroenterol Hepatol, 2002 May, 17(5):606-616

283 Molybdenum. Barceloux DG; J Toxicol Clin Toxicol, 1999, 37(2):231-37 Review

284 Assessment of Molybdenum Toxicity in Humans. Vyskocil A et al; J Appl Toxicol, 1999 May-Jun, 19(3):185-92 Review

285 Case Report of Acute Human Molybdenum Toxicity from a Dietary Molybdenum Supplement. Momcilovic B; Arh Hig Rada Toksikol, 1999 Sep, 50(3):289-97

Chapter 7 – Herbs

1 Biotechnology Turns to Ancient Remedies in Quest for Sources of New Therapies. Mack A; The Scientist, 11[1]:1, 1997 Jan 6

2 Discrimination among Three Species of Medicinal Scutellaria Plants using RAPD Markers. Hosokawa K et al; Planta Med, 2000 Apr, 66(3):270-72

3 Extract from Scutellaria baicalensis Attenuates Oxidant Stress in Cardiomyocytes. Shao ZH et al; J Mol Cell Cardiol, 1999 Oct, 31(10):1885-95

4 Free Radical Scavenging and Antioxidant Activities of Flavonoids Extracted from the Radix of Scutellaria

baicalensis. Gao Z et al; Biochim Biophys Acta, 1999 Nov 16, 1472(3):643-50

5   Baicalin Promoted the Repair of DNA Single Strand Breakage Caused by H2O2 in Cultured NIH3T3 Fibroblasts. Chen X et al; Biol Pharm Bull, 2003 Feb, 26(2):282-84

6   Effect of an Extract of Baikal Skullcap (Scutelleria baicalensis) on Succinic acid Oxidation by the Brain Mitochondria in Rats with Hypoxia. Saifutdinov RR et al; Eksp Klin Farmakol, 1998 Sep-Oct, 61(5):27-29

7   Modulating Effects of Preparations of Baikal Skullcap (Scutellaria baicalensis) on Erythron Reactions under Conditions of Neurotic Exposures. Dygai AM et al; Eksp Klin Farmakol, 1998 Jan-Feb, 61(1):37-39

8   Search for New Anti-Ulcer Agents from Plants in Siberia and the Far East. Amosova EN et al; Eksp Klin Farmakol, 1998 Nov-Dec, 61(6):31-35

9   Flavonoid Baicalein Attenuates Activation-Induced Cell Death of Brain Microglia. Suk K et al; J Pharmacol Exp Ther, 2003 May, 305(2):638-45

10   Anti-Inflammatory Properties and Inhibition of Leukotriene C4 Biosynthesis in Vitro by Flavonoid Baicalein from Scutellaria baicalensis Roots. Butenko IG et al; Agents Actions, 1993, 39 Spec No:C49-51

11   Oldenlandia diffusa and Scutellaria barbata Augment Macrophage Oxidative Burst and Inhibit Tumor Growth. Wong BY et al; Cancer Biother Radiopharm, 1996 Feb, 11(1):51-56

12   Inhibition of HIV Infection by Baicalin–A Flavonoid Compound Purified from Chinese Herbal Medicine. Li BQ et al; Cell Mol Biol Res, 1993, 39(2):119-24

13   Screening for Antimycotic Properties of 56 Traditional Chinese Drugs. Blaszczyk T et al; Phytother Res, 2000 May, 14(3):210-12

14   Anticancer Activity of Scutellaria baicalensis and its Potential Mechanism. Ye F et al; J Altern Complement Med, 2002 Oct, 8(5):567-72

15   Baicalein and Baicalin are Potent Inhibitors of Angiogenesis: Inhibition of Endothelial Cell Proliferation, Migration and Differentiation. Liu JJ et al; Int J Cancer, 2003 Sep 10, 106(4):559-65

16   Effect of Scutellaria baicalensis Extract on the Immunologic Status of Patients with Lung Cancer Receiving Antineoplastic Chemotherapy. Smol'ianinov ES et al; Eksp Klin Farmakol, 1997 Nov-Dec, 60(6):49-51

17   Stimulating Property of Turnera diffusa and Pfaffia paniculata Extracts on the Sexual-Behavior of Male Rats. Arletti R et al; Psychopharmacology (Berl), 1999 Mar, 143(1):15-19

18   Study of the Anti-Hyperglycemic Effect of Plants used as Antidiabetics. Alarcon-Aguilara FJ et al; J Ethnopharmacol, 1998 Jun, 61(2):101-10

19   Hydration of Sickle Erythrocytes using a Herbal Extract (Pfaffia Paniculata) in Vitro. Ballas SK; Br J Haematol, 2000 Oct, 111(1):359-62

20   Therapy of Degenerative Diseases of the Musculoskeletal System with South African Devil's Claw. Wegener T; Wien Med Wochenschr,1999, 149(8-10):254-57 Review

21   Anti-inflammatory and Analgesic Effects of an Aqueous Extract of Harpagophytum procumbens. Lanhers MC et al; Planta Med, 1992 Apr, 58(2):117-23

22   Anti-Inflammatory and Analgesic Effects of Harpagophytum procumbens and Harpagophytum zeyheri. Baghdikian B et al; Planta Med, 1997 Apr, 63(2):171-76

23   Devil's Claw (Harpagophytum procumbens): No Evidence for Anti-Inflammatory Activity in the Treatment of Arthritic Disease. Whitehouse LW et al; Can Med Assoc J, 1983 Aug 1, 129(3):249-51

24   Harpagophytum procumbens: No Evidence for NSAID-like Effect on Whole Blood Eicosanoid Production in Human. Moussard C et al; Prostaglandins Leukot Essent Fatty Acids, 1992 Aug, 46(4):283-86

25   Role of Stomachal Digestion on the Pharmacological Activity of Plant Extracts, using as an Example Extracts of Harpagophytum procumbens. Soulimani R et al; Can J Physiol Pharmacol, 1994 Dec, 72(12):1532-36

26   Randomized Double-Blind Pilot Study Comparing Doloteffin and Vioxx in the Treatment of Low Back Pain. Chrubasik S et al; Rheumatology (Oxford), 2003 Jan, 42(1):141-48.

27   Harpagophytum procumbens: Cardiovascular Activity. Circosta C et al; J Ethnopharmacol, 1984 Aug, 11(3):259-74

28   Harpagophytum procumbens: Effects on Hyperkinetic Ventricular Arrhythmias by Reperfusion. Costa De Pasquale R et al; J Ethnopharmacol, 1985 May, 13(2):193-99

29   Potential Interactions between Alternative Therapies and Warfarin. Heck AM et al; Am J Health Syst Pharm, 2000 Jul 1, 57(13):1221-27

30   Increased Production of Antigen-Specific Immunoglobulins G and M following in Vivo Treatment with the Medicinal Plants Echinacea angustifolia and Hydrastis canadensis. Rehman J et al; Immunol Lett, 1999 Jun 1, 68(2-3):391-95

31   Berberine. Altern Med Rev, 2000 Apr, 5(2):175-77

32   Berberine Sulfate Inhibits Tumor-Promoting Activity of Teleocidin in Two-Stage Carcinogenesis on Mouse Skin. Nishino H et al; Oncology, 1986, 43(2):131-34

33   Antitubercular Natural Products: Berberine from the Roots of Commercial Hydrastis canadensis Powder*. Gentry EJ et al; J Nat Prod, 1998 Oct, 61(10):1187-93

34   Contribution to our Knowledge of Ginseng. Hu SY; Am J Chin Med, 1977 Spring, 5(1):1-23

35   Antioxidant Properties of a North American Ginseng Extract. Kitts DD et al; Mol Cell Biochem, 2000 Jan, 203(1-2):1-10

36   Panax quinquefolium Saponins Protects Low Density Lipoproteins from Oxidation. Li J et al; Life Sci, 1999, 64(1):53-62

37   Panax quinquefolium Inhibits Thrombin-Induced Endothelin Release in Vitro. Yuan CS et al; Am J Chin Med, 1999, 27(3-4):331-38

38   Ginsenoside Rb1 Regulates ChAT, NGF and trkA mRNA Expression in the Rat Brain. Salim KN et al; Brain Res Mol Brain Res, 1997 Jul, 47(1-2):177-82

39   Effects of Ginsenoside Rb1 on Central Cholinergic Metabolism. Benishin CG et al; Pharmacology, 1991, 42(4):223-29

40   Modulation of American Ginseng on Brainstem GABAergic Effects in Rats. Yuan CS et al; J Ethnopharmacol, 1998 Oct, 62(3):215-22

41   Gut and Brain Effects of American Ginseng Root on Brainstem Neuronal Activities in Rats. Yuan CS et al; Am J Chin Med, 1998, 26(1):47-55

42   American Ginseng (Panax quinquefolius) Reduces Postprandial Glycemia in Nondiabetic Subjects and Subjects with Type 2 Diabetes Mellitus. Vuksan V et al; Arch Intern Med, 2000 Apr 10, 160(7):1009-13

43   Quinqueginsin, a Novel Protein with Anti-Human Immunodeficiency Virus, Antifungal, Ribonuclease and Cell-Free Translation-Inhibitory Activities from American Ginseng Roots. Wang HX et al; Biochem Biophys Res Commun, 2000 Mar 5, 269(1):203-08

44   In Vitro Effects of Echinacea and Ginseng on Natural Killer and Antibody-Dependent Cell Cytotoxicity in Healthy Subjects and Chronic Fatigue Syndrome or Acquired Immunodeficiency Syndrome Patients. See DM et al; Immunopharmacology, 1997 Jan, 35(3):229-35

45   pS2 Expression Induced by American Ginseng in MCF-7 Breast Cancer Cells. Duda RB et al; Ann Surg Oncol, 1996 Nov, 3(6):515-20

46   American Ginseng and Breast Cancer Therapeutic Agents Synergistically Inhibit MCF-7 Breast Cancer Cell Growth. Duda RB et al; J Surg Oncol, 1999 Dec, 72(4):230-39

47   Ginseng, Sex Behavior, and Nitric Oxide. Murphy LL et al; Ann N Y Acad Sci, 2002 May, 962:372-77

48   Herbal Medicinals: Selected Clinical Considerations Focusing on Known or Potential Drug-Herb Interactions. Miller LG; Arch Intern Med, 1998 Nov 9, 158(20):2200-11 Review

49   Myocardial Protective Effect of an Anthraquinone-Containing Extract of Polygonum multiflorum ex Vivo. Yim TK et al; Planta Med, 1998 Oct, 64(7):607-11

50   Myocardial Protection against Ischaemia-Reperfusion Injury by a Polygonum multiflorum Extract Supplemented 'Dang-Gui Decoction for Enriching Blood'. Yim TK et al; Phytother Res, 2000 May, 14(3):195-99

51   Polygonum multiflorum Extracts Improve Cognitive Performance in Senescence Accelerated Mice. Chan YC et al; Am J Chin Med, 2003, 31(2):171-79

52   Vasorelaxants from Chinese Herbs, Emodin and Scoparone, Possess Immunosuppressive Properties. Huang HC et al; Eur J Pharmacol, 1991 Jun 6, 198(2-3):211-13

53   Moderate Inhibition of Mutagenicity and Carcinogenicity of Benzo[a]pyrene, 1,6-Dinitropyrene and 3,9-Dinitrofluoranthene by Chinese Medicinal Herbs. Horikawa K et al; Mutagenesis, 1994 Nov, 9(6):523-26

54   Morphological Observation of Effect of Bee Pollen on Intercellura Lipofuscin in NIH Mice. Liu X et al; Chung Kuo Chung Yao Tsa Chih, 1990 Sep, 15(9):561-63, 578

55   Effect of Bee Pollen Extract on Glutathione System Activity in Mice Liver Under X-ray Irradiation. Bevzo VV et al; Ukr Biokhim Zh, 1997 Jul-Aug, 69(4):115-17

56   Indices of the Antioxidant System and the Status of the Cerebral Blood Supply in Patients with an Ischemic Stroke on Apitherapy. Samoliuk VA; Lik Sprava, 1995 Jan-Feb, (1-2):68-70

57   Phytotherapy in Chronic Prostatitis. Shoskes DA; Urology, 2002 Dec, 60(6 Suppl):35-37 Review

58   Immunomodulatory Effect of Honeybee Flower Pollen Load. Dudov IA et al; Ukr Biokhim Zh, 1994 Nov-Dec, 66(6):91-93

59   Anaphylactic Reaction after Ingestion of Bee Pollen. Geyman JP; J Am Board Fam Pract, 1994 May-Jun, 7(3):250-52

60   Acute Hypersensitivity to Ingested Processed Pollen. Prichard M et al; Aust N Z J Med, 1985 Jun, 15(3):346-47

61   Hypereosinophilia, Neurologic, and Gastrointestinal Symptoms after Bee-Pollen Ingestion. Lin FL et al; J Allergy Clin Immunol, 1989 Apr, 83(4):793-96

62   Scientific Basis for the Reputed Activity of Valerian. Houghton PJ; J Pharm Pharmacol, 1999 May, 51(5):505-12

63   Biological Activity of the Sum of the Valepotriates Isolated from Valeriana alliariifolia. Dunaev VV et al; Farmakol Toksikol, 1987 Nov-Dec, 50(6):33-37

64   Critical Evaluation of the Effect of Valerian Extract on Sleep Structure and Sleep Quality. Donath F et al; Pharmacopsychiatry, 2000 Mar, 33(2):47-53

65   Effect of Valerian Extract on Sleep Polygraphy in Poor Sleepers. Schulz H et al; Pharmacopsychiatry, 1994 Jul, 27(4):147-51

66   Double Blind Study of a Valerian Preparation. Lindahl O et al; Pharmacol Biochem Behav, 1989 Apr, 32(4):1065-66

67   Influence of Valerian Treatment on "Reaction Time, Alertness and Concentration" in Volunteers. Kuhlmann J et al; Pharmacopsychiatry, 1999 Nov, 32(6):235-41

68   Efficacy and Tolerability of Valerian Extract LI 156 Compared with Oxazepam in The Treatment Of Non-Organic Insomnia. Ziegler G et al; Eur J Med Res, 2002 Nov 25, 7(11):480-86

69   Effect of Valepotriates (Valerian Extract) in Generalized Anxiety Disorder: A Randomized Placebo-Controlled Pilot Study. Andreatini R et al; Phytother Res, 2002 Nov, 16(7):650-54

70   Safety of Herbal Medicines in the Psychiatric Practice. Boniel T et al; Harefuah, 2001 Aug, 140(8):780-3, 805 Review

71   Mechanism of Action of St John's Wort in Depression. Butterweck V; CNS Drugs, 2003, 17(8):539-62 Review

72   St John's Wort for Depression. Linde K et al; Cochrane Database Syst Rev, 2000, (2):CD000448 Review

73   Hypericum Extract versus Imipramine or Placebo in Patients with Moderate Depression: Randomised Multicentre Study of Treatment for Eight Weeks. Philipp M et al; BMJ, 1999 Dec 11, 319(7224):1534-38

74   Potential Treatment for Subthreshold and Mild Depression: A Comparison of St. John's Wort Extracts and Fluoxetine. Volz HP et al; Compr Psychiatry, 2000 Mar-Apr, 41(2 Suppl 1):133-37 Review

75   Equivalence of St John's Wort Extract (Ze 117) and Fluoxetine: A Randomized, Controlled Study in Mild-Moderate Depression. Schrader E; Int Clin Psychopharmacol, 2000 Mar, 15(2):61-68

76   High Dose St. John's Wort Extract as a Phytogenic Antidepressant. Kasper S et al; Wien Med Wochenschr, 1999, 149(8-10):191-96 Review

77   St. John's Wort: A New Alternative for Depression? Josey ES et al; Int J Clin Pharmacol Ther, 1999 Mar, 37(3):111-19 Review

78   St John's Wort: Prozac from the Plant Kingdom. Di Carlo G et al; Trends Pharmacol Sci, 2001 Jun, 22(6):292-97 Review

79   Screen of Receptor and Uptake-Site Activity of Hypericin Component of St. John's Wort Reveals Sigma Receptor Binding. Raffa RB; Life Sci, 1998, 62(16):PL265-70

80   Neuropharmacology of St. John's Wort (Hypericum). Bennett DA Jr et al; Ann Pharmacother, 1998 Nov, 32(11):1201-08 Review

81   Inhibition of Synaptosomal Uptake of 3H-L-Glutamate and 3H-GABA by Hyperforin, a Major Constituent of St. John's Wort. Wonnemann M et al; Neuropsychopharmacology, 2000 Aug 1, 23(2):188-197

82   Hyperforin, A Major Antidepressant Constituent of St. John's Wort, Inhibits Serotonin Uptake by Elevating Free Intracellular Na+1. Singer A et al; J Pharmacol Exp Ther, 1999 Sep, 290(3):1363-68

83   Neuroendocrine Evidence for Dopaminergic Actions of Hypericum Extract (LI 160) in Healthy Volunteers. Franklin M et al; Biol Psychiatry, 1999 Aug 15, 46(4):581-84

84   Treatment of Seasonal Affective Disorder (SAD) with Hypericum Extract. Kasper S; Pharmacopsychiatry, 1997 Sep, 30 Suppl 2:89-93

85   St John's Wort: A Potential Therapy for Elderly Depressed Patients? Vorbach EU et al; Drugs Aging, 2000 Mar, 16(3):189-97 Review

86   Treating Depression Comorbid with Anxiety–Results of an Open, Practice-Oriented Study with St John's Wort WS 5572 and Valerian Extract in High Doses. Muller D et al; Phytomedicine, 2003, 10 Suppl 4:25-30

87   Pilot Study of Hypericum perforatum for the Treatment of Premenstrual Syndrome. Stevinson C et al; BJOG, 2000 Jul, 107(7):870-76

88   St. John's Wort Extract: Efficacy for Menopausal Symptoms of Psychological Origin. Grube B et al; Adv Ther, 1999 Jul-Aug, 16(4):177-86

89   Comparison of Hypericum Extracts with Imipramine and Fluoxetine in Animal Models of Depression and Alcoholism. De Vry J et al; Eur Neuropsychopharmacol, 1999 Dec, 9(6):461-68

90   Adverse Effects Profile of the Herbal Antidepressant St. John's Wort (Hypericum perforatum). Ernst E et al; Eur J Clin Pharmacol, 1998 Oct, 54(8):589-94 Review

91   Drug Interactions of Hypericum perforatum (St. John's Wort) are Potentially Hazardous. Baede-van Dijk PA et al; Ned Tijdschr Geneeskd, 2000 Apr 22, 144(17):811-12 Review

92   Inhibition of Platelet MAO-B by Kava Pyrone-Enriched Extract from Piper methysticum (Kava-Kava). Uebelhack R et al; Pharmacopsychiatry, 1998 Sep, 31(5):187-92

93   Piper Methysticum (Kava Kava). Altern Med Rev, 1998 Dec, 3(6):458-60

94   Treatment with Kava–The Root to Combat Stress. Muller B et al; Wien Med Wochenschr, 1999, 149(8-10):197-201 Review

95   Efficacy of Kava Extract for Treating Anxiety. Pittler MH et al; J Clin Psychopharmacol, 2000 Feb, 20(1):84-89

96   Dietary Supplements Used in the Treatment of Depression, Anxiety, and Sleep Disorders. Cauffield JS et al; Lippincotts Prim Care Pract, 1999 May-Jun, 3(3):290-304 Review

97   Kava-Kava Extract in Anxiety Disorders. Scherer J; Adv Ther, 1998 Jul-Aug, 15(4):261-69

98   Kava-Kava Extract LI 150 is as Effective as Opipramol and Buspirone in Generalized Anxiety Disorder. Boerner RJ et al; Phytomedicine, 2003, 10 Suppl 4:38-49

99   Kava Extract for Treating Anxiety. Pittler MH et al; Cochrane Database Syst Rev, 2003, (1):CD003383.

100   Kava-Kava Extract WS 1490 versus Placebo in Anxiety Disorders. Volz HP et al; Pharmacopsychiatry, 1997 Jan, 30(1):1-5

101   Action Profile of D,L-Kavain. Cerebral Sites and Sleep-Wakefulness-Rhythm in Animals. Holm E et al; Arzneimittelforschung, 1991 Jul, 41(7):673-83

102   Psychosomatic Dysfunctions in the Female Climacteric. Clinical Effectiveness and Tolerance of Kava Extract WS 1490. Warnecke G; Fortschr Med, 1991 Feb 10, 109(4):119-22

103   Kava Extracts: Safety and Risks Including Rare Hepatotoxicity. Teschke R et al; Phytomedicine, 2003,10(5):440-46

104   Hepatitis Induced by Kava (Piper methysticum rhizoma). Stickel F et al; J Hepatol, 2003 Jul, 39(1):62-67

105   Kava, Kavapyrones and Toxic Liver Injury. Teschke R; Z Gastroenterol, 2003 May, 41(5):395-404

106 Yohimbine in the Treatment of Erectile Disorder. Riley AJ; Br J Clin Pract, 1994 May-Jun, 48(3):133-36 Review

107 Yohimbine for Erectile Dysfunction. Ernst E et al; J Urol, 1998 Feb, 159(2):433-36 Review

108 Effects of Depression and Antidepressants on Sexual Functioning. Gitlin MJ; Bull Menninger Clin, 1995 Spring, 59(2):232-48 Review

109 Manipulation of Norepinephrine Metabolism with Yohimbine in the Treatment of Autonomic Failure. Biaggioni I et al; J Clin Pharmacol, 1994 May, 34(5):418-23 Review

110 Neuropharmacological and Genetic Study of Panic Disorder. Akiyoshi J; Nihon Shinkei Seishin Yakurigaku Zasshi, 1999 Jul, 19(3):93-99 Review

111 Herb-Drug Interactions. Fugh-Berman A; Lancet, 2000 Jan 8, 355(9198):134-38 Review

112 Kudzu Root: An Ancient Chinese Source of Modern Antidipsotropic Agents. Keung WM et al; Phytochemistry, 1998 Feb, 47(4):499-506 Review

113 Effects of Isoflavones on Alcohol Pharmacokinetics and Alcohol-Drinking Behavior in Rats. Lin RC et al; Am J Clin Nutr, 1998 Dec, 68(6 Suppl):1512S-1515S Review

114 Biochemical Studies of a New Class of Alcohol Dehydrogenase Inhibitors from Radix Puerariae. Keung WM; Alcohol Clin Exp Res, 1993 Dec, 17(6):1254-60

115 Pilot Study Exploring the Effect of Kudzu Root on the Drinking Habits of Patients with Chronic Alcoholism. Shebek J et al; J Altern Complement Med, 2000 Feb, 6(1):45-48

116 Chemical, Pharmacological and Clinical Profile of the East Asian Medical Plant Centella asiatica. Brinkhaus B et al; Phytomedicine, 2000 Oct, 7(5):427-48 Review

117 Total Triterpenic Fraction of Centella asiatica in Chronic Venous Insufficiency and in High-Perfusion Microangiopathy. Incandela L et al; Angiology, 2001 Oct, 52 Suppl 2:S9-13 Review

118 Total Triterpenic Fraction of Centella asiatica in the Treatment of Venous Hypertension. Incandela L et al; Angiology, 2001 Oct, 52 Suppl 2:S61-67

119 Treatment of Edema and Increased Capillary Filtration in Venous Hypertension with Total Triterpenic Fraction of Centella asiatica. De Sanctis MT et al; Angiology, 2001 Oct, 52 Suppl 2:S55-59

120 Hemorrhoids and Varicose Veins. MacKay D; Altern Med Rev, 2001 Apr, 6(2):126-40 Review

121 Evaluation of Treatment of Diabetic Microangiopathy with Total Triterpenic Fraction of Centella asiatica. Cesarone MR et al; Angiology, 2001 Oct, 52 Suppl 2:S49-54

122 Effect of Centella asiatica on Cognition and Oxidative Stress in an Intracerebroventricular Streptozotocin Model of Alzheimer's Disease in Rats. Veerendra Kumar MH et al; Clin Exp Pharmacol Physiol, 2003 May-Jun, 30(5-6):336-42

123 Antioxidant Activity of Centella asiatica on Lymphoma-bearing Mice. Jayashree G et al; Fitoterapia, 2003 Jul, 74(5):431-34

124 Influence of Aloe Vera on Collagen Characteristics in Healing Dermal Wounds in Rats. Chithra P et al; Mol Cell Biochem, 1998 Apr, 181(1-2):71-76

125 Influence of Aloe Vera on Collagen Turnover in Healing of Dermal Wounds in Rats. Chithra P et al; Indian J Exp Biol, 1998 Sep, 36(9):896-901

126 Aloe Vera Leaf Gel. Reynolds T et al; J Ethnopharmacol, 1999 Dec 15, 68(1-3):3-37 Review

127 Antiinflammatory Activity of Extracts from Aloe Vera Gel. Vazquez B et al; J Ethnopharmacol, 1996 Dec, 55(1):69-75

128 Anti-inflammatory Constituents, Aloesin and Aloemannan in Aloe Species and Effects of Tanshinon VI in Salvia Miltiorrhiza on Heart. Yagi A et al; Yakugaku Zasshi, 2003 Jul, 123(7):517-32

129 Influence of Aloe Vera on the Healing of Dermal Wounds in Diabetic Rats. Chithra P et al; J Ethnopharmacol, 1998 Jan, 59(3):195-201

130 Antidiabetic Activity of Aloes. Ghannam N et al; Horm Res, 1986, 24(4):288-94

131 Aloe Vera. Klein AD et al; J Am Acad Dermatol, 1988 Apr, 18(4 Pt 1):714-20 Review

132 Comparative Evaluation of Aloe Vera in the Management of Burn Wounds in Guinea Pigs. Rodriguez-Bigas M et al; Plast Reconstr Surg, 1988 Mar, 81(3):386-89

133   Therapeutic Effects of Aloe Vera on Cutaneous Microcirculation and Wound Healing in Second Degree Burn Model in Rats. Somboonwong J et al; J Med Assoc Thai, 2000 Apr, 83(4):417-25

134   Effect of Aloe Vera Gel to Healing of Burn Wound a Clinical and Histologic Study. Visuthikosol V et al; J Med Assoc Thai, 1995 Aug, 78(8):403-09

135   Management of Psoriasis with Aloe Vera Extract in a Hydrophilic Cream. Syed TA et al; Trop Med Int Health, 1996 Aug, 1(4):505-09

136   Evaluation of Aloe vera Gel Gloves in the Treatment of Dry Skin Associated with Occupational Exposure. West DP et al; Am J Infect Control, 2003 Feb,31(1):40-42

137   Aloe Barbadensis Extracts Reduce the Production of Interleukin-10 after Exposure to Ultraviolet Radiation. Byeon SW et al; J Invest Dermatol, 1998 May, 110(5):811-17

138   Prevention of Ultraviolet Radiation-Induced Suppression of Contact Hypersensitivity by Aloe Vera Gel Components. Lee CK et al; Int J Immunopharmacol, 1999 May, 21(5):303-10

139   Aloe Vera: Magic or Medicine? Atherton P; Nurs Stand, 1998 Jul 1-7, 12(41):49-52, 54 Review

140   Wound Healing. Oral and Topical Activity of Aloe Vera. Davis RH et al; J Am Podiatr Med Assoc, 1989 Nov, 79(11):559-62

141   Upregulation of Phagocytosis and Candidicidal Activity of Macrophages Exposed to the Immunostimulant Acemannan. Stuart RW et al; Int J Immunopharmacol, 1997 Feb, 19(2):75-82

142   Anti-Leukaemic and Anti-Mutagenic Effects of Di(2-ethylhexyl)phthalate Isolated from Aloe Vera. Lee KH et al; J Pharm Pharmacol, 2000 May, 52(5):593-98

143   Vitamin C and Aloe Vera Supplementation Protects from Chemical Hepatocarcinogenesis in the Rat. Shamaan NA et al; Nutrition, 1998 Nov-Dec, 14(11-12):846-52

144   Isozymes of Superoxide Dismutase from Aloe Vera. Sabeh F et al; Enzyme Protein, 1996, 49(4):212-21

145   Anthocyanosides in the Treatment of Retinopathies. Scharrer A et al; Klin Monatsbl Augenheilkd, 1981 May, 178(5):386-89

146   Diabetic Eye Disease. Frank KJ et al; South Med J, 1996 May, 89(5):463-70 Review

147   Effect of Anthocyanins on Human Connective Tissue Metabolism in the Human. Boniface R et al; Klin Monatsbl Augenheilkd, 1996 Dec, 209(6):368-72

148   Effect of Vaccinium myrtillus Anthocyanosides on Ischaemia Reperfusion Injury in Hamster Cheek Pouch Microcirculation. Bertuglia S et al; Pharmacol Res, 1995 Mar-Apr, 31(3-4):183-87

149   Effects of Vaccinium myrtillus Anthocyanosides on Arterial Vasomotion. Colantuoni A et al; Arzneimittelforschung, 1991 Sep, 41(9):905-09

150   Studies on Vaccinium myrtillus Anthocyanosides:Vasoprotective and Antiinflammatory Activity. Lietti A et al; Arzneimittelforschung, 1976, 26(5):829-32

151   Experiences in the Medical Treatment of Progressive Myopia. Politzer M; Klin Monatsbl Augenheilkd, 1977 Oct, 171(4):616-19

152   Effect of Bilberry Nutritional Supplementation on Night Visual Acuity and Contrast Sensitivity. Muth ER et al; Altern Med Rev, 2000 Apr, 5(2):164-73

153   Effect of Anthocyanosides in a Multiple Oral Dose on Night Vision. Zadok D et al; Eye, 1999 Dec, 13 (Pt 6):734-36

154   Potential Mechanisms of Cancer Chemoprevention by Anthocyanins. Hou DX; Curr Mol Med, 2003 Mar, 3(2):149-59 Review

155   Antioxidant Action of Vaccinium myrtillus Extract on Human Low Density Lipoproteins in Vitro. Laplaud PM et al; Fundam Clin Pharmacol, 1997, 11(1):35-40

156   Induction of Apoptosis in Cancer Cells by Bilberry (Vaccinium myrtillus) and the Anthocyanins. Katsube N et al; J Agric Food Chem, 2003 Jan 1, 51(1):68-75

157   Antiulcer Activity of an Anthocyanidin from Vaccinium myrtillus. Magistretti MJ et al; Arzneimittelforschung, 1988 May, 38(5):686-90

158   Evaluation of the Gastric Antiulcerogenic Effects of Solanum nigrum, Brassica oleracea and Ocimum basilicum in Rats. Akhtar MS et al; J Ethnopharmacol, 1989 Nov, 27(1-2):163-76

159   Sulphydryl-Containing Agents: A New Approach to the Problem of Refractory Peptic Ulceration. Salim AS; Pharmacology, 1992, 45(6):301-06

160   Mechanisms for Cytoprotection by Vitamin U from Ethanol-Induced Gastric Mucosal Damage in Rats. Watanabe T et al; Dig Dis Sci, 1996 Jan, 41(1):49-54

161   Sulphydryl-Containing Agents Stimulate the Healing of Duodenal Ulceration in Man. Salim AS; Pharmacology, 1992, 45(3):170-80

162   Sulfhydryl-Containing Agents in the Treatment of Gastric Bleeding Induced by Nonsteroidal Anti-Inflammatory Drugs. Salim AS; Can J Surg, 1993 Feb, 36(1):53-58

163   Role of Sulphydryl-Containing Agents in the Management of Recurrent Attacks of Ulcerative Colitis. Salim AS; Pharmacology, 1992, 45(6):307-18

164   Effects of S-Methylmethionine (Vitamin U) on Experimental Nephrotic Hyperlipidemia. Seri K et al; Arzneimittelforschung, 1979, 29(10):1517-20

165   Urinary Metabolites of Flavonoids and Hydroxycinnamic Acids in Humans after Application of a Crude Extract from Equisetum arvense. Graefe EU et al; Phytomedicine, 1999 Oct, 6(4):239-46

166   Vasorelaxant Activity of Caffeic Acid Derivatives from Cichorium Intybus and Equisetum Arvense. Sakurai N et al; Yakugaku Zasshi, 2003 Jul,123(7):593-98

167   Urolithiasis and Phytotherapy. Grases F et al; Int Urol Nephrol, 1994, 26(5):507-11

168   Seborrhoeic Dermatitis Induced by Nicotine of Horsetails (Equisetum arvense). Sudan BJ; Contact Dermatitis, 1985 Sep, 13(3):201-02

169   Occurrence of Dermatitis in Rats Fed a Cholesterol Diet Containing Field Horsetail (Equisetum arvense). Maeda H et al; J Nutr Sci Vitaminol (Tokyo), 1997 Oct, 43(5):553-63

170   Polymeric Chondroitin Sulfate vs. Monomeric Glucosamine for the Treatment of Osteoarthritis. Menzel EJ; Wien Med Wochenschr, 2000, 150(5):87-90 Review

171   On the Role of Intracellular Physicochemistry in Quantitative Gene Expression during Aging and the Effect of Centrophenoxine. Zs -Nagy I; Arch Gerontol Geriatr, 1989 Nov-Dec, 9(3):215-29 Review

172   Electron Spin Resonance Spectroscopic Demonstration of the Hydroxyl Free Radical Scavenger Properties of Dimethylaminoethanol in Spin Trapping Experiments Confirming the Molecular Basis for the Biological Effects of Centrophenoxine. Nagy I et al; Arch Gerontol Geriatr, 1984 Dec, 3(4):297-310

173   Ethanolamine Analogues Stimulate DNA Synthesis by a Mechanism not Involving Phosphatidylethanolamine Synthesis. Kiss Z et al; FEBS Lett, 1996 Feb 26, 381(1-2):67-70

174   Phosphorylation of Ethanolamine, Methylethanolamine, and Dimethylethanolamine by Overexpressed Ethanolamine Kinase in NIH 3T3 Cells Decreases the Co-Mitogenic Effects of Ethanolamines and Promotes Cell Survival. Malewicz B et al; Eur J Biochem, 1998 Apr 1, 253(1):10-19

175   Cytokine Immunotrapping: An Assay to Study the Kinetics of Production and Consumption or Degradation of Human Interferon-Gamma. Akdis AC et al; J Immunol Methods, 1995 Jun 9, 182(2):251-61

176   Enhancement of Interferon Induction in Mice by Polycationic Modified Polypeptides. Mecs I et al; Acta Virol, 1976 Apr, 20(2):164-66

177   Source Density Analysis of Functional Topographical EEG: Monitoring of Cognitive Drug Action. Dimpfel W et al; Eur J Med Res, 1996 Mar 19, 1(6):283-90

178   Deanol and Methylphenidate in Minimal Brain Dysfunction. Lewis JA et al; Clin Pharmacol Ther, 1975 May, 17(5):534-40

179   Meige's Disease and a Positive Treatment Response with Deanol. Coats ME; Mil Med,1985 Mar, 150(3):152-53

180   Orofacial and Respiratory Tardive Dyskinesia: Potential Side Effects of 2-Dimethylaminoethanol (Deanol)? Haug BA et al; Eur Neurol, 1991, 31(6):423-25

181   Hemiballismus-Hemichorea Treated with Dimethylaminoethanol, Jameson HD et al; Dis Nerv Syst, 1977 Nov, 38(11):931-32

182   Deanol in the Treatment of Tardive Dyskinesia. Casey DE et al; Am J Psychiatry, 1975 Aug, 132(8):864-67

183   Global in Vivo Replacement of Choline by N-Aminodeanol. Testing a Hypothesis about Progressive

Degenerative Dementia: Dynamics of Choline Replacement. Knusel B et al; Pharmacol Biochem Behav, 1990 Dec, 37(4):799-809

184 Effect of Dimethylamino-2-Ethoxyimino-2-Adamantane (CM 54903), a Non-Polar Dimethylaminoethanol Analog, on Brain Regional Cholinergic Neurochemical Parameters. Vezzani A et al; Biochem Pharmacol, 1982 May 1, 31(9):1693-98

185 Mood Alterations during Deanol Therapy. Casey DE; Psychopharmacology (Berl), 1979 Apr 11, 62(2):187-91

186 Alpha-Lipoic Acid in Liver Metabolism and Disease. Bustamante J et al; Free Radic Biol Med, 1998 Apr, 24(6):1023-39 Review

187 Molecular Aspects of Lipoic Acid in the Prevention of Diabetes Complications. Packer L et al; Nutrition, 2001 Oct, 17(10):888-95

188 Thiol Homeostasis and Supplements in Physical Exercise. Sen CK et al; Am J Clin Nutr, 2000 Aug, 72(2 Suppl):653S-69S Review

189 Thiol-based Antioxidants. Deneke SM; Curr Top Cell Regul, 2000, 36:151-80 Review

190 Antioxidant and Prooxidant Activities of Alpha-Lipoic Acid and Dihydrolipoic Acid. Moini H et al; Toxicol Appl Pharmacol, 2002 Jul 1, 182(1):84-90 Review

191 Alpha-Lipoic Acid as a Biological Antioxidant. Packer L et al; Free Radic Biol Med, 1995 Aug, 19(2):227-50 Review

192 Alpha-Lipoic Acid in the Treatment of Diabetic Polyneuropathy in Germany. Ziegler D et al; Exp Clin Endocrinol Diabetes, 1999, 107(7):421-30 Review

193 Effects of Antioxidants on Nerve and Vascular Dysfunction in Experimental Diabetes. Cameron NE et al; Diabetes Res Clin Pract, 1999 Sep, 45(2-3):137-46 Review

194 Alpha-Lipoic Acid as a New Treatment Option for Azheimer Type Dementia. Hager K et al; Arch Gerontol Geriatr, 2001 Jun, 32(3):275-282

195 Advanced Glycation Endproducts Cause Lipid Peroxidation in the Human Neuronal Cell Line SH-SY5Y. Gasic-Milenkovic J et al; J Alzheimers Dis, 2003 Feb, 5(1):25-30

196 Lipoic Acid Improves Survival in Transgenic Mouse Models of Huntington's Disease. Andreassen OA et al; Neuroreport, 2001 Oct 29, 12(15):3371-73

197 Alpha-Lipoic Acid Inhibits TNF-Alpha-Induced NF-Kappab Activation and Adhesion Molecule Expression in Human Aortic Endothelial Cells. Zhang WJ et al; FASEB J, 2001 Nov, 15(13):2423-32

198 Oxidative Stress in the Aging Rat Heart is Reversed by Dietary Supplementation with (R)-(Alpha)-Lipoic Acid. Suh JH et al; FASEB J, 2001 Mar, 15(3):700-06

199 Improved Cardiac Performance after Ischemia in Aged Rats Supplemented with Vitamin E and Alpha-Lipoic Acid. Coombes JS et al; Am J Physiol Regul Integr Comp Physiol, 2000 Dec, 279(6):R2149-55

200 (R)-Alpha-Lipoic Acid Reverses the Age-Associated Increase in Susceptibility of Hepatocytes to Tert-Butylhydroperoxide Both In Vitro and In Vivo. Hagen TM et al; Antioxid Redox Signal, 2000 Fall, 2(3):473-83

201 Oxidative Stress, Exercise, and Antioxidant Supplementation. Urso ML et al; Toxicology, 2003 Jul 15, 189(1-2):41-54 Review

202 Vitamin C as an Antioxidant: Evaluation of its Role in Disease Prevention. Padayatty SJ et al; J Am Coll Nutr, 2003 Feb, 22(1):18-35 Review

203 Ascorbate Regulation and its Neuroprotective Role in the Brain. Rice ME; Trends Neurosci, 2000 May, 23(5):209-16 Review

204 Mitochondria, Oxidative Stress and Aging. Sastre J et al; Free Radic Res, 2000 Mar, 32(3):189-98 Review

205 A Vitamin as Neuromodulator: Ascorbate Release into the Extracellular Fluid of the Brain Regulates Dopaminergic and Glutamatergic Transmission. Rebec GV et al; Prog Neurobiol, 1994 Aug, 43(6):537-65 Review

206 Ascorbate Availability and Neurodegeneration in Amyotrophic Lateral Sclerosis. Kok AB; Med Hypotheses, 1997 Apr, 48(4):281-96 Review

207 Biosynthesis and Regulation of Superoxide Dismutases. Hassan HM; Free Radic Biol Med, 1988, 5(5-6):377-85 Review

208 Ascorbic Acid: Metabolism and Functions of a Multi-Facetted Molecule. Smirnoff N; Curr Opin Plant Biol, 2000 Jun, 3(3):229-35 Review

209 Neuroprotective Approaches in Experimental Models of Beta-Amyloid Neurotoxicity: Relevance to Alzheimer's Disease. Harkany T et al; Prog Neuropsychopharmacol Biol Psychiatry, 1999 Aug, 23(6):963-1008 Review

210 On the Role of Vitamin C and Other Antioxidants in Atherogenesis and Vascular Dysfunction. Frei B; Proc Soc Exp Biol Med, 1999 Dec, 222(3):196-204 Review

211 Role of Natural Antioxidants in Preserving the Biological Activity of Endothelium-Derived Nitric Oxide. Carr A et al; Free Radic Biol Med, 2000 Jun 15, 28(12):1806-14 Review

212 How does Ascorbic Acid Prevent Endothelial Dysfunction? May JM; Free Radic Biol Med, 2000 May 1, 28(9):1421-9 Review

213 Induction of Antioxidant Stress Proteins in Vascular Endothelial and Smooth Muscle Cells: Protective Action of Vitamin C against Atherogenic Lipoproteins. Siow RC et al; Free Radic Res,1999 Oct, 31(4):309-18 Review

214 Hyperglycemia-Induced Latent Scurvy and Atherosclerosis: The Scorbutic-Metaplasia Hypothesis. Price KD et al; Med Hypotheses, 1996 Feb, 46(2):119-29 Review

215 Key Role of Histamine in the Development of Atherosclerosis and Coronary Heart Disease. Clemetson CA; Med Hypotheses, 1999 Jan, 52(1):1-8 Review

216 Vitamin C and Cardiovascular Disease. Ness AR et al; J Cardiovasc Risk, 1996 Dec, 3(6):513-21 Review

217 Vitamin C and Blood Pressure. Ness AR et al; J Hum Hypertens, 1997 Jun, 11(6):343-50 Review

218 Antioxidant Vitamins and the Prevention of Coronary Heart Disease. Adams AK et al; Am Fam Physician, 1999 Sep 1, 60(3):895-904 Review

219 Vitamins E plus C and Interacting Conutrients Required for Optimal Health. A Critical and Constructive Review of Epidemiology and Supplementation Data Regarding Cardiovascular Disease and Cancer. Gey KF; Biofactors, 1998, 7(1-2):113-74 Review

220 Glucose/Insulin System and Vitamin C: Implications in Insulin-Dependent Diabetes Mellitus. Cunningham JJ; J Am Coll Nutr, 1998 Apr, 17(2):105-08 Review

221 Oxidative Stress and Glycemic Regulation. Ceriello A; Metabolism, 2000 Feb, 49(2 Suppl 1):27-29 Review

222 Nonenzymatic Glycosylation of Tissue and Blood Proteins. Emekli N; J Marmara Univ Dent Fac, 1996 Sep, 2(2-3):530-34 Review

223 Micronutrients as Nutriceutical Interventions in Diabetes Mellitus. Cunningham JJ; J Am Coll Nutr, 1998 Feb, 17(1):7-10 Review

224 Potential Preventive Effects of Vitamins for Cataract and Age-Related Macular Degeneration. Jacques PF; Int J Vitam Nutr Res, 1999 May, 69(3):198-205 Review

225 Possible Role for Vitamin C in Age-Related Cataract. van der Pols JC; Proc Nutr Soc, 1999 May, 58(2):295-301 Review

226 Use of Antioxidants in Healing. Martin A; Dermatol Surg, 1996 Feb;22(2):156-60 Review

227 Depletion of Reduced Glutathione, Ascorbic Acid, Vitamin E and Antioxidant Defence Enzymes in a Healing Cutaneous Wound. Shukla A et al; Free Radic Res, 1997 Feb, 26(2):93-101

228 Specific Nutritional Factors in Wound Healing. Thomas DR; Adv Wound Care, 1997 Jul-Aug, 10(4):40-43 Review

229 Role of Vitamins in the Prevention of Osteoporosis. Weber P; Int J Vitam Nutr Res, 1999 May, 69(3):194-97 Review

230 Glucose Transport and Metabolism in Chondrocytes: A Key to Understanding Chondrogenesis, Skeletal Development and Cartilage Degradation in Osteoarthritis. Mobasheri A et al; Histol Histopathol, 2002 Oct, 17(4):1239-67 Review

231 Adult Scurvy. Hirschmann JV et al; J Am Acad Dermatol, 1999 Dec, 41(6):895-906 Review

232   Scurvy: More than Historical Relevance. Oeffinger KC; Am Fam Physician, 1993 Sep 15, 48(4):609-13 Review

233   Vitamin C: Prospective Functional Markers for Defining Optimal Nutritional Status. Benzie IF; Proc Nutr Soc, 1999 May, 58(2):469-76 Review

234   Retroviruses, Ascorbate, and Mutations, in the Evolution of Homo Sapiens. Challem JJ et al; Free Radic Biol Med, 1998 Jul 1, 25(1):130-32 Review

235   Vitamin C and Human Health–A Review of Recent Data Relevant to Human Requirements. Weber P et al; Int J Vitam Nutr Res,1996, 66(1):19-30 Review

236   Biomarkers for Establishing a Tolerable Upper Intake Level for Vitamin C. Johnston CS; Nutr Rev, 1999 Mar, 57(3):71-77 Review

237   Vitamin C Function and Status in Chronic Disease. Jacob RA et al; Nutr Clin Care, 2002 Mar-Apr, 5(2):66-74 Review

238   Antioxidant Vitamins and Prevention of Lung Disease. Menzel DB; Ann N Y Acad Sci, 1992 Sep 30, 669:141-55 Review

239   Assessment of the Roles of Vitamin C, Vitamin E, and Beta-Carotene in the Modulation of Oxidant Stress Mediated by Cigarette Smoke-Activated Phagocytes.

240   Vitamin C Prevents the Acute Atherogenic Effects of Passive Smoking. Valkonen MM et al; Free Radic Biol Med, 2000 Feb 1, 28(3):428-36

241   Role of Vitamins in the Prevention and Control of Anaemia. Fishman SM et al; Public Health Nutr, 2000 Jun, 3(2):125-50 Review

242   Does Vitamin C Act as a Pro-Oxidant under Physiological Conditions? Carr A et al; FASEB J, 1999 Jun, 13(9):1007-24 Review

243   High-Dose Vitamin C: A Risk for Persons with High Iron Stores? Gerster H; Int J Vitam Nutr Res, 1999 Mar, 69(2):67-82 Review

244   Antioxidant Activity and Biologic Properties of a Procyanidin-Rich Extract from Pine (Pinus maritima) Bark, Pycnogenol. Packer L et al; Free Radic Biol Med, 1999 Sep, 27(5-6):704-24 Review

245   Bioflavonoid Effects on the Mitochondrial Respiratory Electron Transport Chain and Cytochrome C Redox State. Moini H et al; Redox Rep, 1999, 4(1-2):35-41

246   Pycnogenol in the Management of Asthma. Hosseini S et al; J Med Food, 2001 Winter, 4(4):201-209

247   Pycnogenol Inhibits the Release of Histamine from Mast Cells. Sharma SC et al; Phytother Res, 2003 Jan, 17(1):66-69

248   Evidence by in Vivo and in Vitro Studies that Binding of Pycnogenols to Elastin Affects its Rate of Degradation by Elastases. Tixier JM et al; Biochem Pharmacol, 1984 Dec 15, 33(24):3933-39

249   Inhibition of Lipogenesis by Pycnogenol. Hasegawa N; Phytother Res, 2000 Sep, 14(6):472-473

250   Antioxidants and Herbal Extracts Protect HT-4 Neuronal Cells against Glutamate-Induced Cytotoxicity. Kobayashi MS et al; Free Radic Res, 2000 Feb, 32(2):115-24

251   Effect of Procyanidins from Pinus maritima on Glutathione Levels in Endothelial Cells Challenged by 3-Morpholinosydnonimine or Activated Macrophages. Rimbach G et al; Redox Rep, 1999, 4(4):171-77

252   Pycnogenol Protects Vascular Endothelial Cells from Beta-Amyloid-Induced Injury. Liu F et al; Biol Pharm Bull, 2000 Jun, 23(6):735-37

253   Endothelium-Dependent Vascular Effects of Pycnogenol. Fitzpatrick DF et al; J Cardiovasc Pharmacol, 1998 Oct, 32(4):509-15

254   Pycnogenol for Diabetic Retinopathy. Schonlau F et al; Int Ophthalmol, 2001, 24(3):161-71 Review

255   Selective Induction of Apoptosis in Human Mammary Cancer Cells (MCF-7) by Pycnogenol. Huynh HT et al; Anticancer Res, 2000 Jul-Aug, 20(4):2417-20

256   Effects of Pycnogenol on the Microsomal Metabolism of the Tobacco-Specific Nitrosamine NNK as a Function of Age. Huynh HT et al; Cancer Lett, 1998 Oct 23, 132(1-2):135-39

257   Inhibition of Smoking-Induced Platelet Aggregation by Aspirin and Pycnogenol. Putter M et al; Thromb Res, 1999 Aug 15, 95(4):155-61

258 Free Radicals and Grape Seed Proanthocyanidin Extract: Importance in Human Health and Disease Prevention. Bagchi D et al; Toxicology, 2000 Aug 7, 148(2-3):187-197 Review

259 Oxygen Free Radical Scavenging Abilities of Vitamins C and E, and a Grape Seed Proanthocyanidin Extract in Vitro. Bagchi D et al; Res Commun Mol Pathol Pharmacol, 1997 Feb, 95(2):179-89

260 Dermal Wound Healing Properties of Redox-Active Grape Seed Proanthocyanidins. Khanna S et al; Free Radic Biol Med, 2002 Oct 15, 33(8):1089-96

261 Molecular Mechanisms of Cardioprotection by a Novel Grape Seed Proanthocyanidin Extract. Bagchi D et al; Mutat Res, 2003 Feb-Mar, 523-524:87-97

262 Novel Proanthocyanidin IH636 Grape Seed Extract Increases in Vivo Bcl-XL Expression and Prevents Acetaminophen-Induced Programmed and Unprogrammed Cell Death in Mouse Liver. Ray SD et al; Arch Biochem Biophys, 1999 Sep 1, 369(1):42-58

263 Cellular Protection with Proanthocyanidins Derived from Grape Seeds. Bagchi D et al; Ann N Y Acad Sci, 2002 May;957:260-70

264 Protective Effects of Grape Seed Proanthocyanidins and Selected Antioxidants against TPA-Induced Hepatic and Brain Lipid Peroxidation and DNA Fragmentation, and Peritoneal Macrophage Activation in Mice. Bagchi D et al; Gen Pharmacol, 1998 May, 30(5):771-76

265 Effectiveness of High-Dose Riboflavin in Migraine Prophylaxis. Schoenen J et al; Neurology, 1998 Feb, 50(2):466-70

266 Feverfew for Preventing Migraine. Pittler MH et al; Cochrane Database Syst Rev 2000;(3):CD002286 Review

267 Feverfew as a Preventive Treatment for Migraine. Vogler BK et al; Cephalalgia, 1998 Dec, 18(10):704-08 Review

268 Prunella vulgaris L.–A Rediscovered Medicinal Plant. Markova H et al; Ceska Slov Farm, 1997 Apr, 46(2):58-63

269 Anti-Allergic and Anti-Inflammatory Triterpenes from the Herb of Prunella vulgaris. Ryu SY et al; Planta Med, 2000 May, 66(4):358-60

270 Antimutagenic Activity of Extracts from Anticancer Drugs in Chinese Medicine. Lee H et al; Mutat Res, 1988 Feb, 204(2):229-34

271 Inhibitory Effects of Rosmarinic Acid on Lck SH2 Domain Binding to a Synthetic Phosphopeptide. Ahn SC et al; Planta Med, 2003 Jul, 69(7):642-646

272 Antioxidative and Free Radical Scavenging Activities of Selected Medicinal Herbs. Liu F et al; Life Sci, 2000 Jan 14, 66(8):725-35

273 Experimental Study of 472 Herbs with Antiviral Action against the Herpes Simplex Virus. Zheng M; Chung Hsi I Chieh Ho Tsa Chih, 1990 Jan, 10(1):39-41, 46

274 Isolation and Characterization of an Anti-HSV Polysaccharide from Prunella vulgaris. Xu HX et al; Antiviral Res, 1999 Nov, 44(1):43-54

275 Anti-HBsAg Herbs Employing ELISA Technique. Zheng MS et al; Chung Hsi I Chieh Ho Tsa Chih, 1990 Sep, 10(9):560-62, 518

276 Extract of Prunella vulgaris Spikes Inhibits HIV Replication at Reverse Transcription in Vitro and Can Be Absorbed from Intestine in Vivo. Kageyama S et al; Antivir Chem Chemother, 2000 Mar, 11(2):157-64

277 Mechanism of Inhibition of HIV-1 Infection in Vitro by Purified Extract of Prunella vulgaris. Yao XJ et al; Virology, 1992 Mar, 187(1):56-62

278 Isolation, Purification, and Partial Characterization of Prunellin, an Anti-HIV Component from Aqueous Extracts of Prunella vulgaris. Tabba HD et al; Antiviral Res, 1989 Jun-Jul, 11(5-6):263-73

279 Screening Test of Crude Drug Extract on Anti-HIV Activity. Yamasaki K et al; Yakugaku Zasshi, 1993 Nov, 113(11):818-24

280 Evaluation of Anti-Inflammatory Activity of Some Swedish Medicinal Plants. Tunon H et al; J Ethnopharmacol, 1995 Oct, 48(2):61-76

281 Characterization of Ursolic Acid as a Lipoxygenase and Cyclooxygenase Inhibitor using Macrophages, Platelets and Differentiated HL60 Leukemic Cells. Najid A et al; FEBS Lett, 1992 Mar 16, 299(3):213-17

282 Calluna vulgaris Extract 5-Lipoxygenase Inhibitor Shows Potent Antiproliferative Effects on Human Leukemia HL-60 Cells. Najid A et al; Eicosanoids, 1992, 5(1):45-51

283 Clinical Observation on the Treatment of Ischemic Heart Disease with Astragalus membranaceus. Li SQ et al; Chung Kuo Chung Hsi I Chieh Ho Tsa Chih, 1995 Feb, 15(2):77-80

284 Action of Astragalus membranaceus on Left Ventricular Function of Angina Pectoris. Lei ZY et al; Chung Kuo Chung Hsi I Chieh Ho Tsa Chih, 1994 Apr, 14(4):199-202, 195

285 Nuclear Cardiology Study on Effective Ingredients of Astragalus membranaceus in Treating Heart Failure. Luo HM et al; Chung Kuo Chung Hsi I Chieh Ho Tsa Chih, 1995 Dec, 15(12):707-09

286 Effects of Astragalus membranaceus on Left Ventricular Function and Oxygen Free Radical in Acute Myocardial Infarction Patients and Mechanism of its Cardiotonic Action. Chen LX et al; Chung Kuo Chung Hsi I Chieh Ho Tsa Chih, 1995 Mar, 15(3):141-43

287 Astragalus membranaceus Stimulates Human Sperm Motility in Vitro. Hong CY et al; Am J Chin Med, 1992, 20(3-4):289-94

288 Memory-Improving Effect of Aqueous Extract of Astragalus membranaceus. Hong GX et al; Chung Kuo Chung Yao Tsa Chih, 1994 Nov, 19(11):687-88, 704

289 Botanical Influences on Cardiovascular Disease. Miller AL; Altern Med Rev, 1998 Dec, 3(6):422-31 Review

290 Randomised Double Blind Placebo Controlled Clinical Trial of a Standardised Extract Of Fresh Crataegus Berries (Crataegisan) in the Treatment of Patients with Congestive Heart Failure NYHA II. Degenring FH et al; Phytomedicine, 2003, 10(5):363-69

291 Effect of Angelica Polysaccharide on Proliferation and Differentiation of Hematopoietic Progenitor Cell. Wang Y et al; Chung Hua I Hsueh Tsa Chih, 1996 May, 76(5):363-66

292 Effects of Different Processed Products of Radix Angelica sinensis on Clearing Out Oxygen Free Radicals and Anti-Lipid Peroxidation. Wu H et al; Chung Kuo Chung Yao Tsa Chih, 1996 Oct, 21(10):599-601, 639

293 Protective Effects of Angelica sinensis Injection on Myocardial Ischemia/Reperfusion Injury in Rabbits. Chen SG et al; Chung Kuo Chung Hsi I Chieh Ho Tsa Chih, 1995 Aug, 15(8):486-88

294 Protective Effect of Angelica Injection on Arrhythmia during Myocardial Ischemia Reperfusion in Rat. Zhuang XX; Chung Hsi I Chieh Ho Tsa Chih, 1991 Jun, 11(6):360-61, 326

295 Protective Effect of Polysaccharides-Enriched Fraction from Angelica Sinensis on Hepatic Injury. Ye YN et al; Life Sci, 2001 Jun 29, 69(6):637-46

296 Study of the Gastrointestinal Protective Effects of Polysaccharides from Angelica sinensis in Rats. Cho CH et al; Planta Med, 2000 May, 66(4):348-51

297 Immunopharmacological Studies of Low Molecular Weight Polysaccharide from Angelica sinensis. Choy YM et al; Am J Chin Med, 1994, 22(2):137-45

298 Using Ligustrazini and Angelica sinensis Treat the Bleomycin-Induced Pulmonary Fibrosis in Rats. Dai L et al; Chung Hua Chieh Ho Ho Hu Hsi Tsa Chih, 1996 Feb, 19(1):26-28

299 Effect of Astragalus Angelica Mixture on Serum Lipids and Glomerulosclerosis in Rats with Nephrotic Syndrome. Lu Y et al; Chung Kuo Chung Hsi I Chieh Ho Tsa Chih, 1997 Aug, 17(8):478-80

300 Gastroduodenal Toxicity of Nonsteroidal Anti-Inflammatory Drugs. Hawkins C et al; J Pain Symptom Manage, 2000 Aug 1, 20(2):140-151

301 Digestive Complications of Aspirin. Hochain P et al; Rev Med Interne, 2000 Mar, 21 Suppl 1:50s-59s Review

302 Treatment of Edematous Disorders with Diuretics. Rasool A et al; Am J Med Sci, 2000 Jan, 319(1):25-37 Review

303 Garlic and Onions: Their Effect on Eicosanoid Metabolism and its Clinical Relevance. Ali M et al; Prostaglandins Leukot Essent Fatty Acids, 2000 Feb, 62(2):55-73 Review

304 Therapeutic Values of Onion (Allium cepa) and Garlic (Allium sativum). Augusti KT; Indian J Exp Biol, 1996 Jul, 34(7):634-40 Review

305 Therapeutic Actions of Garlic Constituents. Agarwal KC; Med Res Rev, 1996 Jan, 16(1):111-24 Review

306 Pleiotropic Effects of Garlic. Siegel G et al; Wien Med Wochenschr, 1999, 149(8-10):217-24 Review

307 Optimization of Allium sativum Solvent Extraction for the Inhibition of In Vitro Growth of Helicobacter

Pylori. Canizares P et al; Biotechnol Prog, 2002 Nov-Dec,18(6):1227-32

308 Protection against Helicobacter pylori and Other Bacterial Infections by Garlic. Sivam GP; J Nutr, 2001 Mar,131(3s):1106S-8S Review

309 Investigation on the Antibacterial Properties of Garlic (Allium Sativum) on Pneumonia Causing Bacteria. Dikasso D et al; Ethiop Med J, 2002 Jul, 40(3):241-49

310 Pharmaceutical Significance of Allium sativum: Antifungal Effects. Sovova M et al; Ceska Slov Farm, 2003 Mar, 52(2):82-87

311 Cancer Preventive Value of Natural, Non-Nutritive Food Constituents. Frohlich RH et al; Acta Med Austriaca, 1997, 24(3):108-13 Review

312 Potential Application of Allium sativum (Garlic) for the Treatment of Bladder Cancer. Lamm DL et al; Urol Clin North Am, 2000 Feb, 27(1):157-62 Review

313 Antiproliferative Effects of Allium Derivatives from Garlic. Pinto JT et al; J Nutr, 2001 Mar, 131(3s):1058S-60S Review

314 Effects of Garlic Components Diallyl Sulfide and Diallyl Disulfide on Arylamine N-Acetyltransferase Activity and 2-Aminofluorene-DNA Adducts in Human Promyelocytic Leukemia Cells. Lin JG et al; Am J Chin Med, 2002, 30(2-3):315-25

315 Garlic-Related Dermatoses. Jappe U et al; Am J Contact Dermat, 1999 Mar, 10(1):37-39 Review

316 Pharmacological Activity of Guarana (Paullinia cupana Mart.) in Laboratory Animals. Espinola EB et al; J Ethnopharmacol, 1997 Feb, 55(3):223-29

317 Effect of Guarana on Exercise in Normal and Epinephrine-Induced Glycogenolytic Mice. Miura T et al; Biol Pharm Bull, 1998 Jun, 21(6):646-48

318 Guarana (Paullinia cupana): Toxic Behavioral Effects in Laboratory Animals and Antioxidants Activity in Vitro. Mattei R et al; J Ethnopharmacol, 1998 Mar, 60(2):111-16

319 Novel Property of an Aqueous Guarana Extract (Paullinia cupana): Inhibition of Platelet Aggregation in Vitro and in Vivo. Bydlowski SP et al; Braz J Med Biol Res, 1988, 21(3):535-38

320 Nettle Sting for Treatment of Base-of-Thumb Pain. Randall C et al; J R Soc Med, 2000 Jun, 93(6):305-09

321 Nettle Sting of Urtica dioica for Joint Pain. Randall C et al; Complement Ther Med, 1999 Sep, 7(3):126-31

322 Antirheumatic Effect of IDS 23, a Stinging Nettle Leaf Extract, on in Vitro Expression of T helper Cytokines. Klingelhoefer S et al; J Rheumatol, 1999 Dec, 26(12):2517-22

323 Plant Extracts from Stinging Nettle (Urtica dioica), an Antirheumatic Remedy, Inhibit the Proinflammatory Transcription Factor NF-kappaB. Riehemann K et al; FEBS Lett, 1999 Jan 8, 442(1):89-94

324 Contact Urticaria due to the Common Stinging Nettle (Urtica dioica)–Histological, Ultrastructural and Pharmacological Studies. Oliver F et al; Clin Exp Dermatol, 1991 Jan, 16(1):1-7

325 Urtica dioica Agglutinin, a New Mitogen for Murine T lymphocytes: Unaltered Interleukin-1 Production but Late Interleukin 2-Mediated Proliferation. Le Moal MA et al; Cell Immunol, 1988 Aug, 115(1):24-35

326 Urtica dioica Agglutinin. A Superantigenic Lectin from Stinging Nettle Rhizome. Galelli A et al; J Immunol, 1993 Aug 15, 151(4):1821-31

327 Urtica dioica Agglutinin, a V beta 8.3-Specific Superantigen, Prevents the Development of the Systemic Lupus Erythematosus-like Pathology of MRL lpr/lpr Mice. Musette P et al; Eur J Immunol, 1996 Aug, 26(8):1707-11

328 Effect of Extracts of the Roots of the Stinging Nettle (Urtica dioica) on the Interaction of SHBG with its Receptor on Human Prostatic Membranes. Hryb DJ et al; Planta Med, 1995 Feb, 61(1):31-32

329 Lignans from the Roots of Urtica dioica and their Metabolites Bind to Human Sex Hormone Binding Globulin (SHBG). Schottner M et al; Planta Med, 1997 Dec, 63(6):529-32

330 Effects of Stinging Nettle Root Extracts and their Steroidal Components on the Na+,K(+)-ATPase of the Benign Prostatic Hyperplasia. Hirano T et al; Planta Med, 1994 Feb, 60(1):30-33

331 Capsaicin: Identification, Nomenclature, and Pharmacotherapy. Cordell GA et al; Ann Pharmacother, 1993 Mar, 27(3):330-36 Review

332 Neuroanatomical Effects of Capsaicin on the Primary Afferent Neurons. Hiura A; Arch Histol Cytol, 2000 Jul,

63(3):199-215 Review

333   Intravesical Neuromodulatory Drugs: Capsaicin and Resiniferatoxin to Treat the Overactive Bladder. Kim DY et al; J Endourol, 2000 Feb, 14(1):97-103 Review

334   Plant Kingdom as a Source of Anti-Ulcer Remedies. Borrelli F et al; Phytother Res, 2000 Dec, 14(8):581-91 Review

335   Anti-tumor Promoting Potential of Selected Spice Ingredients with Antioxidative and Anti-Inflammatory Activities. Surh YJ; Food Chem Toxicol, 2002 Aug, 40(8):1091-97 Review

336   Chemoprotective Properties of Some Pungent Ingredients Present in Red Pepper and Ginger. Surh YJ et al; Mutat Res, 1998 Jun 18, 402(1-2):259-67 Review

337   Capsaicin Inhibits Growth of Adult T-Cell Leukemia Cells. Zhang J et al; Leuk Res, 2003 Mar, 27(3):275-83

338   Antioxidant Activity of Selected Indian Spices. Shobana S et al; Prostaglandins Leukot Essent Fatty Acids, 2000 Feb, 62(2):107-10

339   Scavenging Effects of Ginger on Superoxide Anion and Hydroxyl Radical. Cao ZF et al; Chung Kuo Chung Yao Tsa Chih, 1993 Dec, 18(12):750-51, 764

340   Ginger Extract Consumption Reduces Plasma Cholesterol, Inhibits LDL Oxidation and Attenuates Development of Atherosclerosis in Atherosclerotic, Apolipoprotein E-Deficient Mice. Fuhrman B et al; J Nutr, 2000 May, 130(5):1124-31

341   Protective Action of Ethanolic Ginger (Zingiber officinale) Extract in Cholesterol Fed Rabbits. Bhandari U et al; J Ethnopharmacol, 1998 Jun, 61(2):167-71

342   Inhibitory Effects of [6]-Gingerol, a Major Pungent Principle of Ginger, on Phorbol Ester-Induced Inflammation, Epidermal Ornithine Decarboxylase Activity and Skin Tumor Promotion in ICR Mice. Park KK et al; Cancer Lett, 1998 Jul 17, 129(2):139-44

343   Suppressive Effects of Eugenol and Ginger Oil on Arthritic Rats. Sharma JN et al; Pharmacology, 1994 Nov, 49(5):314-18

344   Ginger (Zingiber officinale) in Rheumatism and Musculoskeletal Disorders. Srivastava KC et al; Med Hypotheses, 1992 Dec, 39(4):342-48

345   Antibacterial Effect of Zingiber officinale and Garcinia kola on Respiratory Tract Pathogens. Akoachere JF et al; East Afr Med J, 2002 Nov, 79(11):588-92

346   Inhibition of Human Pathogenic Fungi by Ethnobotanically Selected Plant Extracts. Ficker CE et al; Mycoses, 2003 Feb, 46(1-2):29-37

347   Chemoprotective Properties of Some Pungent Ingredients Present in Red Pepper and Ginger. Surh YJ et al; Mutat Res, 1998 Jun 18, 402(1-2):259-67 Review

348   Inhibition of Tumor Promotion in SENCAR Mouse Skin by Ethanol Extract of Zingiber officinale Rhizome. Katiyar SK et al; Cancer Res, 1996 Mar 1, 56(5):1023-30

349   Induction of Apoptosis in HL-60 cells by Pungent Vanilloids, [6]-Gingerol and [6]-Paradol. Lee E et al; Cancer Lett, 1998 Dec 25, 134(2):163-68

350   Gastroprotective Activity of Ginger Zingiber officinale in Albino Rats. al-Yahya MA et al; Am J Chin Med, 1989, 17(1-2):51-56

351   Anti-Ulcer Effect in Rats of Ginger Constituents. Yamahara J et al; J Ethnopharmacol, 1988 Jul-Aug, 23(2-3):299-304

352   Effects of Ginger on Gastroduodenal Motility. Micklefield GH et al; Int J Clin Pharmacol Ther, 1999 Jul, 37(7):341-46

353   Zingiber officinale Does Not Affect Gastric Emptying Rate. Phillips S et al; Anaesthesia, 1993 May, 48(5):393-95

354   Influence of Dietary Spices and their Active Principles on Pancreatic Digestive Enzymes in Albino Rats. Platel K et al; Nahrung, 2000 Feb, 44(1):42-46

355   Ginger: History and Use. Langner E et al; Adv Ther, 1998 Jan-Feb, 15(1):25-44 Review

356   Anti-Motion Sickness Mechanism of Ginger. Holtmann S et al; Acta Otolaryngol, 1989 Sep-Oct, 108(3-4):168-74

357 Effects of Ginger on Motion Sickness and Gastric Slow-Wave Dysrhythmias Induced by Circular Vection. Lien HC et al; Am J Physiol Gastrointest Liver Physiol, 2003 Mar, 284(3):G481-89

358 Effects of Ginger on Motion Sickness Susceptibility and Gastric Function. Stewart JJ et al; Pharmacology, 1991, 42(2):111-20

359 Ginger Root against Seasickness. A Controlled Trial on the Open Sea. Grontved A et al; Acta Otolaryngol, 1988 Jan-Feb, 105(1-2):45-49

360 Vertigo-Reducing Effect of Ginger Root. Grontved A et al; ORL J Otorhinolaryngol Relat Spec, 1986, 48(5):282-86

361 Interventions for Nausea and Vomiting in Early Pregnancy. Jewell D et al; Cochrane Database Syst Rev, 2000;(2):CD000145 Review

362 Zingiber officinale (Ginger)–An Antiemetic for Day Case Surgery. Phillips S et al; Anaesthesia, 1993 Aug, 48(8):715-17

363 Ginger Root–A New Antiemetic. The Effect of Ginger Root on Postoperative Nausea and Vomiting after Major Gynaecological Surgery. Bone ME et al; Anaesthesia, 1990 Aug, 45(8):669-71

364 Efficacy of Ginger in Prevention of Post-Operative Nausea and Vomiting after Outpatient Gynecological Laparoscopy. Pongrojpaw D et al; J Med Assoc Thai, 2003 Mar, 86(3):244-50

365 Double-Blind Randomized Controlled Trial of Ginger for the Prevention of Postoperative Nausea and Vomiting. Arfeen Z et al; Anaesth Intensive Care, 1995 Aug, 23(4):449-52

366 Ginger does not Prevent Postoperative Nausea and Vomiting after Laparoscopic Surgery. Eberhart LH et al; Anesth Analg, 2003 Apr, 96(4):995-98

367 Steroidal Saponins from Smilax officinalis. Bernardo RR et al; Phytochemistry, 1996 Sep, 43(2):465-69

368 Role of Phytotherapy in Treating Lower Urinary Tract Symptoms and Benign Prostatic Hyperplasia. Dreikorn K; World J Urol, 2002 Apr,19(6):426-35 Review

369 Association of Benign Prostatic Hyperplasia with Male Pattern Baldness. Oh BR et al; Urology, 1998 May, 51(5):744-48

370 Prostates, Pates, and Pimples. The Potential Medical Uses of Steroid 5 Alpha-Reductase Inhibitors. Tenover JS; Endocrinol Metab Clin North Am, 1991 Dec, 20(4):893-909 Review

371 Saw Palmetto Extracts for Treatment of Benign Prostatic Hyperplasia. Wilt TJ et al; JAMA, 1998 Nov 11, 280(18):1604-09 Review

372 Serenoa repens for Benign Prostatic Hyperplasia. Wilt T et al; Cochrane Database Syst Rev, 2002, (3):CD001423. Review

373 Serenoa repens (Permixon). A Review of its Pharmacology and Therapeutic Efficacy in Benign Prostatic Hyperplasia. Plosker GL et al; Drugs Aging, 1996 Nov, 9(5):379-95 Review

374 Saw Palmetto for the Treatment of Men with Lower Urinary Tract Symptoms. Gerber GS; J Urol, 2000 May, 163(5):1408-12 Review

375 Benign Prostatic Hyperplasia Treated with Saw Palmetto. McPartland JM et al; J Am Osteopath Assoc, 2000 Feb, 100(2):89-96

376 Effects of Long-Term Treatment with Serenoa repens (Permixon) on the Concentrations and Regional Distribution of Androgens and Epidermal Growth Factor in Benign Prostatic Hyperplasia. Di Silverio F et al; Prostate, 1998 Oct 1, 37(2):77-83

377 Effects of a Saw Palmetto Herbal Blend in Men with Symptomatic Benign Prostatic Hyperplasia. Marks LS et al; J Urol, 2000 May, 163(5):1451-56

378 Effect of the Lipidic Lipidosterolic Extract of Serenoa repens (Permixon) on the Ionophore A23187-Stimulated Production of Leukotriene B4 (LTB4) from Human Polymorphonuclear Neutrophils. Paubert-Braquet M et al; Prostaglandins Leukot Essent Fatty Acids, 1997 Sep, 57(3):299-304

379 Serenoa repens (Permixon): A 5alpha-Reductase Types I and II Inhibitor-New Evidence in a Coculture Model of BPH. Bayne CW et al; Prostate, 1999 Sep 1, 40(4):232-41

380 Biologically Active Acylglycerides from the Berries of Saw-Palmetto (Serenoa repens). Shimada H et al; J Nat Prod, 1997 Apr, 60(4):417-18

381 Functional Evaluation of Tadenan on Micturition and Experimental Prostate Growth Induced with Exogenous Dihydrotestosterone. Choo MS et al; Urology, 2000 Feb, 55(2):292-98

382 Antiproliferative Effect of Pygeum africanum Extract on Rat Prostatic Fibroblasts. Yablonsky F et al; J Urol, 1997 Jun, 157(6):2381-87

383 Effect of Pygeum africanum Extract on A23187-Stimulated Production of Lipoxygenase Metabolites from Human Polymorphonuclear Cells. Paubert-Braquet M et al; J Lipid Mediat Cell Signal, 1994 May, 9(3):285-90

384 Efficacy and Acceptability of Tadenan (Pygeum africanum extract) in the Treatment of Benign Prostatic Hyperplasia (BPH). Breza J et al; Curr Med Res Opin, 1998, 14(3):127-39

385 Efficacy of Pygeum africanum Extract in the Medical Therapy of Urination Disorders due to Benign Prostatic Hyperplasia. Barlet A et al; Wien Klin Wochenschr, 1990 Nov 23, 102(22):667-73

386 Pygeum africanum Extracts on the In Vitro Proliferation of Human Prostate Cells. Santa Maria Margalef A et al; Arch Esp Urol, 2003 May, 56(4):369-78

387 Cellular and Molecular Aspects of Bladder Hypertrophy. Levin RM et al; Eur Urol, 1997, 32 Suppl 1:15-21

388 Improved Contractility of Obstructed Bladders after Tadenan Treatment is Associated with Reversal of Altered Myosin Isoform Expression. Gomes CM et al; J Urol, 2000 Jun,163(6):2008-13

389 Effects of Unilateral Ischemia on the Contractile Response of the Bladder: Protective Effect of Tadenan (Pygeum africanum Extract). Chen MW et al; Mol Urol, 1999, 3(1):5-10

390 Hormone-Modulating Herbs: Implications for Women's Health. Wade C et al; J Am Med Womens Assoc, 1999 Fall, 54(4):181-3 Review

391 Therapeutic Efficacy and Safety of Cimicifuga racemosa for Gynecologic Disorders. Liske E; Adv Ther, 1998 Jan-Feb, 15(1):45-53 Review

392 Is Black Cohosh Estrogenic? Mahady GB; Nutr Rev, 2003 May, 61(5 Pt 1):183-86 Review

393 Effectiveness of Cimicifuga racemosa (Black Cohosh) for the Symptoms of Menopause. Lieberman S; J Womens Health, 1998 Jun, 7(5):525-29 Review

394 Clinical and Endocrinologic Studies of the Treatment of Ovarian Insufficiency Manifestations Following Hysterectomy with Intact Adnexa. Lehmann-Willenbrock E et al; Zentralbl Gynakol, 1988, 110(10):611-18

395 Black Cohosh. Kligler B; Am Fam Physician, 2003 Jul 1, 68(1):114-16

396 Influence of Cimicifuga racemosa on the Proliferation of Estrogen Receptor-Positive Human Breast Cancer Cells. Bodinet C et al; Breast Cancer Res Treat, 2002 Nov, 76(1):1-10

397 Growth Inhibition of Human Breast Cancer Cells by Herbs and Phytoestrogens. Dixon-Shanies D et al; Oncol Rep, 1999 Nov-Dec, 6(6):1383-87

398 Chaste Tree (Vitex agnus-castus)–Pharmacology and Clinical Indications. Wuttke W et al; Phytomedicine, 2003 May, 10(4):348-57 Review

399 Fluoxetine versus Vitex agnus castus Extract in the Treatment of Premenstrual Dysphoric Disorder. Atmaca M et al; Hum Psychopharmacol, 2003 Apr, 18(3):191-95

400 Treatment of Premenstrual Syndrome with a Phytopharmaceutical Formulation Containing Vitex agnus castus. Loch EG et al; J Womens Health Gend Based Med, 2000 Apr, 9(3):315-20

401 Vitex agnus castus Essential Oil and Menopausal Balance. Chopin Lucks B; Complement Ther Nurs Midwifery, 2003 Aug, 9(3):157-60

402 Cytotoxicity and Apoptotic Inducibility of Vitex agnus-castus Fruit Extract in Cultured Human Normal and Cancer Cells and Effect on Growth. Ohyama K et al; Biol Pharm Bull, 2003 Jan, 26(1):10-18

403 Herbs of Special Interest to Women. Hardy ML et al; J Am Pharm Assoc (Wash), 2000 Mar-Apr, 40(2):234-42 Review

404 Does Dong Quai have Estrogenic Effects in Postmenopausal Women? Hirata JD et al; Fertil Steril, 1997 Dec, 68(6):981-86

405 Inhibitory Effects of Tetramethylpyrazine and Ferulic acid on Spontaneous Movement of Rat Uterus in Situ. Ozaki Y et al; Chem Pharm Bull (Tokyo), 1990 Jun, 38(6):1620-23

406 Stimulating Action of Carthamus tinctorius, Angelica sinensis and Leonurus sibiricus on the Uterus. Shi M et al; Chung Kuo Chung Yao Tsa Chih, 1995 Mar, 20(3):173-75, 192

407 Perimenopausal Hot Flash: Epidemiology, Physiology, and Treatment. Shaw CR; Nurse Pract, 1997 Mar, 22(3):55-56, 61-66 Review

408 The Day of the Yam. Rosser A; Nurs Times, 1985 May, 1-7;81(18):47

409 Effects of Wild Yam Extract on Menopausal Symptoms, Lipids and Sex Hormones in Healthy Menopausal Women. Komesaroff PA et al; Climacteric, 2001 Jun, 4(2):144-50

410 Inhibition of Oxidative Stress in Blood Platelets by Different Phenolics from Yucca schidigera. Olas B et al; Nutrition, 2003 Jul-Aug, 19(7-8):633-40

411 Effect of Quillaja saponaria Saponins and Yucca schidigera Plant Extract on Growth of Escherichia coli. Sen S et al; Lett Appl Microbiol, 1998 Jul, 27(1):35-38

412 Antiyeast Steroidal Saponins from Yucca schidigera (Mohave yucca), A New Anti-Food-Deteriorating Agent. Miyakoshi M et al; J Nat Prod, 2000 Mar, 63(3):332-38

413 Antimutagenic Effect of Resveratrol against Trp-P-1. Uenobe F et al; Mutat Res, 1997 Feb 3, 373(2):197-200

414 Chemical Modification of Glycyrrhizic Acid as a Route to New Bioactive Compounds for Medicine. Baltina LA; Curr Med Chem, 2003 Jan, 10(2):155-71 Review

415 Licorice Ingestion and Blood Pressure Regulating Hormones. Schambelan M; Steroids, 1994 Feb, 59(2):127-30 Review

416 Liquorice and its Health Implications. Olukoga A et al; J R Soc Health, 2000 Jun, 120(2):83-89 Review

417 Transient Visual Loss after Licorice Ingestion. Dobbins KR et al; J Neuroophthalmol, 2000 Mar, 20(1):38-41

418 My Engagement with Steroids. Biglieri EG; Steroids, 1995 Jan, 60(1):52-58 Review

419 Immunopotentiating Effect of Traditional Chinese Drugs–Ginsenoside and Glycyrrhiza Polysaccharide. Yang G et al; Proc Chin Acad Med Sci Peking Union Med Coll, 1990, 5(4):188-93 Review

420 Glucosamine. Barclay TS et al; Ann Pharmacother, 1998 May, 32(5):574-79 Review

421 Glucosamine Sulfate for Osteoarthritis. da Camara CC, et al; Ann Pharmacother, 1998 May, 32(5):580-87 Review

422 Glucosamine Therapy for Treating Osteoarthritis. Towheed TE et al; Cochrane Database Syst Rev 2001, 1:CD002946 Review

423 Nutraceuticals as Therapeutic Agents in Osteoarthritis. The Role of Glucosamine, Chondroitin Sulfate, and Collagen Hydrolysate. Deal CL et al; Rheum Dis Clin North Am, 1999 May, 25(2):379-95 Review

424 Glucosamine and Chondroitin Sulfate are Effective in the Management of Osteoarthritis. Hungerford DS et al; J Arthroplasty, 2003 Apr, 18(3 Suppl 1):5-9 Review

425 Enhanced Synovial Production of Hyaluronic Acid May Explain Rapid Clinical Response to High-Dose Glucosamine in Osteoarthritis. McCarty MF; Med Hypotheses, 1998 Jun, 50(6):507-10 Review

426 Gonarthrosis–Current Aspects of Therapy with Glucosamine Sulfate. Fortschr Med Suppl, 1998, 183:1-12 Review

427 Anti-Tumor Promotion with Food Phytochemicals: A Strategy for Cancer Chemoprevention. Murakami A et al; Biosci Biotechnol Biochem, 1996 Jan, 60(1):1-8 Review

428 Evaluation of Chemoprevention of Oral Cancer with Spirulina fusiformis. Mathew B et al; Nutr Cancer, 1995, 24(2):197-202

429 Inhibitive Effects of Spirulina on Aberrant Crypts in Colon Induced by Dimethylhydrazine. Chen F et al; Chung Hua Yu Fang I Hsueh Tsa Chih, 1995 Jan, 29(1):13-17

430 Inhibition of Tumor Invasion and Metastasis by Calcium Spirulan, a Novel Sulfated Polysaccharide Derived from a Blue-Green Alga, Spirulina platensis. Mishima T et al; Clin Exp Metastasis, 1998 Aug, 16(6):541-50

431 Novel Glycoprotein Obtained from Chlorella vulgaris Strain CK22 Shows Antimetastatic Immunopotentiation. Tanaka K et al; Cancer Immunol Immunother, 1998 Feb, 45(6):313-20

432 Microcolins A and B, New Immunosuppressive Peptides from the Blue-Green Alga Lyngbya majuscula. Koehn FE et al; J Nat Prod, 1992 May, 55(5):613-19

433 Dose-Dependent Selective Cytotoxicity of Extracts from Marine Green Alga, Cladophoropsis vaucheriae-

formis, against Mouse Leukemia L1210 Cells. Harada H et al; Biol Pharm Bull, 1998 Apr, 21(4):386-89

434   Compound 14-Keto-Stypodiol Diacetate from the Algae Stypopodium flabelliforme Inhibits Microtubules and Cell Proliferation in DU-145 Human Prostatic Cells. Depix MS et al; Mol Cell Biochem, 1998 Oct, 187(1-2):191-99

435   Antitumor and Antiproliferative Effects of an Aqueous Extract from the Marine Diatom Haslea ostrearia (Simonsen) against Solid Tumors: Lung Carcinoma (NSCLC-N6), Kidney Carcinoma (E39) and Melanoma (M96) Cell Lines. Carbonnelle D et al; Anticancer Res, 1999 Jan-Feb, 19(1A):621-24

436   Calcium Spirulan, an Inhibitor of Enveloped Virus Replication, from a Blue-Green Alga Spirulina platensis. Hayashi T et al; J Nat Prod, 1996 Jan, 59(1):83-87

437   Antiviral Activity of Spirulina maxima against Herpes Simplex Virus Type 2. Hernandez-Corona A et al; Antiviral Res, 2002 Dec, 56(3):279-85

438   Inhibition of Enterovirus 71-Induced Apoptosis by Allophycocyanin Isolated from a Blue-Green Alga Spirulina platensis. Shih SR et al; J Med Virol, 2003 May, 70(1):119-25 Review

439   Cyanobacteria a Potential Source of Antiviral Substances against Influenza Virus. Zainuddin EN et al; Med Microbiol Immunol (Berl), 2002 Dec,191(3-4):181-82

440   Anti-HIV Activity of Extracts and Compounds from Algae and Cyanobacteria. Schaeffer DJ et al; Ecotoxicol Environ Saf, 2000 Mar, 45(3):208-27 Review

441   Nutritional Supplementation with Chlorella pyrenoidosa for Patients with Fibromyalgia Syndrome. Merchant RE et al; Phytother Res, 2000 May, 14(3):167-73

442   Exercise and Immune Function: Effect of Ageing and Nutrition. Pedersen BK et al; Proc Nutr Soc, 1999 Aug, 58(3):733-42 Review

443   Free Radicals, Exercise and Antioxidant Supplementation. Kanter M; Proc Nutr Soc, 1998 Feb, 57(1):9-13 Review

444   Vitamin C, Neutrophil Function, and Upper Respiratory Tract Infection Risk in Distance Runners. Peters-Futre EM; Exerc Immunol Rev, 1997, 3:32-52 Review

445   Exercise, Immunology and Upper Respiratory Tract Infections. Peters EM; Int J Sports Med, 1997 Mar, 18 Suppl 1:S69-77 Review

446   Vitamin C and Acute Respiratory Infections. Hemila H et al; Int J Tuberc Lung Dis, 1999 Sep, 3(9):756-61 Review

447   Vitamin C Supplementation and Common Cold Symptoms: Factors Affecting the Magnitude of the Benefit. Hemila H; Med Hypotheses, 1999 Feb, 52(2):171-78 Review

448   Diet as a Risk Factor for Asthma. Weiss ST; Ciba Found Symp, 1997;206:244-57: discussion 253-57 Review

449   Asthma, Inhaled Oxidants, and Dietary Antioxidants. Hatch GE; Am J Clin Nutr, 1995 Mar, 61(3 Suppl):625S-630S Review

450   Asthma and Vitamin C. Bielory L et al; Ann Allergy, 1994 Aug, 73(2):89-96 Review

451   Use of Endogenous Antioxidants to Improve Photoprotection. Steenvoorden DP et al; J Photochem Photobiol B, 1997 Nov, 41(1-2):1-10 Review

452   Ascorbic Acid Metabolism and Cancer in the Human Stomach. Schorah CJ; Acta Gastroenterol Belg, 1997 Jul-Sep, 60(3):217-19 Review

453   Antioxidant Micronutrients and Gastric Cancer. Correa P et al; Aliment Pharmacol Ther, 1998 Feb, 12 Suppl 1:73-82 Review

454   Effect of Antioxidants on the Immune Response of Helicobacter pylori. Akyon Y; Clin Microbiol Infect, 2002 Jul, 8(7):438-41 Review

455   Nutrition and Cancer. Joossens JV et al; Biomed Pharmacother, 1986, 40(4):127-38 Review

456   Nutrition and Stomach Cancer. Kono S et al; Cancer Causes Control, 1996 Jan, 7(1):41-55 Review

457   Role of Ascorbic Acid in Oral Cancer and Carcinogenesis. Chan SW et al; Oral Dis, 1998 Jun, 4(2):120-29 Review

458   Apoptosis-Inducing Activity of Vitamin C and Vitamin K. Sakagami H et al; Cell Mol Biol, 2000 Feb, 46(1):129-43 Review

459 Modulating Factors of Radical Intensity and Cytotoxic Activity of Ascorbate. Sakagami H et al; Anticancer Res, 1997 Sep-Oct, 17(5A):3513-20 Review

460 Prolongation of Survival Times of Terminal Cancer Patients by Administration of Large Doses of Ascorbate. Murata A et al; Int J Vitam Nutr Res Suppl, 1982, 23:103-13

461 Ascorbic Acid in the Prevention and Treatment of Cancer. Head KA; Altern Med Rev, 1998 Jun, 3(3):174-86 Review

462 Medicinal Properties of Echinacea: A Critical Review. Barrett B; Phytomedicine, 2003 Jan, 10(1):66-86 Review

463 Evaluation of Echinacea for Treatment of the Common Cold. Giles JT et al; Pharmacotherapy, 2000 Jun, 20(6):690-97 Review

464 Echinacea for Upper Respiratory Infection. Barrett B et al; J Fam Pract, 1999 Aug, 48(8):628-35 Review

465 The American Coneflower: A Prophylactic Role Involving Nonspecific Immunity. Sun LZ et al; J Altern Complement Med, 1999 Oct, 5(5):437-46

466 Echinacea-Induced Cytokine Production by Human Macrophages. Burger RA et al; Int J Immunopharmacol, 1997 Jul, 19(7):371-79

467 Increased Production of Antigen-Specific Immunoglobulins G and M following in Vivo Treatment with the Medicinal Plants Echinacea angustifolia and Hydrastis canadensis. Rehman J et al; Immunol Lett, 1999 Jun 1, 68(2-3):391-95

468 Macrophage Activation by the Polysaccharide Arabinogalactan Isolated from Plant Cell Cultures of Echinacea purpurea. Luettig B et al; J Natl Cancer Inst, 1989 May 3, 81(9):669-75

469 Cytokine Production in Leukocyte Cultures during Therapy with Echinacea Extract. Elsasser-Beile U et al; J Clin Lab Anal, 1996, 10(6):441-45

470 Natural Killer Cells from Aging Mice Treated with Extracts from Echinacea purpurea are Quantitatively and Functionally Rejuvenated. Currier N et al; Exp Gerontol, 2000 Aug 1, 35(5):627-639

471 Light-Mediated Antifungal Activity of Echinacea Extracts. Binns SE et al; Planta Med, 2000 Apr, 66(3):241-44

472 Effects of Plant Preparations on Cellular Functions in Body Defense. Wildfeuer A et al; Arzneimittelforschung, 1994 Mar, 44(3):361-66

473 Testing for Immunomodulating Effects of Ethanol-Water Extracts of the Above-Ground Parts of the Plants Echinaceae and Rudbeckia. Bukovsky M et al; Cesk Farm, 1993 Oct, 42(5):228-31

474 Toxicity of Echinacea purpurea. Acute, Subacute and Genotoxicity Studies. Mengs U et al; Arzneimittelforschung, 1991 Oct, 41(10):1076-81

475 Echinacea-Associated Anaphylaxis. Mullins RJ; Med J Aust, 1998 Feb 16, 168(4):170-71

476 Effect of Astragalus membranaceus on T-lymphocyte Subsets in Patients with Viral Myocarditis. Huang ZQ et al; Chung Kuo Chung Hsi I Chieh Ho Tsa Chih, 1995 Jun, 15(6):328-30

477 Enhancement of the Immune Response in Mice by Astragalus membranaceus Extracts. Zhao KS et al; Immunopharmacology, 1990 Nov-Dec, 20(3):225-33

478 Effects of Exercise in the Growing Stage in Mice and of Astragalus membranaceus on Immune Functions. Sugiura H et al; Nippon Eiseigaku Zasshi, 1993 Feb, 47(6):1021-31

479 Immunotherapy with Chinese Medicinal Herbs. II. Reversal of Cyclophosphamide-Induced Immune Suppression by Administration of Fractionated Astragalus membranaceus in Vivo. Chu DT et al; J Clin Lab Immunol, 1988 Mar, 25(3):125-29

480 Effects of Astragalus membranaceus and Tripterygium hypoglancum on Natural Killer Cell Activity of Peripheral Blood Mononuclear in Systemic Lupus Erythematosus. Zhao XZ; Chung Kuo Chung Hsi I Chieh Ho Tsa Chih, 1992 Nov, 12(11):669-71, 645

481 Chinese Medicinal Herbs Reverse Macrophage Suppression Induced by Urological Tumors. Rittenhouse JR et al; J Urol, 1991 Aug, 146(2):486-90

482 Effect of Astragalan on Secretion of Tumor Necrosis Factors in Human Peripheral Blood Mononuclear Cells. Zhao KW et al; Chung Kuo Chung Hsi I Chieh Ho Tsa Chih, 1993 May, 13(5):263-65, 259

483 Phytochemicals Potentiate Interleukin-2 Generated Lymphokine-Activated Killer Cell Cytotoxicity against Murine Renal Cell Carcinoma. Wang Y et al; Mol Biother, 1992 Sep, 4(3):143-46

484 In Vitro Potentiation of LAK Cell Cytotoxicity in Cancer and AIDS Patients Induced by F3–a Fractionated Extract of Astragalus membranaceus. Chu DT et al; Chung Hua Chung Liu Tsa Chih, 1994 May, 16(3):167-71

485 Viral Etiology of Chronic Cervicitis and its Therapeutic Response to a Recombinant Interferon. Qian ZW et al; Chin Med J (Engl), 1990 Aug, 103(8):647-51

486 Hepatoprotective Effects of Astraglus Root. Zhang ZL et al; J Ethnopharmacol, 1990 Sep, 30(2):145-49

487 Suppressive Effect of Astragalus membranaceus on Chemical Hepatocarcinogenesis in Rats. Cui R et al; Cancer Chemother Pharmacol, 2003 Jan, 51(1):75-80

488 Effect of Astragalus Polysaccharide on Endotoxin-Induced Toxicity in Mice. Wang LX et al; Yao Hsueh Hsueh Pao, 1992, 27(1):5-9

489 Green Tea (Camellia sinensis) Extract and its Possible Role in the Prevention of Cancer. Brown MD; Altern Med Rev, 1999 Oct, 4(5):360-70 Review

490 Cancer Chemoprevention by Tea Polyphenols through Mitotic Signal Transduction Blockade. Lin JK et al; Biochem Pharmacol, 1999 Sep 15, 58(6):911-15 Review

491 Tea and Tea Polyphenols in Cancer Prevention. Yang CS et al; J Nutr, 2000 Feb, 130(2S Suppl):472S-478S Review

492 Tea Polyphenols: Prevention of Cancer and Optimizing Health. Mukhtar H et al; Am J Clin Nutr, 2000 Jun, 71(6 Suppl):1698S-702S Review

493 Green Tea and Cancer in Humans. Bushman JL; Nutr Cancer, 1998, 31(3):151-59 Review

494 Major Constituent of Green Tea, EGCG, Inhibits the Growth of a Human Cervical Cancer Cell Line, Caski Cells, Through Apoptosis, G(1) Arrest, and Regulation of Gene Expression. Ahn WS et al; DNA Cell Biol, 2003 Mar, 22(3):217-24

495 Molecular Targets for Green Tea in Prostate Cancer Prevention. Adhami VM et al; J Nutr, 2003 Jul,133(7 Suppl):2417S-2424S

496 Green Tea Polyphenols: DNA Photodamage and Photoimmunology. Katiyar SK et al; J Photochem Photobiol B, 2001 Dec 31, 65(2-3):109-14 Review

497 Green Tea and Skin. Katiyar SK et al; Arch Dermatol, 2000 Aug, 136(8):989-94 Review

498 Growth Inhibition of Leukemic Cells by (-)-Epigallocatechin Gallate, the Main Constituent of Green Tea. Otsuka T et al; Life Sci, 1998, 63(16):1397-403

499 Green Tea Polyphenol Epigallocatechin Inhibits DNA Replication and Consequently Induces Leukemia Cell Apoptosis. Smith DM et al; Int J Mol Med, 2001 Jun, 7(6):645-52

500 Green Tea Polyphenols Induce Apoptosis in Vitro in Peripheral Blood T Lymphocytes of Adult T-Cell Leukemia Patients. Li HC et al; Jpn J Cancer Res, 2000 Jan, 91(1):34-40.

501 Anti-Proliferative and Differentiation-Inducing Activities of the Green Tea Catechin Epigallocatechin-3-Gallate (EGCG) on the Human Eosinophilic Leukemia Eol-1 Cell Line. Lung HL et al; Life Sci, 2002 Dec 6, 72(3):257-68

502 Inhibition of the Infectivity of Influenza Virus by Tea Polyphenols. Nakayama M et al; Antiviral Res, 1993 Aug, 21(4):289-99

503 Inhibition of Rotavirus and Enterovirus Infections by Tea Extracts. Mukoyama A et al; Jpn J Med Sci Biol, 1991 Aug, 44(4):181-86

504 Differential Inhibitory Effects of Some Catechin Derivatives on the Activities of Human Immunodeficiency Virus Reverse Transcriptase and Cellular Deoxyribonucleic and Ribonucleic Acid Polymerases. Nakane H et al; Biochemistry, 1990 Mar 20, 29(11):2841-45

505 Tea and Health: The Underlying Mechanisms. Weisburger JH et al; Proc Soc Exp Biol Med, 1999 Apr, 220(4):271-75 Review

506 Microbiological Activity of Whole and Fractionated Crude Extracts of Tea (Camellia sinensis), and of Tea Components. Yam TS et al; FEMS Microbiol Lett, 1997 Jul 1, 152(1):169-74

507 Anti-Helicobacter pylori Activity of Chinese Tea: In Vitro Study. Yee YK et al; Aliment Pharmacol Ther, 2000 May, 14(5):635-38

508 Antibacterial Activity of Camellia sinensis Extracts against Dental Caries. Rasheed A et al; Arch Pharm Res, 1998 Jun, 21(3):348-52

509 Effects of Green Tea Catechins on Membrane Fluidity. Tsuchiya H; Pharmacology, 1999 Jul, 59(1):34-44

510 Cross Sectional Study of Effects of Drinking Green Tea on Cardiovascular and Liver Diseases. Imai K et al; BMJ, 1995 Mar 18, 310(6981):693-96 Review

511 Tea Flavonols in Cardiovascular Disease and Cancer Epidemiology. Hollman PC et al; Proc Soc Exp Biol Med, 1999 Apr, 220(4):198-202 Review

512 Inhibitory Effect of Green Tea Infusion of Hepatotoxicity. Hasegawa R et al; Kokuritsu Iyakuhin Shokuhin Eisei Kenkyusho Hokoku, 1998, (116):82-91 Review

513 How to Reduce the Risk Factors of Osteoporosis in Asia. Kao PC et al; Chung Hua I Hsueh Tsa Chih (Taipei), 1995 Mar, 55(3):209-13 Review

514 Epigallocatechin-3-Gallate Selectively Inhibits Interleukin-1beta-Induced Activation of Mitogen Activated Protein Kinase Subgroup C-Jun N-Terminal Kinase in Human Osteoarthritis Chondrocytes. Singh R et al; J Orthop Res, 2003 Jan, 21(1):102-19

515 Fluoride in Tea–Its Dental Significance. Kavanagh D et al; J Ir Dent Assoc, 1998, 44(4):100-05 Review

516 Anticariogenic Effects of Green Tea. Yu H et al; Fukuoka Igaku Zasshi, 1992 Apr, 83(4):174-80

517 Fluoride Content in Caffeinated, Decaffeinated and Herbal Teas. Chan JT et al; Caries Res, 1996, 30(1):88-92

Chapter 8 – Pituitary

1 Ginkgo–Myth and Reality. Z'Brun A; Schweiz Rundsch Med Prax, 1995 Jan 3, 84(1):1-6 Review

2 Ginkgo biloba Extract (EGb 761). State of Knowledge in the Dawn of the Year 2000. Clostre F; Ann Pharm Fr, 1999 Jul, 57 Suppl 1:1S8-88 Review

3 Value of Ginkgo biloba in Treatment of Alzheimer Dementia. Loew D; Wien Med Wochenschr, 2002, 152(15-16):418-22 Review

4 Clinical Improvement of Memory and Other Cognitive Functions by Ginkgo biloba. Soholm B; Adv Ther, 1998 Jan-Feb, 15(1):54-65 Review

5 Efficacy of Ginkgo biloba on Cognitive Function in Alzheimer Disease. Oken BS et al; Arch Neurol, 1998 Nov, 55(11):1409-15 Review6

6 Herbal Medicines for Psychiatric Disorders. Beaubrun G et al; Psychiatr Serv, 2000 Sep, 51(9):1130-34 Review

7 Ginkgo biloba Extract for Age-Related Macular Degeneration. Evans JR; Cochrane Database Syst Rev, 2000;(2):CD001775 Review

8 Ginkgo biloba in Treatment of Intermittent Claudication. Ernst E; Fortschr Med, 1996 Mar 20, 114(8):85-87 Review

9 Ginkgo biloba for the Prevention and Treatment of Cardiovascular Disease. Mahady GB; J Cardiovasc Nurs, 2002 Jul, 16(4):21-32 Review

10 Mitochondria, Oxidative Stress and Aging. Sastre J et al; Free Radic Res, 2000 Mar, 32(3):189-98 Review

11 Safety of Herbal Medicines in the Psychiatric Practice. Boniel T et al; Harefuah, 2001 Aug, 140(8):780-83, 805 Review

12 Herbal Medicinals: Selected Clinical Considerations Focusing on Known or Potential Drug-Herb Interactions. Miller LG; Arch Intern Med, 1998 Nov 9, 158(20):2200-11 Review

13 Current Perspectives on the Management of Seasonal Affective Disorder. Jepson TL et al; J Am Pharm Assoc (Wash), 1999 Nov-Dec, 39(6):822-89 Review

14 Melatonin: from Biochemistry to Therapeutic Applications. Zawilska JB et al; Pol J Pharmacol, 1999 Jan-Feb, 51(1):3-23 Review

15 Melatonin: A Clock-Output, a Clock-Input. Stehle JH et al; J Neuroendocrinol, 2003 Apr, 15(4):383-89

Review

16 Hormonal and Pharmacological Manipulation of the Circadian Clock: Recent Developments and Future Strategies. Richardson G et al; Sleep, 2000 May 1, 23 Suppl 3:S77-85 Review

17 Hypothalamic Suprachiasmatic Nucleus and Pineal Gland in the Circadian Rhythmic Organization of Mammals. Zhou XJ et al; Sheng Li Ke Xue Jin Zhan, 2001 Apr, 32(2):116-20 Review

18 Endocrine Activity during Sleep. Luboshitzky R; J Pediatr Endocrinol Metab, 2000 Jan, 13(1):13-20 Review

19 Pathophysiology of Human Circadian Rhythms. Copinschi G et al; Novartis Found Symp, 2000, 227:143-57 Review

20 Use of Melatonin for the Treatment of Insomnia. Zisapel N; Biol Signals Recept, 1999 Jan-Apr, 8(1-2):84-89 Review

21 Supplementary Administration of Artificial Bright Light and Melatonin as Potent Treatment for Disorganized Circadian Rest-Activity and Dysfunctional Autonomic and Neuroendocrine Systems in Institutionalized Demented Elderly Persons. Mishima K et al; Chronobiol Int, 2000 May, 17(3):419-32 Review

22 Use of Melatonin in the Treatment of Phase Shift and Sleep Disorders. Skene DJ et al; Adv Exp Med Biol, 1999, 467:79-84 Review

23 Pharmacology and Physiology of Melatonin in the Reduction of Oxidative Stress in Vivo. Reiter RJ et al; Biol Signals Recept, 2000 May-Aug, 9(3-4):160-71 Review

24 Significance of Melatonin in Antioxidative Defense System: Reactions and Products. Tan DX et al; Biol Signals Recept, 2000 May-Aug, 9(3-4):137-59 Review

25 Melatonin Oxidative Stress and Neurodegenerative Diseases. Srinivasan V; Indian J Exp Biol, 2002 Jun, 40(6):668-79 Review

26 Utility of Melatonin in Reducing Cerebral Damage Resulting from Ischaemia and Reperfusion. Cheung RT; J Pineal Res, 2003 Apr, 34(3):153-60

27 Melatonin as a Time-Meaningful Signal in Circadian Organization of Immune Response. Cardinali DP et al; Biol Signals Recept, 1999 Jan-Apr, 8(1-2):41-48 Review

28 MLT and the Immune-Hematopoietic System. Maestroni GJ; Adv Exp Med Biol, 1999, 460:395-405 Review

29 Melatonin and Mammary Pathological Growth. Cos S et al; Front Neuroendocrinol, 2000 Apr, 21(2):133-70 Review

Chapter 9 – Thyroid

1 Epidemiology of Thyroid Disease and Implications for Screening. Wang C et al; Endocrinol Metab Clin North Am, 1997 Mar, 26(1):189-218 Review

2 Managing Thyroid Dysfunction in the Elderly. Mohandas R et al; Postgrad Med, 2003 May, 113(5):54-56, 65-68 Review

3 Rational Use of Thyroid Function Tests. Volpe R; Crit Rev Clin Lab Sci, 1997 Oct, 34(5):405-38 Review

4 Tests of Thyroid Function: Update in the Diagnosis and Management of Thyroid Disease. Meek JC; Compr Ther, 1990 Jul, 16(7):20-27

5 Iodine and Thyroid Function. Schlienger JL et al; Rev Med Interne, 1997, 18(9):709-16 Review

6 Prevention and Management of Iodine-Induced Hyperthyroidism and its Cardiac Features. Dunn JT et al; Thyroid, 1998 Jan, 8(1):101-06 Review

7 Iodine Supplementation: Benefits Outweigh Risks. Delange F et al; Drug Saf, 2000 Feb, 22(2):89-95 Review

8 Iodine-Induced Hyperthyroidism: Occurrence and Epidemiology. Stanbury JB et al; Thyroid, 1998 Jan, 8(1):83-100 Review

9 Hyperthyroidism. Current Treatment Guidelines. Gittoes NJ et al; Drugs, 1998 Apr, 55(4):543-53 Review

10 Graves' Ophthalmopathy. Carter JN; Aust N Z J Ophthalmol, 1990 Aug, 18(3):239-42 Review

11 Coincidence of Hot Thyroid Nodules and Primary Hyperparathyroidism. Klemm T et al; Exp Clin Endocrinol Diabetes, 1999, 107(5):295-98 Review

12 Heart and Thyroid Disease. Aronow WS; Clin Geriatr Med, 1995 May, 11(2):219-29 Review

13   Subclinical Thyroid Disease in the Elderly. Samuels MH; Thyroid, 1998 Sep, 8(9):803-13 Review

14   Diagnosing and Treating Hypothyroidism. Elliott B et al; Nurse Pract, 2000 Mar, 25(3):92-4, 99-105 Review

15   Thyroid Hormone and Cardiovascular Disease. Gomberg-Maitland M et al; Am Heart J, 1998 Feb, 135(2 Pt 1):187-96 Review

16   Thyroid Function and Postmenopause. Schindler AE; Gynecol Endocrinol, 2003 Feb, 17(1):79-85 Review

17   Physiopathology of Iodine Deficiency. Pinchera A et al; Ann Ist Super Sanita, 1998, 34(3):301-05 Review

18   Evaluation and Management of Multinodular Goiter. Hurley DL et al; Otolaryngol Clin North Am, 1996 Aug, 29(4):527-40 Review

19   Therapeutic Options in the Management of Toxic and Nontoxic Nodular Goiter. Freitas JE; Semin Nucl Med, 2000 Apr, 30(2):88-97 Review

20   Thyroid Nodules. Welker MJ et al; Am Fam Physician, 2003 Feb 1, 67(3):559-66 Review

21   Management Strategies for Endemic Goiter in Developing Countries. Kouame P et al; Med Trop (Mars), 1999, 59(4):401-10 Review

22   Maternal Iodine Supplements in Areas of Deficiency. Mahomed K et al; Cochrane Database Syst Rev, 2000;(2):CD000135 Review

23   Iodine Supplementation and the Prevention of Cretinism. Dunn JT et al; Ann N Y Acad Sci, 1993 Mar 15, 678:158-68 Review

24   Role of Iodine in Brain Development. Delange F; Proc Nutr Soc, 2000 Feb, 59(1):75-79 Review

25   Sudden Infant Death Syndrome and Placental Disorders: The Thyroid-Selenium Link. Reid GM et al; Med Hypotheses, 1997 Apr, 48(4):317-24 Review

26   Trace Element Selenium and the Thyroid Gland. Kohrle J; Biochimie, 1999 May, 81(5):527-33 Review

27   Sudden Infant Death Syndrome: Oxidative Stress. Reid GM et al; Med Hypotheses, 1999 Jun, 52(6):577-80 Review

28   Nutrition and Development: Other Micronutrients' Effect on Growth and Cognition. Wasantwisut E; Southeast Asian J Trop Med Public Health, 1997, 28 Suppl 2:78-82 Review

29   Thyroid Function. Arthur JR et al; Br Med Bull, 1999, 55(3):658-68 Review

30   Changes in U.S. Life Expectancy. Statistical Bull; 1994 Jul-Sept; 11-17

Chapter 10 – Pancreas

1   Fatty Acids and Beta Cells. Girard J; Diabetes Metab, 2000 Jun, 26 Suppl 3:6-9 Review

2   Role of Eicosanoids in Biosynthesis and Secretion of Insulin. Pek SB et al; Diabete Metab, 1994 Mar-Apr, 20(2):146-49 Review

3   Metabolic Effects of Omega-3 Fatty Acids in Type 2 (Non-Insulin-Dependent) Diabetic Patients. Pelikanova T et al; Ann N Y Acad Sci, 1993 Jun 14, 683:272-78

4   Diabetic Emergencies: Hypoglycaemia. Lewis R; Accid Emerg Nurs, 1999 Oct, 7(4):190-96 Review

5   Hypoglycaemia Unawareness. Bolli GB; Diabetes Metab, 1997 Sep, 23 Suppl 3:29-35 Review

6   Hypoglycemia–Occurrence, Causes and Hormonal Counterregulatory Mechanisms in Healthy Persons and in Patients with IDDM. Mokan M; Bratisl Lek Listy, 1995 Jun, 96(6):311-16 Review

7   Diabetes Mellitus and Traffic Incidents. Veneman TF; Neth J Med, 1996 Jan, 48(1):24-28 Review

8   Genetics of Type 1 Diabetes Mellitus. Friday RP et al; Diabetes Nutr Metab, 1999 Feb, 12(1):3-26 Review

9   Aetiology of Type 1 Diabetes: An Epidemiological Perspective. Dahlquist G; Acta Paediatr Suppl, 1998 Oct, 425:5-10 Review

10   Novel Insulins: Expanding Options in Diabetes Management. Gerich JE; Am J Med, 2002 Sep, 113(4):339-40 Review

11   New Insulin Replacement Technologies: Overcoming Barriers to Tight Glycemic Control. Leslie CA; Cleve Clin J Med, 1999 May, 66(5):293-302 Review

12   Pharmacological Management of Diabetes. Emilien G et al; Pharmacol Ther, 1999 Jan, 81(1):37-51 Review

13   Importance of Insulin Resistance in the Pathogenesis of Type 2 Diabetes Mellitus. Fujimoto WY; Am J Med,

2000 Apr 17, 108 Suppl 6a:9S-14S Review

14   Type 2 Diabetes Mellitus: The Grand Overview. Ratner RE; Diabet Med, 1998, 15 Suppl 4:S4-7 Review

15   Potential New Treatments for Type 2 Diabetes. Bailey CJ; Trends Pharmacol Sci, 2000 Jul, 21(7):259-65 Review

16   From Obesity to Diabetes: Why, When and Who? Scheen AJ; Acta Clin Belg, 2000 Jan-Feb, 55(1):9-15 Review

17   Type II Diabetes Mellitus. Edelman SV; Adv Intern Med, 1998, 43:449-500 Review

18   Care of Adults with Type 2 Diabetes Mellitus. O'Connor PJ et al; J Fam Pract, 1998 Nov, 47(5 Suppl):S13-22 Review

19   Cardiovascular Disease in Patients with Diabetes. Gaba MK et al; J Assoc Acad Minor Phys, 1999, 10(1):15-22 Review

20   Diabetes, Coagulation and Vascular Events. Nenci GG et al; Recenti Prog Med, 2000 Feb, 91(2):86-90 Review

21   Preserving Renal Function in Adults with Hypertension and Diabetes. Bakris GL et al; Am J Kidney Dis, 2000 Sep, 36(3):646-61

22   Diabetic Neuropathy: Pathophysiology and Prevention of Foot Ulcers. Zangaro GA et al; Clin Nurse Spec, 1999 Mar, 13(2):57-65 Review

23   Experimental Diabetic Neuropathy. Sima AA et al; Diabetologia, 1999 Jul, 42(7):773-88 Review

24   Metabolic Neuropathies. Comi G et al; Curr Opin Neurol, 1998 Oct, 11(5):523-29 Review

25   Diabetic Eye Disease. Frank KJ et al; South Med J, 1996 May, 89(5):463-70 Review

26   Diabetic Retinopathy: Primary Care Physician. Fonseca V et al; South Med J, 1996 Sep, 89(9):839-50 Review

27   Diabetic Retinopathy. Grange JD; Rev Prat, 1996 Sep 15, 46(14):1714-21 Review

28   Lowering the Risk of Visual Impairment and Blindness. Cunha-Vaz J; Diabet Med, 1998, 15 Suppl 4:S47-50 Review

29   Risk Factors in the Progression of Diabetic Nephropathies. Rossing P; Ugeskr Laeger, 2000 Sep 18, 162(38):5057-61 Review

30   Prevention of Microvascular Complications in Diabetic Children and Adolescents. Verrotti A et al; Acta Paediatr Suppl, 1999 Jan, 88(427):35-38 Review

31   Nephropathy in Non-Insulin-Dependent (Type-2) Diabetes Mellitus. Nagy J et al; Orv Hetil, 2000 Mar 19, 141(12):609-14 Review

32   Blood Pressure, Diabetes and Diabetic Nephropathy. Chantrel F et al; Diabetes Metab, 2000 Jul, 26 Suppl 4:37-44 Review

33   Implications of the Hyperinsulinaemia-Diabetes-Cancer Link for Preventive Efforts. Moore MA et al; Eur J Cancer Prev, 1998 Apr, 7(2):89-107 Review

34   Interaction of the Endo- and Exocrine Pancreas. Gyr K et al; Schweiz Med Wochenschr, 1985 Sep 21, 115(38):1299-306 Review

35   Gastrointestinal Involvement in Patients with Diabetes Mellitus: Epidemiology, Pathophysiology, Clinical Findings. Folwaczny C et al; Z Gastroenterol, 1999 Sep, 37(9):803-15 Review

36   Gastrointestinal Complications of Diabetes Mellitus. Vogt M et al; Med Klin, 1999 Jun 15, 94(6):329-37 Review

37   Hypoglycemia in Adults. Virally ML et al; Diabetes Metab, 1999 Dec, 25(6):477-90 Review

38   Symptoms of Hypoglycemia, Thresholds for their Occurrence, and Hypoglycemia Unawareness. Cryer PE; Endocrinol Metab Clin North Am, 1999 Sep, 28(3):495-500 Review

39   Physiology of Glucose Counterregulation to Hypoglycemia. Bolli GB et al; Endocrinol Metab Clin North Am, 1999 Sep, 28(3):467-93 Review

40   Cerebral Energy Metabolism, Glucose Transport and Blood Flow: Changes with Maturation and Adaptation to Hypoglycaemia. Nehlig A; Diabetes Metab, 1997 Feb, 23(1):18-29 Review

41   Reactive Hypoglycemia. Hofeldt FD; Endocrinol Metab Clin North Am, 1989 Mar, 18(1):185-201 Review

42   Regulation of Carbohydrate Metabolism and Response to Hypoglycemia. Butler PC et al; Endocrinol Metab

Clin North Am, 1989 Mar, 18(1):1-25 Review

43 Postprandial Hyperglycemia: Physiopathology, Clinical Consequences and Dietary Management. Scheen AJ et al; Rev Med Liege, 2002 Mar, 57(3):138-41 Review

44 Hypoglycemia Associated with Liver Disease and Ethanol. Arky RA; Endocrinol Metab Clin North Am, 1989 Mar, 18(1):75-90 Review

45 Nutrition Therapy for Hepatic Glycogen Storage Diseases. Goldberg T et al; J Am Diet Assoc, 1993 Dec, 93(12):1423-30 Review

46 Drug-Induced Disorders of Glucose Metabolism. Chan JC et al; Drug Saf, 1996 Aug, 15(2):135-57 Review

47 Hypoglycemia Associated with Renal Failure. Arem R; Endocrinol Metab Clin North Am, 1989 Mar, 18(1):103-21 Review

48 Insulinoma. Grant CS; Surg Oncol Clin N Am, 1998 Oct, 7(4):819-44 Review

49 Newborn Hypoglycemia. Armentrout D et al; J Pediatr Health Care, 1999 Jan-Feb,13(1):2-6 Review

50 Neonatal Hypoglycemia. Brooks C; Neonatal Netw, 1997 Mar, 16(2):15-21 Review

51 Congenital Hyperinsulinism. Meissner T et al; Hum Mutat, 1999, 13(5):351-61 Review

52 Persistent Hyperinsulinemic Hypoglycemia in the Newborn and Infants. de Lonlay-Debeney P et al; Arch Pediatr, 1998 Dec, 5(12):1347-52 Review

53 Long-Term Treatment of Persistent Hyperinsulinaemic Hypoglycaemia of Infancy with Diazoxide. Touati G et al; Eur J Pediatr, 1998 Aug, 157(8):628-33 Review

54 Persistent Hyperinsulinemic Hypoglycemia of Infancy: Long-Term Results. Dacou-Voutetakis C et al; J Pediatr Endocrinol Metab, 1998 Mar, 11 Suppl 1:131-41 Review

55 Role of Hydrophobic Amino Acids in Gurmarin, a Sweetness-Suppressing Polypeptide. Ota M et al; Biopolymers, 1998 Mar, 45(3):231-38

56 Electrophysiological Characterization of the Inhibitory Effect of a Vovel Peptide Gurmarin on the Sweet Taste Response in Rats. Miyasaka A et al; Brain Res, 1995 Apr 3, 676(1):63-68

57 Inhibitory Effect of Gymnemic Acid on Intestinal Absorption of Oleic Acid in Rats. Wang LF et al; Can J Physiol Pharmacol, 1998 Oct-Nov, 76(10-11):1017-23

58 Suppression of Glucose Absorption by Some Fractions Extracted from Gymnema sylvestre Leaves. Shimizu K et al; J Vet Med Sci, 1997 Apr, 59(4):245-51

59 Medicinal Foodstuffs: Inhibitors of Glucose Absorption from the Leaves of Gymnema sylvestre. Yoshikawa M et al; Chem Pharm Bull (Tokyo), 1997 Oct, 45(10):1671-76

60 Overview on the Advances of Gymnema sylvestre: Chemistry, Pharmacology and Patents. Porchezhian E et al; Pharmazie, 2003 Jan, 58(1):5-12 Review

61 Antidiabetic Effect of a Leaf Extract from Gymnema sylvestre in Non-Insulin-Dependent Diabetes Mellitus Patients. Baskaran K et al; J Ethnopharmacol, 1990 Oct, 30(3):295-300

62 Use of Gymnema sylvestre Leaf Extract in the Control of Blood Glucose in Insulin-Dependent Diabetes Mellitus. Shanmugasundaram ER et al; J Ethnopharmacol, 1990 Oct, 30(3):281-94

63 Comparative Effects of Chromium, Vanadium and Gymnema sylvestre on Sugar-Induced Blood Pressure Elevations in SHR. Preuss HG et al; J Am Coll Nutr, 1998 Apr, 17(2):116-23

64 Fecal Steroid Excretion is Increased in Rats by Oral Administration of Gymnemic Acids Contained in Gymnema sylvestre Leaves. Nakamura Y et al; J Nutr, 1999 Jun, 129(6):1214-22

65 4-Hydroxyisoleucine: Effects of Synthetic and Natural Analogues on Insulin Secretion. Broca C et al; Eur J Pharmacol, 2000 Mar 3, 390(3):339-45

66 4-Hydroxyisoleucine: A Novel Amino Acid Potentiator of Insulin Secretion. Sauvaire Y et al; Diabetes, 1998 Feb, 47(2):206-10

67 Glucose-Lowering Effect of Fenugreek in Non-Insulin Dependent Diabetics. Madar Z et al; Eur J Clin Nutr, 1988 Jan, 42(1):51-54

68 Effect of Fenugreek Seeds on Blood Glucose and Serum Lipids in Type I Diabetes. Sharma RD et al; Eur J Clin Nutr, 1990 Apr, 44(4):301-06

69   Effect of Fenugreek Seeds on Blood Lipid Peroxidation and Antioxidants in Diabetic Rats. Ravikumar P et al; Phytother Res, 1999 May, 13(3):197-201

70   Modulation of Some Gluconeogenic Enzyme Activities in Diabetic Rat Liver and Kidney: Effect of Antidiabetic Compounds. Gupta D et al; Indian J Exp Biol, 1999 Feb, 37(2):196-99

71   Alterations in Antioxidant Enzymes and Oxidative Damage in Experimental Diabetic Rat Tissues: Effect of Vanadate and Fenugreek (Trigonellafoenum graecum). Genet S et al; Mol Cell Biochem, 2002 Jul, 236(1-2):7-12

72   Influence of Dietary Spices and Their Active Principles on Pancreatic Digestive Enzymes in Albino Rats. Platel K et al; Nahrung, 2000 Feb, 44(1):42-46

73   Inhibitors of Human and Bovine Trypsin and Chymotrypsin in Fenugreek (Trigonella foenum-graecum) Seeds. Weder JK et al; Z Lebensm Unters Forsch, 1991 Sep, 193(3):242-46

74   Effects of a Fenugreek Seed Extract on Feeding Behaviour in the Rat: Metabolic-Endocrine Correlates. Petit P et al; Pharmacol Biochem Behav, 1993 Jun, 45(2):369-74

75   False Diagnosis of Maple Syrup Urine Disease Owing to Ingestion of Herbal Tea. Sewell AC et al; N Engl J Med, 1999 Sep 2, 341(10):769

76   Etiopathogenesis of Acute Pancreatitis. Karne S et al; Surg Clin North Am, 1999 Aug, 79(4):699-710 Review

77   Acute Pancreatitis: A Multisystem Disease. Agarwal N et al; Gastroenterologist, 1993 Jun, 1(2):115-28 Review

78   Diagnosis and Management of Acute Pancreatitis. Munoz A et al; Am Fam Physician, 2000 Jul 1, 62(1):164-74 Review

79   Management of Severe Acute Necrotising Pancreatitis. Wyncoll DL; Intensive Care Med, 1999 Feb, 25(2):146-56 Review

80   Current Principles of Treatment in Acute Pancreatitis. Puolakkainen P et al; Ann Chir Gynaecol, 1998, 87(3):200-03 Review

81   Chronic Pancreatitis: Diagnosis and Staging. Manes G et al; Ann Ital Chir, 2000 Jan-Feb, 71(1):23-32 Review

82   Chronic Pancreatitis: Pathogenesis and Molecular Aspects. Kleeff J et al; Ann Ital Chir, 2000 Jan-Feb, 71(1):3-10 Review

83   Medical Treatment of Chronic Pancreatitis. Gullo L; Ann Ital Chir, 2000 Jan-Feb;71(1):33-37 Review

84   Is There Still an Indication for Pancreatic Duct Drainage in Chronic Pancreatitis? Ihse I et al; Ann Ital Chir, 2000 Jan-Feb, 71(1):39-42 Review

85   Gastrointestinal Surgery and Gastroenterology. Chronic Pancreatitis: Surgical Aspects. van Gulik TM et al; Ned Tijdschr Geneeskd, 2000 Feb 5, 144(6):268-74 Review

86   Quality of Life and Long-Term Survival after Surgery for Chronic Pancreatitis. Sohn TA et al; J Gastrointest Surg, 2000 Jul-Aug, 4(4):355-65

87   Pancreatic Dysfunction and Treatment Options. Nakamura T et al; Pancreas, 1998 Apr, 16(3):329-36 Review

88   Gastric Acid Suppression and Treatment of Severe Exocrine Pancreatic Insufficiency. DiMagno EP; Best Pract Res Clin Gastroenterol, 2001 Jun, 15(3):477-86 Review

89   Secondary Diabetes in Chronic Pancreatitis. Raue G et al; Z Gastroenterol, 1999 Jun, Suppl 1:4-9 Review

90   Use of Gastric Acid-Inhibitory Drugs–Physiological and Pathophysiological Considerations. Waldum HL et al; Aliment Pharmacol Ther, 1993 Dec, 7(6):589-96 Review

91   Helicobacter Pylori and Peptic Ulcer Disease. Cello JP; AJR Am J Roentgenol, 1995 Feb, 164(2):283-86 Review

92   Management of Helicobacter Pylori Infection in Primary Care. Childs S et al; Fam Pract, 2000 Aug, 17 Suppl 2:S6-11 Review

93   Gastroenterology: Acid Research and Ulcer Therapy. Martinek J et al; Arzneimittelforschung, 1997 Dec, 47(12):1424-35 Review

94   Physiopathology of Helicobacter Pylori Infections. Gschwantler M et al; Acta Med Austriaca, 2000, 27(4):117-21 Review

95   Helicobacter Pylori. One Bacterium and a Broad Spectrum of Human Disease. Pakodi F et al; J Physiol Paris,

2000 Mar-Apr, 94(2):139-52 Review

96 Anxiety and Helplessness in the Face of Stress Predisposes, Precipitates, and Sustains Gastric Ulceration. Overmier JB et al; Behav Brain Res, 2000 Jun 1, 110(1-2):161-74 Review

97 Consensus Conference. Medical Treatment of Peptic Ulcer Disease. Practice Guidelines. Soll AH; JAMA, 1996 Feb 28, 275(8):622-29 Review

98 Cure of Helicobacter Pylori-Associated Ulcer Disease through Eradication. Malfertheiner P et al; Baillieres Best Pract Res Clin Gastroenterol, 2000 Feb, 14(1):119-32 Review

99 Association between Nonsteroidal Anti-Inflammatory Drugs and Upper Gastrointestinal Tract Bleeding/Perforation. Hernandez-Diaz S et al; Arch Intern Med, 2000 Jul 24, 160(14):2093-99 Review

100 How do NSAIDs Cause Ulcer Disease? Wallace JL; Baillieres Best Pract Res Clin Gastroenterol, 2000 Feb, 14(1):147-59 Review

101 Non-Steroidal Anti-Inflammatory Drugs (NSAIDs) and Gastro-Intestinal Toxicity. Shah AA et al; Ir J Med Sci, 1999 Oct-Dec, 168(4):242-45 Review

102 Gastric Mucosa-Associated Lymphoid Tissue Lymphoma. Ahmad A et al; Am J Gastroenterol, 2003 May, 98(5):975-86 Review

103 Gastric MALT Lymphoma, a Malignancy Potentially Curable by Eradication of Helicobacter Pylori. Delchier JC; Gastroenterol Clin Biol, 2003 Mar, 27(3 Pt 2):453-58 Review

104 Acid Reflux on the Esophagus. Mork H; MMW Fortschr Med, 2000 Apr 27, 142(17):26-29 Review

105 New Therapeutic Options in the Treatment of GERD and Other Acid-Peptic Disorders. Based on a Presentation by Duane D. Webb, MD, FACG. Am J Manag Care, 2000 May, 6(9 Suppl):S467-75 Review

106 Management of Gastroesophageal Reflux Disease. Stanghellini V; Drugs Today (Barc), 2003 Mar, 39 Suppl A:15-20 Review

107 Potential Gastrointestinal Effects of Long-Term Acid Suppression with Proton Pump Inhibitors. Laine L et al; Aliment Pharmacol Ther, 2000 Jun, 14(6):651-68 Review

108 Antacids Revisited. Maton PN et al; Drugs, 1999 Jun, 57(6):855-70 Review

109 Nonulcer Dyspepsia. Locke GR; Mayo Clin Proc, 1999 Oct, 74(10):1011-14 Review

110 Epidemiological Evidence on Helicobacter Pylori Infection and Nonulcer or Uninvestigated Dyspepsia. Danesh J et al; Arch Intern Med, 2000 Apr 24, 160(8):1192-98 Review

111 Eradication of Helicobacter Pylori for Non-Ulcer Dyspepsia. Moayyedi P et al; Cochrane Database Syst Rev, 2000; (2):CD002096 Review

112 Initial Management Strategies for Dyspepsia. Delaney BC et al; Cochrane Database Syst Rev,2000; (2):CD001961 Review

113 Update on the Role of Drug Therapy in Non-Ulcer Dyspepsia. Talley NJ; Rev Gastroenterol Disord, 2003 Winter, 3(1):25-30 Review

114 Effect of Lactic Acid Bacteria on Diarrheal Diseases. Heyman M; J Am Coll Nutr, 2000 Apr, 19(2 Suppl):137S-146S Review

115 Lactic Acid Bacteria and the Human Gastrointestinal Tract. Hove H et al; Eur J Clin Nutr, 1999 May, 53(5):339-50 Review

116 Effects of Probiotic Bacteria on Diarrhea, Lipid Metabolism, and Carcinogenesis. de Roos NM et al; Am J Clin Nutr, 2000 Feb, 71(2):405-11 Review

117 Probiotics, Infection and Immunity. Macfarlane GT et al; Curr Opin Infect Dis, 2002 Oct, 15(5):501-06 Review

118 Probiotics in Health Maintenance and Disease Prevention. Drisko JA et al; Altern Med Rev, 2003 Apr, 8(2):143-55

119 Intestinal Bacteria and Ulcerative Colitis. Cummings JH et al; Curr Issues Intest Microbiol, 2003 Mar, 4(1):9-20 Review

120 Intestinal Flora and Mucosal Immune Responses. Heller F et al; Int J Med Microbiol, 2003 Apr, 293(1):77-86 Review

121 Use of Probiotics in the Treatment of Inflammatory Bowel Disease. Hart AL et al; J Clin Gastroenterol, 2003

Feb, 36(2):111-19 Review

122   Common Complementary and Alternative Therapies for Yeast Vaginitis and Bacterial Vaginosis. Van Kessel K et al; Obstet Gynecol Surv, 2003 May, 58(5):351-58 Review

123   Role of Yoghurt in the Prevention of Colon Cancer. Perdigon G et al; Eur J Clin Nutr, 2002 Aug, 56 Suppl 3:S65-68 Review

124   Role of Probiotics in the Management of Patients with Food Allergy. Vanderhoof JA et al; Ann Allergy Asthma Immunol, 2003 Jun, 90(6 Suppl 3):99-103

125   Lactose Intolerance and Consumption of Milk and Milk Products. Sieber R et al; Z Ernahrungswiss, 1997 Dec, 36(4):375-93 Review

Chapter 11 – Liver

1   Formaldehyde and Hepatotoxicity. Beall JR et al; J Toxicol Environ Health, 1984, 14(1):1-21 Review

2   Regulation of Hepatic Glutathione Metabolism and its Role in Hepatotoxicity. Kretzschmar M; Exp Toxicol Pathol, 1996 Jul, 48(5):439-46 Review

3   Glutathione Metabolism and its Role in Hepatotoxicity. DeLeve LD et al; Pharmacol Ther, 1991 Dec, 52(3):287-305 Review

4   Mitochondrial Changes Associated with Glutathione Deficiency. Meister A; Biochim Biophys Acta, 1995 May 24, 1271(1):35-42 Review

5   Glutathione Deficiency Increases Hepatic Ascorbic Acid Synthesis in Adult Mice. Martensson J et al; Proc Natl Acad Sci U S A, 1992 Dec 1, 89(23):11566-68

6   Glutathione Depletion: Its Effects on Other Antioxidant Systems and Hepatocellular Damage. Comporti M et al; Xenobiotica, 1991 Aug, 21(8):1067-76 Review

7   Role of Oxidative Stress in the Selective Toxicity of Dieldrin in the Mouse Liver. Bachowski S et al; Toxicol Appl Pharmacol, 1998 Jun, 150(2):301-09

8   Pentachlorophenol-Induced Oxidative DNA Damage in Mouse Liver and Protective Effect of Antioxidants. Sai-Kato K et al; Food Chem Toxicol, 1995 Oct, 33(10):877-82

9   Spermatogenic Disturbance Induced by Di-(2-Ethylhexyl) Phthalate is Significantly Prevented by Treatment with Antioxidant Vitamins in the Rat. Ishihara M et al; Int J Androl, 2000 Apr, 23(2):85-94

10   Vitamin C in CCl4 Hepatotoxicity. Ademuyiwa O et al; Hum Exp Toxicol, 1994 Feb, 13(2):107-09

11   Alcohol-Induced Generation of Lipid Peroxidation Products in Humans. Meagher EA et al; J Clin Invest, 1999 Sep, 104(6):805-13

12   Oxidative Stress in Viral and Alcoholic Hepatitis. Loguercio C et al; Free Radic Biol Med, 2003 Jan 1, 34(1):1-10 Review

13   Management of Acetaminophen Toxicity. Larsen LC et al; Am Fam Physician, 1996 Jan, 53(1):185-90 Review

14   Influence of Ascorbic Acid Esters on Acetaminophen-Induced Hepatotoxicity in Mice. Mitra A et al; Toxicol Lett, 1988 Nov, 44(1-2):39-46

15   Comparison of the Effects of Ascorbyl Palmitate and L-ascorbic Acid on paracetamol-Induced Hepatotoxicity in the Mouse. Jonker D et al; Toxicology, 1988 Nov 30, 52(3):287-95

16   Humoral and Cellular Indices of Nonspecific Resistance in Viral Hepatitis A and Ascorbic Acid. Vasil'ev VS et al; Ter Arkh, 1989, 61(11):44-46

17   Ascorbic Acid Level and the Indicators of Cellular Immunity in Patients with Hepatitis A during Pathogenetic Therapy. Vasil'ev VS et al; Vopr Pitan, 1988 Jul-Aug, (4):31-34

18   Vitamin C Prophylaxis for Posttransfusion Hepatitis: Lack of Effect in a Controlled Trial. Knodell RG et al; Am J Clin Nutr, 1981 Jan, 34(1):20-23

19   Oxidative Stress in Chronic Hepatitis C: Not just a Feature of Late Stage Disease. Jain SK et al; J Hepatol, 2002 Jun, 36(6):805-11

20   Retroviruses, Ascorbate, and Mutations in the Evolution of Homo sapiens. Challem JJ et al; Free Radic Biol Med, 1998 Jul 1, 25(1):130-32 Review

21 Milk Thistle (Silybum marianum) for the Therapy of Liver Disease. Flora K et al; Am J Gastroenterol, 1998 Feb, 93(2):139-43 Review

22 Plants Used in the Treatment of Liver Disease. Luper S; Altern Med Rev, 1998 Dec, 3(6):410-21 Review

23 St. Mary's Thistle: An Overview. Laekeman G et al; J Pharm Belg, 2003, 58(1):28-31 Review

24 Biochemical Bases of the Pharmacological Action of the Flavonoid Silymarin and of its Structural Isomer Silibinin. Valenzuela A et al; Biol Res, 1994, 27(2):105-12

25 Advances in Pharmacological Studies of Silymarin. Rui YC; Mem Inst Oswaldo Cruz, 1991, 86 Suppl 2:79-85 Review

26 Alcohol and Liver Fibrosis–Pathobiochemistry and Treatment. Schuppan D et al; Z Gastroenterol, 1995 Sep, 33(9):546-50 Review

27 Liver-Protective Action of Silymarin Therapy in Chronic Alcoholic Liver Diseases. Feher J et al; Orv Hetil 1989, Dec 17, 130(51):2723-27 Review

28 Insulin Resistance: Lifestyle and Nutritional Interventions. Kelly GS; Altern Med Rev,2000 Apr, 5(2):109-32 Review

29 Oxidative Stress in the Liver and Biliary Tract Diseases. Feher J et al; Scand J Gastroenterol Suppl, 1998, 228:38-46 Review

30 Immunomodulator Effect of Silymarin Therapy in Chronic Alcoholic Liver Diseases. Deak G et al; Orv Hetil, 1990 Jun 17, 131(24):1291-92, 1295-96 Review

31 Treatment of Amanita Mushroom Poisoning. Parish RC et al; Vet Hum Toxicol, 1986 Aug, 28(4):318-22 Review

32 Experimental Basis for the Therapy of Amanita phalloides. Floersheim GL; Schweiz Med Wochenschr, 1978 Feb 11, 108(6):185-97 Review

33 Silymarin as a Potential Hypocholesterolaemic Drug. Skottova N et al; Physiol Res, 1998, 47(1):1-7 Review

34 Earlier Charcoal Haemoperfusion in Fulminant Hepatic Failure. Gimson AE et al; Lancet, 1982 Sep 25, 2(8300):681-83

35 Biochemical Correlates of Reversal of Hepatic Coma Coated with Charcoal Hemoperfusion. Gelfand MC et al; Trans Am Soc Artif Intern Organs, 1978, 24:239-42

36 Reduction of Diazepam Serum Half Life and Reversal of Coma by Activated Charcoal in a Patient with Severe Liver Disease. Traeger SM et al; J Toxicol Clin Toxicol, 1986, 24(4):329-37

37 Haemoperfusion through Activated Charcoal in Dogs with Fulminant Liver Failure. Horak J et al; Digestion, 1980, 20(1):22-30

38 In-vitro Assessment of the Removal of Phenols by ACAC Hemoperfusion. Kaziuka EN et al; Int J Artif Organs, 1979 Jul, 2(4):215-21

39 Efficacy of Charcoal Hemoperfusion in Paraquat Poisoning. Tabei K et al; Artif Organs, 1982 Feb, 6(1):37-42

40 Model for Theophylline Overdose Treatment with Oral Activated Charcoal. Radomski L et al; Clin Pharmacol Ther, 1984 Mar, 35(3):402-08

41 Prevention of T-2 Toxin-Induced Morphologic Effects in the Rat by Highly Activated Charcoal. Bratich PM et al; Arch Toxicol, 1990, 64(3):251-53

42 Misadventures with Activated Charcoal and Recommendations for Safe Use. Mauro LS et al; Ann Pharmacother, 1994 Jul-Aug, 28(7-8):915-24 Review

43 Frequency of Complications Associated with the Use of Multiple-Dose Activated Charcoal. Dorrington CL et al; Ann Emerg Med, 2003 Mar, 41(3):370-77

44 Peroral Application of Synthetic Activated Charcoal in USSR. Nikolaev VG; Biomater Artif Cells Artif Organs, 1990, 18(4):555-68 Review

45 Adverse Effects of Superactivated Charcoal Administered to Healthy Volunteers. Sato RL et al; Hawaii Med J, 2002 Nov, 61(11):251-53

46 Environmental Pollution and Allergy. Ring J et al; Ann Allergy Asthma Immunol, 2001 Dec, 87(6 Suppl 3):2-6 Review

47 Antioxidant Vitamins and Prevention of Lung Disease. Menzel DB; Ann N Y Acad Sci, 1992 Sep 30, 669:141-

55 Review

48   Synergistic Mechanisms in Carcinogenesis by Polycyclic Aromatic Hydrocarbons and by Tobacco Smoke. Rubin H; Carcinogenesis, 2001 Dec, 22(12):1903-30 Review

49   Toxicology of the Synthetic Antioxidants BHA and BHT in Comparison with the Natural Antioxidant Vitamin E. Kahl R et al; Z Lebensm Unters Forsch, 1993 Apr, 196(4):329-38 Review

50   Cytotoxicity of Propyl Gallate and Related Compounds in Rat Hepatocytes. Nakagawa Y et al; Arch Toxicol, 1995, 69(3):204-08

51   Effect of Ascorbic Acid on the Hepatotoxicity due to the Daily Intake of Nitrate, Nitrite and Dimethylamine. Garcia Roche MO et al; Nahrung, 1987, 31(2):99-104

52   Food Heating and the Formation of Heterocyclic Aromatic Amine and Polycyclic Aromatic Hydrocarbon Mutagens/Carcinogens. Knize MG et al; Adv Exp Med Biol, 1999, 459:179-93 Review

53   Carcinogenic Heterocyclic Amines in Model Systems and Cooked Foods: Formation, Occurrence and Intake. Skog KI et al; Food Chem Toxicol, 1998 Sep-Oct, 36(9-10):879-96 Review

54   Excitotoxins in Foods. Olney JW; Neurotoxicology, 1994 Fall, 15(3):535-44 Review

55   Saccharin Mechanistic Data and Risk Assessment: Urine Composition, Enhanced Cell Proliferation, and Tumor Promotion. Whysner J et al; Pharmacol Ther, 1996, 71(1-2):225-52 Review

56   Assessment of the Carcinogenicity of the Nonnutritive Sweetener Cyclamate. Ahmed FE et al; Crit Rev Toxicol, 1992, 22(2):81-118 Review

57   Evaluation of Certain Food Additives and Contaminants. World Health Organ Tech Rep Ser, 1997, 868:1-69

58   Functional Relationship between Artificial Food Colors and Hyperactivity. Rose TL; J Appl Behav Anal, 1978 Winter, 11(4):439-46

59   Synergistic Effects of Food Colors on the Toxicity of 3-Amino-1,4-Dimethyl-5H-Pyrido[4,3-b]Indole (Trp-P-1) in Primary Cultured Rat Hepatocytes. Ashida H et al; J Nutr Sci Vitaminol (Tokyo), 2000 Jun, 46(3):130-36

60   Reproductive Toxicity of Erythrosine in Male Mice. Abdel Aziz AH et al; Pharmacol Res, 1997 May, 35(5):457-62

61   DNA Damage Induced by Red Food Dyes Orally Administered to Pregnant and Male Mice. Tsuda S et al; Toxicol Sci, 2001 May, 61(1):92-99

62   Immunotoxicity of the Colour Additive Caramel Colour III. Houben GF et al; Toxicology, 1994 Aug 12, 91(3):289-302 Review

63   Aldehydes: Occurrence, Carcinogenic Potential, Mechanism of Action and Risk Assessment. Feron VJ et al; Mutat Res, 1991 Mar-Apr, 259(3-4):363-85 Review

64   Reaction of Furfural and Methylfurfural with DNA. Shahabuddin; Food Chem Toxicol, 1991 Oct, 29(10):719-21

65   Time- and Dose-Dependent Development of Potassium Bromate-Induced Tumors in Male Fischer 344 Rats. Wolf DC et al; Toxicol Pathol, 1998 Nov-Dec, 26(6):724-29

66   Two-Year Toxicity and Carcinogenicity Study of Methyleugenol in F344/N Rats and B6C3F(1) Mice. Johnson JD et al; J Agric Food Chem, 2000 Aug, 48(8):3620-32

67   Ninety-Day Feeding Study in Fischer-344 Rats of Highly Refined Petroleum-Derived Food-Grade White Oils and Waxes. Smith JH et al; Toxicol Pathol, 1996 Mar-Apr, 24(2):214-30

68   Final Report on the Safety Assessment of Benzyl Alcohol, Benzoic Acid, and Sodium Benzoate. Nair B; Int J Toxicol, 2001, 20 Suppl 3:23-50

69   Safety Assessment of Propyl Paraben. Soni MG et al; Food Chem Toxicol, 2001 Jun, 39(6):513-32 Review

70   Methyldibromoglutaronitrile (Euxyl K400). Jackson JM et al; J Am Acad Dermatol, 1998 Jun, 38(6 Pt 1):934-37

71   Fate and Effects of the Surfactant Sodium Dodecyl Sulfate. Singer MM et al; Rev Environ Contam Toxicol, 1993, 133:95-149

72   Mutagenicity of Azo Dyes: Structure-Activity Relationships. Chung KT; Mutat Res, 1992 Sep, 277(3):201-20 Review

73   Genotoxic Hazards of Azo Pigments and Other Colorants Related to 1-Phenylazo-2-Hydroxynaphthalene. Moller P et al; Mutat Res, 2000 Jan, 462(1):13-30 Review

74   Effect of Inhalation of Hair Spray on the Rat Respiratory System. Pages G et al; Bull Eur Physiopathol Respir, 1986 Jan-Feb, 22(1):9-14

75   Acute Exposure to Hair Bleach Causes Airway Hyperresponsiveness in a Rabbit Model. Mensing T et al; Eur Respir J, 1998 Dec, 12(6):1371-74

76   Toxic Effects of Potassium Bromate and Thioglycolate on Vestibuloocular Reflex Systems of Guinea Pigs and Humans. Young YH et al; Toxicol Appl Pharmacol, 2001 Dec 1, 177(2):103-11

77   Embryotoxicity of Zinc Pyrithione, Antidandruff Chemical, in Fish. Goka K; Environ Res, 1999 Jul, 81(1):81-83

78   Evaluation of Health Risks Caused by Musk Ketone. Schmeiser HH et al; Int J Hyg Environ Health, 2001 May, 203(4):293-99 Review

79   Developmental Toxicity Studies of Four Fragrances in Rats. Christian MS et al; Toxicol Lett, 1999 Dec 20, 111(1-2):169-74

80   Acute Hepatotoxicity of the Polycyclic Musk 7-Acetyl-1,1,3,4,4,6-Hexamethyl-1,2,3,4-Tetrahydronaphtaline (AHTN). Steinberg P et al; Toxicol Lett, 1999 Dec 20, 111(1-2):151-60

81   AHTN and HHCB Show Weak Estrogenic–But No Uterotrophic Activity. Seinen W et al; Toxicol Lett, 1999 Dec 20, 111(1-2):161-68

82   Photosensitivity Associated with Antibacterial Agents. Wainwright NJ et al; Drug Saf, 1993 Dec, 9(6):437-40 Review

83   Effects of Sanguinarium, Chlorhexidine and Tetracycline on Neutrophil Viability and Functions in Vitro. Agarwal S et al; J Periodontal Res, 1997 Apr, 32(3):335-44

84   Cytotoxicity of Sanguinarine Chloride to Cultured Human Cells from Oral Tissue. Babich H et al; Pharmacol Toxicol, 1996 Jun, 78(6):397-403

85   Effect of Sodium Hypochlorite and Chlorhexidine on Cultured Human Periodontal Ligament Cells. Chang YC et al; Oral Surg Oral Med Oral Pathol Oral Radiol Endod, 2001 Oct, 92(4):446-50

86   Chlorhexidine Mouthwash-Induced Fixed Drug Eruption. Moghadam BK et al; Oral Surg Oral Med Oral Pathol, 1991 Apr, 71(4):431-34 Review

87   Triclosan: Cytotoxicity, Mode of Action, and Induction of Apoptosis in Human Gingival Cells in Vitro. Zuckerbraun HL et al; Eur J Oral Sci, 1998 Apr, 106(2 Pt 1):628-36

88   Pustular Allergic Contact Dermatitis to Isoconazole Nitrate. Lazarov A et al; Am J Contact Dermat, 1997 Dec, 8(4):229-30 Review

89   Assessment of the In Vivo Genotoxicity of 2-Hydroxy 4-Methoxybenzophenone. Robison SH et al; Environ Mol Mutagen, 1994, 23(4):312-17

90   Chemical Oxidation and DNA Damage Catalysed by Inorganic Sunscreen Ingredients. Dunford R et al; FEBS Lett, 1997 Nov 24, 418(1-2):87-90

91   Aplastic Anemia Associated with Canthaxanthin Ingested for 'Tanning' Purposes. Bluhm R et al; JAMA, 1990 Sep 5, 264(9):1141-42

92   Immunotoxicity of 180-Day Exposure to Polydimethylsiloxane (Silicone) Fluid, Gel and Elastomer and Polyurethane Disks in Female B6C3F1 Mice. Bradley SG et al; Drug Chem Toxicol, 1994, 17(3):221-69

93   Nail Polish Removers: Are They Harmful? Kechijian P; Semin Dermatol, 1991 Mar, 10(1):26-28

94   Gamma Butyrolactone Poisoning and its Similarities to Gamma Hydroxybyric Acid. Rambourg-Schepens MO et al; Vet Hum Toxicol, 1997 Aug 39(4):234-35 Review

95   Toxicology of Acetonitrile. Hashimoto K; Sangyo Igaku, 1991 Nov, 33(6):463-74 Review

96   Reactive Chemicals and Cancer. Blair A et al; Cancer Causes Control, 1997 May, 8(3):473-90 Review

97   Common Commercial Cosmetic Products Induce Arthritis in the DA Rat. Sverdrup B et al; Environ Health Perspect, 1998 Jan, 106(1):27-32

98   Toxic Effects of Air Freshener Emissions. Anderson RC et al; Arch Environ Health, 1997 Nov-Dec, 52(6):433-41

99 OTC Pharmaceuticals and Genotoxicity Testing. Muller L et al; Arch Toxicol Suppl, 1995, 17:312-25 Review

100 Nonsteroidal Anti-Inflammatory Drug-Associated Toxicity of the Liver, Lower Gastrointestinal Tract, and Esophagus. Bjorkman D; Am J Med, 1998 Nov 2, 105(5A):17S-21S Review

101 Nonnarcotic Analgesics. McGoldrick MD et al; Ann Pharmacother, 1997 Feb, 31(2):221-27 Review

102 Fetal Consequences and Risks Attributed to the Use of Prescribed and Over-The-Counter (OTC) Preparations during Pregnancy. Kacew S; Int J Clin Pharmacol Ther, 1994 Jul, 32(7):335-43 Review

103 Assessment of the Genotoxic Risk from Laxative Senna Products. Brusick D et al; Environ Mol Mutagen, 1997, 29(1):1-9 Review

104 Insights into the Mechanism of Action of Benzoyl Peroxide as a Tumor Promoter. Rudra N et al; Indian J Physiol Pharmacol, 1997 Apr, 41(2):109-15.

105 Hepatic Side-Effects of Antibiotics. Westphal JF et al; J Antimicrob Chemother, 1994 Mar, 33(3):387-401 Review

106 Hepatic Diseases Caused by Drugs. Lammert F et al; Schweiz Rundsch Med Prax, 1997 Jul 16, 86(29-30):1167-71 Review

107 Photomutagenicity of Fluoroquinolones and Other Drugs. Gocke E et al; Toxicol Lett, 1998 Dec 28, 102-103:375-81 Review

108 Hepatotoxicity of Anesthetics and Other Central Nervous System Drugs. Holt C et al; Gastroenterol Clin North Am, 1995 Dec, 24(4):853-74 Review

109 Adverse Reactions to New Anticonvulsant Drugs. Wong IC et al; Drug Saf, 2000 Jul, 23(1):35-56 Review

110 Chlorinated Methanes and Liver Injury. Plaa GL; Annu Rev Pharmacol Toxicol, 2000, 40:42-65 Review

111 Cardiac Toxicity of Anabolic Steroids. Sullivan ML et al; Prog Cardiovasc Dis, 1998 Jul-Aug, 41(1):1-15 Review

112 Acitretin in Psoriasis: An Overview of Adverse Effects. Katz HI et al; J Am Acad Dermatol, 1999 Sep, 41(3 Pt 2):S7-S12 Review

113 Drug-Induced Pneumonitis: The Role of Methotrexate. Zisman DA et al; Sarcoidosis Vasc Diffuse Lung Dis, 2001 Oct, 18(3):243-52 Review

114 Side Effects of Chemotherapy and Combined Chemohormonal Therapy in Women with Early-Stage Breast Cancer. Partridge AH et al; J Natl Cancer Inst Monogr, 2001, (30):135-42 Review

115 Drug-Induced Hepatic Diseases. Biour M et al; Pathol Biol (Paris), 1999 Nov, 47(9):928-37 Review

116 Drug-Induced Hepatic Disorders: Incidence, Management and Avoidance. Dossing M et al; Drug Saf, 1993 Dec, 9(6):441-49 Review

117 Potential Risks and Prevention: Fatal Adverse Drug Events. Kelly WN; Am J Health Syst Pharm, 2001 Jul 15, 58(14):1317-24 Review

118 Adverse Drug Events in Hospitalized Patients. Excess Length of Stay, Extra Costs, and Attributable Mortality. Classen DC et al; JAMA, 1997 Jan 22-29, 277(4):301-06

119 Neurotoxicity Risk of Selected Hydrocarbon Fuels. Ritchie GD et al; J Toxicol Environ Health B Crit Rev, 2001 Jul-Sep, 4(3):223-312 Review

120 Carcinogenic Potential of Gasoline. Raabe GK; Environ Health Perspect, 1993 Dec, 101 Suppl 6:35-38 Review

121 New Evidence Regarding the Relationship of Gasoline Exposure to Kidney Cancer and Leukemia. Enterline PE; Environ Health Perspect,1993 Dec, 101 Suppl 6:101-03 Review

122 Toxicological and Epidemiological Evidence for Health Risks from Inhaled Engine Emissions. Mauderly JL; Environ Health Perspect, 1994 Oct, 102 Suppl 4:165-71 Review

123 Toxicology and Human Health Effects Following Exposure to Oxygenated or Reformulated Gasoline. Ahmed FE; Toxicol Lett, 2001 Sep 15, 123(2-3):89-113 Review

124 Manganese in the U.S. Gasoline Supply. Frumkin H et al; Am J Ind Med, 1997 Jan, 31(1):107-15

125 Toxicity of Benzene and its Metabolism and Molecular Pathology in Human Risk Assessment. Yardley-Jones A et al; Br J Ind Med, 1991 Jul, 48(7):437-44 Review

126 Plasticizer Diethylhexyl Phthalate Induces Malformations by Decreasing Fetal Testosterone Synthesis during Sexual Differentiation in the Male Rat. Parks LG et al; Toxicol Sci, 2000 Dec, 58(2):339-49

127 Carcinogenicity of Di(2-Ethylhexyl) Phthalate (DEHP) in Perspective. Kluwe WM et al; J Toxicol Environ Health, 1983 Jul, 12(1):159-69

128 Potential Health Effects of Phthalate Esters in Children's Toys. Wilkinson CF et al; Regul Toxicol Pharmacol, 1999 Oct, 30(2 Pt 1):140-55 Review

129 Two Episodes of Ethylene Oxide Poisoning. Lin TJ et al; Kaohsiung J Med Sci, 2001 Jun, 17(7):372-76

130 Health Impact of Polychlorinated Dibenzo-p-Dioxins. Mukerjee D; J Air Waste Manag Assoc, 1998 Feb, 48(2):157-65 Review

131 Toxic Encephalopathy Associated with Use of DEET Insect Repellents: A Case Analysis of its Toxicity in Children. Briassoulis G et al; Hum Exp Toxicol, 2001 Jan, 20(1):8-14 Review

132 Pesticide-Induced Oxidative Stress. Banerjee BD et al; Rev Environ Health, 2001 Jan-Mar, 16(1):1-40 Review

133 Toxic Threats to Neurologic Development of Children. Schettler T et al; Environ Health Perspect, 2001 Dec, 109 Suppl 6:813-16 Review

134 Fate and Effects of Diazinon. Larkin DJ et al; Rev Environ Contam Toxicol, 2000, 166:49-82 Review

135 Genetic Toxicity of Malathion. Flessel P et al; Environ Mol Mutagen, 1993, 22(1):7-17 Review

136 Organophosphates and Their Impact on the Global Environment. Satoh T et al; Neurotoxicology, 2000 Feb-Apr, 21(1-2):223-27 Review

137 Variation of Pesticide Residues in Fruits and Vegetables and the Associated Assessment of Risk. Hamey PY et al; Regul Toxicol Pharmacol, 1999 Oct, 30(2 Pt 2):S34-41 Review

138 Pesticide Exposure: Human Cancers on the Horizon. Jaga K et al; Rev Environ Health, 1999 Jan-Mar, 14(1):39-50 Review

139 Mechanistic Model Predicts a U-Shaped Relation of Radon Exposure to Lung Cancer Risk Reflected in Combined Occupational and US Residential Data. Bogen KT; Hum Exp Toxicol, 1998 Dec, 17(12):691-96 Review

140 Neurotoxicology and Pathology of Organomercury, Organolead, and Organotin. Chang LW; J Toxicol Sci, 1990 Dec, 15 Suppl 4:125-51 Review

141 Low-Level Lead Exposure and Children's Intelligence from Recent Epidemiological Studies in the U.S.A. and Other Countries. Koike S; Nippon Eiseigaku Zasshi, 1997 Oct, 52(3):552-61 Review

142 Perspectives on Lead Toxicity. Lockitch G; Clin Biochem, 1993 Oct, 26(5):371-81 Review

143 Toxicology of Mercury. Clarkson TW; Crit Rev Clin Lab Sci, 1997 Aug, 34(4):369-403 Review

144 Amalgam–Resurrection and Redemption: The Medical Mythology of Anti-Amalgam. Wahl MJ; Quintessence Int, 2001 Oct, 32(9):696-710 Review.

145 Documented Clinical Side-Effects to Dental Amalgam. Ziff MF; Adv Dent Res, 1992 Sep, 6:131-34 Review

146 Aluminum–Occurrence and Toxicity for Organisms. Ochmanski W et al; Przegl Lek, 2000, 57(11):665-68 Review

147 Comparison of Pediatric Poisoning Hazards: An Analysis of 3.8 Million Exposure Incidents. Litovitz T et al; Pediatrics, 1992 Jun, 89(6 Pt 1):999-1006

148 Prevention of Nickel Contact Dermatitis. Gawkrodger DJ et al; Contact Dermatitis, 1995 May, 32(5):257-65 Review

149 Mechanisms of Nephrotoxicity from Metal Combinations. Madden EF et al; Drug Chem Toxicol, 2000 Feb, 23(1):1-12 Review

150 Metal Toxicity and the Respiratory Tract. Nemery B; Eur Respir J, 1990 Feb, 3(2):202-19 Review

151 Food-Related Illness and Death in the United States. Mead PS et al; Emerg Infect Dis, 1999 Sep-Oct, 5(5):607-25 Review

152 Infectious Diarrhea. Goodman L et al; Dis Mon, 1999 Jul, 45(7):268-99 Review

153 Microbial Food Borne Pathogens. Salmonella. Ekperigin HE et al; Vet Clin North Am Food Anim Pract, 1998 Mar, 14(1):17-29 Review

154 Staphylococcus aureus Small Colony Variants . von Eiff C et al; Int J Clin Pract Suppl, 2000 Dec, (115):44-49 Review

155 Characteristics and Molecular Biology of Verotoxin Produced by Enterohemorrhagic Escherichia coli. Iijima Y et al; Nippon Rinsho,1997 Mar, 55(3):646-50

156 Botulinum Toxin: From Poison to Drug. Kreyden OP et al; Hautarzt, 2000 Oct, 51(10):733-37 Review

157 Toxigenic Fungi. Pitt JI et al; Med Mycol, 2000, 38 Suppl 1:17-22 Review

158 Chemistry and Biology of Aflatoxin B(1). Smela ME et al; Carcinogenesis, 2001 Apr, 22(4):535-45 Review

159 Prevention of Nephrotoxicity of Ochratoxin A, Food Contaminant. Creppy EE et al; Toxicol Lett, 1995 Dec, 82-83:869-77 Review

160 Dietary Soya Lecithin Decreases Plasma Triglyceride Levels and Inhibits Collagen- and ADP-induced Platelet Aggregation. Brook JG et al; Biochem Med Metab Biol, 1986 Feb, 35(1):31-39

161 Effects of Long-Term Ingestion of Soya Phospholipids on Serum Lipids in Humans. Tompkins RK et al; Am J Surg, 1980 Sep, 140(3):360-64

162 Cholesterol-Lowering and HDL-Raising Properties of Lecithinated Soy Proteins in Type II Hyperlipidemic Patients. Sirtori CR et al; Ann Nutr Metab, 1985, 29(6):348-57

163 Lecithin has No Effect on Serum Lipoprotein, Plasma Fibrinogen and Macro Molecular Protein Complex Levels in Hyperlipidaemic Men. Oosthuizen W et al; Eur J Clin Nutr, 1998 Jun, 52(6):419-24

164 Soy Lecithin Reduces Plasma Lipoprotein Cholesterol and Early Atherogenesis in Hypercholesterolemic Monkeys and Hamsters. Wilson TA et al; Atherosclerosis, 1998 Sep, 140(1):147-53

165 Evidence that Polyunsaturated Lecithin Induces a Reduction in Plasma Cholesterol Level and Favorable Changes in Lipoprotein Composition in Hypercholesterolemic Rats. Jimenez MA et al; J Nutr, 1990 Jul, 120(7):659-67

166 Comparison of the Effects of Feeding Linoleic Acid-Rich Lecithin or Corn Oil on Cholesterol Absorption and Metabolism in the Rat. O'Mullane JE et al; Atherosclerosis, 1982 Oct, 45(1):81-90

167 Cholesterol-Lowering Effect of Soyabean Lecithin in Normolipidaemic Rats by Stimulation of Biliary Lipid Secretion. Polichetti E et al; Br J Nutr, 1996 Mar, 75(3):471-78

168 Influence of Dietary Soybean and Egg Lecithins on Lipid Responses in Cholesterol-Fed Guinea Pigs. O'Brien BC et al; Lipids, 1988 Jul. 23(7):647-50

169 Hyperlipoproteinaemia and Atherosclerosis in Rabbits fed Low-Level Cholesterol and Lecithin. Hunt CE et al; Br J Exp Pathol, 1985 Feb, 66(1):35-46

170 Overview of Reverse Cholesterol Transport. Tall AR; Eur Heart J, 1998 Feb, 19 Suppl A:A31-35 Review

171 Reverse Cholesterol Transport: Its Contribution to Cholesterol Catabolism in Normal and Disease States. Loh KC et al; Can J Cardiol, 1996 Oct, 12(10):944-50 Review

172 Lecithin-Cholesterol Acyltransferase: Role in Lipoprotein Metabolism, Reverse Cholesterol Transport and Atherosclerosis. Santamarina-Fojo S et al; Curr Opin Lipidol, 2000 Jun, 11(3):267-75 Review

173 Antiatherogenic Role of High-Density Lipoprotein Cholesterol. Kwiterovich PO; Am J Cardiol, 1998 Nov 5, 82(9A):13Q-21Q Review

174 Emerging Importance of HDL Cholesterol in Developing High-Risk Coronary Plaques in Acute Coronary Syndromes. Viles-Gonzalez JF et al; Curr Opin Cardiol, 2003 Jul, 18(4):286-94

175 Hypocholesterolemic Statins. Evaluation and Prospects. Dairou F; Presse Med, 1994 Sep 24, 23(28):1304-10

176 Comparison of Properties of Four Inhibitors of 3-Hydroxy-3-Methylglutaryl-Coenzyme A Reductase. Blum CB; Am J Cardiol, 1994 May 26, 73(14):3D-11D Review

177 Atorvastatin (Lipitor). Carpentier Y et al; Rev Med Brux, 1999 Oct, 20(5):427-33 Review

178 Quantifying Effect of Statins on Low Density Lipoprotein Cholesterol, Ischaemic Heart Disease, and Stroke. Law MR et al; BMJ, 2003 Jun 28, 326(7404):1423 Review

179 Pharmacogenomics and Pharmacogenetics of Cholesterol-Lowering Therapy. Schmitz G et al; Clin Chem Lab Med, 2003 Apr, 41(4):581-89 Review

180 Statins as Potential Therapeutic Agents in Neuroinflammatory Disorders. Stuve O et al; Curr Opin Neurol, 2003 Jun, 16(3):393-401

181 Use of In Vivo Models to Study the Role of Cholesterol in the Etiology of Alzheimer's Disease. Burns M et al; Neurochem Res, 2003 Jul, 28(7):979-86 Review

182 Defining Patient Risks from Expanded Preventive Therapies. Tolman KG; Am J Cardiol, 2000 Jun 22, 85(12A):15E-9E Review

183 Hepatotoxicity of Hydroxy-Methyl-Glutaryl-Coenzyme A Reductase Inhibitors. Ballare M et al; Minerva Gastroenterol Dietol, 1992 Jan-Mar, 38(1):41-44

184 Proteomics to Display Lovastatin-Induced Protein and Pathway Regulation in Rat Liver. Steiner S et al; Electrophoresis, 2000 Jun, 21(11):2129-37

185 Statin-Associated Myopathy. Thompson PD et al; JAMA, 2003 Apr 2, 289(13):1681-90 Review

186 In Vitro Myotoxicity of the 3-Hydroxy-3-Methylglutaryl Coenzyme A Reductase Inhibitors, Pravastatin, Lovastatin, and Simvastatin. Masters BA et al; Toxicol Appl Pharmacol, 1995 Mar, 131(1):163-74

187 Carcinogenicity of Lipid-Lowering Drugs. Newman TB et al; JAMA, 1996 Jan 3, 275(1):55-60 Review

188 Cholesterol Based Antineoplastic Strategies. Lenz M et al; Anticancer Res, 1997 Mar-Apr, 17(2A):1143-46

189 Phase I Study of Lovastatin, an Inhibitor of the Mevalonate Pathway, in Patients with Cancer. Thibault A et al; Clin Cancer Res, 1996 Mar, 2(3):483-91

190 Phase I-II Trial of Lovastatin for Anaplastic Astrocytoma and Glioblastoma Multiforme. Larner J et al; Am J Clin Oncol, 1998 Dec, 21(6):579-83

191 Statins as Anticancer Agents. Chan KK et al; Clin Cancer Res, 2003 Jan, 9(1):10-19 Review

192 Choline: An Important Nutrient in Brain Development, Liver Function and Carcinogenesis. Zeisel SH; J Am Coll Nutr, 1992 Oct, 11(5):473-81 Review

193 Lecithin and Choline in Human Health and Disease. Canty DJ et al; Nutr Rev, 1994 Oct, 52(10):327-39 Review

194 Membrane Breakdown in Acute and Chronic Neurodegeneration: Focus on Choline-Containing Phospholipids. Klein J; J Neural Transm, 2000, 107(8-9):1027-63 Review

195 Reappraising Neurotransmitter-Based Strategies. Moller HJ; Eur Neuropsychopharmacol, 1999 Apr, 9 Suppl 2:S53-59 Review

196 Choline and Human Nutrition. Zeisel SH et al; Annu Rev Nutr, 1994, 14:269-96 Review

197 Choline: A Nutrient Involved in the Regulation of Cell Proliferation, Cell Death, and Cell Transformation. Zeisel SH; Adv Exp Med Biol, 1996, 399:131-41 Review

198 Inositol–Clinical Applications for Exogenous Use. Colodny L et al; Altern Med Rev, 1998 Dec, 3(6):432-47 Review

199 Inositol Lipid Cycle and Autonomous Nuclear Signalling. Cocco L et al; Adv Enzyme Regul, 1996, 36:101-14 Review

200 Inositol Phosphates - Intracellular Signalling. Irvine R et al; Curr Biol, 1996 May 1, 6(5):537-40 Review

201 Metabolism and Function of Myo-Inositol and Inositol Phospholipids. Holub BJ; Annu Rev Nutr, 1986, 6:563-97 Review

202 Inositol Trisphosphate and Calcium: Two Interacting Second Messengers. Berridge MJ; Am J Nephrol, 1997, 17(1):1-11 Review

203 Nutritional Significance, Metabolism, and Function of Myo-Inositol and Phosphatidylinositol in Health and Disease. Holub BJ; Adv Nutr Res, 1982, 4:107-41 Review

204 Inositol for Respiratory Distress Syndrome in Preterm Infants. Howlett A et al; Cochrane Database Syst Rev, 2000, (2):CD000366 Review

205 Gallstones, from Gallbladder to Gut. Management Options for Diverse Complications. Agrawal S et al; Postgrad Med, 2000 Sep 1, 108(3):143-6, 149-53 Review

206 Physical and Metabolic Factors in Gallstone Pathogenesis. Donovan JM; Gastroenterol Clin North Am, 1999 Mar, 28(1):75-97 Review

207 Pathogenesis of Gallstones. Dowling RH; Aliment Pharmacol Ther, 2000 May, 14 Suppl 2:39-47 Review

208 Gallstone Formation. Local Factors. Ko CW et al; Gastroenterol Clin North Am, 1999 Mar, 28(1):99-115

Review

209 Clinical Correlates of Gallstone Composition: Distinguishing Pigment from Cholesterol Stones. Diehl AK et al; Am J Gastroenterol, 1995 Jun, 90(6):967-72 Review

210 Pregnancy and the Biliary Tract. Gilat T et al; Can J Gastroenterol, 2000 Nov, 14 Suppl D:55D-59D Review

211 Gall-Bladder Motor Function in Obesity. Petroni ML; Aliment Pharmacol Ther, 2000 May, 14 Suppl 2:48-50 Review

212 Alcohol, Wine, and Health. de Lorimier AA; Am J Surg, 2000 Nov, 180(5):357-61 Review

Chapter 12 – Correcting Dis-ease

1 Use of Pantothenic Acid Preparations in Treating Patients with Viral Hepatitis A. Komar VI; Ter Arkh, 1991, 63(11):58-60

2 Multiple Sclerosis: Fat-Oil Relationship. Swank RL. Nutrition, 1991 Sep-Oct, 7(5):368-76

3 Molecular Aspects of Pathogenesis in Osteoarthritis: The Role of Inflammation. Hedbom E et al; Cell Mol LifeSci, 2002 Jan, 59(1):45-53 Review

4 Osteoarthritis: A Problem of Joint Failure. Nuki G; Z Rheumatol, 1999 Jun, 58(3):142-47 Review

5 Osteoarthritis. Pathogenesis, Clinical Features and Treatment. Veje K et al; Ugeskr Laeger, 2002 Jun 10, 164(24):3173-79 Review

6 Molecular Pathology and Pathobiology of Osteoarthritic Cartilage. Aigner T et al; Cell Mol Life Sci, 2002 Jan, 59(1):5-18 Review

7 Osteoarthritis Overview. Birchfield PC; Geriatr Nurs, 2001 May-Jun, 22(3):124-30 Review

8 Aging, Articular Cartilage Chondrocyte Senescence and Osteoarthritis. Martin JA et al; Biogerontology, 2002, 3(5):257-64 Review

9 Glucosamine Sulfate for Osteoarthritis. da Camara CC, et al; Ann Pharmacother, 1998 May, 32(5):580-87 Review

10 Role of Cytokines in Osteoarthritis Pathophysiology. Fernandes JC et al; Biorheology, 2002, 39(1-2):237-46 Review

11 Arthrosis–A Single or Many Diseases? Watt I; Radiologe, 2000 Dec, 40(12):1134-40 Review

12 Role of Anti-Inflammatory Drugs in the Treatment of Osteoarthritis. Dougados M; Clin Exp Rheumatol, 2001 Nov-Dec, 19(6 Suppl 25):S9-14 Review

13 Glucosamine. Barclay TS et al; Ann Pharmacother, 1998 May, 32(5):574-79 Review

14 Glucosamine Therapy for Treating Osteoarthritis (Cochrane Review). Towheed TE et al; Cochrane Database Syst Rev 2001, 1:CD002946 Review

15 Nutraceuticals as Therapeutic Agents in Osteoarthritis. The Role of Glucosamine, Chondroitin Sulfate, and Collagen Hydrolysate. Deal CL et al; Rheum Dis Clin North Am, 1999 May, 25(2):379-95 Review

16 Polymeric Chondroitin Sulfate vs. Monomeric Glucosamine for the Treatment of Osteoarthritis. Menzel EJ; Wien Med Wochenschr, 2000, 150(5):87-90 Review

17 Enhanced Synovial Production of Hyaluronic Acid May Explain Rapid Clinical Response to High-Dose Glucosamine in Osteoarthritis. McCarty MF; Med Hypotheses, 1998 Jun, 50(6):507-10 Review

18 Gonarthrosis–Current Aspects of Therapy with Glucosamine Sulfate. Fortschr Med Suppl, 1998, 183:1-12 Review

19 Potential Effects of Nutrition including Additives on Healthy and Arthrotic Joints. Basic Dietary Constituents. Wilhelmi G; Z Rheumatol, 1993 May-Jun, 52(3):174-79 Review

20 Potential Influence of Nutrition with Supplements on Healthy and Arthritic Joints. Nutritional Quantity, Supplements, Contamination. Wilhelmi G; Z Rheumatol, 1993 Jul-Aug, 52(4):191-200 Review

21 Zinc Status in Human Immunodeficiency Virus Infection. Baum MK et al; J Nutr, 2000 May, 130(5S Suppl):1421S-23S Review

22 Capsaicin: Identification, Nomenclature, and Pharmacotherapy. Cordell GA et al; Ann Pharmacother, 1993 Mar, 27(3):330-36 Review

23   Ginger (Zingiber officinale) in Rheumatism and Musculoskeletal Disorders. Srivastava KC et al; Med Hypotheses, 1992 Dec, 39(4):342-48

24   Pathology and Progression of Intra-Articular Inflammation in Rheumatoid Arthritis. Geiler G; Verh Dtsch Ges Pathol, 1996, 80:46-57 Review

25   Update on Synovitis. Szekanecz Z et al; Curr Rheumatol Rep, 2001 Feb, 3(1):53-63 Review

26   Follow-Up and Prognosis in Chronic Polyarthritis. Mau W et al; Versicherungsmedizin, 1999 Sep 1, 51(3):115-21 Review

27   Uncoupling of Inflammatory and Destructive Mechanisms in Arthritis. van den Berg WB; Semin Arthritis Rheum, 2001 Apr, 30(5 Suppl 2):7-16 Review

28   Blocking the Effects of IL-1 in Rheumatoid Arthritis Protects Bone and Cartilage. Abramson SB et al; Rheumatology (Oxford), 2002 Sep, 41(9):972-80 Review

29   NF-Kappa B in Rheumatoid Arthritis: A Pivotal Regulator of Inflammation, Hyperplasia, and Tissue Destruction. Makarov SS; Arthritis Res, 2001, 3(4):200-06 Review

30   Involvement of Receptor Activator of NFkappaB Ligand and Tumor Necrosis Factor-Alpha in Bone Destruction in Rheumatoid Arthritis. Romas E et al; Bone, 2002 Feb, 30(2):340-46 Review

31   Nutritional Modulation of Cytokine Biology. Grimble RF; Nutrition, 1998 Jul-Aug, 14(7-8):634-40 Review

32   Antioxidants in Nutrition and their Importance in the Anti-/Oxidative Balance in the Immune System. Biesalski HK et al; Immun Infekt, 1995 Oct, 23(5):166-73 Review

33   Immunonutrition: the Role of Omega-3 Fatty Acids. Alexander JW; Nutrition, 1998 Jul-Aug, 14(7-8):627-33 Review

34   N-3 Fatty Acid Supplements in Rheumatoid Arthritis. Kremer JM; Am J Clin Nutr, 2000 Jan, 71(1 Suppl):349S-51S Review

35   Effects of Dietary N-3 Polyunsaturated Fatty Acids on Neutrophils. Sperling RI; Proc Nutr Soc, 1998 Nov, 57(4):527-34 Review

36   Osteoporosis in Rheumatoid Arthritis–Significance of Alfacalcidol in Prevention and Therapy. Schacht E; Z Rheumatol, 2000, 59 Suppl 1:10-20 Review

37   1,25-Dihydroxyvitamin D3–A Hormone with Immunomodulatory Properties. Lemire J; Z Rheumatol, 2000, 59 Suppl 1:24-27 Review

38   Vitamin E in Therapy of Rheumatic Diseases. Sangha O et al; Z Rheumatol, 1998 Aug, 57(4):207-14 Review

39   Use and Safety of Elevated Dosages of Vitamin E in Adults. Machlin LJ; Int J Vitam Nutr Res Suppl, 1989, 30:56-68 Review

40   Importance of Dietary Gamma-Linolenic Acid in Human Health and Nutrition. Fan YY et al; J Nutr, 1998 Sep, 128(9):1411-14 Review

41   Evening Primrose Oil and Borage Oil in Rheumatologic Conditions. Belch JJ et al; Am J Clin Nutr, 2000 Jan, 71(1 Suppl):352S-56S Review

42   Antirheumatic Effect of IDS 23, a Stinging Nettle Leaf Extract, on in Vitro Expression of T helper Cytokines. Klingelhoefer S et al; J Rheumatol, 1999 Dec, 26(12):2517-22

43   Plant Extracts from Stinging Nettle (Urtica dioica), an Antirheumatic Remedy, Inhibit the Proinflammatory Transcription Factor NF-kappaB. Riehemann K et al; FEBS Lett, 1999 Jan 8, 442(1):89-94

44   Inhibitory Effects of [6]-Gingerol, a Major Pungent Principle of Ginger, on Phorbol Ester-Induced Inflammation, Epidermal Ornithine Decarboxylase Activity and Skin Tumor Promotion in ICR Mice. Park KK et al; Cancer Lett, 1998 Jul 17, 129(2):139-44

45   Suppressive Effects of Eugenol and Ginger Oil on Arthritic Rats. Sharma JN et al; Pharmacology, 1994 Nov, 49(5):314-18

46   Ginger (Zingiber officinale) in Rheumatism and Musculoskeletal Disorders. Srivastava KC et al; Med Hypotheses, 1992 Dec, 39(4):342-48

47   Rheumatoid Arthritis and Metal Compounds–Perspectives on the Role of Oxygen Radical Detoxification. Aaseth J et al; Analyst, 1998 Jan, 123(1):3-6 Review

48   Therapeutic Effects of Organic Germanium. Goodman S; Med Hypotheses, 1988 Jul, 26(3):207-15 Review

49   Glutathione Reductase Activity, Riboflavin Status, and Disease Activity in Rheumatoid Arthritis. Mulherin DM et al; Ann Rheum Dis, 1996 Nov, 55(11):837-40

50   Protection by Vitamin B2 against Oxidant-Mediated Acute Lung Injury. Seekamp A et al; Inflammation, 1999 Oct, 23(5):449-60

51   Acute Ethanol Exposure Alters Hepatic Glutathione Metabolism in Riboflavin Deficiency. Dutta P et al; Alcohol, 1995 Jan-Feb, 12(1):43-47

52   Multiple Sclerosis: Epidemiology, Molecular Pathology and Therapy. Steck AJ et al; Schweiz Med Wochenschr, 1999 Nov 20, 129(46):1764-68 Review

53   Early Intervention with Immunomodulatory Agents in the Treatment of Multiple Sclerosis. Jeffery DR; J Neurol Sci, 2002 May 15, 197(1-2):1-8 Review

54   Evolving Concepts in the Pathogenesis of Multiple Sclerosis and their Therapeutic Implications. Rudick RA; J Neuroophthalmol, 2001 Dec, 21(4):279-83 Review

55   Pathogenesis of Tissue Injury in MS Lesions. Trapp BD et al; J Neuroimmunol, 1999 Jul 1, 98(1):49-56 Review

56   Neuroimmunology of Multiple Sclerosis: Possible Roles of T and B Lymphocytes in Immunopathogenesis. O'Connor KC et al; J Clin Immunol, 2001 Mar, 21(2):81-92 Review

57   Immunopathogenesis of the Multiple Sclerosis Lesion. Markovic-Plese S et al; Curr Neurol Neurosci Rep, 2001 May, 1(3):257-62 Review

58   Neuropathology in Multiple Sclerosis: New Concepts. Lassmann H; Mult Scler, 1998 Jun, 4(3):93-98 Review

59   Cytokine Storm in Multiple Sclerosis. Link H; Mult Scler, 1998 Feb, 4(1):12-15 Review

60   Interleukin-10 and the Interleukin-10 Receptor. Moore KW et al; Annu Rev Immunol, 2001, 19:683-765 Review

61   Role of Th1 and Th2 Cells in Autoimmune Demyelinating Disease. Nagelkerken L; Braz J Med Biol Res, 1998 Jan, 31(1):55-60 Review

62   Imbalance between Th1 And Th2-like Cytokines in Patients with Autoimmune Diseases–Differential Diagnosis between Th1 Dominant Autoimmune Diseases and Th2 Dominant Autoimmune Diseases. Ishida H et al; Nippon Rinsho, 1997 Jun, 55(6):1438-43 Review

63   Matrix Metalloproteinases, Tumor Necrosis Factor and Multiple Sclerosis. Chandler S et al; J Neuroimmunol, 1997 Feb, 72(2):155-61 Review

64   Matrix Metalloproteinases: Multifunctional Effectors of Inflammation in Multiple Sclerosis and Bacterial Meningitis. Leppert D et al; Brain Res Brain Res Rev, 2001 Oct, 36(2-3):249-57 Review

65   Matrix Metalloproteinases and Neuroinflammation in Multiple Sclerosis. Rosenberg GA; Neuroscientist, 2002 Dec, 8(6):586-95 Review

66   Pathological Abnormalities in the Normal-Appearing White Matter in Multiple Sclerosis. Allen IV et al; Neurol Sci, 2001 Apr, 22(2):141-44 Review

67   Beta-Interferons in Multiple Sclerosis: Comparative Trials and Potential Individual Selection in Different Types of the Disease Course. Boiko AN et al; Zh Nevrol Psikhiatr Im S S Korsakova, 2002, Suppl:65-71 Review

68   Role of Autoimmunity in Multiple Sclerosis. Chabas D et al; Pathol Biol (Paris), 2000 Feb, 48(1):25-46 Review

69   Multiple Sclerosis. Keegan BM et al; Annu Rev Med, 2002, 53:285-302 Review

70   Vitamin D and Multiple Sclerosis. Hayes CE et al; Proc Soc Exp Biol Med, 1997 Oct, 216(1):21-27 Review

71   Exogenous Lipids in Myelination and Myelination. Di Biase A et al; Kao Hsiung I Hsueh Ko Hsueh Tsa Chih, 1997 Jan, 13(1):19-29 Review

72   Protective Effects of Omega-6 Fatty Acids in Experimental Autoimmune Encephalomyelitis (EAE) in Relation to Transforming Growth Factor-Beta 1 (TGF-Beta1) Up-Regulation and Increased Prostaglandin E2 (PGE2) Production. Harbige LS et al; Clin Exp Immunol, 2000 Dec, 122(3):445-52

73   Use of Gamma Linolenic Acid in the Prevention and Treatment of Diabetic Neuropathy. Jamal GA; Diabet Med, 1994 Mar, 11(2):145-49 Review

74   Effect of (n-3) Polyunsaturated Fatty Acids on Cytokine Production and their Biologic Function. Meydani SN; Nutrition, 1996 Jan, 12(1 Suppl):S8-14 Review

75   Multiple Sclerosis and Vitamin B12 Metabolism. Reynolds EH; J Neuroimmunol, 1992 Oct, 40(2-3):225-30 Review

76   Folate, Vitamin B12, and Neuropsychiatric Disorders. Bottiglieri T; Nutr Rev, 1996 Dec, 54(12):382-90 Review

77   Morbidity and Mortality in Systemic Lupus Erythematosus. Marai I et al; Harefuah, 2001 Dec, 140(12):1177-80 Review

78   Natural Killer Cells in Connective Tissue Disorders. Sibbitt WL Jr et al; Clin Rheum Dis, 1985 Dec, 11(3):507-Review

79   Role of NK Cells and TGF-beta in the Regulation of T-Cell-Dependent Antibody Production in Health and Autoimmune Disease. Horwitz DA et al; Microbes Infect, 1999 Dec, 1(15):1305-11 Review

80   Effects of Astragalus membranaceus and Tripterygium hypoglancum on Natural Killer Cell Activity of Peripheral Blood Mononuclear in Systemic Lupus Erythematosus. Zhao XZ; Chung Kuo Chung Hsi I Chieh Ho Tsa Chih, 1992 Nov, 12(11):669-71, 645

81   Natural Killer Cells and Autoimmunity. Grunebaum E et al; Immunol Res, 1989, 8(4):292-304 Review

82   Clinical Implication of IL-10 in Patients with Immune and Inflammatory Diseases. Ishida H; Rinsho Byori, 1994 Aug, 42(8):843-52 Review

83   Cytokines and Lupus. Emilie D et al; Ann Med Interne (Paris), 1996, 147(7):480-84 Review

84   Interleukin 10 in Disseminated Lupus Erythematosus. Viallard JF et al; J Soc Biol, 2002;196(1):19-21 Review

85   Lupus Erythematosus and Nutrition. Brown AC; J Ren Nutr, 2000 Oct, 10(4):170-83 Review

86   Diet and Lupus. Leiba A et al; Lupus, 2001, 10(3):246-48 Review

87   Potential Application of Allium sativum (Garlic) for the Treatment of Bladder Cancer. Lamm DL et al; Urol Clin North Am, 2000 Feb, 27(1):157-62 Review

88   American Coneflower: A Prophylactic Role Involving Nonspecific Immunity. Sun LZ et al; J Altern Complement Med, 1999 Oct, 5(5):437-46

89   Natural Killer Cells from Aging Mice Treated with Extracts from Echinacea purpurea are Quantitatively and Functionally Rejuvenated. Currier N et al; Exp Gerontol, 2000 Aug 1, 35(5):627-639

90   In Vitro Effects of Echinacea and Ginseng on Natural Killer and Antibody-Dependent Cell Cytotoxicity in Healthy Subjects and Chronic Fatigue Syndrome or Acquired Immunodeficiency Syndrome Patients. See DM et al; Immunopharmacology, 1997 Jan, 35(3):229-35

91   Aloe Barbadensis Extracts Reduce the Production of Interleukin-10 after Exposure to Ultraviolet Radiation. Byeon SW et al; J Invest Dermatol, 1998 May, 110(5):811-17

92   Urtica dioica Agglutinin, a New Mitogen for Murine T lymphocytes: Unaltered Interleukin-1 Production but Late Interleukin 2-Mediated Proliferation. Le Moal MA et al; Cell Immunol, 1988 Aug, 115(1):24-35

93   Urtica dioica Agglutinin. A Superantigenic Lectin from Stinging Nettle Rhizome. Galelli A et al; J Immunol, 1993 Aug 15, 151(4):1821-31

94   Urtica dioica Agglutinin, a V beta 8.3-Specific Superantigen, Prevents the Development of the Systemic Lupus Erythematosus-like Pathology of MRL lpr/lpr Mice. Musette P et al; Eur J Immunol, 1996 Aug, 26(8):1707-11

95   Vitamin E and Immunity. Moriguchi S et al; Vitam Horm, 2000, 59:305-36 Review

96   Zinc: An Overview. Prasad AS; Nutrition 1995, Jan-Feb, 11(1 Suppl):93-99 Review

97   Copper and Immunity. Percival SS; Am J Clin Nutr, 1998 May, 67(5 Suppl):1064S-1068S Review

98   Selenium and Immune Function. Kiremidjian-Schumacher L et al; Z Ernahrungswiss, 1998, 37 Suppl 1:50-56 Review

99   MLT and the Immune-Hematopoietic System. Maestroni GJ; Adv Exp Med Biol, 1999, 460:395-405 Review

100   Fibromyalgia. What Is It and How Do We Treat It? Littlejohn G; Aust Fam Physician, 2001 Apr, 30(4):327-33

101   Fibromyalgia Syndrome. Matsumoto Y; Nippon Rinsho, 1999 Feb, 57(2):364-69 Review

102   Evidence for Metabolic Abnormalities in the Muscles of Patients with Fibromyalgia. Park JH et al; Curr Rheumatol Rep, 2000 Apr, 2(2):131-40 Review

103   Treating Fibromyalgia. Millea PJ et al; Am Fam Physician, 2000 Oct 1, 62(7):1575-82, 1587 Review

104   Fibromyalgia Syndrome: A Comprehensive Approach to Identification and Management. Leslie M; Clin Excell Nurse Pract, 1999 May, 3(3):165-71 Review

105   Management of Fibromyalgia-Associated Syndromes. Silver DS et al; Rheum Dis Clin North Am, 2002 May, 28(2):405-17 Review

106   Adult Growth Hormone Deficiency in Patients with Fibromyalgia. Bennett RM; Curr Rheumatol Rep, 2002 Aug, 4(4):306-12 Review

107   Trauma and Fibromyalgia: Is There an Association and What Does It Mean? White KP et al; Semin Arthritis Rheum, 2000 Feb, 29(4):200-16 Review

108   Association of Silicone-Gel Breast Implant Rupture and Fibromyalgia. Brown SL et al; Curr Rheumatol Rep, 2002 Aug, 4(4):293-98 Review

109   Exercise for Treating Fibromyalgia Syndrome. Busch A et al; Cochrane Database Syst Rev, 2002 (3):CD003786 Review

110   Pain Treatment with Acupuncture for Patients with Fibromyalgia. Targino RA et al; Curr Pain Headache Rep, 2002 Oct, 6(5):379-83 Review

111   Serotonergic Agents in the Treatment of Fibromyalgia Syndrome. Miller LJ et al; Ann Pharmacother, 2002 Apr, 36(4):707-12 Review

112   Nutritional Supplementation with Chlorella pyrenoidosa for Patients with Fibromyalgia Syndrome. Merchant RE et al; Phytother Res, 2000 May, 14(3):167-73

113   Chronic Fatigue Syndrome. Kakumanu S et al; J Am Osteopath Assoc, 1999 Oct, 99(10 Su Pt 1):S1-5 Review

114   Chronic Fatigue Syndrome: New Insights and Old Ignorance. Evengard B et al; J Intern Med, 1999 Nov, 246(5):455-69 Review

115   Evidence for and Pathophysiologic Implications of Hypothalamic-Pituitary-Adrenal Axis Dysregulation in Fibromyalgia and Chronic Fatigue Syndrome. Demitrack MA et al; Ann N Y Acad Sci, 1998 May 1, 840:684-97 Review

116   Stress-Associated Immune Modulation: Relevance to Viral Infections and Chronic Fatigue Syndrome. Glaser R et al; Am J Med, 1998 Sep 28, 105(3A):35S-42S Review

117   Natural Killer Cells and Natural Killer Cell Activity in Chronic Fatigue Syndrome. Whiteside TL et al; Am J Med, 1998 Sep 28, 105(3A):27S-34S Review

118   Altered Glucocorticoid Regulation of the Immune Response in the Chronic Fatigue Syndrome. Visser JT et al; Ann N Y Acad Sci, 2000, 917:868-75 Review

119   Eicosanoids and Essential Fatty Acid Modulation in Chronic Disease and the Chronic Fatigue Syndrome. Gray JB et al; Med Hypotheses, 1994 Jul;43(1):31-42 Review

120   Food Use and Health Effects of Soybean and Sunflower Oils. Meydani SN et al; J Am Coll Nutr, 1991 Oct, 10(5):406-28 Review

121   Post-Viral Fatigue Syndrome, Viral Infections in Atopic Eczema, and Essential Fatty Acids. Horrobin DF; Med Hypotheses, 1990 Jul, 32(3):211-7 Review

122   Essential Fatty Acids and Immune Response. Hwang D; FASEB J, 1989 Jul, 3(9):2052-61 Review

123   Neuroendocrinology of Chronic Fatigue Syndrome and Fibromyalgia. Parker AJ et al; Psychol Med, 2001 Nov, 31(8):1331-45

124   Interactions of Retinoid Binding Proteins and Enzymes in Retinoid Metabolism. Napoli JL; Biochim Biophys Acta, 1999 Sep 22, 1440(2-3):139-62 Review

INDEX

Page numbers in **bold type** indicate scientific medical literature.

I

Imbalance (functional imbalance), 11, 25, 62, 72, 73, 74, 76, 77, 85, 107, 125, 151, 153, 156, 157, 164, 204, 207, 209, 211, 213, 214, 215, 219, 238, 240, 264, 305, 306, 313, 388, 402, 403, 404, 406, 407, 409, 410, 413, 428-430

Imipramine (antidepressant), **230**

Immune function and system, 2, 4, 7-14, 19-21, 22, 23, 25, 26, 33, 48-54, *see also* lymphatic system.

Immune exhaustion, 11, 19-21, 164, 292, 304-305, 406, 408, 412, 420-421, 424-426, 430

Immunosuppression, immunosuppressive activity 10, **68, 117, 119, 140,** 163, **186,** 213, **222,** 264, **275, 297, 300, 303, 384, 448, 450**

Leukocytes (white blood cells), 10, 12, 19, **20,** 20, **244, 256,** 264, **296, 297, 299,** 405

Lymphocytes and other effectors

B-lymphocyte (B-cell), 10, 19, 20, 21, **45, 88, 90, 109, 133, 135, 141, 162, 187, 277, 290, 299,** 415, 430, **439, 440, 441, 444, 445, 448, 449, 450, 455, 456**

Antibodies, 20, 40, **51, 78, 81, 88, 90, 128, 133, 183, 187, 290, 301,** 335, **336, 341, 371, 377, 444, 448,** *see also* antigens.

Immunoglobulins (antibody proteins), 20, **78, 324, 407, 439**

Immunoglobulin A (IgA), **213, 297, 363**

Immunoglobulin E (IgE), **128**

Immunoglobulin G (IgG), **213, 223**

Immunoglobulin M (IgM), **223, 363**

Basophil (histamine), 20

Mast cell, **20, 242, 258, 277, 370,** *see also* connective tissue.

Cytokines (non-antibody proteins), 111, **117, 126, 127, 129, 136, 141, 162, 183, 184, 242, 272, 297, 299, 300, 354, 436, 439, 440, 441, 444, 445, 446, 448, 449, 450**

Interferon, 83, **187, 248, 275, 290, 300, 301,** 366, **444, 445**

Interleukins (IL)

IL-1, **141, 299, 300, 436, 440, 441, 445, 446**

IL-2, **81,** 180, **183,** 262, **275, 301, 318, 449, 450**

IL-4, **141, 441, 445**

IL-6, **141, 299, 441, 445**

IL-10, **141, 242, 300, 363, 441, 444, 445, 449**

IL-12, **141, 441, 445, 449**

Lympokines/LAK cells, **275, 301**

Tumor necrosis factor (TNF), **141, 184, 275, 300, 301, 394, 436, 437, 440, 441, 442, 444, 445, 446**

Eicosanoids (part of immune/inflammatory response), **101,** 107, **108, 110, 126, 127, 128, 188, 272,** 415, 430, **441, 449, 455**

Prostaglandins (PG), 47, **91, 101,** 107, **108 109, 110, 111, 126, 127,** 144, **188, 212, 272, 280, 291, 359, 373, 436, 441, 455**

PGE group, **91, 109, 110, 111, 212, 359, 436, 441, 455**

Leukotrienes, 107, **108, 111, 128, 258, 263, 212, 258, 263, 280, 284**

Thromboxanes, 107, **108**

Eosinophil (histamine), 20, **46, 224, 303**

Macrophage, 20, **98, 114, 127, 128, 140, 162, 187, 190, 212, 242, 258, 275, 290, 299, 300, 301, 354, 393, 439, 441, 445, 450**

Monocyte, 20, **141, 251, 255, 299, 441, 445**

Neutrophil (bacteria), **20, 51, 78, 113, 180, 181, 186, 296, 354, 378, 407**

NF-kappaB/RANKL, **277, 440, 441**

NK-cell (cancer, viruses), **20, 51,** 107, **110, 116, 127, 187, 190, 221, 275, 290, 299, 300, 301, 378, 381,** 426, 430, **448, 449, 450, 455, 456**

Phagocyte, 20, **78, 88, 180, 189, 190, 290, 297, 299, 300, 301, 407**

TGF-beta (Transforming Growth Factor-beta), **41, 444, 448**

T-lymphocyte (T-cell), 10, 19-20, 21, **45, 51, 81,** 107, **109, 110, 116, 127, 128, 133, 140, 162,** 163, **180, 181, 183, 187, 212, 242, 262, 263, 275, 277, 278, 279, 295, 301, 303,** 305, **318, 369, 371, 394,** 405, 415, 430, **439, 441, 444, 448, 449, 450, 455, 456**

Th1, **141, 275, 318,** 430, **439, 440, 441, 444, 445, 448, 449, 450**

Th2, **111, 128, 141, 394,** 430, **441, 444, 445, 448, 449, 450**

CD4/CD8, **116, 135, 263, 278, 371, 439, 440, 444, 448, 449**

T-suppressor cell, **187, 450, 456**

Immunity

Cellular immunity, 20, **88,** 107, **116, 140, 301,** 430, **441, 449, 450, 455, 456**

Humoral immunity, 20, **88, 223,** 430, **449**

37, 57, 62, 69, 95, 103, 145, 202, 306, 309, 321, 331, 332, 334, 402, 403

Raw materials, *see* nutrition.

End products, *see* specific hormones, neuro-transmitters, and other effectors.

RDA (recommended daily allowance), 113, **186**

Reactive oxygen species (ROS), **112**, **117**, **121-122**, **165**, **169**, **170**, **178**, **179**, **180**, **190**, **245**, **250**, **251**, **258**, **259**, **302**, **317**, **368**, *see also* free radicals.

Red blood cells (erythrocytes), 12, 20, **44**, 68, 78, **79**, **81**, **87**, **109**, **130**, 160, 166, **167**, **169**, **172**, **178**, **182**, **262**, 264, 265, 266, **270**, 365, **378**, 405, **442**, **445**, *see also* blood.

Erythropoiesis (red blood cell production), **167**, **168**, **212**, **222**, **270**, **271**, **383**

Redox of metals, **165**, **176**, **179**, **182**, **184**, *see also* trace metals, metal mismanagement.

Red Root, 319, 350, 351, 352, 399

Reflux esophagitis, *see* GERD.

Reishi mushroom, 293

Renal function, *see* kidneys.

Renin, renin-angiotensin-aldosterone system, **289**, **290**, **455**

Reproductive health, **45**, **47**, **114**, **132**, 166, **176**, **191**, **213**, **381**, **382**, 384, *see also* sexual function.

Respiratory distress, **224**, **355**, **379**, *see also* breath/breathing *and* lungs.

Respiratory distress syndrome (RDS) in infants, **397**, *see also* infants.

Restless leg syndrome, 385, 388, *see also* muscles.

Retardation: fetal, infant and child

Retarded growth/stunted growth, **26**, **87**, **118**, **131**, **135**, **140**, **159**, 166, **185**, 321, 327, **327**, **341**, **347**, **377**, *see also* growth, physical.

Mental retardation, **44**, **178**, 321, 327, **327**

Retina, 80, 83, **116**, **178**, **186**, **244**, **259**, 314, **316**, **338**, 342, *see also* eyes.

Retinitis pigmentosa (RP), **132-133**, *see also* eyes.

Retinol, *see* Vitamin A.

Retinopathy, **52**

Diabetic retinopathy, **3**, **80**, **112**, **116**, 144, **237**, **244**, **255**, **259**, 314, 330, 332, 335, **337**, **338**, 342, 345, 349

Retinopathy of premature newborns, **108**, **118**, **397**

Rheumatism, 216, 407

Rheumatoid arthritis (RA), 1, 11, **79**, **111**, **117**, **127**, **128**, 141, 144, **180**, **190**, **277**, **278**, **280**, **380**, 402,

404, 407, 428, **439-442**, 442-443 *see also* arthritis.

Riboflavin, *see* Vitamin B2.

Rice, 35, **65**

Brown rice (whole grain), 63, 64, 65, **66**, 70, **86**, 91, 432

White rice, 63, 64, **86**, 395

Rickets, 137, **138**, **139**, **140**, **141**, 144

Ringing/noise in the ears, **314**, **325**, 374, *see also* hearing.

RNA (ribonucleic acid), *see* nucleic acids.

ROS, *see* reactive oxygen species.

Rose hips, 36, 252, 253, 296

Rosemary, 261, 294

Rutin, **50**, 64, **244**, 253

Rye, 63, 64, **66**, **67**

S

Saccharin, **376**

SAD (seasonal affective disorder), **231**, 315, 316, **316**, **317**, *see also* mood.

Safflower oil, 24, 96, 106

Saffron, 237, 238, 293, 429

Sage, 217, 218, 238, 302, 433

Salicylic acid, 209, 271

Salmon, 53, 105, 124, 128, **130**, 273, 282, 332, 349, 353

Salmonella, 100, 362, **383**, **384**

Salt, salt balance in the body (Na ⇌ K), 17, 18, 28, 156, 272, 273, 276, 358, 385, 386-387, 388

Table salt (NaCl), 18, 273, 276, **322**, 322, 323, 328, 387

Salt substitute (KCl), 273, 276, 387

SAMe (S-adenosylmethionine), **42**, 46, **172**, **173**, 374, 375

Saponins, 48, **52**, **282**, **287**, **346**, **347**

Sardines, 247

Sarsaparilla, 265, 281, 282, **282**, 343

Saturated fats, *see* fats.

Savoy Cabbage, 343

Saw Palmetto Berries, 265, 282, **283-284**; 206, 343

Scar tissue and injury, 8, 16, 31-32

Schwann cells, **250**, *see also* myelin sheath.

Schizophrenia, **91**, **109**, **130**, **135**, **139-140**, 144

Scleroderma, **141**, 434, **448** *see also* skin.

Wheat grass, 293

White blood cells (leukocytes), 10, 12, 19, **20**, 20, **244**, **256**, 264, **296**, **297**, **299**, 405, *see also* blood *and* immune system.

White Willow Bark, 209, 265, 271

Whole grains, whole-grain cereals, 63-65, **65-67**; 2, 62, 68, 70, 71, 73, 74, 75, 76, 77, 82, 84, 85, **86**, 89, 91, 93, 94, 148, 203, 213, 220, 224, 240, 246, 262, 331, 342, 364, 395, 410, 431, 432

Williams syndrome (hypervitaminosis D), **143**

Willow Bark, 209, 265, 271

Wilson's disease, 177, **177**, **178**

Wine, red wine, **49**, 390

Wintertime blues, *see* seasonal affective disorder.

Withdrawal, *see* addiction.

Wood Betony, 218, 228, 312

Workaholism, 13-14

Worry and fear, 17, 232, **233**, 402

Wounds, wound healing, **26**, **78**, **118-119**, **123**, **183**, **184**, **237**, **241**, **242**, **247**, **256**, **260**, 385, 386, 412, **444**, *see also* healing.

Woundwort, 239, 261, 262, **262-263**, 265, 276, 281, 293, 305, 358, 424, 433

Wrinkling, **242**, *see also* skin.

X

'X' therapeutic action (1X, 2X, 3X), 69-72

Xanthine (xanthurenic acid), **80**, 196, **197**

Xanthine oxidase, **164**, **196**, **197**, **198**

Xanthophylls (yellow-pigment fruits and vegetables), **118**, **255**

Xerophthalmia, 130, **131**, *see also* eyes.

Xerosis, **256**, *see also* skin.

Y

Yams, 120

Wild Yam, 266, 287, **287**

Yarrow, 294, 319, 342, 342, 345, 415

Yeast (food), *see* nutritional yeast.

Yeast infection, Candida, 11, **68**, **212**, **242**, **288**, **300**, **363**, 424, 435, *see also* fungus.

Yellow Dock, 240

Yohimbe/yohimbine, 219, 234-235, **235**

Yogurt, 361-362, **362**, **363**; 100, 353, 358, 388, 391

Yucca, 264, 266, 288, **288**, 293

Z

Zeaxanthin, **51**, 345, *see also* eyes.

Zinc, 181, **182-186**; 82, 107, **119**, **149**, **150**, 153, 154, 155, 156, 157, 163-164, **165**, 169, **170**, **174**, **176**, 177, **178**, **179**, **181**, **189**, 240, **256**, 305, 349, 405, 424, 430, 431, 432, **437**, **442**, **444**, **449**, **450**, *see also* copper-zinc superoxide dismutase (CuZnSOD).

Zinc gluconate lozenges, 163-164, **183**, 213

Zirconium, 194, **194**; 154, 155, 156, 157, 192, 193, 199, 333, 415, 432

Zocor (simvastatin), **393**, **394**

Zone, "in the zone", 94, 364